Atrial Fibrillation
Mechanisms and Management

Atrial Fibrillation
Mechanisms and Management

Editors

Rodney H. Falk, M.D., M.R.C.P. (U.K.), F.A.C.C.
Director of Clinical Cardiology
Boston City Hospital
Associate Professor of Medicine
Boston University School of Medicine
Boston, Massachusetts

Philip J. Podrid, M.D., F.A.C.C.
Director, Arrhythmia Service
University Hospital
Associate Professor of Medicine
Boston University School of Medicine
Boston, Massachusetts

Raven Press 🙤 New York

Raven Press, Ltd., 1185 Avenue of the Americas, New York, New York 10036

© 1992 by Raven Press, Ltd. All rights reserved. This book is protected by copyright. No part of it may be reproduced, stored in a retrieval system, or transmitted, in any form or by any means, electronic, mechanical, photocopy, or recording, or otherwise, without the prior written permission of the publisher.

Made in the United States of America

Library of Congress Cataloging-in-Publication Data

Atrial fibrillation : mechanisms and management / editors, Rodney H. Falk,
    Philip J. Podrid.
        p.   cm.
    Includes bibliographical references and index.
    ISBN 0-88167-831-7
    1. Atrial fibrillation   I. Falk, Rodney, H.   II. Podrid, Philip J.
    [DNLM: 1. Atrial Fibrillation—physiopathology.   2. Atrial
Fibrillation—therapy.   WG 330 A8818]
    RC685.A72A89   1992
    616.1′28—dc20
    DNLM/DLC
    for Library of Congress   91-27955
                                                                        CIP

The material contained in this volume was submitted as previously unpublished material, except in the instances in which credit has been given to the source from which some of the illustrative material was derived.

Great care has been taken to maintain the accuracy of the information contained in the volume. However, neither Raven Press nor the editors can be held responsible for errors or for any consequences arising from the use of the information contained herein.

Materials appearing in this book prepared by individuals as part of their official duties as U.S. Government employees are not covered by the above-mentioned copyright.

9 8 7 6 5 4 3 2 1

For Joni
and for Leora, Avital, and Shira
—Rodney H. Falk

For Vivian
—Philip J. Podrid

Contents

Contributing Authors

Maurits A. Allessie *Department of Physiology, University of Limburg and The Interuniversity Cardiology Institute, 6200 MD Maastricht, The Netherlands*

J. Edwin Atwood *Cardiology Division, Department of Medicine, Stanford University, Stanford, California 94305; Palo Alto Veterans Administration Hospital, 3801 Miranda Avenue, Palo Alto, California 94304*

Saroja Bharati *Congenital Heart and Conduction System Center, The Heart Institute for Children, Christ Hospital and Medical Center, 4440 West 95th Street, Oak Lawn, Illinois 60453; Department of Pathology, Rush Medical College, Rush University, Rush-Presbyterian-St. Luke's Medical Center, 1753 West Congress Parkway, Chicago, Illinois 60612*

Philippe Coumel *Department of Cardiology, Hôpital Lariboisière, 2 rue Ambroise-Paré, 75010 Paris, France*

Kim A. Eagle *Cardiac Unit, Massachusetts General Hospital, Fruit Street, Boston, Massachusetts 02114*

Rodney H. Falk *Division of Cardiology, The Talbot Building, Boston City Hospital, 818 Harrison Avenue, Boston, Massachusetts 02118; Boston University School of Medicine, Boston, Massachusetts 02118*

Therese Fuchs *Cardiology Section, The Talbot Building, Boston City Hospital, 818 Harrison Avenue, Boston, Massachusetts 02118*

A. P. M. Gorgels *Department of Cardiology, Academic Hospital Maastricht, University of Limburg, Annadel 624, P.O. Box 5800, 6202 AZ Maastricht, The Netherlands*

Gerard M. Guiraudon *Cardiac Investigation Unit, University Hospital, 339 Windermere Road, London, Ontario, Canada N6A 5A5*

Michiel J. Janse *Department of Clinical and Experimental Cardiology, Academisch Medisch Centrum, Meibergdreef 9, 1105 AZ Amsterdam, The Netherlands*

William B. Kannel *Department of Medicine, University Hospital, Section of Preventive Medicine and Epidemiology, Evans Memorial Department of Clinical Research, Boston University School of Medicine, 720 Harrison Avenue, Boston, Massachusetts 02118*

Charles R. Kerr *Division of Cardiology, Department of Medicine, University of British Columbia, 2211 Wesbrook Mall, Vancouver, British Columbia, Canada V6T 2B5*

George J. Klein *Cardiac Investigation Unit, University Hospital, 339 Windermere Road, London, Ontario, Canada N6A 5A5*

Michael S. Lauer *Section of Cardiology, Lahey Clinic Medical Center, 41 Mall Road, Burlington, Massachusetts 01805*

Richard A. Leather *Division of Cardiology, Department of Medicine, University of British Columbia, 2211 Wesbrook Mall, Vancouver, British Columbia, Canada V6T 2B5*

James W. Leitch *Cardiac Investigation Unit, University Hospital, 339 Windermere Road, London, Ontario, Canada N6A 5A5*

Maurice Lev *Congenital Heart and Conduction System Center, The Heart Institute for Children, Christ Hospital and Medical Center, 4440 West 95th Street, Oak Lawn, Illinois 60453; Departments of Pathology and Medicine and Pediatrics, Rush Medical College, Rush University, Rush-Presbyterian-St. Luke's Medical Center, 1753 West Congress Parkway, Chicago, Illinois 60612*

J. T. Lie *Department of Pathology and Laboratory Medicine, Mayo Medical School and Mayo Clinic, 200 First Street Southwest, Rochester, Minnesota 55905*

Frits L. Meijler *The Interuniversity Cardiology Institute of the Netherlands, 52 Catharijnesingel, 3501 GC Utrecht, The Netherlands*

Palle Petersen *Department of Neurology, University Hospital, Rigshospitalet, 9 Blegdamsveg, DK-2100 Copenhagen, Denmark*

Philip J. Podrid *Arrhythmia Service, University Hospital, 88 East Newton Street, Boston, Massachusetts 02118; Boston University School of Medicine, Boston, Massachusetts 02118*

Arthur Pollak *Division of Cardiology, The Talbot Building, Boston City Hospital, 818 Harrison Avenue, Boston, Massachusetts 02118; Boston University School of Medicine, Boston, Massachusetts 02118*

Charles Pollick *Echocardiography Laboratory, Vancouver General Hospital, 855 West 12th Avenue, Vancouver, British Columbia, Canada V5Z 1M9; Department of Medicine, University of British Columbia, 920 West 10th Avenue, Vancouver, British Columbia, Canada V5S 1G4*

L. M. Rodriguez *Department of Cardiology, Academic Hospital Maastricht, University of Limburg, Annadel 624, P.O. Box 5800, 6202 AZ Maastricht, The Netherlands*

Mårten Rosenqvist *Division of Cardiology, Department of Medicine, Karolinska Hospital, 113 22 Stockholm, Sweden*

Melvin M. Scheinman *Department of Medicine, University of California, San Francisco, 505 Parnassus Avenue, San Francisco, California 94143*

Ross J. Simpson, Jr. *Cardiology Section, CB #7075, Burnett-Womack Building, University of North Carolina at Chapel Hill, Chapel Hill, North Carolina 27599*

J. L. R. M. Smeets *Department of Cardiology, Academic Hospital Maastricht, University of Limburg, Annadel 624, P.O. Box 5800, 6202 AZ Maastricht, The Netherlands*

H. J. J. Wellens *Department of Cardiology, Academic Hospital Maastricht, University of Limburg, Annadel 624, P.O. Box 5800, 6202 AZ Maastricht, The Netherlands*

Fred H. M. Wittkampf *Heart Lung Institute, University Hospital Utrecht, P.O. Box 85500, 3508 GA Utrecht, The Netherlands*

Philip A. Wolf *Department of Neurology, Boston University School of Medicine, Section of Preventive Medicine and Epidemiology, Evans Memorial Department of Clinical Research, University Hospital, 720 Harrison Avenue, Boston, Massachusetts 02118*

Raymond Yee *Cardiac Investigation Unit, University Hospital, 339 Windermere Road, London, Ontario, Canada N6A 5A5*

Foreword

While I write this foreword, the United States is riveted on the topic of atrial fibrillation since President Bush has just become the most famous patient with this disorder. As President Eisenhower's infarction did much to educate the general public about the pathophysiology of coronary artery disease, so will President Bush's arrhythmia call attention to atrial fibrillation.

Atrial fibrillation is a major clinical problem and is probably the most frequently occurring cardiac rhythm disturbance, next to premature atrial and ventricular systoles. One to two million Americans may have chronic nonvalvular atrial fibrillation. Considering that it is the most common cardiac disorder leading to systemic emboli and the most common cardiogenic cause of stroke, atrial fibrillation looms as a major rhythm disturbance. In older age groups, the chance of developing atrial fibrillation over two decades is 2 percent. Thus, given the magnitude of the problem, it is fitting that an entire book be devoted to this arrhythmia.

The editors have enticed a group of clinical scientists to contribute their expertise to a variety of topics. This book begins with the pathology of atrial fibrillation and continues through the basic electrophysiology, epidemiology, and associated/precipitating factors. The remaining half of the book discusses the therapeutic issues revolving around atrial fibrillation. They are mainly three: systemic emboli and anticoagulation; conversion to and maintenance of sinus rhythm; and control of the ventricular response during atrial fibrillation. Each of these issues is dealt with in great depth in chapters written by the editors as well as by the invited experts. These well written chapters have important clinical implications that should help in the complex decision-making involved in caring for patients with intermittent and chronic, nonvalvular and valvular atrial fibrillation.

I am pleased to have been asked to write a foreword for such an important book. I am certain the reader will enjoy and learn from these chapters as much as I did.

Douglas P. Zipes, M.D.
Professor of Medicine
Indiana University
*   School of Medicine*
Senior Research Associate
Krannert Institute of Cardiology
Indianapolis, Indiana

Preface

Atrial fibrillation is the most common sustained arrhythmia seen and treated by internists and cardiologists, yet, remarkably, it is one of the least studied disorders of cardiac rhythm. In the past, each subspecialty viewed the arrhythmia from a different perspective. Pathologists described multiple organ infarctions in patients dying of diseases associated with the arrhythmia and neurologists described the high prevalence of atrial fibrillation in groups of patients presenting with stroke. For the cardiologist or internist, however, it was considered a relatively benign arrhythmia, which, because of mild or absent symptoms, was often ignored or inadequately treated. Even the most common etiology of the arrhythmia was debated—while many textbooks list coronary artery disease as the most common cause, epidemiologic studies, such as the Framingham Heart Study, and large studies of coronary disease patients, such as the Coronary Artery Surgery Study, found this not to be so.

The treatment of atrial fibrillation has, until very recently, undergone little change. For example, the majority of patients with the arrhythmia still receive the same drug, digoxin, which has been used for more than two centuries. Yet digoxin is often not the best therapy, may sometimes be ineffective, and may occasionally aggravate paroxysmal atrial fibrillation. Although it has been recognized for 50 years that embolic stroke is a devastating complication of atrial fibrillation in the setting of rheumatic heart disease, it is only in the past 3 years that definitive trials have demonstrated that patients with nonvalvular atrial fibrillation have a high incidence of stroke, which can be safely and dramatically reduced by anticoagulation.

Much of what has been learned and written about atrial fibrillation in recent years is scattered throughout the general, cardiology, and neurology literature. This book represents an attempt to bring this knowledge together and to survey in detail the current understanding of atrial fibrillation and its treatment. The need for such a book appeared obvious to us, and the positive response with which the authors greeted our invitation to contribute was gratifying, confirming our initial impression. We have been fortunate to obtain contributions from leading authorities in the field who describe the latest developments in understanding the mechanisms of the arrhythmia, the risk factors for its development, the prevention of thromboembolic complications, and the medical and nonmedical treatment options. Each chapter describes a topic in detail, and in the final chapter, we have summarized many clinical aspects in an overview that can stand alone as a guide to management of atrial fibrillation. Thus, the book should be of interest to a wide range of physicians who see and treat patients with this common arrhythmia.

It is a comprehensive volume, which, we believe, provides an informative, readable, and, most important, practical guide to this long-neglected arrhythmia.

Rodney H. Falk
Philip J. Podrid

Acknowledgments

The authors wish to acknowledge all those who have helped to bring this book together. First of all, we are extremely grateful to our contributors, whose enthusiasm in responding and precision in writing made our task so enjoyable.

Carol Hudson, Carol Antonelli, Janet Clare, and Don Davies are to be commended and thanked for their expert administrative and secretarial assistance and their ability to meet seemingly impossible deadlines without complaint. Margo Mitchell, R.N., Nancy Battinelli, R.N., and Bob Brayboy, R.N., our clinical and research nurses, are an ongoing source of help. Lisa Berger of Raven Press was constantly available throughout the development and production of this book and her advice contributed greatly to its formation. Paula Edelsack, project editor, was, again, always available and cheerfully dealt with our multitude of questions and last-minute changes.

Finally, our heartfelt thanks go to our wives, Joni Kaplan Falk and Vivian Rubinstein Podrid. Without their encouragement and support this book never would have been completed. We thank them for their abundant patience during the long hours of writing and editing.

Atrial Fibrillation
Mechanisms and Management

*Atrial Fibrillation: Mechanisms
and Management*, edited by
R. H. Falk and P. J. Podrid.
Raven Press, Ltd., New York © 1992.

1

Pathology of Atrial Fibrillation: Insights from Autopsy Studies

*J. T. Lie and †Rodney H. Falk

*Department of Pathology and Laboratory Medicine, Mayo Medical School and Mayo
Clinic, Rochester, Minnesota 55905; †Division of Cardiology, Boston City Hospital,
Boston, Massachusetts 02118 and Boston University School of Medicine,
Boston, Massachusetts 02118*

OVERVIEW

Atrial fibrillation, considered to be "the grandfather of cardiac arrhythmias" (1,2), occurs in 0.4% of the adult population and in as many as 2% to 4% of those 60 years of age or older (3,4). In the Framingham study of 5,191 men and women, 30 to 62 years old at entry and followed over 22 years, the overall incidence of atrial fibrillation was 2%. The incidence rose sharply with age but did not differ significantly between the genders (5).

Atrial fibrillation may be paroxysmal (transient) or persistent (chronic); the transient type often precedes the chronic variety. Most patients suffering from atrial fibrillation have one or more forms of underlying heart disease, but the arrhythmia can also occur as an independent entity, which has been referred to as lone atrial fibrillation (LAF) (6). The prevalence of LAF varies considerably in published series because of different diagnostic criteria and definitions of LAF. Godtfredsen (7) found a 5% and 0.6% prevalence of LAF in patients with paroxysmal and persistent atrial fibrillation, respectively. Others have reported 25% LAF in paroxysmal atrial fibrillation (8) and 25% to 30% in persistent atrial fibrillation (5), a five- to 50-fold difference compared with the findings of Godtfredsen (7). Patients diagnosed as having LAF may actually have clinically inapparent or occult cardiac disease, and this is more likely among the ambulatory population (5,8) than the hospital population (7).

In a study of 1,212 patients with all types of atrial fibrillation (7), the survival was almost identical in paroxysmal and persistent atrial fibrillation as well as between the different main etiologic groups. In a collective series of 4,602 cases reviewed by Petersen and Godtfredsen (4), the 1-year mortality ranged from 0.2% to 16%. The higher mortality rates were seen in elderly hospitalized patients with persistent atrial fibrillation, whereas younger asymptomatic patients with paroxysmal atrial fibrillation had a better prognosis.

Atrial fibrillation has long been recognized as a risk factor for stroke, although arguments regarding "cause or effect" have persisted until very recently (9), and questions have repeatedly been posed as to the clinical significance of nonrheumatic atrial fibrillation, and the prevalence and significance of clinically unsuspected embolization. The pathologist is in a unique position to answer many of the questions raised by clinicians. Despite the inherent limitation of autopsy studies, which only examine fatal cases of a specific disease (or of entities occurring in the setting of another fatal disease), much can be learned from detailed pathologic examination particularly when case controls are used. In patients with atrial fibrillation autopsy studies have clarified such questions as the prevalence of intra-atrial thrombus, the relation of atrial fibrillation to atherosclerosis, the prevalence of systemic and cerebral embolism, and localized factors associated with arrhythmia.

Although most pathologic studies related to atrial fibrillation have concentrated on a specific disease entity and its relationship to atrial fibrillation (e.g., mitral stenosis and coronary disease) or have described histopathologic abnormalities in atrial fibrillation without detailing gross anatomical changes, much can be gleaned from them. In this chapter we review the published data on the anatomy of the heart in patients with atrial fibrillation and discuss these findings in relation to current cardiologic and neurologic concepts of the arrhythmia.

PATHOLOGY OF ATRIAL FIBRILLATION

Atrial fibrillation is an arrhythmia of many etiologies, some with and some without demonstrable cardiac abnormalities (Table 1). Epidemiologic studies suggest that only 5% to 15% of patients with sustained or paroxysmal atrial fibrillation have no apparent associated heart disease (10), although subtle abnormalities of cardiac function may have gone undetected in these population-based studies.

The morphologic changes identified at autopsy in the hearts of patients with atrial fibrillation are varied and include atrial dilation, acute or chronic atrial myocardial injury, and fibrosis of the sinoatrial node or internodal fibers (11). The marked increase in incidence of atrial fibrillation with increasing age may be due not only to an increased prevalence of predisposing diseases but also to age-related changes in the heart. These include a gradual loss of nodal fibers and an increase of fibrous and adipose tissue in the sinoatrial node. Some degree of atrial dilation also occurs with aging (11,12). Focal myocardial fibrosis, unrelated to coronary artery disease, occurs with increasing frequency with advancing age and correlates poorly with significant coronary disease (13). This may, in part, contribute to decreased ventricular compliance of the aging heart, resulting in the atrial dilation, which occurs in older hearts and which may predispose to fibrillation (14). In a study by one of the authors, 237 hearts from patients aged 90 to 105 years old (39% men) were examined (12). Atrial dilation and decreased ventricular size was frequently seen. Focal deposits of amyloid, primarily confined to the interstitial area of atrial myocardium, were present in 66% of subjects, one-third of whom had extensive involvement. These, and other "normal" concomitants of aging such as mitral annular calcification, may predispose to atrial fibrillation (15).

The true prevalence of atrial fibrillation in specific disease states may not necessarily be reflected in the type of patients coming to autopsy. For example, patients with acute myocardial infarction experiencing transient atrial fibrillation may represent those with larger infarcts who are more likely to die. Nevertheless, two large autopsy series of patients in whom atrial fibrillation has been the central theme of study provide a useful insight into the pathology of this disorder.

TABLE 1. *Causes of atrial fibrillation*

With demonstrable morphologic cardiac abnormalities
1. Changes related to pressure elevation in the atria
   - Atrioventricular valve abnormalities (rheumatic and nonrheumatic)
   - Semilunar valve abnormalities (rheumatic and nonrheumatic)
   - Intracardiac thrombi or tumors
   - Myocardial disease (cardiomyopathies)
   - Systemic or pulmonary hypertension
2. Coronary heart disease and its sequelae
3. Inflammatory or infiltrative atrial disease
   - Myocarditis (noninfective or infective)
   - Amyloidosis
   - Sarcoidosis
   - Metastases
   - Hemachromatosis
4. Atrial fibrosis related to aging
5. Pericarditis or postcardiotomy syndrome
6. Cardiac trauma

Without demonstrable morphologic cardiac abnormalities
1. Intoxications (carbon monoxide, alcohol, drugs, chemicals)
2. Increased sympathetic activity
   - Anxiety
   - Hyperthyroidism
   - Pheochromocytoma
   - Alcohol, caffeine, or drugs
3. Increased parasympathetic activity
4. Idiopathic

Aberg (16), in 1969, published details of 693 patients with atrial fibrillation who had died at either of two Swedish hospitals between 1955 and 1964. These patients represented 18.5% of all hospital deaths during that period. Of these patients 642 (92.6%) underwent autopsy. The author reviewed autopsy reports with reference, among other features, to the type of heart disease present. The most common association was prior myocardial infarction (32%), followed by coronary disease without infarction (15.6%), rheumatic heart disease (14.8%), and hypertensive heart disease (13.2%). Miscellaneous causes accounted for the 18% and included malignancy, infection, uremia, and idiopathic etiologies. This study, while indicating the prevalence of various etiologies of atrial fibrillation in an autopsy population, was based on a retrospective review of autopsy records and did not give details of specific pathologic abnormalities in the heart other than thrombi.

A more detailed study from England describes the findings in 100 consecutive patients with atrial fibrillation who underwent autopsy in a 1-year period (11). Subjects were divided into those with short-term atrial fibrillation (less than 2 weeks) or long-term fibrillation (4 weeks–10 years). Distinct differences in etiology and gross and microscopic pathology were found in the two groups. In the short-term group pericarditis accounted for 13 of the 26 cases, followed by pulmonary emboli in seven, and acute myocardial infarction in four. The etiology of pericarditis was malignant in six of the 13 cases, and an additional two cases were considered to have malignancies related to the arrhythmia. In contrast, the most common etiology in 74 patients with chronic atrial fibrillation was ischemic heart disease, which occurred in 25 of 74 (33.8%) cases. Of note, this was associated with left ventricular failure in all 25. The 49 remaining cases consisted of rheumatic valve disease (24%), cor pulmonale (13.5%), hypertension with left ventricular failure (9.4%), and lone "senile" atrial fibrillation (8.1%). Carcinoma was less common than in the short-term group (four patients) and the remaining three had miscellaneous cardiac conditions.

For patients with recent-onset atrial fibrillation, right atrial volume was usually considerably increased, particularly in those patients with pulmonary embolism, whereas left atrial volume was less consistently increased. In contrast, biatrial enlargement was common in the chronic arrhythmia. Marked differences in atrial fibrosis were found between groups with acute and chronic fibrillation, with extensive degrees of fibrosis present in many patients in the latter group but little or no change in the former. The six subjects classified as having LAF were all over 80 years of age without any cardiac abnormality other than in the atrium. Isolated atrial dilation with or without internodal tract fibrosis was the typical finding in LAF with sinoatrial nodal architecture lying "at the extreme lower limit of the normal morphologic range."

Thus, although the etiologic factors causing atrial fibrillation are varied, it appears that chronic atrial fibrillation is associated with a common spectrum of atrial changes including dilation and fibrosis.

ATRIAL FIBRILLATION IN CORONARY HEART DISEASE

Acute myocardial infarction is an undisputed cause of atrial fibrillation. However, the role of chronic coronary heart disease as a risk factor for atrial fibrillation represents one of the most controversial aspects of the etiology of this arrhythmia. Although considered the leading cause of atrial fibrillation by some authors (17), others have questioned the role played by coronary disease in the development of chronic atrial fibrillation (18). The Coronary Artery Surgery Study (CASS) found only a 0.6% prevalence of chronic atrial fibrillation in more than 18,000 patients undergoing coronary angiography. This was positively associated with older age, mitral regurgitation, and congestive heart failure (19). The Framingham epidemiology study suggested similar risk factors (20).

Autopsy studies of coronary disease suffer from a selection bias toward more severe disease and/or recent infarction. As implied by the CASS study, these are a group of patients in whom atrial fibrillation may be disproportionately represented. Nevertheless important data may be derived from them. Early autopsy studies relevant to patients with atrial fibrillation tend to concentrate either on subjects with rheumatic heart disease or on the prevalence of intracardiac thrombi. Beer and Ghitman (21) reviewed 1,000 autopsies over a 10-year period and found 295 with "arteriosclerotic heart disease." Fifty-two of these had artrial fibrillation during life. The authors found thromboemboli arising from the atrium to be uncommon. However, their definition of atherosclerotic disease was imprecise and their figures should be interpreted with caution.

As indicated above, Davies and Pomerance (11) suggested that prior left ventricular failure is a major risk factor for atrial fibrillation. Other autopsy studies have disputed this finding. Hinton et al. (22) noted a 91% prevalence of prior myocardial infarction in patients with atrial fibrillation at autopsy. However, they found no difference in the prevalence of congestive heart failure between patients with atrial fibrillation and coronary disease and a control group with coronary disease without atrial fibrillation (approximately 25% in both groups). Those without atrial fibrillation did, however, tend to include a higher proportion of patients with recent myocardial infarction. In the autopsy series of patients with atrial fibrillation published by Aberg (16), patients with prior myocardial infarction outnumbered those with coronary disease and no infarction by 2:1. The latter group was almost equal in number by patients with rheumatic heart disease. Since the prevalence of ischemic heart disease in the general population greatly exceeds that of rheumatic heart disease, it is clear that the latter is a much stronger predisposing factor for atrial fibrillation than coronary disease.

The mechanisms producing atrial fibrillation in both acute myocardial infarction and chronic coronary disease include congestive heart failure and atrial infarction (23). Occasionally, mitral regurgitation secondary to ischemic damage of a papillary muscle may contribute to the arrhythmia (Fig. 1). Indeed, this and atrial infarction may be the only structural abnormalities in a group of patients with atrial fibrillation that are clearly related to coronary disease.

In summary, autopsy studies of patients with coronary artery disease and atrial fibrillation have concentrated on the prevalence of systemic emboli and/or atrial thrombi. Epidemiologic studies suggest that, other than patients with acute myocardial infarction, the association between coronary artery disease and atrial fibrillation is relatively weak. Thus, the relatively high proportion of patients in autopsy series with atrial fibrillation who had significant coronary disease probably indicates that the arrhythmia is a marker of more severe disease, a suggestion that is supported by the majority of studies (11,18–20).

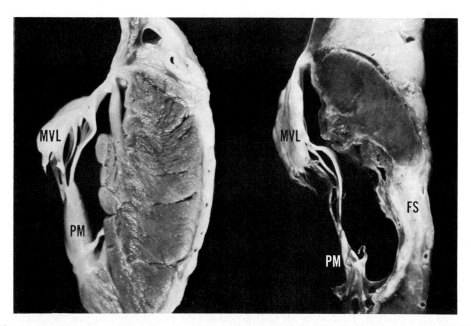

FIG. 1. Anatomy of mitral valve apparatus. Normally (*left*) the mitral valve leaflet (MVL) is securely anchored to the stout papillary muscle (PM), which in turn is supported at its base by the intact muscular ventricular wall. In frail mitral valve apparatus (*right*), the mitral valve leaflet droops and becomes incompetent due to loss of mechanical support postmyocardial infarction. The papillary muscle is atrophic, and the muscular ventricular wall is replaced by a noncontractile, full-thickness fibrous scan (FS).

MITRAL VALVE DISEASE

Atrial fibrillation occurs as a complication of virtually every known form of cardiac disease, but it has a tendency to develop in specific conditions, of which mitral valve disease is the most noteworthy (24) (Fig. 2). Both mitral stenosis and mitral regurgitation occur in rheumatic heart disease, whereas mitral valve prolapse is nowadays probably the most common cause of mitral regurgitation in developed countries.

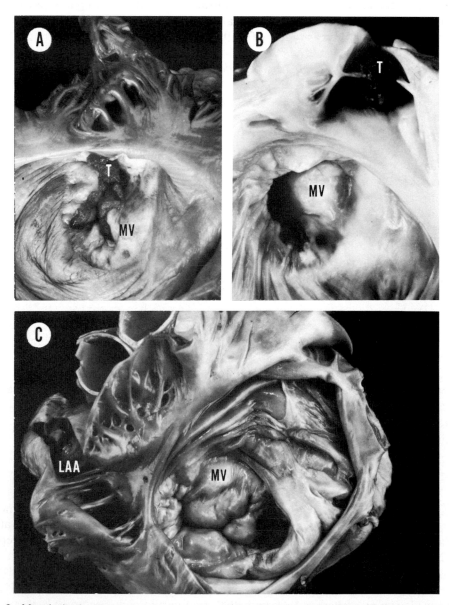

FIG. 2. Morphologic spectrum of mitral valve (MV) abnormalities associated with atrial fibrillation. **A:** With thrombotic endocarditis (T). **B:** With mural thrombus (T) in atrial appendage. **C:** With prolapsed leaflets, dilated atrium, and distended left atrial appendage (LAA).

Atrial fibrillation has been estimated to occur in about 40% of patients with mitral stenosis and in 75% of patients with significant mitral regurgitation (25). Although mitral regurgitation is a more powerful predictor of atrial fibrillation than mitral stenosis, clinical studies suggest that advancing age and duration of mitral stenosis are important contributory factors. Probst et al. (25) found a stepwise increase in the incidence of atrial fibrillation with age in patients with mitral stenosis. They also found no significant difference in mitral valve area, pulmonary artery or wedge pressure, or total pulmonary vascular resistance in patients with mitral stenosis with or without atrial fibrillation.

In a retrospective study of 101 cases of mitral stenosis undergoing autopsy at Boston City Hospital between January 1945 and June 1949, Graham et al. (26) noted a mean age at death of 52 years. Atrial fibrillation was present before death in 52% of patients with mild mitral stenosis and in 62% with severe mitral stenosis. In patients with a history of congestive heart failure and rheumatic involvement limited to the mitral valve, atrial fibrillation was "twice as common as sinus rhythm." Thromboembolism was significantly associated with the presence of atrial fibrillation.

Stone and Feil (27) studied 100 cases of "advanced" mitral stenosis coming to autopsy between 1920 and 1933. Atrial fibrillation was present in 53% of 94 cases in which the rhythm had been documented. They noted five cases of subacute bacterial endocarditis, none of which occurred in patients with atrial fibrillation. The apparent negative correlation of bacterial endocarditis and atrial fibrillation in patients with valve disease had previously been noted by other investigators (28,29). Indeed, Rothschild et al. (28) found only one case of atrial fibrillation among 109 cases of endocarditis. This is partly attributable to the relative rarity of bacterial endocarditis in pure mitral stenosis but may also suggest that a high degree of blood turbulence predisposes to endocarditis.

In autopsy series of patients dying between 1955 and 1974, consisting only of patients with atrial fibrillation, rheumatic heart disease was present in 14.7% to 28.9% (11,17,22). The prevalence of rheumatic heart disease had decreased considerably since the studies quoted above, although rheumatic heart disease still represents a significant cause of atrial fibrillation. Naturally the most obvious pathologic features of patients with rheumatic heart disease is the valvular involvement and associated atrial enlargement. As with other conditions, the onset of atrial fibrillation may result in a progressive increase in size of the atrium (30). The atrial enlargement may be extreme in mitral regurgitation. The prevalence of thromboembolism, both clinically apparent and silent, is great with atrial fibrillation and rheumatic heart disease and is considered in detail in the next section.

THROMBUS AND THROMBOEMBOLISM IN ATRIAL FIBRILLATION

Patients with rheumatic heart disease and atrial fibrillation have long been known to be at an increased risk of stroke. The association between nonrheumatic atrial fibrillation and thromboembolic stroke has, however, been a much less accepted association by the cardiology community, although epidemiologic, neurologic, and pathologic studies have indicated an association for many years. Indeed, it is only very recently, as a result of the three large trials of anticoagulation in nonvalvular atrial fibrillation published in 1989 and 1990, that cardiologists seem to have finally accepted the significant risks of chronic atrial fibrillation (31–33). In this section we examine data regarding the prevalence of atrial thrombi in patients with valvular or nonvalvular heart disease and atrial fibrillation derived from autopsy studies and discuss the findings relevant to systemic thromboembolism.

Ball Thrombus and Atrial Fibrillation

The first description of left atrial thrombus predated that of atrial fibrillation by almost 100 years. In 1809, Burns (34) differentiated endocardial thrombi from post-mortem clots and other intracardiac tumors. Although an exceedingly rare form of atrial thrombus, a large, rounded intracavitary atrial clot, termed a ball thrombus, exemplifies some of the features necessary for the development of intra-atrial thrombosis (Fig. 3). The term was first used by Wood in 1814 (35) when he described the case of a 15-year-old girl whose chief complaint was fainting spells occurring three or four times a day. After the patient died, the clinical diagnosis of mitral stenosis was confirmed at autopsy, and a spherical thrombus, 1.5 inches in diameter, was also found in the dilated left atrium.

Intracardiac ball thrombi are rare, with an estimated autopsy incidence of about one in 3,000 (2,36–41). Read et al. (40) were the last to have searched the literature and found about 60 reported cases up to 1955, and only seven additional cases have been reported since then (2). The peak age incidence among the reported cases was the fifth decade, with a 3:1 female predominance. The 15-year-old girl described by Wood (35) was probably the youngest patient known and an 86-year-old woman reported by Garvin (36) was probably the oldest.

Mitral stenosis and atrial fibrillation are present in the great majority (although not all) of cases, suggesting that this combination is particularly thrombogenic. Indeed, patients with mitral stenosis develop marked atrial dilation but have stagnant atrial flow due to obstructed flow through the mitral orifice; this is in contrast to patients with mitral regurgitation in whom the left atrium may become enormous yet who may be partially protected against atrial thrombosis by turbulent blood flow produced by the high pressure systolic regurgitant jet (42).

A mobile left atrial thrombus with a fixed-base or a free-floating ball thrombus, which intermittently obstructs the mitral valve orifice, has been detected clinically with increased frequency with the advent of echocardiography (43–45). Once detected, removal of the ball thrombus by surgical extraction is advisable and should be done with a sense of urgency, lest we witness the consequence of "hole-in-one" sudden death (41) from an abrupt and complete occlusion of the mitral valve orifice that could occur at any time.

Sites and Precipitating Factors of Atrial Thrombi

While ball thrombus is the most extreme example of intracardiac thrombus, it is also the most rare. The majority of thrombi are small and are often hidden within the left atrial appendage—a trabeculated structure that, in the fibrillating atrium, is doubtless a haven for stagnant blood and thus a fertile ground for thrombus formation. In 1930 Harvey and Levine (46) reviewed 2,091 autopsies performed between 1913 and 1929 and found 111 (5.3%) with intracardiac thrombi. Thrombi were limited to the ventricle in 35 (32%) cases, and the remaining patients had either atrial thrombi alone or both atrial and ventricular thrombi. An atypical finding compared with other studies was the predominance of right over left atrial thrombi in a ratio

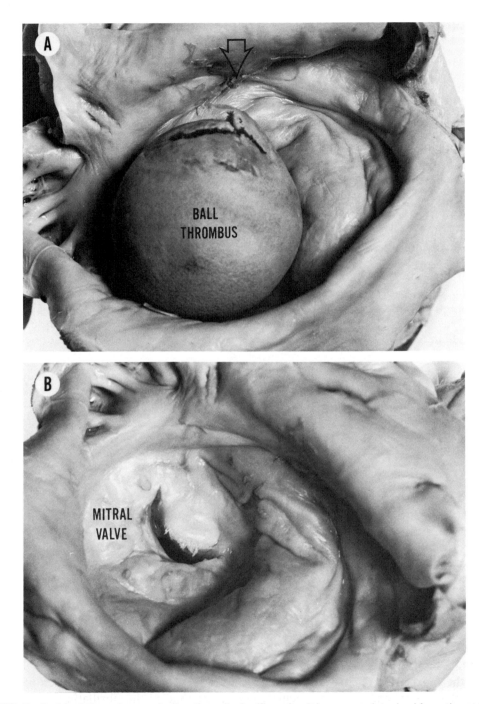

FIG. 3. A: A ball thrombus occluding the mitral orifice after it becomes detached from the atrial wall (*arrow*). **B:** Removal of the ball thrombus reveals a fish mouth-shaped stenotic mitral orifice.

of 2:1. Patients with a history of atrial fibrillation had a greater likelihood of atrial thrombi than those with sinus rhythm.

Weiss and Davis (47), in 1933, reviewed 5,215 autopsies performed at Boston City Hospital over the preceding 25-year period to determine those in whom the cause of death was rheumatic heart disease. One hundred and sixty-four patients were identified, and atrial fibrillation had occurred in 74 of 131 (57%) in whom the cardiac rhythm has been determined. "Auricular thrombi" were present in 28 patients (17%), 88% of whom had AF. Of note was the finding that 48 subjects (29.2%) had evidence of arterial embolization, which was multiple in 23 subjects. Cerebral infarction was the cause of death in 22 patients. The authors examined the question as to whether active carditis played a role in the formation of atrial thrombi and concluded that this was less common in patients dying with atrial thrombi compared with those without. They concluded that there was no evidence that active atrial inflammation predisposed to thrombi but, rather, that the stagnation of blood due to atrial fibrillation was the prime factor. Similar findings regarding the prevalence of thromboembolism in rheumatic heart disease with atrial fibrillation were reported by Stone and Feil (27) and Garvin (36). The latter author noted an equal prevalence of right and left atrial thrombi.

Paul Dudley White and co-workers (48), in 1951, published a more detailed study of 194 patients with rheumatic heart disease and systemic emboli seen in their clinical practice. One hundred and seventy-four (90%) had atrial fibrillation at the time of embolization. They stressed the considerable discrepancy between clinical and autopsy documentation of emboli and described the pathologic findings in 39 of the patients (of a total of 137 deaths) who subsequently died and were autopsied. Twenty-five of the autopsied patients had atrial thrombi, and all 25 had been in atrial fibrillation. Thrombi occurred with equal frequency in the left atrial appendage and the posterior left atrial wall. Of the total of 194 patients, death was due to an embolic cause in 78 patients, usually from cerebral embolism, but a few died of mesenteric or renal emboli. Nonfatal emboli to the extremities were also frequent.

In a similar study by Graham et al. (26) in 1951, atrial thrombi were also shown to correlate with a history of atrial fibrillation. Of 101 patients with mitral stenosis, 61 had been in atrial fibrillation, 30 of whom had atrial thrombi (again, evenly distributed between the left atrial appendage and the posterior wall). This contrasted with three of 40 patients in sinus rhythm. Peripheral emboli had occurred in 49 patients (of whom atrial fibrillation had been present in 76%). Only 31 of these subjects had visible atrial thrombi, suggesting that complete dislodgement may have occurred in many patients. Brain, kidney, and peripheral vessels were the most common site of emboli. Right atrial thrombi were found in nine patients, all of whom were in atrial fibrillation. Pulmonary infarction was common in patients with either atrial fibrillation or sinus rhythm, but this was attributed primarily to pulmonary emboli arising from a peripheral venous source.

In the large series of autopsies reviewed by Aberg (16), 20.8% of 642 patients with a history of atrial fibrillation had thrombi in one or more atrium compared with 2.3% of controls in sinus rhythm. Of patients with valvular atrial fibrillation, 30% had left atrial thrombi compared with 14% with a nonvalvular etiology of arrhythmia. The proportions of right atrial thrombi in atrial fibrillation and sinus rhythm were 9% and 2.6%, respectively. The distribution of atrial thrombi favored the left atrial appendage in a ratio of 2:1 over the free wall. However, for the valvular group the distribution was equal, whereas in the nonvalvular group the appendage thrombi outnumbered those in the body by a ratio of 3:1. Arterial emboli were documented with equal prevalence in the valvular and nonvalvular group with an overall prevalence of 44% compared with 19% of controls.

Viewing the problem from another angle, Hoxie and Coggin (49) examined autopsy reports of 205 consecutive patients with evidence of renal infarction at postmortem examination. Heart disease was present in 75% of cases, and the predominant cause of embolism was considered to be bacterial endocarditis, atrial fibrillation, or myocardial infarction. Renal infarction was often unsuspected in life, and 69% of patients had evidence of infarction in other organs.

In a relatively recent large pathologic study performed to examine the etiology of atrial fibrillation on the incidence of system embolism, Hinton et al. (22) noted that splenic and renal emboli were very common and usually clinically silent. They limited their investigation to the effects of symptomatic arterial embolism and found a prevalence of 41% in atrial fibrillation with mitral valve disease and 35% in atrial fibrillation with ischemic heart disease, compared with 7% of controls with sinus rhythm and ischemic heart disease. The most common site was the brain, followed by mesenteric artery, renal arteries, coronary arteries, and large arteries of the limbs. Emboli were often multiple. They concluded that, contrary to the conventional teaching at the time, nonrheumatic atrial fibrillation was a significant risk factor for thromboemboli and that a clinical trial of anticoagulation in nonvalvular atrial fibrillation would be of value. Of note, such a trial was instituted 10 years later by one of the report's authors and conclusively proved the initial impressions based on autopsy data (33).

CONCLUSIONS

From the above studies certain conclusions may be drawn. Atrial fibrillation is a clearly demonstrable risk factor for intra-atrial thrombosis and thromboembolism, a clinical observation recognized for many years in patients with rheumatic heart disease. In atrial fibrillation of nonrheumatic origin associated with other organic heart disease (most commonly ischemic heart disease), atrial thrombi and thromboemboli appear almost as frequently as they do in rheumatic disease. However, a pattern of atrial thrombus distribution emerges that suggests that in nonvalvular disease the most common site by far is the left atrial appendage, whereas the appendage and posterior wall are equally affected in mitral stenosis.

One can only postulate why the difference in thrombus distribution between rheumatic and nonrheumatic atrial fibrillation, if real, occurs. Whether a similar distribution is present uniformly in life is not known, and it is possible that clots in the atrial body occur primarily in more severely ill patients later coming to autopsy. Transthoracic echocardiography, which visualizes the atrial appendage poorly, is, in skilled hands, reasonably sensitive for the diagnosis of left atrial thrombi in the body of the atrium, and a recent series, confirmed by surgical observation, indicates that this site of thrombus formation is not uncommon in mitral valve disease (50). It may be postulated that patients with mitral stenosis have a greater degree of stagnant blood in the atrium when in atrial fibrillation compared with nonrheumatic patients, as a result of the larger atrial size in combination with outlet obstruction. This may predispose to intracavitary thrombi. In contrast, nonvalvular patients with atrial fibrillation may have adequate atrial blood turbulence to prevent thrombi, except in the atrial appendage (51). It is feasible that the greater prevalence of atrial body in thrombi in mitral stenosis may, in part, account for the very high thromboembolic risk when atrial fibrillation develops.

Almost all the patients in the studies quoted in this chapter were receiving no long-term anticoagulation. Since anticoagulation is increasingly used prophylactically in patients with atrial fibrillation, it is likely that the prevalence of atrial thrombosis and its complications will be markedly reduced. In addition, the relative rarity of thrombi in the body of the left atrium, as reported in series of patients studied by transesophageal echocardiography, may reflect the low prevalence of rheumatic disease and/or the use of anticoagulation in patients with mitral valve disease and atrial fibrillation.

In summary, autopsy examination of the heart has played an important role in understanding the clinicopathologic correlations in patients with atrial fibrillation. Long before the current interest in anticoagulation in nonvalvular atrial fibrillation, pathologists had noted the high thromboembolic event rate in both valvular and nonvalvular atrial fibrillation alike. They recognized that asymptomatic embolism of the brain was common—a fact that has recently been confirmed in living patients (52), and they urged that trials of anticoagulation be performed in nonvalvular disease (16,22). The intimate involvement of clinicians with pathologists in the early, classic studies of rheumatic heart disease (26,46–48) led to the formation of many recommendations still in place today. Such cooperative interdisciplinary studies are, unfortunately, less common today but could no doubt shed further light into the serious complications of this common and fascinating arrhythmia.

REFERENCES

1. Selzer A. Atrial fibrillation revisited. *N Engl J Med* 1982;306:1044–1045.
2. Lie JT. Atrial fibrillation and left atrial thrombus: an insufferable odd couple. *Am Heart J* 1988;116:1374–1377.
3. Ostrander LD Jr, Brandt RL, Kjelsberg MO, Epstein FH. Electrocardiographic findings among the adult population of a total natural community. Tecumseh, Michigan. *Circulation* 1965;31:888–898.
4. Petersen P, Godtfredsen J. Atrial fibrillation—a review of course and prognosis. *Acta Med Scand* 1984;216:5–9.
5. Kannel WB, Abbott RD, Savage DD, McNamara PM. Epidemiologic features of chronic atrial fibrillation: the Framingham study. *N Engl J Med* 1982;306:1018–1022.
6. Evans W, Swan P. Lone atrial fibrillation. *Br Heart J* 1954;16:189–194.
7. Godtfredsen J. *Atrial fibrillation. Etiology, course and prognosis: a follow-up study of 1212 cases.* Copenhagen: Munksgaard, 1975.
8. Takahashi N, Seki A, Imataka K, Fujii J. Clinical features of paroxysmal atrial fibrillation: an observation of 94 patients. *Jpn Heart J* 1981;22:143–149.
9. Bucknall CA, Morris GK, Mitchell JRA. Physicians' attitudes to four common problems: hypertension, atrial fibrillation, transient ischemic attacks and angina pectoris. *Br Med J* 1986;293:739–742.
10. Brand FN, Abbott RD, Kannell WB, Wolf PA. Characteristics and prognosis of lone atrial fibrillation. *JAMA* 1985;254:3449–3453.
11. Davies MJ, Pomerance A. Pathology of atrial fibrillation in man. *Br Heart J* 1972;34:520–525.
12. Lie JT, Hammond PI. Pathology of the senescent heart: anatomic observations on 237 autopsy studies of patients of 90 to 105 years old. *Mayo Clin Proc* 1988;63:552–564.
13. Anderson KR, St. John-Sutton MG, Lie JT. Histopathological types of cardiac fibrosis in myocardial disease. *J Pathol* 1979;128:79–85.
14. Manyari DE, Patterson C, Johnson D, Melendez L, Kotuk WJ, Cape RDT. Atrial and ventricular arrhythmias in asymptomatic elderly subjects. Correlation with left atrial size and left ventricular mass. *Am Heart J* 1990;119:1069–1076.
15. Aronow WS, Schmoetz KS, Koenigsberg M. Correlation of atrial fibrillation with presence or

absence of mitral annular calcium in 604 persons older than 60 years. *Am J Cardiol* 1987;59:1213–1214.

16. Aberg H. Atrial fibrillation. 1. A study of atrial thrombosis and systemic embolism in a necropsy material. *Acta Med Scand* 1969;185;373–379.

17. Marriott HJL, Myerburg RF. Recognition of arrhythmias and conduction abnormalities. In: Hurst WJ, ed. *The heart*. New York: McGraw-Hill, 1986;433–475.

18. Haddad AH, Prehkov VK, Dean DC. Chronic atrial fibrillation and coronary artery disease. *J Electrocardiol* 1978;11:67–69.

19. Cameron A, Schwartz MJ, Kronmal RA, Kosinski AS. Prevalence and significance of atrial fibrillation in coronary artery disease (CASS registry). *Am J Cardiol* 1988;61:714–717.

20. Kannel WB, Abbott RD, Savage DD. Coronary heart disease and atrial fibrillation: the Framingham study. *Am Heart J* 1983;106:389–396.

21. Beer DT, Ghitman B. Embolization from the atria in arteriosclerotic heart disease. *JAMA* 1961;177:287–291.

22. Hinton RC, Kistler JP, Fallon JT, Friedlich AL, Fisher CM. Influence of etiology of atrial fibrillation on incidence of systemic embolism. *Am J Cardiol* 1977;40:509–513.

23. Soderstrom N. Myocardial infarction and mural thrombosis in the atria of the heart. *Acta Med Scand* 1948;suppl:217.

24. Morris DC, Hurst JW. Atrial fibrillation. *Curr Probl Cardiol* 1980;5:1–51.

25. Probst P, Goldschlager N, Selzer A. Left atrial size and atrial fibrillation in mitral stenosis: factors influencing their relationship. *Circulation* 1973;48:1282–1287.

26. Graham GK, Taylor JA, Ellis LB, Greenberg DJ, Robbins SL. Studies in mitral stenosis: a correlation of postmortem findings with the clinical course in the disease in one hundred and one cases. *Arch Intern Med* 1951;88:532–547.

27. Stone SS, Feil HS. Mitral stenosis: a clinical and pathological study of 100 cases. *Am Heart J* 1933;9:53–62.

28. Rothschild MA, Sachs B, Libman E. The disturbances of the cardiac mechanism in subacute bacterial endocarditis and rheumatic fever. *Am Heart J* 1927;2:356–374.

29. Fulton MN, Levine SA. Subacute bacterial endocarditis, with special reference to the valvular lesions and previous history. *Am J Med Sci* 1932;183:60–77.

30. Sanfillipo AJ, Abascal VM, Sheehan M, et al. Atrial enlargement as a consequence of atrial fibrillation. A prospective echocardiographic study. *Circulation* 1990;82:792–797.

31. Special Report. Preliminary report of the Stroke Prevention in Atrial Fibrillation Study. *N Engl J Med* 1990;322:863–868.

32. Petersen P, Boysen G, Godtfredsen J, Andersen ED, Andersen B. Placebo-controlled, randomized trial of warfarin and aspirin for prevention of thromboembolic complications in chronic atrial fibrillation. The Copenhagen AFASAK Study. *Lancet* 1989;1:175–179.

33. The Boston Area Anticoagulation Trial for Atrial Fibrillation Investigators. The effect of low-dose warfarin on the risk of stroke in patients with nonrheumatic atrial fibrillation. *N Engl J Med* 1990;323:1505–1511.

34. Burns A. Observations on formation of polypi of the heart. In: *Diseases of the heart*. Edinburgh: Bryce, 1809.

35. Wood W. Letter enclosing the history and dissection of a case in which a foreign body was found within the heart. *Edinb Med Surg J* 1814;10:50–54.

36. Garvin CF. Mural thrombi in the heart. *Am Heart J* 1941;21:713–720.

37. Evans W, Benson R. Mass thrombus of the left auricle. *Br Heart J* 1948;10:39–47.

38. Evans ME. Ball thrombus of the heart. *Br Heart J* 1948;10:34–38.

39. Radding RS. Ball thrombus of the right auricle. *Br Heart J* 1948;11:653–657.

40. Read JL, Porter RR, Russi S, Kriz JR. Occlusive auricular thrombi. *Circulation* 1955;12:250–258.

41. Lie JT, Ertman ML. "Hole-in-one" sudden death: mitral stenosis and left atrial ball thrombus. *Am Heart J* 1976;91:798–804.

42. Daley R, Franks R. Massive dilatation of the left auricle. *Q J Med* 1949;18:81–92.

43. Sunagawa K, Orita Y, Tanaka S, Kikuchi Y, Nakamura M, Hirata T. Left atrial ball thrombus diagnosed by two-dimensional echocardiography. *Am Heart J* 1980;100:89–94.

44. Furukawa K, Katsume H, Masukubo H, Inoue D. Echocardiographic findings of floating thrombus in left atrium. *Br Heart J* 1980;44:599–601.

45. Dent RG, Dick JPR, Cory-Pearce R. Left atrial ball valve thrombus: treatable cause of clinical deterioration a patient with mitral stenosis. *Br Heart J* 1984;49:400–402.

46. Harvey EA, Levine SA. A study of uninfected mural thrombi of the heart. *Am J Med Sci* 1930;180:365–372.

47. Weiss S, Davis D. Rheumatic heart disease, III. Embolic manifestations. *Am Heart J* 1933;9:45–52.

48. Daley R, Mattingley TW, Holt CL, Bland EF, White PD. Systemic arterial embolism in rheumatic heart disease. *Am Heart J* 1951;42:566–581.

49. Hoxie HJ, Coggin CB. Renal infarction. Statistical study of 205 cases and a detailed report of an unusual case. *Arch Intern Med* 1940;65:587–594.
50. Bansal RC, Heywood T, Applegate PM, Jetzy KR. Detection of left atrial thrombi by two-dimensional echocardiography and surgical correlation in 148 patients with mitral valve disease. *Am J Cardiol* 1989;64:243–246.
51. Pollick C, Taylor D. Assessment of left atrial appendage function by transesophageal echocardiography: implications for the development of thrombus. *Circulation* 1991;84:223–231.
52. Feinberg WM, Seeger JF, Carmody RF, Anderson DC, Hart RG, Pearce LA. Epidemiologic features of asymptomatic cerebral infarction in patients with nonvalvular atrial fibrillation. *Arch Intern Med* 1990;250:2340–2344.

Atrial Fibrillation: Mechanisms and Management, edited by
R. H. Falk and P. J. Podrid.
Raven Press, Ltd., New York © 1992.

2

Histology of the Normal and Diseased Atrium

*Saroja Bharati and †Maurice Lev

*Congenital Heart and Conduction System Center, The Heart Institute for Children,
Christ Hospital and Medical Center, Oak Lawn, Illinois 60453
and Departments of *†Pathology, and †Medicine and Pediatrics, Rush Medical College,
Rush University, Rush-Presbyterian-St. Luke's Medical Center, Chicago, Illinois 60612*

For almost 100 years, there has been considerable interest generated in the exact pathologic change or anatomic substrate for the development of atrial fibrillation. Are there specific structural changes in the atria that are responsible for this arrhythmia? This question has intrigued both cardiologists and pathologists, since, in a very broad perspective, one may answer the question positively (yes) and negatively (no) because both are in essence true. The normal structure of the atria is *not* present in cases of atrial fibrillation. Therefore, the answer is "yes," there are structural changes in the atrial musculature. However, are these changes in the atria specific for atrial fibrillation? The answer here is "no"; the structural changes are rather *general*, not specific, and rather diffuse in nature. Various pathologic changes in the atria may alter the normal atrial musculature to such an extent that it may result in atrial fibrillation clinically.

When dealing with the subject of atrial fibrillation pathologically, it is mandatory to consider that part of the conduction system that is related to the atria. In a broader perspective, in our opinion, the distal conduction system and the entire heart should also be studied in cases of atrial fibrillation. Although rarely "isolated" atrial disease (disease without involvement of the ventricles) can give rise to atrial fibrillation clinically, in the majority of instances changes are present in the entire heart, including the conduction system, which may influence its occurrence.

In order to understand the histologic abnormalities in atrial fibrillation, it is only appropriate that one first understands the normal anatomy of the atria at the gross and histologic levels. This includes the approaches to the sinoatrial (SA) node and the SA node, the approaches to the atrioventricular (AV) node and the AV node, the atrial preferential pathways, and Bachmann's bundle.

The gross and histologic structures of the atria are different from those of the ventricles. In various pathologic states, the atria are often more involved than the ventricles. We will therefore present the normal anatomy and histology of the atria at various ages and then will present its pathology in atrial fibrillation.

THE NORMAL ANATOMY OF THE ATRIA

At the gross level, the right atrium internally presents the entry of the superior and inferior vena cava and coronary sinus. The entry of the superior vena cava is at an angle, while that of the inferior vena cava is in the inferodistal end of the right atrium. The eustachian and the thebesian valves guard the entry of the inferior vena cava and the coronary sinus, respectively. The triangle of Koch is situated between the coronary sinus and the medial leaflet of the tricuspid valve. The limbus fossae ovalis is more or less in the center of the right side of the atrial septum. The presence of the limbus indicates that this chamber is the right atrium. The tubercle of Lower extends from the proximal end of the limbus on to the septum proximally. The right atrial appendage is a broad structure with a wide mouth.

The left atrium receives the pulmonary veins proximally. Either each individual pulmonary vein enters separately, or the pulmonary veins join together to form one pulmonary vein in its entry into the atrium. This chamber presents the upturned septum primum. The left atrial appendage is an irregularly curved structure with a narrow mouth.

AGE-RELATED CHANGES IN THE NORMAL ATRIA (1–3)

Right Atrium

At about 6 months gestation, small zones of grayish-white opacity appear on the limbus and extend toward the superior and inferior venae cavae. At term, a slight opacity appears over the posterior crest and at the base of the anterior tricuspid leaflet. By the end of the first year, the gross pattern resembles that of the adult. Thickened endocardium is found over the limbus and adjacent to the venae cavae, with a lesser thickening over the posterior and anterior crests. By the end of the first decade, zones of opacity become plaque-like, while the appendage, pectinate muscles, and orifice of the coronary sinus and the area above the medial tricuspid leaflet remain translucent. In the second decade, a thickening becomes apparent at the base of the posterior tricuspid leaflet. In the fourth and fifth decades, small fat spots appear in the septum and in the region of the AV node. In later decades, there is accentuation of the plaques of thickening with some whitening, especially on the limbus (Fig. 1) and around the caval orifices. Fat at the gross level is present beyond the age of 35 at the junction of the superior vena cava with the right atrium, atrial septum, and along the AV sulcus on both sides.

Left Atrium

Here the endocardial thickening is diffuse. The earliest opacities appear on the posterior wall, at the orifices of the pulmonary veins, and at the orifice of the appendage. At 7 months gestation, there is a coalescence of these zones. At birth, the posterior atrial myocardium is markedly opaque, with occasional superimposed white plaques. With closure of the foramen ovale, the septum primum rapidly becomes thick and opaque, and by the end of the first year, most of the endocardium

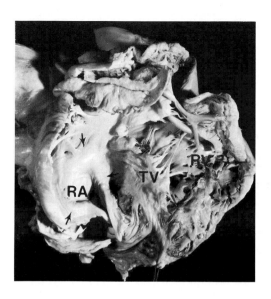

FIG. 1. Right atrial and right ventricular view of the heart from an aged person showing the thickened atrial septum. RA, right atrium; RV, right ventricle; TV, tricuspid valve. *Arrows* point to the thickened atrial septum.

shows some degree of opacity. However, there is a relatively translucent area above the anterior leaflet of the mitral valve. By 20 years of age, plaque formation with pronounced corrugation of the endocardium is constant in the posterior wall, accompanied by similar corrugation at the orifice of the appendage and pulmonary veins. Thereafter, there is general augmentation of the thickening, especially at the anulus of the mitral valve until the sixth decade. This may be associated with calcification and fatty infiltration, which may be evident at a gross level. At this time, the endocardium is thick, grayish-white with zones of pronounced wrinkling. Fat spots may be noticed in the fifth and sixth decades with a thickened atrial septum (Fig. 2).

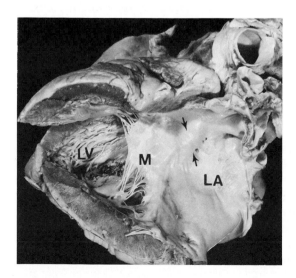

FIG. 2. Left atrial and left ventricular view of the same heart showing the thickened atrial septum. LA, left atrium; LV, left ventricle; MV, mitral valve. *Arrows* point to the thickened atrial septum. Note the aging changes of the mitral valve.

HISTOLOGY OF THE ENDOCARDIUM IN VARIOUS AGE GROUPS

In general, in both atria, at birth, in some areas, the simplest type of endocardium is seen. This consists of an endothelial lining, beneath which there is a delicate elastic layer that rests on a small amount of connective tissue. However, in most parts of the atria, beneath the endothelial lining, there is a fibroelastic core or subendocardium. From birth on, this basic structure is altered by focal or diffuse areas of proliferation of smooth muscle cells and/or elastic fibers, and/or collagen fibers. We call this process *endocardial hypertrophy*. This process is more diffuse in the left atrium and focally more marked in the right atrium. By maturity, there are increases in elastic and collagenous fibers in the subendocardium and in the extent of endocardial hypertrophy. With time, sclerotic changes set in. They consist of fragmentation, coarse clumping and zoning of elastic fibers, dissolution of distinct endocardial layers, vacuolization and atrophy of endocardial muscle with replacement by collagen and elastic fibers, and irregularity in staining of the reticular and glycoprotein components of the basement membranes. With time, in the subendocardium, there is a loosening of previous compact structures and elastification of subendocardial fat, accompanied by focal irregularities in the basement membranes of the elastic fibers. In several areas of sclerosis, small amounts of sudanophilic material appear in the elastic fibers, in smooth muscle, and in ground substance of the endocardium. Metachromasia and calcium deposits are conspicuously absent in most of the endocardium.

Right Atrium

Endocardial hypertrophy is noted in the eighth month and is more pronounced at birth. This hypertrophy is elastic or musculoelastic except in the region of the inferior vena cava, where it is fibroelastic. Early endocardial sclerosis is already seen at birth. The maximal amount of hypertrophy and sclerosis is seen in the limbus, where it is occasionally accompanied by metachromasia. By the fifth year, the process of endocardial hypertrophy is maximal in the septal, anterior, and posterior walls and commences also focally in the posterior crest, the pectinate muscles, and the appendage. Retrogressive changes become pronounced at the end of the first decade. In the second decade, fatty metamorphosis is noted in the limbus and at points in the anterior and posterior walls. Collagen plaques in the hypertrophic zones become manifest in the third decade. In the fourth decade, hypertrophic and sclerotic changes in previously uninvolved areas of the atrium occur. In the fifth decade, atrophy of smooth muscle layers is seen, and in the sixth decade, increased sclerotic changes are seen (Fig. 3A).

Left Atrium

By the eighth month of gestation, the basic structure is established so that there is diffuse thickening of the endocardium. The subendocardium contains more elastic tissue than the right atrium, and the endocardial hypertrophy is greater and more diffuse. Already in fetal life, there is a tendency for a loss of distinction between various endocardial strata, and early retrogressive changes are already noted.

In the first year of life, the left atrial endocardium becomes much thicker than that

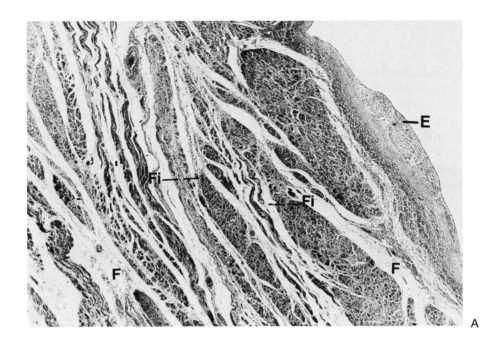

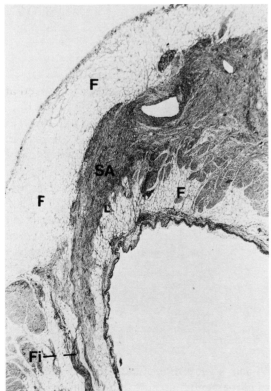

FIG. 3. A: Photomicrograph of the right atrium from an aged individual. Gomori trichrome stain, ×45. E, thickened endocardium; Fi, fibrosis of the myocardium; F, fatty infiltration. **B:** Approaches to the SA node and the SA node showing marked fatty metamorphosis and fibrosis from an elderly with normal aging. Weigert-van Gieson stain, ×37.5. F, fat; SA, sinoatrial node; Fi, fibrosis.

of the right atrium, especially in the posterior wall. Considerable lamination is noted in the hypertrophic zones. Retrogressive changes are more intense than in the right atrium. As in the right atrium, maximal hypertrophic changes are seen at 5 years of age. The hypertrophy is mostly elastic in the inner part, with smooth muscle being seen in the deeper region. At all times, the hypertrophy is more marked in the posterior than in the anterior wall, but retrogressive changes are already considerable in the anterior wall as well. In the second decade, endocardial hypertrophy of the appendage becomes more accentuated. In the third decade, rugosity of the posterior wall becomes more intense. In the fourth decade, the entire atrium is the seat of hypertrophy and sclerosis, more intense than in the right atrium, with collagen replacement being frequent. The maximal retrogressive changes are seen in the sixth decade.

MYOCARDIUM OF ATRIA

Atrial myocardium is more loosely arranged than ventricular myocardium, and there is a greater amount of connective tissue in the former. The reticular nets or the basement membranes of the myocardial fibers in the atria show a somewhat different pattern than those of the ventricles. At birth, they are similar in thickness. In late fetal life, thick collagen fibers and occasional short elastic fibers are seen in the myocardium of the right atrium. The normal orientation of the myocardial fibers is chaotic in the left atrium. On the other hand, the orientation of the myocardial fibers is relatively smooth in the limbic margin in the right atrium. In the left atrial myocardium, collagen fibers are less conspicuous. Only minimal fine elastic fibers are seen in the interstitial blood vessels of the myocardium. This is in contrast to the more prominent elastic endocardium in this chamber. In the first decade relatively more elastic tissue is seen in atrial myocardium of both sides.

By age 20, fatty metamorphosis is constant in atrial myocardial interstitial tissue, more in the right atrium than in the left. In both, numerous elastic fibers are seen in atrial myocardium. In the third decade, elastic tissue in the myocardium is more prominent, especially in the right atrium, and fatty metamorphosis becomes diffuse on both sides. By middle age, fat replacement or penetration in the right atrial myocardium becomes more pronounced. In the fourth and fifth decades, collagenization and elastic fibers become abundant in the atrial myocardial interstitium in the right atrium (Fig. 3A), while both atria show a relatively greater increase in interstitial tissue with elastification of fat tissue. In old age, there is atrophy of musculature of the left atrium.

EPICARDIUM

Gross Changes

Before birth, the epicardium is thickened over the SA nodal region and over Wenckebach's bundle and the posterior wall of the left atrium. By maturity, there is a marked increase in epicardial opacity over the SA nodal region.

At birth, there is a fat pad between the aorta, the right atrium, and the right ventricle. Fat also is present in the right AV groove anteriorly. After birth, fat occasionally appears in the SA nodal region. With advancing age, fat appears at entry of the pulmonary veins and the superior vena cava, posteriorly. Fat also extends from the left circumflex artery upward on the left atrium. Fat is thus commonly seen beyond the age of 35 (sometimes earlier) at the region of the SA node and its approaches, Bachmann's bundle, along the AV sulcus anteriorly and posteriorly accompanying the right and left circumflex coronary arteries. By the fifth decade, there is a confluence of regions of fat accumulation.

Microscopic Changes

The epicardium over the atria is thicker than that over ventricles. In the newborn period, the lamina propria is covered by a single layer of mesothelial cells. In both atria, beneath this layer, there is an extremely thin elastic layer. The epicardium over the right atrium is more compact than that over the left atrium. In the first decade, the lamina propria becomes more prominent with an increase in both elastic and collagen components.

In the second decade, there is an increase in collagen and fat in the epicardium. By maturity, fine elastic fibers are seen dispersed through the collagen layer. Beneath the lamina propria, adipose tissue is prominent. Elastic fibers are more pronounced over the right atrium. In the fourth decade, pericardial "milk spots" are occasionally seen.

From middle age upward, epicardial plaques are seen with increased frequency. The majority of these show accumulation of inflammatory cells, usually lymphocytes. The right atrial epicardium is thicker than that of the other chambers.

THE CONDUCTION SYSTEM IN THE ATRIA (4–6)

The conduction system in the atria consists of the SA node and its approaches, the atrial preferential pathways, the AV node and its approaches, and Bachmann's bundle.

Sinoatrial Node

This lies in the sulcus terminalis and extends from the junction of the superior vena cava and the right atrial appendage upward to the hump of the atrial appendage and downward toward the intercaval band. It consists of fusiform cells with a smaller diameter than that of the atrial cells and shorter in length, arranged in a serpiginous manner, with a tendency toward following the longitudinal diameter of the sulcus terminalis. The cytoplasm stains lighter than that of atrial cells, the myofibrils are fewer in number, and the cells contain striations. Intercalated discs are not noted. The cells are surrounded by a thick mass of collagen and copious elastic fibers. Nerve ganglia are situated around the SA node, but only nerve fibers are in the node. On electron microscopy, the SA nodal cells have scant myofibrils arranged chaotically, with few mitochondria. There is no transverse tubular system. Tight junctions are rare, but fasciae adherentes and desmosomes are present.

Approaches to the Sinoatrial Node

These consist of transitional cells characteristic of both nodal and atrial working cells. Wenckebach's bundle consists of large cells with copious cytoplasm.

Atrial Preferential Pathways

These are the superior middle and inferior pathways. They occupy the entire atrial septum and consist of large Purkinje-like cells, working atrial cells, and small node-like cells.

Bachmann's Bundle

This is present on the roof of the atria connecting the right and the left atria. It consists of the same type of cells present in the atria.

Approaches to the Atrioventricular Node

These consist of cells that may be smaller in diameter than that of the atrial cells or the same size. They are relatively loosely arranged with spaces intervening with the presence of the AV nodal artery and nerve ganglia.

Atrioventricular Node

This is situated between the right side of the central fibrous body and the medial leaflet of the tricuspid valve. The cells are smaller in diameter and in length than atrial or ventricular cells. They contain fewer cross-striated myofibrils. The nuclei are oval, the cytoplasm is light staining, and intercalated discs are present. Between the parenchymal cells are sheath cells. Copious collagen and elastic fibers are noted. Nerve ganglia are present outside the node, and nerve fibers are seen in the node. On electron microscopy, the myofibrils are scant, as are the mitochondria, and both are irregularly distributed. The cells contain no transverse tubular system. Tight junctions are scarce.

The remainder of the conduction system will not be described here, since the thrust of this chapter concerns the atria.

THE PATHOLOGY OF THE ATRIA

The pathology of the atria may be described according to the various atrial arrhythmias that may be present. The various atrial arrhythmias that have been found clinically in our autopsied material are very extensive. Certainly the basic pathologic changes in the atria that are found may produce various different arrhythmias at various times. The pathologic changes include congenital abnormalities of the atria and the conduction system in the atria, and acquired pathologic change in the atria and the conduction system such as fibrosis, infiltrative diseases, coronary artery disease, fatty metamorphosis, acute and chronic inflammation, and tumor formation. The conduction system in the atria that may be involved includes the SA node and its approaches, the left and right atrial myocardium, the approaches to the AV node, the AV node, Bachmann's bundle, Wenckebach's bundle, and the eustachian and thebesian valves. We will not include in our discussion the central fibrous body, the right atrial left ventricular part of the membranous septum, and the mitral and tricuspid valves. However, we wish to emphasize that changes in these regions (congenital or acquired) may be associated with varying types of atrial arrhythmias including atrial fibrillation.

The arrhythmias that have been noted are atrial fibrillation and flutter, atrial tachycardia, tachycardia-bradycardia or sick sinus syndrome, a combination of atrial flutter with AV block, atrial standstill (transient or persistent), multifocal atrial tachycardia, junctional (nodal) rhythm, marked variation in atrial depolarization complexes, slow and erratic atrial rate, idiopathic familial atrial cardiomyopathy with conduction block, prolonged A-H time, prolonged sinus node recovery time, prolonged effective and functional refractory period, unstable cardiac rhythm, depression of junctional pacemaker, and familial atrial arrhythmias. We will not discuss AV block unless the block is produced in the atria, completely or in part.

The literature reveals that only occasionally has work been done in which a specific arrhythmia has been studied as such in many clinical cases. We will deal with this type of work first, then we will discuss cases from our own work in which atrial arrhythmias were present, associated with our conduction system findings.

Atrial Fibrillation and Flutter

The earlier work was reviewed by Yater (7). He quoted a large number of previous authors (8–32).

In atrial fibrillation these authors found either changes in the SA node, AV node, or the nerves supplying these structures, myocarditis in the right atrium, dilation of the atria, pathology in the bundle of His, or no changes in the conduction system.

Yater (7) studied 145 cases of atrial fibrillation, seven cases of flutter, and two cases of paroxysmal tachycardia. These were in cases of rheumatic fever, thyroid disease, hypertension, coronary disease, and syphilis. Histology was done in 29 of these. In the histologic examination, he took one block of the SA node and one block containing the AV node, bundle, and the beginning of the bundle branches. These he fixed in formaldehyde and embedded in celloidin. Sections were taken for examination 1 mm apart in these blocks. The controls consisted of 35 normal hearts. Yater found no distinctions between his cases of fibrillation and his controls to account for atrial fibrillation.

After Yater's work there was lapse of some years before the subject of atrial fibrillation was reinvestigated.

Davies and Pomerance (33) studied 100 patients with atrial fibrillation with anatomic findings, including the conduction system. In 26 patients the fibrillation was present only in the last 2 weeks of life, and in 74 patients it persisted for 1 month to 10 years. Where it had developed in the last 2 weeks, dilatation of the atria was common, and the SA node and internodal tracts were normal. Where it was long term, the nodal artery showed stenosis, and there was loss of muscle in the SA node and internodal tracts. The pathologic conditions found in these cases were chronic rheumatic heart disease, ischemic heart disease, hypertension, and cor pulmonale. In some aged patients, the fibrillation was associated with the loss of muscle fibers in the SA node. The atrial preferential tracts showed no specific histologic features. They quoted Hudson (34,35), who found damage to the SA node in auricular fibrillation, James (36–39), who found damage in the internodal pathways, Laas (40), who mentioned atrial dilatation, and Lippestad and Marton (41), who found occlusion of the SA nodal artery.

In their work, Davies and Pomerance estimated the atrial volume by weighing atrial wax casts, and they studied coronary angiocardiograms in many cases. The SA node and internodal tracts were quantitatively assessed for the amount of muscle and fibrous tissue by point counting, using slides stained by picro-Mallory stains. They studied a combination of coronary artery angiograms and serial blocks of nodal tissues within the atria.

In the short-term fibrillation group, they found (a) the right atrial volume was increased, (b) a large number of cases associated with pulmonary embolism, (c) the left atrial volume was less consistently elevated, and (d) the majority showed *no* muscle loss in the SA node and internodal tracts. In the long-term fibrillation group, they found

1. the left and right atrial volume was increased,
2. severe damage to the SA node, with loss of muscle fibers in the SA node,
3. fibrous thickening and obliteration of the pericardial sac were present,
4. an increase in fibrosis of the internodal tracts,
5. no evidence of active inflammation,
6. no Aschoff bodies were identified,
7. stenosis or occlusion of the SA nodal artery was present,
8. thrombosis in the left atrial appendage was seen in 46 cases,
9. cerebral infarction was present in 19,
10. half of the patients had acute pericarditis.

Davies and co-workers (42) stated that in atrial fibrillation there were (a) a reduction in the number of myocardial cells in the SA node, (b) a generalized loss of atrial myocardial cells in the approaches to the SA node, (c) an increase in adipose tissue in the internodal myocardium, (d) occasional deposition of amyloid in the atrial myocardium, and (e) atrial dilatation. Atrial fibrillation was associated with ischemic heart disease, mitral valve disease (especially of the rheumatic variety), thyrotoxicosis, prolapsed mitral valve with regurgitation, acute myocardial infarction, pulmonary embolism, acute pericarditis, and secondary tumors of the atria. The factors involved in the production of atrial fibrillation were atrial dilatation and SA nodal disease with muscle loss, and fibrosis and disruption of the atrial muscle.

In the subsequent years, we and others have studied single or groups of cases pathologically of atrial fibrillation, including conduction system studies.

From our work and review of the literature the classification outlined in Table 1 may be considered for atrial fibrillation. This is by no means a complete one.

Normal Aging

As we have discussed in detail, the normal aging changes of the atrial myocardium eventually result in loss of myocardial fibers with increase in fatty metamorphosis and connective tissue in the SA and AV nodes and their approaches (Fig. 3A, B). Thus it is not surprising to find that atrial fibrillation is the most common type of cardiac arrhythmia in the elderly. We believe that the loss of myocardial cells (atrophy) in part, with increase in fat and fibrous tissue, probably alters the transmission of the impulse from the SA node to the AV node and may result in atrial fibrillation. Although we find atrophy of some of the atrial myocardial cells, this is usually associated with atrial enlargement. There is a tendency for the size of both atria to be

TABLE 1. *Classification of atrial fibrillation*

I. Normal aging
II. Acquired
   A. Hypertensive heart disease
   B. Coronary artery disease
   C. Postoperative heart disease
      1. Atrial septum defect—any type
      2. Mustard procedure
      3. Senning
      4. Atrial septectomy—Blalock-Hanlon procedure
      5. Coronary artery bypass surgery
   D. Rheumatic heart disease—mitral stenosis
   E. Infiltrative disease of the heart
      1. Fat
      2. Amyloid
      3. Sarcoid
   F. Alcohol
III. Arrhythmias associated with atrial fibrillation
   A. Familial arrhythmias with AV block
   B. Preexcitation
   C. Congenital AV block in the middle aged
   D. Sick sinus syndrome—tachycardia-bradycardia syndrome
IV. Congenital
   A. Idiopathic dilatation of the right atrium
   B. Atrial septal defect—any type of long-standing duration
   C. Ebstein's anomaly
   D. Tumors
      1. Lipoma of the atrial septum
      2. Myxoma
      3. Rhabdomyoma
   E. Congenital anomalies of the AV junction—atrio-Hisian fibers
V. Miscellaneous
   A. Thyrotoxicosis
   B. Myotonia dystrophica
   C. Kearns-Sayre syndrome
   D. Hypertrophic cardiomyopathy
   E. Any disease that affects the atria to a moderate-considerable extent

larger than normal. This probably is due to the varying types of myocardial fibers in the atrium. Some are hypertrophied, some atrophied, and some show varying stages of degenerative changes. This, in association with an increase in fatty metamorphosis, probably results in the enlargement of the atria. It is also of interest that the atrial myocardium exhibits large spaces in between the above described myocardial fibers (Fig. 3A). At the light level, we are unable to define what might have occupied the space. It might represent the lymphatics or other biochemical phenomena with fluid components.

The constant increase in fat and fibrosis (connective tissue) with aging may be one of the reasons that atrial fibrillation in the elderly gradually progresses with time, starting with intermittent forms of atrial fibrillation and eventually progressing to a permanent form of atrial fibrillation.

REPRESENTATIVE CASES

The following examples are taken from representative cases of patients with atrial fibrillation and illustrate the variety of pathologic states and histopathologic abnormalities that may predispose to atrial fibrillation.

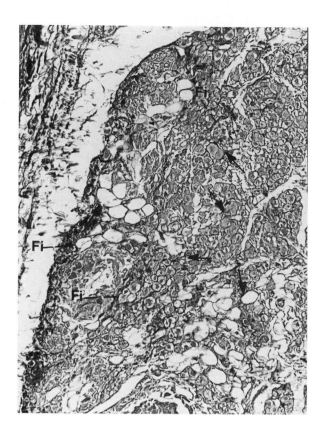

FIG. 4. Atrial myocardium infiltrated with amyloid and fibrosis. Weigert-van Gieson stain, ×150. *Arrows* point to amyloid. Fi, fibrosis.

Senile Amyloidosis Associated with the Extremely Aged

Senile amyloidosis is seen in those over the age of 80. This is a form of primary amyloidosis that is seen with senility and affects the atrial myocardium more than the ventricular myocardium. Amyloid infiltrates the interstitium and compresses the surrounding myocardial fibers. The SA node and its approaches may be the seat amyloid. Amyloid may also involve the SA nodal artery as well as the small blood vessels (arterioles) of the atrium. Thus, the blood supply to the SA node and its approaches and the atrial myocardium (the atrial preferential pathways) may be compromised, resulting in varying types of tachyarrhythmia or bradyarrhythmia.

Figure 4 is an illustration of atrial myocardium in an 83-year-old male with bundle branch block who in addition had atrial fibrillation (44). There was a history of hypertension without other cardiovascular manifestations. The SA node and the approaches to the SA and AV nodes were infiltrated with amyloid and showed arteriolosclerosis. The AV node revealed moderate fibrosis and the atrial myocardium was considerably replaced by amyloid.

Hypertensive Heart Disease

Hypertensive heart disease is associated with increased incidence of supraventricular arrhythmias and atrial fibrillation (45). In hypertensive heart disease there are usually hypertrophy and enlargement of the left atrium more than the right atrium.

This may be associated with moderate or severe coronary artery disease. There is left ventricular hypertrophy often with associated hypertrophy of the entire heart. Pathologically there is severe small vessel disease (arteriolosclerosis) in the SA node and its approaches, in the approches to the AV node with associated increase in fat and fibroelastosis of the above structures and in part of the AV node. There is also fibro-fatty degenerative changes of the distal part of the conduction system in many cases. This is accompanied by the usual aging changes of the summit of the ventricular septum, which consists of the sclerosis of the left side of the cardiac skeleton (Fig. 5).

Rosen et al. (44) found cardiac arteriolosclerosis and cardiac amyloidosis in an 81-year-old male with a history of hypertension, heart failure, atrial flutter, and left bundle branch block. The SA node showed marked arteriolosclerosis with fibrosis. Amyloidosis, fat, and marked vacuolar degeneration were seen in the approaches to the SA and AV node. The AV node showed moderate arteriolosclerosis and fibroelastosis. The main left bundle branch was replaced by fibroelastic tissue. The atria and the ventricles were the seat of degenerative changes with amyloidosis, arteriolosclerosis of a moderate to marked degree.

Figure 6 demonstrates changes found in the heart of a 78-year-old male with a history of hypertension and heart failure who presented with Mobitz type II 2:1 AV block with left bundle branch block. Electrophysiologically the site of block was distal to the His bundle recording site and, in addition, there was a mildly prolonged A-H interval (145 msec). The patient developed atrial fibrillation and died 3 years later of progressive congestive heart failure.

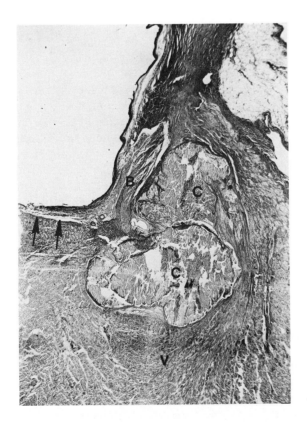

FIG. 5. Summit of the ventricular septum showing the sclerosis of the left side of the cardiac skeleton and calcification pressing on the branching bundle and the left bundle branch with fibrosis, from an aged individual with hypertensive heart disease. Weigert-van Gieson stain, ×37.5. C, calcific mass; V, ventricular septum; B, bundle branching part. *Arrow* points to left bundle branch.

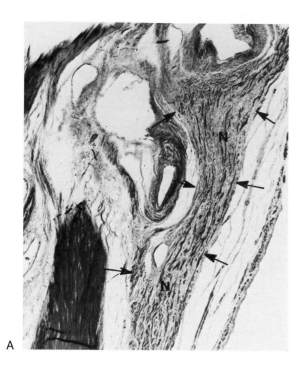

A

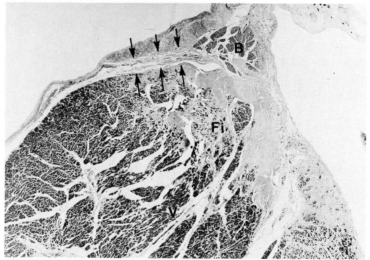

B

FIG. 6. Photomicrographs from a case of hypertensive heart disease with type II and 2:1, 2° AV block with left bundle branch block that progressed to atrial fibrillation. Gomori trichrome stain. **A:** Fibroelastosis of the AV node, ×45. **B:** Branching bundle with fibrosis of the left bundle branch, ×30. **C:** Fibrosis of the right bundle branch, ×120. *Arrows* point to AV node in A, to fibrosis of the left bundle branch in B, and fibrosis of the right bundle branch in C. N, AV node; B, bundle; V, ventricular septum with fibrosis; Fi, fibrosis. (From ref. 46, with permission.) (*Figure continues.*)

Pathologically there were marked fatty infiltration of the SA node with loss of cells and arteriolosclerosis of the node and its approaches, with acute degenerative changes of some cells and hypertrophy of other cells. There were marked fibroelastosis of the AV node (Fig. 6A) and its approaches, arteriosclerosis, and thickening of AV nodal artery. Both bundle branches showed marked fibrosis (Fig. 6B, C) as did the summit of the ventricular septum (Fig. 6B), which also showed marked fibrosis and arteriosclerosis.

In summary, atrial fibrillation has a tendency to occur more frequently with hypertension than with normotension and this may be accelerated with increasing age.

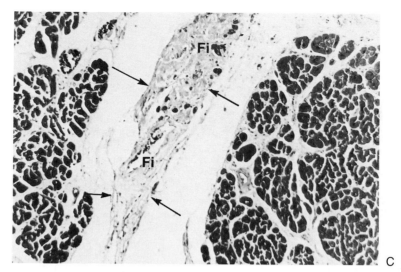

FIG. 6. *Continued.*

Although the anatomic substrate may be present in the atria and the SA and AV nodes, there is often distinct conduction system disease peripherally as well. Thus, bundle branch block, especially left bundle branch block, may be present clinically with atrial fibrillation in the elderly.

Coronary Artery Disease

Coronary artery disease is a common cause of atrial fibrillation, which may occur either in the acute or chronic forms of myocardial infarction (47).

Acute Coronary Insufficiency

Although atrial fibrillation may be seen in anteroseptal as well as in posteroseptal infarction, it is more common in the latter. The anatomic substrate for atrial fibrillation is frequently atrial infarction with or without infarction of the SA node. This is usually associated with AV block and infarction of the AV node. The AV nodal artery may be markedly thickened, narrowed (Fig. 7A), or occluded.

Figure 7 shows the findings in an elderly black male studied by Lev et al. (48) (Case 1), who, in addition to coronary disease, had atrial fibrillation and flutter. The following findings were present: (a) the SA node showed focal fibroelastosis with focal absence of nodal cells and focal infiltration of mononuclear cells; (b) the approaches to the SA node revealed an infiltration of mononuclear cells with fibrosis and hemorrhage; (c) the approaches to the AV node showed a recent infarct with fibroelastosis; (Fig. 7B); (d) the AV node was the seat of necrosis with infiltration of mononuclear cells and neutrophils. Arteriolosclerosis was also in evidence (Fig. 7A).

Chronic Coronary Insufficiency

Atrial fibrillation may be related to chronic coronary insufficiency (47), and a representative case is described below (49).

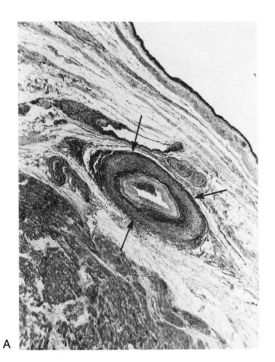

A

FIG. 7. A: Approaches to the AV node showing marked thickening of the AV nodal artery with narrowing. Weigert-van Gieson stain, ×60. *Arrows* point to thickened artery. **B:** Approaches to the AV node and the AV node showing focal necrosis of the node and a recent infarct of the approaches, from a case of coronary artery disease with acute posterior wall infarction that progressed to atrial fibrillation and flutter. Hematoxylin-eosin stain, ×150. A, approaches to the AV node; N, AV node. (From ref. 48, with permission.)

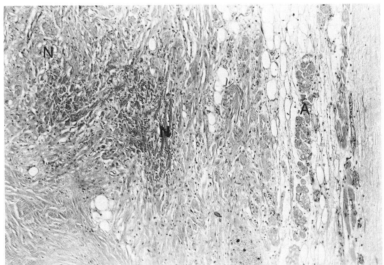

B

This was a 51-year-old male with severe coronary artery disease and previous myocardial infarction who had atrial fibrillation and bundle branch block (49). The SA node was not available for study. The approaches to the AV node showed marked acute degeneration and early necrosis of cells. The AV node and its approaches revealed proliferation of sheath cells and an infiltration of mononuclear cells and arteriolosclerosis (Fig. 8A). Fibrosis of the bundle, the bundle branches, and old scars of the ventricular septum was seen (Fig. 8B).

Although we have discussed the occurrence of atrial fibrillation individually, as seen in normal aging phenomena, hypertensive heart disease, and coronary artery

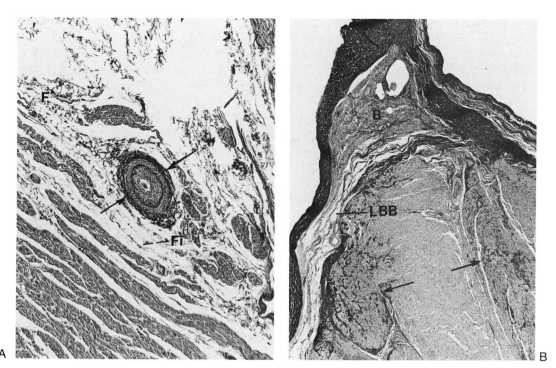

FIG. 8. A,B: Photomicrographs from a case of chronic coronary artery disease with previous myocardial infarction with 1° AV block, left bundle branch block, and development of atrial fibrillation showing **A:** the atrial myocardium with arteriolosclerosis fat and fibrosis. Weigert-van Gieson stain, ×45. F, fat; Fi, fibrosis. *Arrows* point to the arteriolosclerosis. **B:** Branching bundle showing fibrosis, partial disruption of the left bundle branch, and old scars of the myocardium. Weigert-van Gieson stain, ×30. B, bundle; LBB, left bundle branch. *Arrows* point to the fibrotic scars in the ventricular septum.

disease, it is understood that such artificial separation is only arbitrary. It is common knowledge that along with normal aging (beyond 65 to 70 years) there is a frequent association of coronary artery disease with or without hypertensive heart disease. This may also be complicated by diabetes. The pathologic substrate, however, is not distinct for any particular entity discussed.

Postoperative Heart Disease

Atrial fibrillation is known to occur in postoperative cases of various types of congenital cardiac malformations. Among them are atrial septal defect of the fossa ovalis type (50), Mustard (51) or Senning procedures for complete transposition, and atrial septectomy procedure (Blalock-Hanlon procedure). In the Mustard procedure, the entire atrial septum is removed and a prosthetic baffle is placed in the atrial septum. In the Senning procedure, several cuts are made in the atrial septum to create flaps of the atrial wall. These flaps are then refashioned. Thus, in both procedures the atrial septum is considerably altered following surgery.

Pathologically, these areas are replaced by fibrosis, fat, and chronic inflammatory cells. In addition, there is practically no continuity of the AV node with the surrounding atrial musculature.

Bharati and Lev (50) studied a 16-year-old male who developed atrial fibrillation 6 years after surgery for atrial septal defect. The conduction system revealed the following: (a) the SA nodal artery was thickened; (b) the approaches to the SA node revealed sutures and foreign body reactions, fibrosis, and neuritis; (c) the atrial preferential pathways showed fibrosis with involvement of nerves; (d) the approaches to the AV node revealed fatty metamorphosis, as did the AV node, accompanied by fibrosis. It is thus clear that fat and fibrosis in the atrial septum and in the SA nodal area with or without sutures, or foreign body reaction, form the anatomic base for the development of atrial fibrillation following various types of surgery in the atrial septum. It is also important to keep in mind that these changes are almost always associated with hypertrophy and enlargement of the right atrium. In atrial septal defect, the atrial arrhythmias that were present before surgery may get worse in some cases following the closure of the defect.

Atrial Fibrillation Following Coronary Artery Bypass Surgery

Although this is seen quite commonly, the anatomic base, to the best of our knowledge, has not been worked out (52). The cause may include surgical injury to the SA nodal area, postoperative pericarditis, abrupt beta-blocker withdrawal, or inadequate atrial protection during cardiopulmonary bypass. Older patients (mean age 65 ± 8 years) were found to be at greater risk for the development of atrial dysrhythmias (52).

Infiltrative Diseases of the Heart

Atrial fibrillation may occur in infiltrative diseases of the heart such as amyloidosis and sarcoidosis.

Bharati et al. (53) examined the heart of a patient with paroxysmal atrial tachycardia (53-year-old male), who, at electrophysiological study, was found to have prolonged atrial effective and functional refractory periods. The SA node showed a slight infiltration of amyloid, amyloid in the arterioles, and marked fatty metamorphosis in the periphery of the node. The approaches to the SA node revealed a marked infiltration of amyloid. The myocardium showed fatty metamorphosis with necrosis of the myocardium and arteriolar narrowing. The atrial preferential pathways likewise presented marked amyloid infiltration in the myocardium and epicardium, with severe degeneration of muscle cells, atrophy of some of these cells (Fig. 9), and marked fatty metamorphosis with necrosis of myocardium. The arterioles were infiltrated with amyloid, and the small arterioles were narrowed. The approaches to the AV node revealed a marked infiltration with amyloid and marked arteriolosclerosis. The AV node in the periphery showed marked fatty metamorphosis, acute necrosis, and a moderate infiltration of amyloid.

Alcohol

It has been demonstrated that the consumption of alcohol, especially in the elderly, triggers the onset of atrial fibrillation. This probably is related to the degenerative changes and associated fatty metamorphosis of the atrial myocardium, the SA and AV nodes, and their approaches.

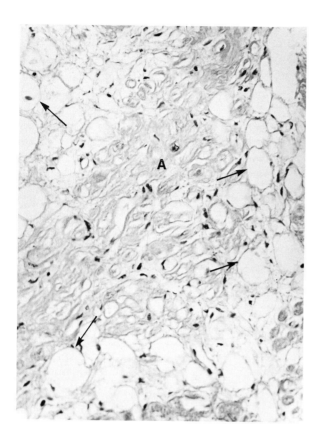

FIG. 9. Atrial myocardium from a case of primary amyloidosis with paroxysmal atrial tachycardia with 2:1 AV block, showing marked degeneration of muscle cells surrounded by amyloid rings. Hematoxylin-eosin stain, ×300. A, atrial myocardium. *Arrows* point to amyloid rings.

OTHER CONDUCTION SYSTEM ABNORMALITIES ASSOCIATED WITH ATRIAL FIBRILLATION

Familial Atrial Arrhythmias with Atrioventricular Block

The familial association of AV block with atrial fibrillation and flutter and the frequent occurrence of such combinations has been previously stressed (54). These authors reported a family with a syndrome of atrial flutter or fibrillation with advanced or complete AV block involving four members in two generations. Less serious arrhythmias were documented in another 15 members. The inheritance appeared to be autosomal dominant with varying degrees of expression.

Atrial biopsy in one of the family members, a 40-year-old female who had atrial flutter with advanced AV block proximal to the His bundle, revealed marked degeneration and necrosis of atrial muscle (Fig. 10).

Preexcitation

Atrial fibrillation is frequently present in the preexcitation syndrome (55). The Kent bundle (anomalous AV pathway) may conduct in a retrograde fashion and may be responsible for initiation of atrial fibrillation.

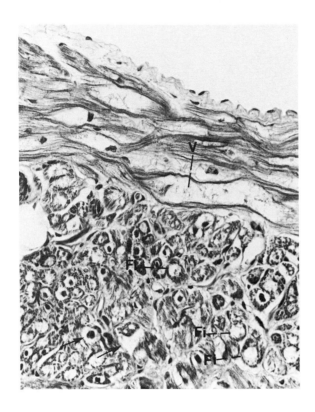

FIG. 10. Atrial biopsy from a case of familial atrial fibrillation or flutter with advanced or complete AV block showing vacuolar degeneration, fatty infiltration, and hypertrophy of atrial cells with early necrosis. Gomori trichrome stain, ×375. V, vacuolar degeneration; F, fatty metamorphosis. *Arrows* point to early necrosis.

Congenital Atrioventricular Block in the Elderly

Atrial fibrillation and/or flutter may be associated with congenital AV block of long-standing duration. We studied two such cases (56,57). In a 49-year-old male with atrial fibrillation, complete AV block, and an escape rhythm with wide QRS complexes, there were a lack of connection between the atrial septum and the peripheral conduction system and almost total replacement, by fat, of the AV node and its approaches. The atria (Fig. 11) showed considerable fibrosis, and there was fatty infiltration of the bundle and the bundle branches. In addition, there was marked sclerosis of the summit of the ventricular system, more marked on the right side.

In the second case, a 57-year-old female with a history of AV block, of 42 years duration, and atrial flutter, the AV node was absent with marked fatty infiltration of the approaches to the AV node and the atria. In addition, there were considerable fibrosis of the SA node, focal fibrosis of the left bundle branch with endocardial sclerosis, and calcification of the atria. The ventricular myocardium showed acute and chronic degenerative changes.

Thus both cases demonstrated a lack of connection between the atria and the peripheral conduction system with extensive fatty changes of the atrial muscle and absence of the AV node. In addition, varying types of degenerative changes were present in the atria and the peripheral conduction system. It is presumed that with advancing age, the sclerosis of the summit of the ventricular system was hastened by progression of abnormal physiologic events (chronic bradycardia with resultant diastolic overloading of the ventricles). The marked fatty infiltration of the atria

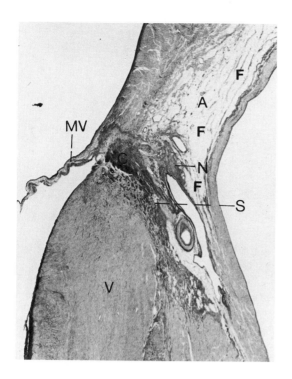

FIG. 11. Photomicrograph from a case of congenital AV block of long-standing duration with atrial fibrillation showing marked fatty infiltration of the approaches to the AV node and the AV node with fibrosis of the node. Weigert-van Gieson stain, × 17. A, approaches to the AV node replaced by fat; F, fat; N, AV node replaced by fat and fibrosis and almost isolated from the atrial muscle; MV, mitral valve; V, ventricular septum; S, right side of the ventricular septum. (From ref. 56, with permission.)

probably was responsible for atrial flutter and fibrillation seen on the electrocardiogram.

Tachycardia-Bradycardia Syndrome

This is characterized by atrial fibrillation followed by atrial arrest. Kaplan et al. (58) reported on the histopathology of two patients with this syndrome. In one case, a 74-year-old male, the SA node showed severe narrowing of the arterioles with acute degeneration and necrosis, fibroblastic proliferation, fatty metamorphosis, and focal fibrinoid necrosis. The approaches to the SA node revealed fibrosis and elastosis, arteriolosclerosis, chronic pericarditis, and degeneration of the nerve trunks. The approaches to the AV node showed acute and chronic inflammation with fatty metamorphosis, arteriolosclerosis, sclerosis, and slight narrowing of the ramus septi fibrosi, mononuclear infiltration, and proliferation of fibroblasts. The AV node revealed chronic inflammation with proliferation of sheath cells. Arteriolosclerosis and necrosis of the right atrium and atrial septum, with inflammation of the nerve ganglia, were also present.

CONGENITAL HEART DISEASE

Atrial Septal Defect

Defects in the atrial septum, either fossa ovalis (secundum) ostium primum or sinus venosus type, may result in atrial fibrillation, particularly in later life. Usually these defects are large in nature. Chronic atrial fibrillation in these cases does not disappear after surgical closure of the defect, and occasionally the arrhythmias may actually worsen following surgery.

Idiopathic Dilatation of the Right Atrium

Idiopathic dilatation of the right atrium or congenital aneurysm of the right atrium, especially in infancy and childhood, may cause intractable atrial arrhythmias. This may be associated with atrial fibrillation.

Ebstein's Anomaly

Atrial fibrillation may be seen in this entity with or without preexcitation.

Tumors of the Heart

We have seen various tumors of the AV node, such as coelotheliomas, and left atrial myxomas produce various atrial arrhythmias. The arrhythmias are not different from those produced by other causes.

CONGENITAL ANOMALIES OF THE ATRIOVENTRICULAR JUNCTION

Atrio-Hisian Connection

Muscular connection either from the right or left atrium may enter the central fibrous body and join the penetrating part of the AV bundle.

Bharati et al. (59) studied a 59-year-old female with atrial fibrillation. The SA node was the seat of fatty metamorphosis and fibrosis of nerves. The AV node was almost completely separated from the atrial myocardium by fat and presented marked fibroelastosis and a moderate infiltration of mononuclear cells. The atrial septum showed fatty metamorphosis, as did the approaches to the AV node. There was an atrio-Hisian connection. This connection could have initiated the atrial fibrillation, which in turn could have resulted in atrial stretch and fatty infiltration and might have caused the progression of atrial fibrillation.

MISCELLANEOUS CAUSES

Atrial fibrillation is known to occur in neuromuscular disorders such as myotonia dystrophica (60,61), fascioscapulomuscular dystrophy (62), hypertrophic cardiomyopathy (63,64), and Kearns-Sayre syndrome (65).

Figure 12 is an example of the abnormality found in a case of Kearns-Sayre syndrome accompanied by atrial fibrillation (65). We found that (a) the SA node was the seat of fatty infiltration with marked degeneration and fat necrosis and (b) the

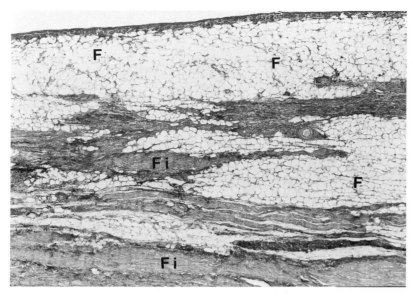

FIG. 12. Approaches to the SA node showing marked fatty metamorphosis and fibrosis from a case of Kearns-Sayre syndrome with atrial fibrillation. Weigert-van Gieson stain, ×45. F, fat; Fi, fibrosis.

approaches to the SA and AV nodes and the atrial preferential pathways showed fatty metamorphosis, with fibrosis. Marked fatty metamorphosis with degeneration and necrosis of muscle cells was also noted. The AV node was likewise the seat of marked fatty metamorphosis with fibrosis.

SUMMARY

It is thus clear that structural abnormalities of the atrial musculature to a varying degree are almost always present in cases of atrial fibrillation. These changes may be in the form of fatty metamorphosis, fibrosis, necrosis, acute and chronic inflammation, and tumor infiltration of the atrial musculature or the SA and AV nodes. In other cases there may be thickening of the ramus septi fibrosi and the ramus ostii cavae superioris, due to arteriolosclerosis of these structures with or without occlusion of these vessels. However, the same kind of pathologic changes may not only be responsible for atrial fibrillation, but for other types of atrial arrhythmias such as atrial tachycardia, multifocal atrial tachycardia, paroxysmal supraventricular tachycardia, and chronic bradycardia-tachycardia syndromes.

Since the structural abnormalities are almost always present in the atrial musculature, it is assumed that these changes were responsible for atrial fibrillation. However, it is very important to keep in mind that associated biochemical, metabolic, and physiologic changes, abnormal neural responses, hormonal imbalances, emotions, and other unknown factors may also be responsible in triggering atrial fibrillation, particularly in patients with preexisting histologic abnormalities.

REFERENCES

1. Lev M, McMillan JB. Aging changes in the heart. In: Bourne GH, ed. *Structural aspects of aging.* London: Pitman Medical, 1961;325–349.
2. McMillan JB, Lev M. The aging heart: I. Endocardium. *J Gerontol* 1959;14:268–283.
3. McMillan JB, Lev M. The aging heart. Myocardium and epicardium. In: Shock NW, ed. *Biological aspects of aging.* New York: Columbia University Press, 1962;163–173.
4. Lev M, Bharati S. Anatomic basis for impulse generation and atrioventricular transmission. In: Narula OS, ed. *His bundle electrocardiography and clinical electrophysiology.* Philadelphia: FA Davis, 1975;1–17.
5. Lev M, Bharati S. A method of study of the pathology of the conduction system for electrocardiographic and His bundle electrogram correlations. *Anat Rec.* 1981;201:43–49.
6. Bharati S, Lev M. Morphology of the sinus and atrioventricular nodes and their innervation. In: Mazgalev T, Dreifus LS, Michelson EL, eds. *Electrophysiology of the sinoatrial and atrioventricular nodes: in progress in clinical and biological research.* New York: Alan R. Liss 1988;3–14.
7. Yater WM. Pathologic changes in auricular fibrillation and in allied arrhythmias. *Arch Intern Med* 1929;43:808–838.
8. Schonberg S. Ueber Veranderungen im Sinusgebiet des Herzens bei chronischer Arrhythmie. *Z Pathol* 1909;2:153.
9. Hedinger E. Ueber Herzbefunde bei Arrhythmia perpetua. *Z Pathol* 1910;5:296–321.
10. Koch W. Zur pathologischen Anatomie der Rhythmusstorungen des Herzens. *Berl klin Wochenschr* 1910;1:1108–1112.
11. Draper G. Pulsus irregularis perpetuus with fibrosis of the sinus node. *Heart* 1911;3:13–21.
12. Cohn AE. A case of bradycardia with post-mortem examination. *Heart* 1911;3:23–31.
13. Freund HA. Klinische and pathologisch-anatomische Untersuchungen uber Arhythmia perpetua, *Dtsch Arch Klin Med* 1912;106:1–32.
14. Falconer AW, Dean G. Observations on a case of heart block associated with intermittent attacks of auricular fibrillation. *Heart* 1911;3:247–254.
15. Cohn AE, Lewis T. Auricular fibrillation and complete heart block: a description of a case of Adams-Stokes syndrome, including the post-mortem examination. *Heart* 1912;4:15–30.
16. Angyan. Kammerautomatie und VorhoFlimmern. *Virchows Arch Pathol Anat* 1913;213:170–176.
17. Falconer AW, Dean G. Observations on a case of auricular fibrillation with slow ventricular action. *Heart* 1912;4:87–95.
18. Price FW, Mackenzie I. Auricular fibrillation and heart block in diphtheria. *Heart* 1911–1912;3:233–242.
19. Hume WE. A polygraphic study of four cases of diphtheria. *Heart* 1913;5:25–44.
20. Berger. Anatomische Untersuchungen des Herzens bei Pulsus irregularis perpetuus. *Dtsch Arch Klin Med* 1913;112:287–301.
21. Cohn AE. The post-mortem examination of horses' hearts from cases of auricular fibrillation. *Heart* 1913;112:221–224.
22. Cohn AE, Heard JD. A case of auricular fibrillation, with a postmortem examination. *Arch Intern Med* 1913;11:630–640.
23. Sutherland GA, Coombs CF. A case of acute rheumatic carditis and auricular fibrillation in a child. *Heart* 1913;5:15–20.
24. Romeis B. Beitrage zur Arrhythmia perpetua. *Dtsch Arch Klin Med* 1914;114:580–604.
25. Jarisch A. Zur pathologischen Anatomie des Pulsus irregularis perpetuus. *Dtsch Arch Klin Med* 1914;115:331–376.
26. Hochhaus, Dreesen. Vorkommen und Bedeutung von anatomischen Veranderungen des Herzmuskels bei Herzschwache. *Festschr. d. Akad. f. prakt. med. zu Coln.* 1915;384–419.
27. Thorel C. Pathologie der Kreislauforgane des Menschen: I. Anatomie des Herzens. *Ergeb Allg Pathol Pathol Anat* 1915;17:690–718.
28. Wilkinson KD, Butterfield HG. Paroxysmal heart block with paroxysmal auricular fibrillation. *Heart* 1914–1915;6:3–9.
29. Floystrup G. Studies on the pathogenesis of auricular fibrillation. *Acta Med Scand* 1922;56:12–32.
30. Mönckeberg JG, Herz. In: Henke F, Lubarsch O, eds. *Handbuch der speziellen pathologischen Anatomie und Histologie,* vol. 2. Berlin: Julius Springer, 1924;502–524.
31. Frothingham C. The auricles in cases of auricular fibrillation. *Arch Intern Med* 1925;36:437–443.
32. Condorelli L. Sull'importanza delle lesioni infiammatorie del plesso sottoepicardico dell'orecchietta destra nella patogenesi di alcune turbe del ritimo cardiaco. *Riforma Med* 1928;44:613–616.
33. Davies MJ, Pomerance A. *Pathology of atrial fibrillation in man. Br Heart J* 1972;34:520–525.
34. Hudson REB. The human pacemaker and its pathology. *Br Heart J* 1960;22:153–167.
35. Hudson REB. *Cardiovascular pathology.* London: Edward Arnold, 1965.

36. James TN. Morphology of the human atrioventricular node with remarks pertinent to its electrophysiology. *Am Heart J* 1961;62:756–771.
37. James TN. Arrhythmias and conduction disturbances in acute myocardial infarction. *Am Heart J* 1962;64:416–426.
38. James TN. The connecting pathways between the sinus node and AV node and between the right and the left atrium in the human heart. *Am Heart J* 1963;66:498–508.
39. James TN, Hershey EA. Experimental studies on the pathogenesis of atrial arrhythmias in myocardial infarction. *Am Heart J* 1962;63:196–211.
40. Laas E. Das Arrythmieherz. *Zentralbl Alleg Pathol* 1962;103:552–576.
41. Lippestad CT, Marton PF. Sinus arrest in proximal right coronary artery occlusion. *Am Heart J* 1967;74:551–556.
42. Davies MJ, Anderson RH, Becker AE. Chapter 8. In: *The conduction system of the heart: pathology of atrial arrhythmias.* London: Butterworths, 1983;203–215.
43. Manyari DE, Patterson C, Johnson D, Melendez L, Kostuk WJ, Cape RDT. Atrial and ventricular arrhythmias in asymptomatic active elderly subjects: correlation with left atrial size and left ventricular mass. *Am Heart J* 1990;119:1069–1076.
44. Rosen KM, Rahimtoola SH, Bharati S, Lev M. Bundle branch block with intact atrioventricular conduction. *Am J Cardiol* 1973;32:782–793.
45. Celentano A, Galderisi M, Mureddu GF, Garofalo M, Tammaro P, de Divitiis O. Arrhythmias, hypertension and the elderly: Holter evaluation. *J Hypertens* 1988;6(suppl):S29–S32.
46. Bharati S, Lev M, Dhingra RC, Chuquimia R, Towne WD, Rosen KM. Electrophysiologic and pathologic correlations in two cases of chronic second degree atrioventricular block with left bundle branch block. *Circulation* 1975;52:221–229.
47. Lev M, Bharati S. The conduction system in coronary artery disease. In: Donosco E, Lipski J, eds. *Acute myocardial infarction.* 1977;1–16.
48. Lev M, Kinare SG, Pick A. The pathogenesis of atrioventricular block in coronary disease. *Circulation* 1970;42:409–425.
49. Bharati S, Lev M, Dhingra R, Wu D, Aruguete J, Mir J, Rosen KM. Pathologic correlations in three cases of bilateral bundle branch disease with unusual electrophysiologic manifestations in two cases. *Am J Cardiol* 1976;38:508–518.
50. Bharati S, Lev M. Conduction system in sudden unexpected death a considerable time after repair of atrial septal defect. *Chest* 1988;94:142–148.
51. Bharati S, Molthan ME, Veasy G, Lev M. Conduction system in two cases of sudden death two years after the Mustard procedure. *J Thorac Cardiovasc Surg* 1979;77:101–108.
52. Crosby LH, Pifalo WB, Woll KR, Burkholder JA. Risk factors for atrial fibrillation after coronary artery bypass grafting. *Am J Cardiol* 1990;66:1520–1522.
53. Bharati S, Lev M, Denes P, et al. Infiltrative cardiomyopathy with conduction disease and ventricular arrhythmia: electrophysiologic and pathologic correlations. *Am J Cardiol* 1980;45:163–172.
54. Amat-Y-Leon F, Racki AJ, Denes P, et al. Familial atrial dysrhythmia with AV block; intracellular microelectrode, clinical electrophysiologic, and morphologic observations. *Circulation* 1974;50:1097–1104.
55. Paul T, Guccione P, Garson A Jr. Relation of syncope in young patients with Wolff-Parkinson-White syndrome to rapid ventricular response during atrial fibrillation. *Am J Cardiol* 1990;65:318–321.
56. Bharati S, Rosen KM, Strasberg B, Rigby E, Lev M. Anatomic substrate for congenital atrioventricular block in middle-aged adults. *PACE* 1982;5:860–869.
57. Lev M, Benjamin JE, White PD. A histopathologic study of the conduction system in a case of complete heart block of 42 years' duration. *Am Heart J* 1958;55:198–214.
58. Kaplan BM, Langendorf R, Lev M, Pick A. Tachycardia-bradycardia syndrome (so-called "sick sinus syndrome"). *Am J Cardiol* 1973;31:497–508.
59. Bharati S, Scheinmann MM, Morady F, Hess DS, Lev M. Sudden death after catheter-induced atrioventricular junctional ablation. *Chest* 1985;88:883–889.
60. Cannon PJ. The heart and lungs in myotonic muscular dystrophy. *Am J Med* 1962;32:765–775.
61. Church SC. The heart in myotonia atrophica. *Arch Intern Med* 1967;119:176–181.
62. Woelfel A, Cascio W, Smith SW. Cerebral embolization in two young patients with fascioscapulohumeral muscular dystrophy and atrial dysrhythmias. *Am Heart J* 1989;118:632–633.
63. Ohkawa S, Suguira M, Fizuka T, Shimada H, Okada R. Three cases of idiopathic cardiomegaly in the aged, with special references to the morphological specificity and to the conduction system. *Jpn Heart J* 1971;12:305.
64. James TN, Marshall TK. De subitaneis mortibus. Asymmetrical hypertrophy of the heart. *Circulation* 1975;51:1149.
65. Gallastegui J, Hariman RJ, Handler B, Lev M, Bharati S. Cardiac involvement in the Kearns-Sayre syndrome. *Am J Cardiol* 1987;60:385–388.

Atrial Fibrillation: Mechanisms and Management, edited by
R. H. Falk and P. J. Podrid.
Raven Press, Ltd., New York © 1992.

3

Experimental Observations in Atrial Fibrillation

*Michiel J. Janse and †Maurits A. Allessie

*Department of Clinical and Experimental Cardiology, Academisch Medisch Centrum,
1105 AZ Amsterdam, The Netherlands; †Department of Physiology, University of Limburg
and The Interuniversity Cardiology Institute, 6200 MD Maastricht, The Netherlands*

CELLULAR ELECTROPHYSIOLOGY OF THE ATRIUM

Atrial myocardium differs from ventricular myocardium, both with respect to morphological and electrophysiological characteristics. Atrial cells have a smaller diameter and a less prominent T-tubule system than ventricular tissue. Also, atrial cells have more side-to-side connections than ventricular cells. The transmembrane potential of mammalian atrial cells shares several properties with that of ventricular myocardial cells and cells of the His-Purkinje system. Resting membrane potential is large, action potential upstroke is rapid, there is a marked overshoot, and recovery of excitability closely follows the time course of repolarization (1). Action potential duration is usually shorter in atrial cells than in cells distal to the atrioventricular node. Possibly the most conspicuous difference between atrial and ventricular cells is their reaction to acetylcholine. Whereas the action potential of both His-Purkinje and ventricular myocardial cells remains largely unaffected, action potential duration of atrial cells shortens markedly, while action potential upstroke and resting potential show no appreciable change (2). Two different types of action potentials have been distinguished in atrial tissue, including human atria: action potentials with a distinct plateau and triangularly shaped action potentials, without a plateau (2–5). The "plateau" action potential fibers were thought to arise from specialized fibers (3–5). Such "plateau" action potentials have been described as showing diastolic depolarization (3), which was another argument favoring their specialized nature. There is some confusion regarding the specialized nature of these fibers in the normal atria. On the one hand, histological identification of the very cell from which action potentials were recorded from rabbit and canine atria showed that action potentials with a marked plateau as well as triangularly shaped action potentials both originated from ordinary atrial myocardial cells (6). An example is shown in Fig. 1. Recordings of atrial transmembrane potentials were made from an isolated right atrial preparation from the rabbit, which was perfused via both right and left coronary arteries. Recordings were made with flexibly mounted microelectrodes, which was necessary because of the vigorous contractions of such a perfused preparation (some move-

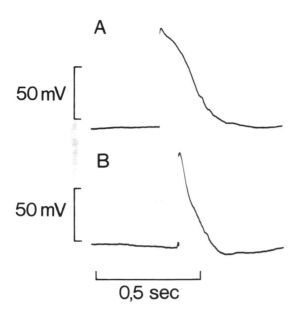

FIG. 1. Two simultaneously recorded transmembrane potentials from an arterially perfused right atrial preparation from the rabbit heart. Note presence of a plateau in **A,** absence of a plateau in **B.** See text for discussion.

ment artifacts are visible in the repolarization phase). In this experiment, an action potential with a plateau (Fig. 1A) was recorded from the crista terminalis, and simultaneously, an action potential without a plateau (Fig. 1B) was recorded from the anterior limbus of the fossa ovalis. Immediately after these recordings were made, the preparation was fixed by perfusion of glutaraldehyde through the coronary arteries while the microelectrodes remained in the tissue. After fixation, the microelectrodes were withdrawn. The appropriate tissue blocks were serially sectioned in 4-μm sections, and the microelectrode track identified. Figure 2 shows the very cell recorded from to obtain the action potential with the plateau. Although this cell is damaged, all surrounding cells are ordinary atrial cells. The same was true for the cell that generated the "spike-like" action potential B (not shown). In no instance was diastolic depolarization observed (6).

On the other hand, subsidiary atrial pacemaker cells, showing diastolic depolarization (but no plateau) originated from cells in the eustachian ridge that morphologically resembled cells in the sinoatrial node (7,8). To complicate matters even further, potentials recorded from isolated preparations of diseased human atria obtained from patients suffering from paroxysmal atrial arrhythmias, frequently had low resting potentials and action potentials had a low amplitude and upstroke velocity ("depressed action potentials") (4,9). It is known that normal myocardium may exhibit automatic activity when resting membrane potential is decreased. In other words, pacemaker activity is not necessarily associated with morphological specialization.

With respect to atrial fibrillation, several electrophysiological abnormalities have been reported. When transmembrane potentials were recorded from tissue from fibrillating human atria, either from atria of normal size or from dilated atria, resting potentials were significantly reduced compared to resting potentials from cells in nonfibrillating atria (4). The functional significance of this finding would be that, because of the decrease in upstroke velocity and action potential amplitude as a consequence of the low resting membrane potential, conduction velocity decreases. As will be discussed later, this is a factor favoring the occurrence of reentry. Attuel

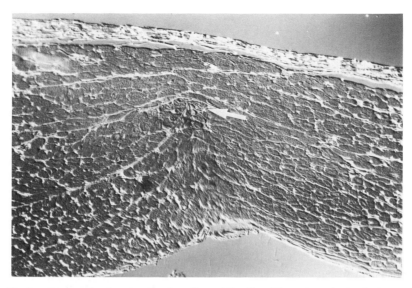

FIG. 2. Photomicrograph showing the location of the tip of the microelectrode (*arrow*) used to record action potential A of Fig. 1. Although the very cell recorded from is damaged, hampering identification, all surrounding cells are ordinary atrial myocardial cells.

and colleagues (10) were the first to report on an intriguing abnormality observed in patients vulnerable to atrial arrhythmias, including fibrillation. In these patients there was no, or hardly any, adaptation of the atrial refractory period to changes in heart rate. At the most rapid rates investigated (cycle lengths in the order of 350–400 msec), the range of refractory period durations was similar to that of normal patients (approximately from 160–250 msec). However, upon slowing of heart rate no prolongation of the refractory period was observed so that at cycle lengths between 800 to 1,000 msec, the refractory periods of the atria of arrhythmic patients were much shorter than those of normals. These findings were largely supported by a later study, in which action potentials from isolated atria were recorded at different pacing rates (11). Again, a poor adaptation of both action potential duration and refractory period to heart rate was found. Moreover, the effective refractory period was usually shorter in atrial tissue obtained from patients with atrial fibrillation than from normal atrial preparations, except at short cycle lengths where, because of postrepolarization refractoriness, refractory periods were longer. In partially depolarized fibers, the recovery kinetics of both the fast and the slow inward currents are markedly delayed (12). This results in a prolongation of the refractory period to such extent that, although repolarization is completed, recovery of excitability has not. This phenomenon is commonly called postrepolarization refractoriness. In addition, it was found that in the atrial fibrillation group, the proportion of triangular action potentials was much greater than in the control group (97% vs 23%). As also found in other studies, a higher percentage of partially depolarized cells occurred. Finally, dispersion of action potential duration was much greater in the atrial fibrillation group than in the control group. Increased dispersion in refractoriness was also found by direct measurements during cardiac surgery in patients with chronic atrial fibrillation (13).

These findings do not quite agree with those of a study in a group of patients with atrial fibrillation in the setting of sinus node dysfunction (14). These patients had longer refractory periods (and also a greater dispersion of refractory periods) than control patients. These findings were not unique to atrial fibrillation but were also present in patients with sinus node dysfunction without fibrillation (14). A possible explanation for the different findings regarding refractory period duration may be differences in pacing protocol and in patient population.

Coumel and co-workers (15) first described the role of vagal activity in some patients with atrial fibrillation. It may be speculated that in such patients abnormal shortening of action potential duration and refractory period occurs under the influence of vagal stimulation. In the absence of enhanced vagal activity (and in the absence of atrial fibrillation), refractory periods might be prolonged. Further investigations on the influence of heart rate and vagal activity on duration and dispersion of refractory periods are clearly needed.

On the basis of present knowledge, the following electrophysiological abnormalities seem to be important for the genesis of atrial fibrillation: (a) the presence of cells with low resting membrane potentials and depressed action potentials that propagate slowly and may exhibit the phenomenon of postrepolarization refractoriness; (b) an increased dispersion of refractory periods; (c) relatively short refractory periods over a wide range of cycle lengths. As will be discussed later, these three factors are of crucial importance for the occurrence and maintenance of reentrant excitation.

IS THERE A SPECIALIZED ATRIAL CONDUCTION SYSTEM?

Possibly no controversy in cardiology is of longer standing than that concerning the existence of specialized internodal pathways since it dates from the time when sinoatrial and atrioventricular nodes were discovered.

The significance of specialized atrial conduction pathways for the genesis of atrial arrhythmias, i.e., atrial flutter, was formulated by Pastelin et al. (16) as follows: "The greater conduction velocity in the loops of specialized tissue than in atrial muscle makes a flutter movement possible without the necessity for a physical obstacle." The question we shall address is whether specialized pathways exist in the atria.

As discussed in greater detail elsewhere (17), Thorel in 1909 claimed to have demonstrated that the sinoatrial and atrioventricular nodes were connected via a tract of "Purkinje-like" cells. One year later, a lengthy debate at a meeting of the Deutsche Pathologische Gesellschaft in which, among others, Aschoff, Hering, Mönckeberg, and Mackenzie participated, resulted in the consensus that the tissue between the two nodes consisted of plain atrial myocardium (18). Since that time, the debate has never really stopped. It is far beyond the scope of this chapter to review the extensive literature on this subject. With reference to an earlier review (17), our view remains that discrete tracts of morphologically specialized fibers that connect sinoatrial and atrioventricular nodes have yet to be demonstrated. This does not eliminate the possibility that single, morphologically "specialized" cells are scattered between ordinary atrial cells. One paper describes no fewer than five different species of such specialized atrial cells (19). Their role, if any, in determining conduction is unclear. We have already mentioned that different types of action potentials can be recorded from atrial cells, and the "plateau" action potentials are often referred to as "Purkinje-like," suggesting fast conduction. However, to quote Hoffman: "It is troubling to learn that in a single part of the atrium there may be as many as six different cell types, even though six different types of transmembrane potentials have not been recorded from the same areas" (20). We know that action potentials with and without a plateau can be generated by ordinary atrial myocardial cells (6) and that, for example, afterdepolarizations, which can lead to triggered activity, can be found in cells that morphologically cannot be distinguished from ordinary atrial myocardium (21). The fact that action potentials with different characteristics can be recorded from cells that are morphologically the same, does not, of course, rule out the possibility that special types of action potentials can be produced by morphologically specialized cells.

The reason why some cells produce plateau type action potentials and others do not is not clear, but the extent of coupling to other cells may be a factor. When a particular cell in a multicellular preparation is in electrotonic contact with other cells, current flow provided by these cells when they are depolarized may prolong the action potential. When such electrotonic contact is less developed, repolarization may begin earlier (22). Horibe (23) found that "the thicker the musculature, the larger the action potential and the more remarkable the plateau."

One of the arguments in favor of the specialized nature of plateau action potential type fibers is their reported resistance to high extracellular potassium concentrations (24–26). Superfusion of isolated preparations with high K$^+$ solutions or infusion of KCl in intact animals (27) results in cessation of atrial activity in some areas, whereas in thicker bundles, such as the crista terminalis or interatrial band (Bachmann's bundle), atrial activity continues. The issue of whether this is due to the presence of specialized cells or to the special architecture of the thick muscle bundles is not completely settled. It has yet to be demonstrated that the K$^+$ resistant cells are morphologically different. Possibly, in superfused preparations, diffusion of K$^+$ into thicker bundles takes longer than in thinner parts of the atria. In arterially perfused atrial tissue, the possibility exists that the safety factor for propagation is larger in thicker bundles, where well-coupled cells are arranged parallel to each other, so that propagation may continue even when depressed action potentials arise from reduced resting potential levels. We found that plateau action potentials were just as susceptible to high K$^+$ as other atrial cells in that action potential amplitude and upstroke velocity were reduced (6). Our own, unpublished, experience with isolated atrial preparations exposed to high K$^+$ solutions is that it was impossible to arrive at a steady-state situation. At critical K$^+$ concentrations, atrial activity changes over a period of several minutes. Initially, electrograms are no longer recorded from the appendages; later, block occurs between the distal crista terminalis and proximal atrioventricular node. Still later, activity also becomes undetectable in the crista terminalis.

PREFERENTIAL CONDUCTION PATHWAYS

The controversy concerning specialized atrial pathways is, in our view, largely semantic. A much more important issue is whether there are routes in the atria where propagation occurs more rapidly than elsewhere. Lewis (28), who was the first to study the spread of atrial activity, is often credited with advocating the concept that once an impulse is initiated in the sinus node, it excites the atria in a radial fashion. However, not only does his figure of atrial activation (Fig. 3) show a deviation of the

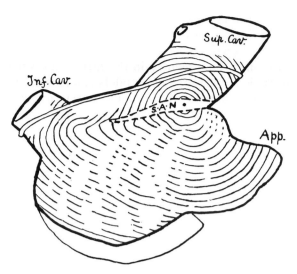

FIG. 3. Diagram by Sir Thomas Lewis illustrating his findings of the spread of activation in the dog right atrium. See text for details. (From ref. 28.)

isochrones along the crista terminalis, indicating a more rapid conduction along that structure, he also wrote: "such variation as exists in the rate of travel along various lines in the auricle is fully accounted for by the simple anatomical arrangement of the tissue." Many subsequent studies in which spread of atrial activity was mapped demonstrated conclusively that preferential conduction occurs along well-developed muscle bundles, such as crista terminalis and interatrial band (for references, see ref. 17). One reason for preferential conduction along certain pathways from the sinoatrial to the atrioventricular node is the presence of "holes" in the atrium (caval veins, coronary sinus ostium, fossa, or foramen ovale) that force the impulse to take precisely the routes it can be shown to follow. In addition, the geometric arrangement of ordinary atrial fibers can explain directional differences in conduction velocity. Conduction velocity in the direction parallel to fiber orientation (longitudinal conduction) is two to three times higher than in the direction perpendicular to the long axis (transverse conduction) (29,30). This is explained by the higher axial resistance in the transverse direction (30). This characteristic of cardiac muscle, in which biophysical properties vary according to the direction in the cardiac syncytium in which they are measured, is called anisotropy.

ANISOTROPIC REENTRY

Spach and co-workers (31,32) were the first to show that anisotropic features of atrial muscle may result in reentrant excitation, even when that tissue generates normal transmembrane action potentials and refractory periods are uniform. In atrial preparations, an appropriately timed impulse induced in the crista terminalis blocked in the longitudinal direction and propagated slowly in the transverse direction, eventually reentering the area of block. The explanation for the longitudinal block was that the safety factor for conduction in the direction parallel to fiber orientation is lower than in the direction perpendicular to it because of the greater load provided by the unexcited tissue ahead due to the lower axial resistance in the longitudinal direction. A distinction can be made between uniform and nonuniform anisotropy.

In the latter, present in aged and diseased atria, the deposition of connective tissue caused extremely slow and fragmented conduction, particularly in the transverse direction (31,32).

Whereas in experimental studies of anisotropic reentry in the atria, only single reentrant beats were observed, anisotropic reentry in other models can lead to sustained tachycardia. These models include healing and healed myocardial infarction in canine hearts (33) and rabbit ventricles where the endocardial and midmural regions are destroyed by freezing (34,35). In both experimental models, only a thin ("two-dimensional") rim of surviving subepicardial muscle remains, exhibiting both uniform and nonuniform anisotropy. In addition, anisotropic reentry has been studied in computer models (36). An important characteristic of sustained anisotropic reentry is the presence of a gap of full excitability between the crest of the circulating wavefront and its refractory tail. The reentrant wavefront propagates clockwise, or counterclockwise, around a line of block that is oriented parallel to the long-fiber axis. Conduction velocity in the reentrant circuit is not uniform; it is fast in the two longitudinal limbs and slow at the two pivoting points, where conduction is in the transverse direction. At the pivoting points of anisotropic reentry, the slowly conducting wavefront encounters a sudden increase of axial current load when it tries to excite the longitudinal limb of the circuit. At the transition from transverse to longitudinal conduction, this sudden increase of the electrotonic load leads to a temporary halt of propagation. The returning longitudinal limb of the circuit will not be activated until a larger part of the wavefront has rotated around the pivoting point. This mismatch between the excitatory current generated by the cells at the pivoting point and the axial current load imposed on these cells by the fibers beyond the pivoting point will create an excitable gap because it causes a conduction delay of about 30 msec after the cells in the longitudinal limb have recovered their excitability. Microelectrode recordings during anisotropic reentry showed that at the pivoting points the cells showed a step-like depolarization preceding the action potential upstroke that resulted in a local conduction delay of about 30 msec. As a result of this, action potential duration was prolonged, so that at the U-turns of the circuit the fibers did not reach their resting potential and the next depolarization occurred during the last part of phase 3 of the action potential. In the longitudinal limbs, however, two successive action potentials were separated by periods of about 30 msec during which the fibers were at resting potential and were fully excitable (34). In a schematic diagram (Fig. 4), these characteristics are illustrated.

As already mentioned, sustained anisotropic reentry has not yet been unequivocally demonstrated in the atria, although the importance of geometric discontinuities for reentrant circuits in atrial flutter has been recognized (37). Anisotropic reentry is, however, likely to occur in the atria in view of the "two-dimensional" anisotropic structure of atrial myocardium.

MAPPING OF ATRIAL ACTIVITY DURING ATRIAL FIBRILLATION

Moe (38) developed the so-called multiple wavelet hypothesis to explain the characteristics of atrial fibrillation. According to this hypothesis, fibrillation is maintained by the presence of a number of independent wavelets that travel randomly through the myocardium around multiple islets or strands of refractory tissue. Each wavelet may accelerate or decelerate when it encounters tissue in a more or less

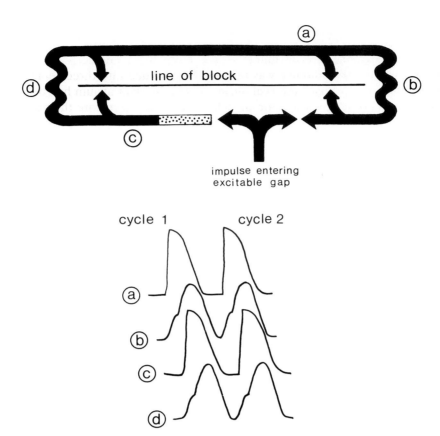

FIG. 4. Schematic representation of an anisotropic reentrant circuit. The line of block is parallel to fiber orientation. The part of the circuit that is absolutely refractory is black, the part that is relatively refractory is stippled, and the part that is fully excitable is white. Conduction parallel to the long fiber axis (longitudinal conduction) is fast; conduction perpendicular to it (transverse conduction) is slow. Only the two longitudinal limbs of the circuit have an excitable gap, as shown by the schematic drawings of the action potentials in both longitudinal limbs (a and c) and at the two pivoting points of transverse conduction (b and d). In the last two action potentials, there is no diastolic interval separating repolarization phase and upstroke of the next action potential, whereas this is present in cells a and c. Therefore, an impulse originating outside the circuit can penetrate the excitable gap only in the longitudinal limbs. It will be conducted retrogradely and collide with the oncoming reentrant wavefront. Depending on the state of recovery of the tissue in the antegrade direction, the penetrating impulse may continue in the circuit (resetting or entrainment) or block.

advanced state of recovery of excitability. They may collide with each other, divide, extinguish, or combine with other wavelets and will continuously fluctuate in size and change direction of propagation. Maintenance of fibrillation will depend on the number of wavelets present. With only a small number of wavelets, they may at a certain moment die out or fuse into a single wavefront, leading to resumption of sinus rhythm or to atrial flutter.

The multiple wavelet hypothesis has been tested experimentally by recordings from electrodes spread at regular distances of 3 mm on the endocardial surface of right and left atria of isolated canine hearts perfused according to the Langendorff technique (39). Simultaneous recordings could be made from 192 recording sites.

Atrial fibrillation was induced by a single premature stimulus while acetylcholine (which shortens the atrial refractory period) was continuously administered to the perfusion fluid. During maintained fibrillation, the presence of multiple independent wavelets was demonstrated. The width of the wavelets could be as small as a few millimeters, but broad wavefronts propagating uniformly over large segments of the atria were observed as well. Each individual wavelet existed only for a short time, no longer than a few hundred milliseconds. Excitation of a wavelet could be caused by fusion or collision with another wavelet, by reaching the border of the atria, or by meeting refractory tissue. New wavelets could be formed by division of a wave at a local area of conduction block or by an offspring of a wave traveling toward the other atrium. The major difference between the excitation patterns observed and those in the computer model of Moe and co-workers (38,40) was that the number of wavelets was much smaller. It was estimated that the critical number of wavelets in both atria to maintain fibrillation was between four and six.

Figure 5 shows a series of activation maps of atrial fibrillation in these hearts. The upper part shows the pattern of excitation of the right atrium, the lower part that of the left atrium. The right and left atria were mapped consecutively and therefore cannot be directly time-aligned. Each series of maps covers a time window of about half a second. In panel A (time zero was chosen arbitrarily), three independent wavelets are present. One wavelet (smallest arrow) travels down the septum and is extinguished at time 30 at the atrioventricular junction. The other two waves originally propagated in opposite directions, the middle one downward along the medial wall, the right wave upward to the tip of the appendage. At time 20, the two waves collided. The right wave, finding its way to the appendage suddenly blocked, changed its direction of propagation by 180° and continued its course as a narrow wavelet in the lateral wall until it died out at the AV ring at time 80. In panel B, the large activation wave at the end of panel A is split into smaller wavelets. One wavelet (lower arrow in panel B) encounters an area in the posterior wall of the atrium that obviously has not yet recovered its excitability, resulting in a 180° clockwise turn. At time 170, this turning wavelet died out at the atrial border. A second wavelet (counterclockwise arrow in panel B) entered the lateral wall and made a full 360° turn in the anterior part of the lateral wall. As shown in panel C, this wavelet created a closed local reentrant circuit that continued for another revolution, although size and location of the circuit changed (compare counterclockwise arrows in panels B and C). Panel C shows two other remarkable phenomena. First, at time 180, a new impulse appeared at the site indicated by the asterisk. The origin of this impulse cannot be explained as a combination of any of the wavelets propagating in the right atrium and most probably is a wavelet coming from the left atrium. The second noteworthy event is indicated by the four small arrows, illustrating what may happen if two narrow wavelets collide. Instead of mutual extinction, we see something that may be described as "clash and go," because after the collision the two colliding wavefronts diverge in opposite directions with a 90° change in course. The events in panel C lead to the presence of three clearly separated narrow wavelets in panel D. The right one is an offspring of the circuit around the appendage, which had ceased to exist. The other two are the result of the "clash and go" phenomenon. After the right wavelet died out at time 260 at the AV ring, only two wavefronts were left in panel D. These two remaining wavelets were simultaneously extinguished by the coincidental combination of reaching the AV ring and refractory tissue at time 290. This sudden disappearance of multiple wavelets in the right atrium did *not* result in

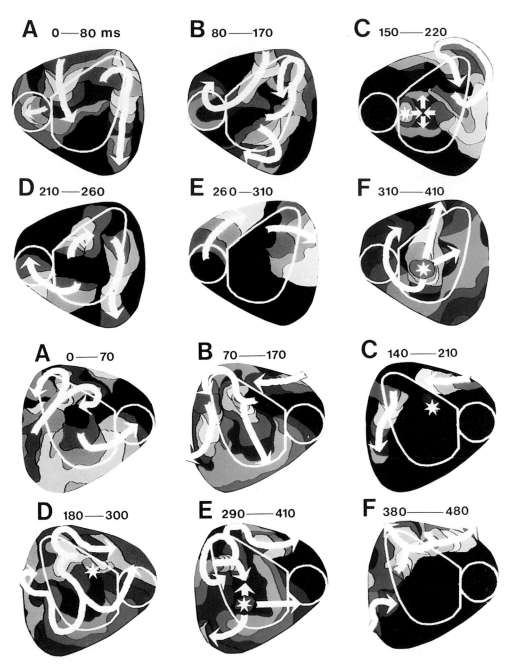

FIG. 5. Consecutive activation maps covering the spread of activation in the right and left atria during half a second of stable atrial fibrillation in the canine heart. The recordings of right and left atria were not made simultaneously and therefore cannot be time-aligned. The endocardial activation is plotted in a two-dimensional plane. This was done by making a virtual cut in the inferior atrium from the AV ring to the tip of the appendage and unfolding the lateral and medial atrial walls. The propagation of impulse is visualized by color coded isochrones of 10 msec. The general direction of wavelets is indicated by *white arrows. Asterisks* indicate sites of origin of "new" impulses coming from the other atrium. See text for discussion. (From ref. 39, with permission.)

termination of fibrillation. Some 20 msec after the right atrium had become electrically silent, a new impulse, which most likely was an offspring from a left atrial wavelet penetrated the right atrium (asterisk in panel F). The activation pattern of panel F shows that this impulse was immediately divided into three separate wavelets. Obviously, the 20-msec interval during which the right atrium had been electrically silent was not long enough for all right atrial fibers to restore their excitability. The new impulse therefore most likely encountered islands of refractory tissue and, accordingly, fragmented into multiple wavelets. (An "anisotropic" reason for conduction block at this time cannot be ruled out.)

The lower half of Fig. 5 shows the fibrillatory process of the left atrium. In general, the activation pattern is similar to that of the right atrium. Frequent entries of "new" impulses from the right atrium were seen (asterisks in panels C, D, and E) and the ever-changing pattern of multiple wavelet reentry is present here as well.

In patients with Wolff-Parkinson-White syndrome who underwent cardiac surgery, atrial fibrillation was induced by programmed electrical stimulation, and epicardial mapping was performed using an epicardial electrode containing 240 unipolar electrodes at 2.5 m distances (41). In essence, the findings were similar to those obtained in the canine heart. In the human atria, maintenance of electrically induced atrial fibrillation is based on multiple wandering wavelets. Wavelets reentering themselves were rarely seen. Most often, wavelets reexcited areas that shortly before had been activated by another wavefront. Thus far, it has been impossible to arrive at an estimate of the minimal number of simultaneously present wavelets necessary to sustain fibrillation. In view of the larger size of the atria in humans, this number may be larger than that in the canine atria.

THE WAVELENGTH AND INDUCIBILITY OF ATRIAL FIBRILLATION

It has been recognized for a long time (42) that during reentrant rhythms, the conduction time of the reentrant impulse traveling around an area of block must be long enough to allow fibers proximal to the zone of block to recover their excitability. The wavelength for circus movement reentry has been defined as the distance traveled by the depolarization wave during the refractory period: wavelength = conduction velocity × refractory period (43). When the wavelength is short, because of depressed conduction, shortening of refractory periods, or both, small areas of conduction block may already be sufficient for the establishment of reentrant circuits. Since conduction block is more likely to occur in small areas than in a large segment of atrial myocardium, it is to be expected that inducibility of atrial fibrillation depends on wavelength. If wavelength during fibrillation is long, fewer wavelets can circulate through the atria and fibrillation may be self-terminating. If wavelength is short, a greater number of wavelets will be present, and fibrillation will tend to be stable and long-lasting. Wavelength is therefore also important for maintenance of fibrillation.

In conscious dogs in which multiple electrodes for recording and stimulation had been attached to both atria, refractory periods and conduction velocity were measured. To change wavelength, a variety of drugs (acetylcholine, propafenone, lidocaine, ouabain, quinidine, sotalol) were administered, and refractory period, conduction velocity, and their product were correlated with the induction of atrial arrhythmias during premature stimulation (44). In all dogs ($n = 19$), atrial arrhyth-

mias ($n = 549$) could be induced by single premature stimuli including atrial fibrillation ($n = 208$). Although at shorter refractory periods, a relatively high incidence of
atrial fibrillation was observed, prolongation of the refractory period did not always
prevent atrial fibrillation. In fact, the predictive power of refractory period duration
alone or conduction velocity alone for induction of arrhythmias was poor. In contrast, wavelength correlated very well with inducibility of atrial arrhythmias. In Fig.
6, the correlation between induction of atrial fibrillation and refractory period, conduction velocity and wavelength of the provoking premature impulse is plotted. The
critical wavelength where atrial arrhythmias (repetitive responses or flutter) started
to occur was 12 cm, the critical wavelength for atrial fibrillation was 8 cm. The
values of premature beats that did not induce an arrhythmia are plotted with open
symbols, those that induced atrial fibrillation with filled symbols. Because of the use
of a variety of drugs, values for refractory period and conduction velocity varied
widely (see also Table 1). It can be seen that atrial fibrillation could be induced over
a wide range of refractory periods (between 50 and 150 msec) and over a wide range
of conduction velocities (50–140 cm/sec). For each of these parameters there is a
wide overlap between the population of "no arrhythmias" and "fibrillation." When,
however, wavelength was used as a criterion, there was a clear separation between
both populations. Although these findings were obtained in healthy dogs in which
electrophysiological properties of the atria were acutely altered by the administration

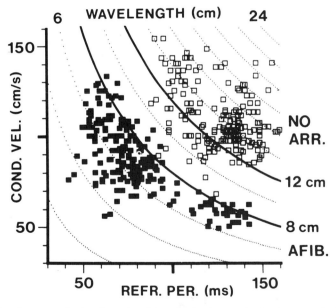

FIG. 6. Relation between induction of atrial arrhythmias and refractory period, and conduction
velocity and wavelength of the initiating premature beat. The refractory period is plotted on the
abscissa and the conduction velocity on the ordinate. Because the wavelength is the product
of refractory period and conduction velocity, "isowavelength" curves at 12 and 8 cm are drawn.
Because of the natural dispersion in electrophysiological properties and the different effects of
a wide variety of administered drugs, a wide range of refractory periods and conduction velocities was achieved. Different responses, i.e., either no arrhythmias or atrial fibrillation, were
obtained over a wide range of conduction velocities and refractory periods. However, wavelength discriminated well between the two types of response. (Modified from ref. 44.)

TABLE 1. *Effects of several cardioactive drugs on refractory period, conduction velocity, and wavelength at left part of Bachmann's bundle*

		Regular rhythm				Earliest premature beat				Maximal pacing rate		
	n	RP (msec)	CV (cm/sec)	WL (cm)		RP (msec)	CV (cm/sec)	WL (cm)	n	RP (msec)	CV (cm/sec)	WL (cm)
Control	18	114 ± 7	127 ± 10	14.5 ± 1.7		8.0 ± 7	82 ± 6	6.6 ± 0.5	13	89 ± 5	89 ± 14	7.9 ± 1.2
Propafenone	5	148 ± 12[a]	99 ± 8[a]	14.6 ± 1.0		116 ± 17[a]	59 ± 5[a]	6.8 ± 0.6	5	109 ± 4[a]	69 ± 10[b]	7.5 ± 1.1
Lidocaine	11	147 ± 11[a]	118 ± 9[b]	17.2 ± 1.7[a]		123 ± 12[a]	61 ± 8[a]	7.3 ± 0.7[a]	11	120 ± 6[a]	72 ± 14[c]	8.7 ± 1.7
Quinidine	14	153 ± 9[a]	115 ± 10[b]	17.7 ± 1.6[a]		120 ± 11[a]	76 ± 10	9.1 ± 1.3[a]	9	129 ± 10[a]	90 ± 11	11.7 ± 1.9[a]
d-Sotalol	4	161 ± 19[a]	123 ± 4	19.9 ± 2.6[a]		119 ± 5[a]	81 ± 5	9.6 ± 0.9[a]	4	121 ± 7[a]	90 ± 10	10.9 ± 1.5[a]
Ouabain	11	107 ± 5[c]	124 ± 8	13.3 ± 0.8[c]		81 ± 6	81 ± 9	6.6 ± 1.1				

[a] p < 0.001.
[b] p < 0.01.
[c] p < 0.05.
RP, refractory period; CV, conduction velocity; WL, wavelength.

of drugs, and extrapolation to spontaneous fibrillation in diseased atria must be made with caution, we suggest that it might be useful to describe part of the antiarrhythmic properties of antiarrhythmic drugs in terms of changes of wavelength, rather than in terms of alterations in refractory period alone or conduction velocity alone.

THE ROLE OF THE SINUS NODE IN ATRIAL FIBRILLATION

A number of experimental studies produced evidence for a possible role of the sinus node in atrial fibrillation. Thus, destruction of the sinus node, by crushing the node or by infusion of trichloroacetic acid into the sinus node artery (45,46), either made induction of atrial fibrillation impossible or drastically reduced its incidence. Similar results were obtained when spontaneous impulse formation in the sinus node was abolished by perfusion of hypertonic solutions (47). When, however, this maneuver only led to sinus bradycardia, atrial fibrillation often occurred spontaneously. In experiments on isolated rabbit right atrial preparations superfused with hypokalemic solutions, atrial fibrillation often occurred immediately after a sinus impulse (48). Thus, these observations suggested that the sinus node could be instrumental in inducing atrial fibrillation.

To obtain more direct information about the possible role of the sinus node, detailed activation maps of the sinus node area were made, and multiple microelectrode recordings were obtained during atrial fibrillation in isolated Langendorff-perfused preparations from giant rabbits (49). Figure 7 shows a map of the sinus node area during half a second of atrial fibrillation. Shaded areas represent tissue where no activity was recorded during the respective time frame; double bars indicate conduction block. The maps show that in the isolated perfused rabbit heart, electrically induced atrial fibrillation is also based on multiple wavelet reentry. The wavelets enter the region of the sinus node from different directions, but the major input is the region of the superior atrial septum, which is contiguous with the bundle of Bachmann. About 60% of the fibrillatory impulses entered the sinus node area from this region. Since the bundle of Bachmann is the major connection between the left and right atria, this suggests that the left atrium is a major source of input. A conspicuous feature was that the intercaval region close to the inferior caval vein was electrically silent during most of the time. Occasionally, the activation pattern suggested that an excitation wave originated in the sinus node.

Figure 8, finally, shows intracellular recordings from the sinus node area during atrial fibrillation. The fibers were located at a distance of 0.0, 0.2, and 1.2 mm from the crista terminalis. In the atrium (upper trace), low-amplitude potentials of brief duration were frequently interposed between well-developed atrial action potentials and represented local conduction block. In the border zone, the average rate of responses was about half the fibrillation rate in the atrium. The variation in action potential configuration was high and markedly influenced by electrotonic potentials. In the center of the sinus node, the response rate was reduced again. The average cycle length was in fact hardly shorter than that during normal sinus rhythm. Less than one in five fibrillation waves penetrated into the center of the sinus node. This high degree of protection prevented the automatic fibers in the center of the sinus node to be overdrive suppressed. Therefore, spontaneous diastolic depolarization was still present, which incidentally led to spontaneous impulse formation. This in-

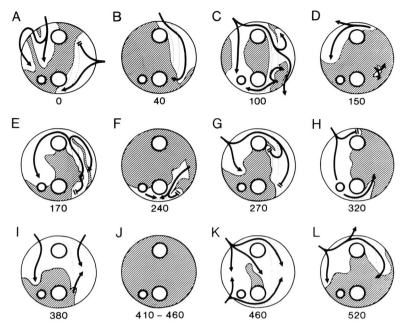

FIG. 7. The atrial spread of excitation during half a second of atrial fibrillation in the region of the sinus node. The *large circles* represent the orifices of superior and inferior caval veins, the *small circles* that of the coronary sinus. *Arrows* in each frame depict propagation of subsequent fibrillatory wavelets; *shaded areas* are zones of conduction block. During atrial fibrillation, the sinus node area was continuously bombarded by fibrillating wavelets coming from different directions. (Modified from ref. 49.)

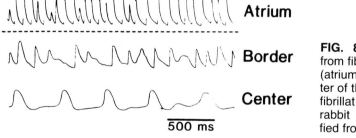

Atrium

Border

Center

500 ms

FIG. 8. Intracellular recordings from fibers in the crista terminalis (atrium), the border, and the center of the sinus node during atrial fibrillation of an isolated giant rabbit heart preparation. (Modified from ref. 49.)

dicates that the sinus node can indeed play a role in the maintenance of atrial fibrillation by providing an impulse during a period of "electrical silence" due to the extinction of multiple fibrillation wavelets.

CONCLUDING REMARKS

The evidence available at the moment warrants the statement that atrial fibrillation is caused by multiple wavelet reentry. Some factors predisposing to atrial fibrillation have been identified: presence of cells with low resting membrane potentials and depressed action potentials; relatively short refractory periods over a wide range of cycle lengths; increased dispersion of refractory periods. Further studies, especially on the role of altered activity of the autonomic nervous system and its influence on cellular electrophysiologic parameters, are clearly needed.

The concept of a critical wavelength for reentrant atrial arrhythmias suggests that it may be useful to study the effects of antiarrhythmic drugs in terms of their effects on wavelengths. Drugs that increase wavelengths, preferably by an increase of both the refractory period and conduction velocity, would be the most effective against atrial fibrillation. Further studies are needed to complete our insight in the interactions between changes in cellular electrophysiology (shortened refractory periods; diminution of rate-dependent changes in refractoriness; impaired conduction) and changes in microanatomy (development of collagenous septae; electrical uncoupling) to result in conditions promoting reentry. Such studies will allow a better understanding of the relative importance of wavelengths and structural inhomogeneities in the genesis of atrial fibrillation.

REFERENCES

1. Fozzard HA, Friedlander IR. Cellular electrophysiology. In: MacFarlane PW, Veitch Lawrie FD, eds. *Comprehensive electrocardiology.* New York: Pergamon Press, 1989;79–100.
2. Hoffman BF, Cranefield PF. *Electrophysiology of the heart.* New York: McGraw-Hill, 1960; 42–74.
3. Gelband H, Bush HL, Rosen MR, et al. Electrophysiological properties of isolated preparations of human atrial myocardium. *Circ Res* 1972;30:293–300.
4. Rosen MR, Bowman FO, Mary-Rabine L. Atrial fibrillation: the relationship between cellular electrophysiologic and clinical data. In: Kulbertus HE, Olsson SB, Schlepper M, eds. *Atrial fibrillation.* Mölndal: AB Hässle, 1982;62–69.
5. Hogan PM, Davis LD. Evidence of specialized fibers in the canine right atrium. *Circ Res* 1968;23:387–396.
6. Tranum-Jensen J, Janse MJ. Fine structural identification of individual cells subjected to microelectrode recording in perfused cardiac preparations. *J Mol Cell Cardiol* 1982;14:233–247.
7. Rubinstein DS, Lipsius SL. Mechanism of automaticity in subsidiary pacemakers from cat right atrium. *Circ Res* 1989;64:648–657.
8. Rubinstein DS, Fox LM, McNulty JA, et al. Electrophysiology and ultrastructure of eustachian ridge from cat right atrium: a comparison with SA node. *J Mol Cell Cardiol* 1987;19:965–976.
9. Hordof AJ, Spotnitz A, Mary-Rabine L, et al. Electrophysiologic properties and response to pharmacologic agents of fibers of diseased human atria. *Circulation* 1976;54:774–779.
10. Attuel P, Childers R, Cauchemer B, et al. Failure in rate adaptation of the atrial refractory period: its relationship to vulnerability. *Int J Cardiol* 1982;2:179–197.
11. Le Heuzey JY, Boutjdir M, Gagey S, et al. Cellular aspects of atrial vulnerability. In: Attuel P, Coumel P, Janse MJ, eds. *The atrium in health and disease.* Mount Kisco, NY: Futura, 1989; 81–94.
12. Gettes LS, Reuter H. Slow recovery from inactivation of inward currents in mammalian fibers. *J Physiol (Lond)* 1974;240:703–725.
13. Ramdat Misier A, Opthof T, Van Hemel N, et al. Dispersion in "refractoriness" in patients with recurrent paroxysmal atrial fibrillation (abstract). *Eur Heart J* 1990;11(suppl):238.
14. Luck JC, Engel TR. Dispersion of atrial refractoriness in patients with sinus node dysfunction. *Circulation* 1979;60:404–412.
15. Coumel P, Attuel P, Lavallee JP, et al. Syndrome d'arythmie auriculaire d'origine vasale. *Arch Mal Coeur* 1978;71:645–651.
16. Pastelin G, Mendez R, Moe GK. Participation of atrial specialized conduction pathways in atrial flutter. *Cir Res* 1978;42:386–393.
17. Janse MJ, Anderson RH. Specialized internodal atrial pathways—fact or fiction? *Eur J Cardiol* 1974;2:117–136.
18. Bericht über die Verhandlungen der XIV Tagung der Deutschen Pathologischen Gesellschaft in Erlangen von 4–6. April 1910. *Zentralbl Allg Pathol* 1910;21:433–443.
19. Sherf L, James TN. Fine structure of cells and their histological organization with internodal pathways of the heart: clinical and electrocardiographic implications. *Am J Cardiol* 1979;44: 345–369.

20. Hoffman BF. Fine structure of internodal pathways. *Am J Cardiol* 1979;44:385–386.
21. Wit AL, Fenoglio JJ Jr, Hordof AJ, et al. Ultrastructure and transmembrane potential of cardiac muscle in the human anterior mitral valve leaflet. *Circulation* 1979;59:1284–1294.
22. Mendez C, Moe GK. Some characteristics of transmembrane potentials of AV nodal cells during propagation of premature beats. *Circ Res* 1966;19:993–1010.
23. Horibe H. Studies on the spread of right atrial activation by means of intracellular microelectrodes. *Jpn Circ J* 1961;25:583–593.
24. Hogan PM, Davis LO. Evidence for specialized fibers in the canine right atrium. *Circ Res* 1968;23:387–394.
25. Wagner ML, Lazzara R, Weiss RM, et al. Specialized conducting fibers in the interatrial band. *Circ Res* 1966;18:502–510.
26. DeMello WC, Hoffman BF. Potassium ions and electrical activity of specialized cardiac fibers. *Am J Physiol* 1960;199:1125–1132.
27. Vassalle M, Hoffman BF. The spread of sinus activation during potassium administration. *Circ Res* 1965;17:285–293.
28. Lewis T. *Lectures on the heart*. New York: Paul Hoeber, 1915.
29. Roberts DE, Hersch LT, Scher AM. Influence of cardiac fiber orientation on wavefront voltage, conduction velocity and tissue resistivity in the dog. *Circ Res* 1979;44:701–712.
30. Clerc L. Directional differences in impulse spread in trabecular muscle from mammalian heart. *J Physiol (Lond)* 1976;255:335–346.
31. Spach MS, Miller WT Jr, Dolber PC, et al. The functional role of structural complexities in the propagation of depolarization in the atrium of the dog. Cardiac conduction disturbances due to discontinuities of effective axial resistivity. *Circ Res* 1982;50:175–191.
32. Spach MS, Dolber PC. Relating extracellular potentials and their derivatives to anisotropic propagation at a microscopic level in human cardiac muscle. Evidence for electrical uncoupling of side-to-side fiber connections with increasing age. *Circ Res* 1986;58:356–371.
33. Dillon S, Allessie MA, Ursell PC, et al. Influence of anisotropic tissue structure on reentrant circuits in the subepicardial border zone of subacute canine infarcts. *Circ Res* 1988;63:182–206.
34. Schalij MJ, Allessie MA, Lammers WJ, et al. Reentry in anisotropic ventricular myocardium (abstract). *Circulation* 1987;76:IV–113.
35. Allessie MA, Schalij MJ, Kirchhof CJHJ, et al. Experimental electrophysiology and arrhythmogeneity. Anisotropy and ventricular tachycardia. *Eur Heart J* 1989;10(suppl E):2–8.
36. Van Capelle FJL, Allessie MA. Computer simulation of anisotropic impulse propagation. Characteristics of action potentials during re-entrant arrhythmias. In: Goldbeter A, ed. *Theoretical models for cell to cell signalling*. New York: Academic Press, 1989;577–588.
37. Boineau JP, Schuessler RB, Cain ME, et al. Activation maps during normal atrial rhythms and atrial flutter. In: Zipes DP, Jalife J, eds. *Cardiac electrophysiology, from cell to bedside*. Philadelphia: WB Saunders, 1990;537–548.
38. Moe GK. On the multiple wavelet hypothesis of atrial fibrillation. *Arch Int Pharmacodyn Ther* 1962;140:183–188.
39. Allessie MA, Lammers WJEP, Bonke FIM, et al. Experimental evaluation of Moe's multiple wavelet hypothesis of atrial fibrillation. In: Zipes DP, Jalife J, eds. *Cardiac arrhythmias*. Orlando: Grune and Stratton, 1985;265–276.
40. Moe GK, Rheinboldt WC, Abildskov JA. A computer model of atrial fibrillation. *Am Heart J* 1964;67:200–220.
41. Allessie MA, Brugada J, Boersma L, et al. Mapping of atrial fibrillation in man (abstract). *Eur Heart J* 1990;11(suppl):5.
42. Mines GR. On circulating excitations in heart muscles and their possible relation to tachycardia and fibrillation. *Trans R Soc Can* 1914;4:43–52.
43. Wiener N, Rosenblueth A. The mathematical formulation of the problem of conduction of impulses in a network of connected excitable elements, specifically in cardiac muscle. *Arch Inst Cardiol Met* 1946;16:205–265.
44. Rensma PL, Allessie MA, Lammers WJEP, et al. The length of the excitation wave as an index for the susceptibility to reentrant atrial arrhythmias. *Circ Res* 1988;62:395–410.
45. Azuma K, Shinmura H, Shimiza K, et al. Significance of the sino-atrial node on mechanism of occurrence of atrial fibrillation. *Jpn Heart J* 1972;13:84–98.
46. Nadeau RA, Roberge FA, Billette J. Role of the sinus node in the mechanism of cholinergic atrial fibrillation. *Circ Res* 1970;27:129–138.
47. Chiba S, Suzuki Y, Hashimoto K. Atrial fibrillation induced by infusion of hypertonic solutions into the canine sinus node artery in situ. *J Pharmacol Exp Ther* 1969;167:274–281.
48. Sano T, Suzuki F, Sato S. Sinus node impulses and atrial fibrillation. *Circ Res* 1967;21:507–513.
49. Kirchhof CJHJ. *The sinus node and atrial fibrillation*, Thesis. Maastricht: Datawyse/University of Limburg, 1989.

Atrial Fibrillation: Mechanisms and Management, edited by
R. H. Falk and P. J. Podrid.
Raven Press, Ltd., New York © 1992.

4

Role of the Atrioventricular Node in Atrial Fibrillation

*Frits L. Meijler and †Fred H. M. Wittkampf

*The Interuniversity Cardiology Institute of the Netherlands,
3501 DG Utrecht, The Netherlands; †Heart Lung Institute, University Hospital
Utrecht, 3508 GA Utrecht, The Netherlands*

Atrial fibrillation is probably the most common cardiac arrhythmia in humans, particularly in the elderly (1–3). The irregularity and inequality of the heart beat first described by Hering in 1903 were, and remain, the landmark of the clinical diagnosis of atrial fibrillation (4,5). Sir Thomas Lewis (6) observed the gross irregularity of the arrhythmia and stated "the pauses betwixt the heart beats bear no relationship to one another." Thanks to work of Lewis (7), Mackenzie (8), Wenckebach (9), and others, the clinical syndrome of atrial fibrillation became well established, and gradually the pathophysiological mechanisms involved were also recognized (10). In 1915 Einthoven and Korteweg (11) studied the effect of heart cycle duration on the size of the carotid pulse and concluded that the strength of the heart beat was related to the duration of the preceding cycle.

Animals, as well as humans, may develop atrial fibrillation (12,13). Indeed, Lewis (7) observed the arrhythmia in a horse and used this observation to determine that the irregular pulse noticed in humans was due to fibrillation of the atria.

Until the 1950s, observations on atrial fibrillation were limited to its etiologic, clinical, and surface ECG manifestations. The beginning of the computer era enabled several groups of investigators to analyze the ventricular rhythm during atrial fibrillation in a more quantitative fashion (14–16). The results of these studies were fascinating and allowed for the development of theories and speculations on the behavior of the atrioventricular (AV) node during atrial fibrillation. Sophisticated computer techniques also allowed Moe and co-workers (17,18) to simulate atrial electrical activity during atrial fibrillation, and they formulated the so-called "multiple wavelet" theory, which was subsequently supported by experimental evidence (19).

Parallel to the growing insight into the electrical behavior of the atria during atrial fibrillation and into the corresponding ventricular rhythm, sophisticated experimental methods were designed to study AV nodal electrophysiology in a variety of circumstances, including induced atrial fibrillation (20,21).

This chapter reexamines some of the established concepts of AV nodal function and, in the light of comparative physiology of the AV node and some specific clinical observations during atrial fibrillation, demonstrates inexplicable flaws in the current theories of AV nodal function. Based on our observations, we postulate that the AV node, rather than acting as an intrinsic part of the cardiac conduction system, is primarily a pacemaker subject to electrotonic influences from other areas in the heart.

DEFINITION

Atrial fibrillation has been defined by a WHO/ISFC Task Force (22) as "an irregular, disorganized, electrical activity of the atria. P waves are absent and the baseline consists of irregular wave forms which continuously change in shape, duration, amplitude and direction. In the absence of advanced or complete AV block, the resulting ventricular response is totally irregular (random)." This definition is applicable to routine medical practice, when we are usually satisfied that the atria are fibrillating if the ventricular arrhythmia fills the criterion of being totally irregular (random).

Several investigators have studied the electrical activity of the atria during atrial fibrillation (23,24). Using signal analysis of the atrial electrogram for the study of atrial fibrillation (25), we found a random rhythm with a rate between 300 and 600 per minute. However, not only does the sequence of the recorded atrial signals display a random pattern during atrial fibrillation, the form and strength of the recorded signals also fail to show any repetition (23,24). Thus, the AV node receives or is surrounded by impulses that are random in time and almost certainly also in form and strength.

THE VENTRICULAR RHYTHM

The random pattern of the ventricular rhythm during atrial fibrillation can be demonstrated by means of a serial autocorrelogram (SAC), as illustrated on the right-hand side of Fig. 1. The SAC is obtained by the measurement of the duration of the RR intervals. Each RR interval duration is correlated with itself, then with the duration of the next RR interval and subsequently with RR interval durations that are a given number of RR intervals ahead. Correlation coefficient number 0 is the result of correlating the duration of each RR interval with itself and consequently equals +1. Correlation coefficient 1 is the result of correlating the duration of each RR interval with the next and its value depends on the measure of relation between the two sets of RR interval durations. Similarly, correlation coefficient 10 represents the relation between the durations of all RR intervals that are 10 intervals apart, 20 represents all those that are 20 intervals apart, and so forth. In a random process all correlation coefficients greater than 0 have values that are statistically not significantly different from 0, and, consequently, if in a SAC the values of successive correlation coefficients of the RR interval durations do not differ from 0, that rhythm may be called random. In Fig. 1, derived from a single patient with atrial fibrillation before and after the administration of digitalis (26), it can be seen that before and after digitalis the correlation coefficients do not differ from 0 and thus the ventricular rhythm under both circumstances is, by definition, random. The histogram (left side of Fig. 1) shows a difference in ventricular rate produced by digitalis, but the degree

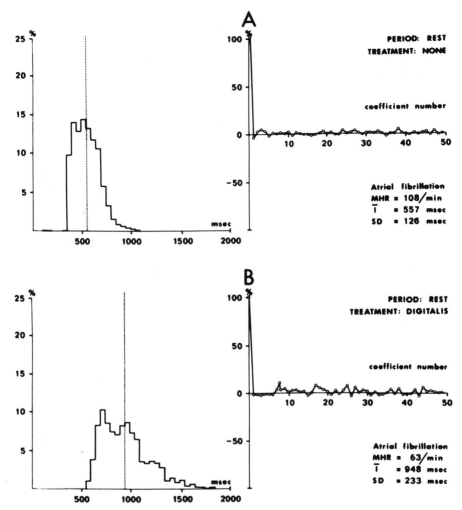

FIG. 1. Histogram and serial autocorrelogram (SAC) of a patient with atrial fibrillation without (**A**) and with (**B**) digitalis treatment. The SAC is unchanged, thus the ventricular rhythm remains random despite change in form and shift to the right of the histogram. For further details, see text. (From ref. 26, with permission.)

of irregularity expressed as the so-called dispersion of RR intervals (27) or coefficient of variation (28) remains constant. We will return to this in later sections of this chapter.

The ventricular rhythm in atrial fibrillation can also be described as a renewal process or as a "point process without memory." A point process is a process in which the duration of the event—the R wave for instance—is short compared with the interval between events. Well-known examples of point processes are the emissions from a radioactive source, the action potentials of a nerve fiber, coal mining disasters, and wars (29). Also in atrial fibrillation the duration of a forthcoming RR interval can never be predicted. After each event the process starts anew, totally disregarding its past.

Another way to display the ventricular rhythm during atrial fibrillation makes use of a so-called "interval plot" (Fig. 2). In this form of display the duration of each RR interval is plotted against its sequential number. The RR interval plot does not contain information that is not present in the histogram, but it illustrates well the functional refractory period (FRP) of the AV junction as well as the maximal duration of the RR intervals of that particular patient at the time the recording was obtained.

We realized (26) that if the AV node has a role to play in determining the random nature of the ventricular rhythm during atrial fibrillation, it would have to be a limited one, since pharmacological (Fig. 1) or physical interventions that affect the ventricular rate during atrial fibrillation do not interfere with the irregularity of the ventricular rhythm. Therefore, there can be little doubt that the primary cause of the randomly irregular ventricular rhythm must reside in the fibrillating atria.

CONCEALED AND DECREMENTAL CONDUCTION

The random ventricular response during atrial fibrillation occurs at a much slower rate than the rate of the electrical impulses produced by the fibrillating atria. The slow ventricular response and its persistent randomness have been explained by concealed conduction in the AV node and its refractory period. In 1948, Langendorf (30) introduced the term "concealed conduction" into clinical electrocardiography. The WHO/ISFC Task Force (22) defined concealed conduction as: "Partial penetration of an impulse into the AV conduction system or a pacemaker-myocardial junction, which exerts an influence on subsequent impulse formation or conduction or both." The term has recently been redefined by Fisch (31) as "the presence of incomplete conduction coupled with an unexpected behaviour of the subsequent impulse." Con-

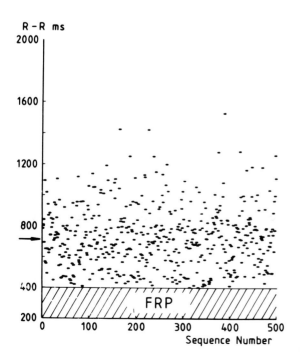

FIG. 2. Interval plot of 500 RR intervals of a human patient with atrial fibrillation. Each *dot* represents one RR interval. The *arrow* indicates the median RR interval. For further details, see text. (From ref. 100, with permission.)

cealed conduction or block is a concept, something that one cannot see but that has to be inferred from the aftereffect of a blocked impulse. Concealed conduction in the AV node during atrial fibrillation may, among others, result from decremental conduction (32). Hoffman and Cranefield (33) described decremental conduction as "a type of conduction in which the properties of the fiber change along its length in such a manner that the action potential becomes progressively less effective as a stimulus to the unexcited portion of the fiber ahead of it."

In 1965, Langendorf et al. (34) postulated that concealed conduction in the AV junction could explain the characteristics of the ventricular rate and rhythm during atrial fibrillation. Several subsequent investigators, using models of experimentally induced atrial fibrillation were able to demonstrate decremental conduction in the node during this arrhythmia and with this the concept of concealed conduction within the AV node as an explanation of the rate and complexity of the rhythm of the ventricles became well established (35,36). The effects of drugs such as digitalis (37), quinidine (38), and beta-blockers (39) on the ventricular rate in atrial fibrillation could be explained by this theory, although the sometimes observed regularizing effect of verapamil and other calcium antagonists remains less well understood (40).

The majority of investigators were satisfied with the concealed conduction concept, although Grant (41) in 1956 and James and his group (42) in 1977 suggested alternate explanations based on the theory that atrial impulses may modify an intrinsic pacemaking function of the AV node rather than being directly, albeit more slowly, conducted through it.

THE ATRIOVENTRICULAR NODE AS A PACEMAKER

The concept of the AV node as an unprotected pacemaker is not new. Again, it was Lewis (43) who in 1925 postulated that AV nodal function could be interpreted in another fashion than as conduction: "The structure of the A-V node and its similarities to the S-A node has suggested the last as the ventricular pacemaker, and it has been thought that a new and distinct wave may start in this after each systole of the auricle." It is clear that in this statement, Lewis considers AV nodal function during sinus rhythm or at least during organized "auricular" activity.

In 1929, two Dutch physicists (44), Van der Pol and Van der Mark, proposed that the heart beat could be viewed as a relaxation oscillator. A relaxation oscillator is best described as a condenser that is periodically discharged by the ignition of a neon tube. An important characteristic of an oscillator is that it can be synchronized by external (electric) forces.

Van der Tweel et al. (45) showed that the sinus node as well as the AV node of an isolated rat heart can be synchronized in the same way as a relaxation oscillator. Many years later we demonstrated that the function of the canine AV node can be described as a periodically perturbed biological oscillator (46). Perturbation and/or synchronization of an oscillator can be electrophysiologically translated into entrainment of a pacemaker (47).

Segers et al. (48) first referred to possible synchronization of the AV nodal pacemaker resulting in a fixed temporal relation between the atria and the ventricles to explain an isorhythmic dissociation during complete heart block. Jalife and Michaels (49) defined entrainment as the coupling of a self-sustained oscillatory system (such as a pacemaker) to an external forcing oscillation with the result that either both oscillations have the same frequency, or both frequencies are related in a harmonic fashion. Winfree (50) defined entrainment as "the locking of one rhythm to another, with N cycles of the one matching M cycles of the other."

A possible electrophysiological mechanism responsible for entrainment or synchronization of pacemaker cells is an alteration of the rate of their phase-4 depolarization. It can thus be made plausible that during sinus rhythm, the AV node, like the SA node, behaves as an oscillator or pacemaker that is entrained by the atrial depolarization sparked by sinoatrial (SA) firing (51) (Fig. 3).

Cohen et al. (52) developed a quantitative model along these lines to describe the ventricular response during atrial fibrillation as well. Electrotonic modulation of phase-4 depolarization of a pacemaker cell equivalent by randomly occurring atrial impulses of random strength and duration and coming from random directions could thus explain the (slower) random ventricular response during atrial fibrillation. This model is an agreement with the concealed conduction concept in the sense that nontransmitted atrial impulses contribute to the transmission of one of the atrial impulses (Fig. 4).

However, during atrial fibrillation the AV node need not necessarily be a pacemaker with spontaneous phase-4 depolarization to be electrotonically modulated by the atrial impulses. In segments with stable resting membrane potentials, nonconducted impulses can exert an inhibitory effect on the electrotonically mediated transmission of subsequent impulses or facilitate propagation when two subthreshold potentials occur in close succession (53). In principle both mechanisms can explain the irregular ventricular response from an irregular atrial input, as in atrial fibrillation.

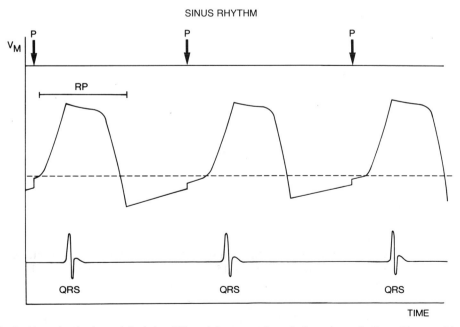

FIG. 3. Hypothetical model of the AV nodal pacemaker during sinus rhythm. The ventricular rate and PR interval depend on the sinus rate and the slope of phase-4 depolarization of the AV nodal pacemaker. During sinus rhythm or any other organized atrial rhythm, the electrotonic effect of the atrial excitations is constant. Varying PR intervals during sinus arrhythmias, long PR intervals of atrial extrasystoles, or, for instance, concealed conduction of a nontransmitted P wave can be explained by this model. (From ref. 51, with permission.)

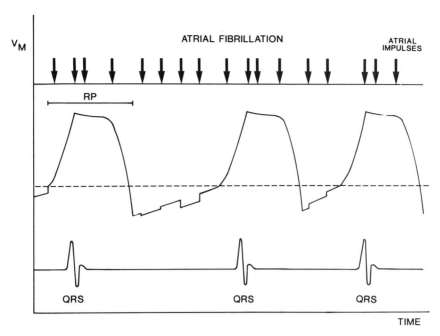

FIG. 4. Hypothetical model of the AV nodal pacemaker during atrial fibrillation. Depending on strength, timing, and direction of the atrial impulses, diastolic depolarization can be speeded up or slowed down (hyperpolarization) during atrial fibrillation. This explains why the RR intervals vary randomly. This model is an extension of the model of Cohen et al. (52). RP, refractory period; VM, voltage of hypothetical monophasic action potential. (From ref. 51, with permission.)

COMPARATIVE ASPECTS OF ATRIOVENTRICULAR NODAL FUNCTION

Sinus Rhythm

As early as 1913, Waller (54) studied comparative physiology and drew attention to the differences in the "auriculo-ventricular" interval in dogs, humans, and horses. Clark (55) in 1927 studied PR intervals in animals of different sizes and noted the small differences between PR intervals compared to the differences in body size. A systematic listing of PR intervals versus body size shows a comparatively short PR interval in hearts of large mammals and a long PR interval in hearts of small mammals (35,56). Despite differences in detail, the overall architecture and microstructure of all mammalian hearts are essentially similar. Whether the source is the mouse or the whale, cardiac muscle is composed of individual cells that are relatively uniform in diameter, approximately 10 to 15 μm (57). This similarity applies to the morphology of the mammalian AV node-His system as well. Both macroscopically and microscopically the structural arrangement of the mammalian AV conduction system tends to be similar, while the size of the heart varies greatly from species to species (58).

Conduction velocity depends largely on cell (fiber) diameter (59,60). Assuming a more or less constant cell-to-cell resistance, it is unlikely that with increasing length or diameter of the His bundle and bundle branches the known conduction velocity of approximately 2.5 m/sec will increase significantly (61). However, Pressler (62) found a substantial difference of conduction velocity in Purkinje fibers in cats and sheep, although not enough to explain the small difference in PR interval between, for instance, a rat and an elephant (56).

These observations suggest that in a large mammalian heart such as the elephant or whale the contribution to the AV conduction delay by the AV node or other components of the AV conduction system may be different from that of the heart in smaller mammals such as the human, dog, or rabbit. For example, in the adult blue whale with His bundles that may be well over 1 m in length from their origin at the distal end of the AV node to their terminal ventricular ramifications, approximately 400 msec will be required for the impulse to cover that distance, assuming a conduction velocity of about 2.5 m/sec. The PR interval in the elephant or a small whale does not exceed 400 msec (56,63,64).

Therefore the AV node, although anatomically present in large mammals and physically larger than in smaller mammals (65), would not be expected to impose a substantial delay on AV transmission during normal sinus rhythm, even if conduction velocity in the His bundles was greater than 2.5 m/sec. Figure 5 shows the PR intervals in a variety of mammals plotted against the third root of heart weight (66). This demonstrates an S-shaped relationship when very small to very large animals are plotted. Unfortunately, despite our attempts, we have been unable to obtain and measure the ECG and PR interval in one of the largest of all mammals, the gray whale (67,68).

If indeed, as can be inferred from Fig. 5, in larger mammals the contribution of the AV nodal delay to the PR interval is proportionately less than in smaller animals, it is difficult to explain the mismatch between the PR interval and heart weight from accepted theories of decremental conduction in the AV node (35). This assertion led us to hypothesize that the PR interval and the well-tuned AV nodal synchrony may not be a simple matter of a varying and reduced conduction velocity through the AV junction. An alternative theory may be found, such as the entrainment of an AV nodal pacemaker by the excitation of the atrial myocardium (51) (Fig. 3).

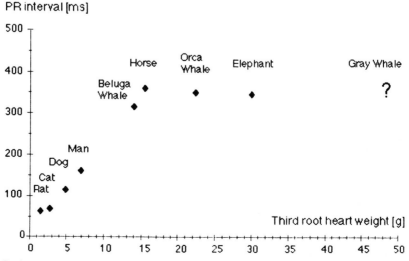

FIG. 5. S-shape relationship between PR interval and third root of heart weight. Values obtained from Altman and Dittmer (100). (From ref. 67, with permission.)

Atrial Fibrillation

Veterinarians are well aware of the frequent occurrence of atrial fibrillation in large dogs (12) (usually with mitral valve disease) and horses (13,69,70). Indeed, as mentioned earlier, the relationship between fibrillating atria and a totally irregular ventricular rhythm was first demonstrated by Lewis (7) in 1912 in a horse. Moe's (18) multiple wavelet theory states that atrial fibrillation is maintained by the presence of a number of independent wavelets that wander randomly through the myocardium around islets or strands of refractory tissue. In order for atrial fibrillation to be maintained, Moe's theory requires a critical mass of atrial tissue. It is of interest that, in keeping with Moe's hypothesis, spontaneous atrial fibrillation is hardly ever observed in smaller mammals (69). Figure 6 demonstrates a once-in-a-lifetime observation: the interval plot, SAC, and histogram of the ventricular rhythm of a kangaroo with atrial fibrillation. This observation lends further credence to the concept that atrial fibrillation may occur in the heart of any mammal if Moe's conditions are fulfilled (17,18), i.e., a sufficient number of cells involved and/or a sufficient degree of electrical inhomogeneity.

Figure 7 shows median RR interval duration versus log body mass in kilograms in dogs, humans, and horses with spontaneous atrial fibrillation. It can be seen that the differences in ventricular rates between the three species as compared with the differences in body weight are small (70). The dog, human, and horse with atrial fibrillation may have ventricular cycles that can be similar despite the fact that a horse heart is 50 to 100 times as large as that of a dog. In dogs, as in humans, the ventricular rhythm is random. In horses, depending on the ventricular rate, a certain degree of periodicity may occasionally be present. Based on our observations we concluded

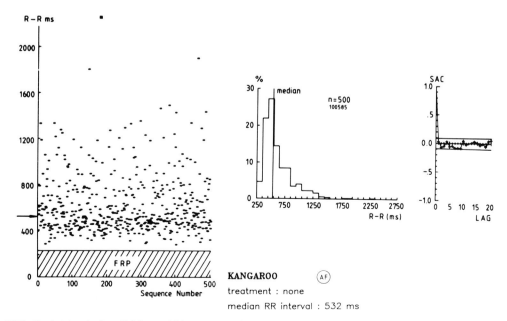

KANGAROO (AF)
treatment : none
median RR interval : 532 ms

FIG. 6. Interval plot, SAC, and histogram of a kangaroo with atrial fibrillation. FRP, functional refractory period. The *arrow* indicates the median RR interval. For further details, see text. (From ref. 101, with permission.)

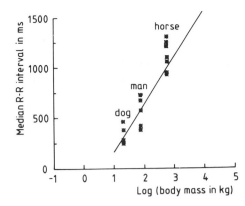

FIG. 7. Median RR intervals of dogs, humans, and horses with atrial fibrillation versus log body weight. For further details, see text. (From ref. 28, with permission.)

that this could be caused by autonomic nerve interference with AV junctional electrophysiological properties elicited by the very long RR intervals that often occur (4 sec and longer) and are associated with a concomitant drop in blood pressure (71).

THE ATRIOVENTRICULAR NODE AS A GATEKEEPER IN ATRIAL FIBRILLATION

According to current opinion, during atrial fibrillation the ventricles are protected against high atrial rates and ventricular fibrillation by the AV node (25,72–74,76). Thus the AV node may be considered as a guard or a gatekeeper, allowing some impulses to pass while preventing many other impulses from entering the gate.

The classical theory that during atrial fibrillation the AV node behaves as a gatekeeper by means of concealed and decremental conduction, allowing some atrial impulses to be propagated to the ventricles, while others are prevented from propagation, has been challenged by several investigators (41,42,52,77–80). However, the metaphor of the AV node as gatekeeper may still be a good one, depending on how the function of the gatekeeper is described. A gatekeeper may consider all subjects that want to pass the gate and then select one or more that will be admitted. He may also guard his gate by only letting pass subjects with certain properties (e.g., a valid passport), while others not having such a passport are not even considered. Moreover, the gatekeeper can also set a time limit (a refractory period) within which no subject, even one with a valid passport, is allowed to pass the gate. So the gatekeeper may have several means of selecting subjects (or impulses during atrial fibrillation) for passage through the gate (AV node). This can be summarized as follows:

1. An impulse may be allowed to pass following a number of blocked impulses. The blocked impulses have influenced the gatekeeper's behavior either by their number, their properties, or both.
2. Only impulses that fulfill certain qualifications of form, strength, or direction are able to pass. These are not affected by impulses that did not meet the preconditioned requirements.
3. The gatekeeper allows impulses (with specified properties) to pass, but only after a prespecified period following a previously allowed impulse, dependent on the conditions of the gate (refractory period).

4. The requirements for passage, and thus the behavior of the gatekeeper, may change when circumstances change as, for instance, under the influence of autonomic nerve control or drug action.
5. The gatekeeper may apply a combination of selection criteria, for instance 1 and 3, or 2 and 3, while adaptation to varying circumstances will lead to inclusion of condition 4.

The informed reader will recognize that the gatekeeper who allows the passage of impulses according to selection criterion 1 makes use of a concealed conduction mechanism. To establish which of the gatekeeper functions agree(s) best with the actual behavior of the ventricles during atrial fibrillation, we describe and try to analyze a number of observations made over the years in patients with this arrhythmia.

THE COMPENSATORY PAUSE IN ATRIAL FIBRILLATION AND THE EFFECT OF VENTRICULAR PACING

A compensatory pause following a premature ventricular depolarization during sinus rhythm is a well-recognized electrocardiographic phenomenon. Langendorf (81), Pritchett et al. (82), and others (83) have demonstrated that the ventricular cycle is lengthened after a ventricular extrasystole even in the presence of atrial fibrillation. Langendorf (81) termed this phenomenon the "compensatory pause in atrial fibrillation" and believed that it was caused by lengthening of the AV nodal refractory period due to retrograde concealed conduction into the AV node of the spontaneous or artificially induced ventricular extrasystole. However, both Moore and Spear (84) and Akhtar and co-workers (85) have subsequently shown that properly timed retrograde concealed conduction into the AV node facilitates rather than slows AV anterograde conduction. A substantial number of atrial impulses normally delayed and blocked within the AV node would be potential candidates for facilitated propagation following concealed retrograde penetration of a ventricular extrasystole into the AV node. Facilitation of anterograde transmission could never be observed after ventricular extrasystoles in the presence of atrial fibrillation, nevertheless lengthening of the refractory period of the AV node is not likely to explain the compensatory pause in atrial fibrillation.

In recently published work (86) we postulated that the duration of the (compensatory) pause after single ventricular extrasystoles may be caused by two different mechanisms, depending on the time of the extrasystole relative to the preceding "normally propagated" QRS complex.

1. Relatively early, retrogradely conducted ventricular extrasystoles (RS = interval between R wave and extrastimulus = 660 msec) cause the histogram of the postextrasystolic RR intervals (SR in Fig. 8) to shift 300 msec to the right without a change in the shape of the histogram when compared with the histogram of the "normal" RR intervals (Fig. 8). Thus, a ventricular extrasystole that has reached the AV node has the same effect on the timing of the next AV nodal discharge as an impulse reaching the AV node from the atrial side. This can be explained by penetration of the ventricular impulse into the AV nodal region, causing a resetting of its timing cycle or of the periodic discharge of a pacemaker.

2. Retrograde conduction of extrasystoles occurring later in the ventricular cycle

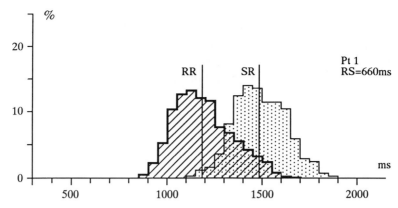

FIG. 8. Histograms of the spontaneous RR intervals (RR) and of the "compensatory pauses" (SR) after properly timed ventricular extrasystoles (RS) in a patient with atrial fibrillation. S stands for the ventricular extrastimulus. The similarity of both histograms should be noted. For further details, see text.

will simply intercept anterograde impulses below the AV node, resulting in a completely different postextrasystolic histogram (86) (not shown in Fig. 8).

If one properly timed ventricular extrasystole is able to penetrate into the AV node and reset the discharge of an AV nodal pacemaker or timing cycle of an activation source, it follows that continued ventricular pacing at an appropriate rate may continuously activate and reset the AV node (77). In Fig. 9 the effect of right ventricular (RV) pacing with decreasing pacing intervals in a patient with atrial fibrillation is shown in an interval plot. It can be seen that, as expected, at a pacing interval of 1,000 msec all RR intervals over 1,000 msec are abolished. However, at the same

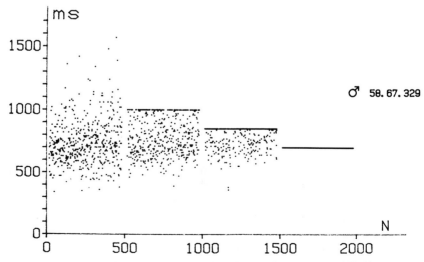

FIG. 9. Successive RR intervals in a patient with atrial fibrillation before (first 500 cycles) and during pacing on the right ventricle with a pacing interval of 1,000, 850, and 700 msec (cycles 500–2,000). At a pacing interval of 700 msec (last 500 cycles), all anterograde "conduction" has ceased and the rhythm has become regular. (From ref. 60, with permission.)

time the number of short RR intervals diminishes. This becomes even more evident at a pacing interval of 850 msec, and at 700 msec all anterograde transmission is blocked despite the fact that the pacing intervals are almost twice as long as the shortest RR intervals before ventricular pacing.

This observation fits well with the theory that repetitive RV pacing (or an accelerated ventricular rhythm) may cause overdrive suppression of an AV nodal pacemaker or continuously reset the timing cycle of an activation source inside the AV node, making it impenetrable for atrial impulses and resulting in total anterograde block. This observation can also be explained on the basis of overdrive suppression of conduction (87).

SCALING IN ATRIAL FIBRILLATION

Another fundamental quality of the ventricular rhythm in patients with atrial fibrillation is the maintenance of its degree of irregularity (relative variability) or dispersion of RR intervals expressed as a constant coefficient of variation (CV) (28) at varying ventricular rates. This remarkable phenomenon is at odds with the principle of scaling (26,88), a term generally used for the linkage between atrial and ventricular rates in atrial fibrillation.

Schmidt-Nielsen (89) defines the term scaling for his studies on animal size as follows: "Scaling deals with the structural and functional consequences of changes in size or scale among otherwise similar organisms."

Scaling of a rhythm cannot so simply be defined. It implies, among other things, that one can scale up or down resulting in a higher or lower rate, respectively. In case of scaling of a rhythm, the so-called scaling factor is the ratio between the rates of the scaled (up or down) rhythms. For instance, the scaling factor in atrial flutter with a 3:1 block is 3, because the atrial rate is three times the ventricular rate. In this case it concerns the conversion of one (high rate) regular rhythm of the atria into another regular rhythm of the ventricles. During a regular rhythm like atrial flutter, scaling only affects the rate, while during an irregular rhythm, e.g., atrial fibrillation, scaling affects both rate and degree of irregularity. Thus, in order to determine whether the AV node indeed scales down the atrial rhythm, not only the rate but also the irregularity of the atrial and ventricular rhythm have to be quantified. We therefore use the CV, which is the ratio between the standard deviation (SD) and the average cycle length (CL). Thus $CV = SD/CL$. It can easily be seen that at $SD = 0$, the CV becomes 0 as well, which implies a strictly regular rhythm.

When two irregular rhythms with different rates have the same CV, their degree of irregularity or relative variability is the same. With a constant scaling factor N, the average CL of the transmitted impulses would increase by the same factor N.

However, variations in the intervals between the atrial impulses during a randomly irregular rhythm like atrial fibrillation will partly compensate each other, and consequently summation of N atrial intervals would not increase the SD of the resulting average ventricular CL with a factor N, but of necessity with the square root of N (90). Therefore, in case of a scaling process, the relative variability (the CV) of such a scaled-down rhythm must decrease. This principle is used in the so-called atomic clock to obtain extremely stable intervals. The greater the scaling factor, the more precise the clock. When we now return to the definition of Schmidt-Nielsen (89), a change in rate of otherwise similarly irregular rhythms paradoxically proves that scaling has not taken place.

If in patients with atrial fibrillation scaling would take place, a greater scaling factor would result in a ventricular rhythm with a lesser irregularity. It follows that a slower ventricular rhythm would have to be less irregular (smaller CV) than a fast ventricular rhythm. That this is not the case is demonstrated in Fig. 1. Despite the lower ventricular rate due to digitalis treatment, the CV remains the same.

Wittkampf et al. (80), including the data of Kirsh et al. (88), studied the relative variability expressed as the CV of the atrial and ventricular rhythms in 100 patients with atrial fibrillation under a variety of circumstances (Fig. 10) known to modulate AV nodal function and to result in rate changes of the ventricular rhythms. They found that, irrespective of the ventricular rates, the CV remained almost constant (in the order of 0.23), and thus the relative variability (degree of irregularity or dispersion of RR intervals) of all ventricular rhythms of all patients remained the same.

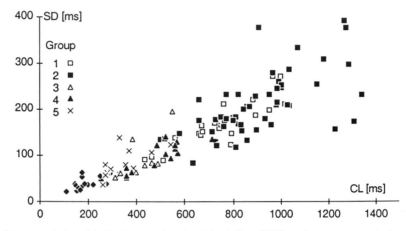

FIG. 10. Linear relationship between standard deviation (SD) and average cycle length (CL) of all rhythms of the five patient groups with atrial fibrillation in Table 1. In case of scaling, the relationship would follow a square root function (see Fig. 11). The group numbers relate to the five groups described in the text and in Table 1.

TABLE 1. *Details of the five groups of patients with atrial fibrillation*

Group	N	CL (msec)	SD (msec)	CV (%)
1	18	186 ± 50	39 ± 13	21 ± 6
2	25	724 ± 177	164 ± 50	23 ± 3
3	51	910 ± 202	210 ± 67	23 ± 6
4	10	419 ± 78	92 ± 45	22 ± 8
5	13	508 ± 101	102 ± 28	20 ± 3
Total	117			22 ± 5

Group 1, atrial rate and rhythm of discrete local deflections in the right atrium as recorded with an electrode catheter; group 2, ventricular rate and rhythm at rest without medication; group 3, ventricular rate and rhythm at rest with various drugs (most often digitalis); group 4, ventricular rate and rhythm during moderate exercise without medication; group 5, ventricular rate and rhythm during moderate exercise with medication.

In each of these groups of rhythms the atrial and ventricular coefficients of variation (CV) were calculated as the ratio between the standard deviation (SD) and average cycle length (CL) of successive intervals. The outcome of the analyses is shown here and in Fig. 10.

CL, group mean of average ventricular cycle lengths; SD, group mean of standard deviations of ventricular cycle length; CV, group mean of coefficients of variation. All values are expressed ± standard deviation. For further details, see text.

These data indicate that a scaling process does not take place in the AV node. In Fig. 11 we give a schematic representation of a scaled (down) rhythm compared with the actual situation.

In patients with Wolff-Parkinson-White syndrome (WPW), atrial fibrillation, and transmission via the bypass, we found that the ratio between SD and average CL = CV is also constant (see solid diamonds in Fig. 10, not indicated in legend or Table 1). So the degree of irregularity of the ventricular rhythm in patients with atrial fibrillation seems an inherent property of the arrhythmia for which no other obvious explanation is currently available than that its source resides in the atria.

The preservation of relative variability of all atrial and ventricular rhythms in patients with atrial fibrillation proves that there is no scaling process operative in the AV node and therefore supports the notion that concealed conduction as traditionally conceived does not explain the slow(er) ventricular rhythm in those patients. Concealed conduction requires that an atrial impulse is selected for propagation because other blocked atrial impulses had gradually broken down the impediments for propagation. According to current thinking the conversion of a high atrial rate into a slower ventricular rate is being effected by concealed conduction. We conclude that atrial impulses are not selected by decremental conduction or otherwise to be conducted through the AV junction, but that the randomly irregular atrial electrical activity imparts, by whatever mechanism, to cells within the AV node a similar irregular behavior, albeit on a different time scale.

THE EFFECT OF DIGITALIS IN ATRIAL FIBRILLATION

Figure 1 demonstrates that digitalis has a dramatic effect on ventricular rate and histogram during atrial fibrillation, while the ventricular rhythm remains random. The mean ventricular rate decreases from 108 beats/min before digitalis, to 63 beats/min during treatment. The mean RR interval increases from 557 to 948 msec and, most important, the FRP of the AV node-His/Purkinje system as represented by the time between the Y axis and the beginning of the histogram increases from 350 msec (no digitalis) to 550 msec. The decrease in mean ventricular rate is caused not only

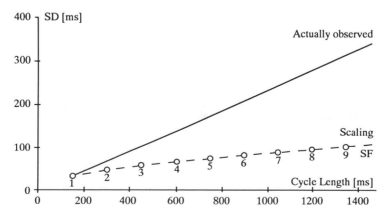

FIG. 11. Schematic representation of a scaled rhythm (hypothetical) versus the real-life situation.

by the increase in FRP, but also, and to a major extent, by an increase of RR intervals longer than 1,000 msec.

Finally, it is of interest to note that the SD of the mean becomes considerably larger at the lower heart rate during digitalis treatment. However, as mentioned above, the ratio between SD and the mean RR interval (the CV) remains constant: $126/557 = 0.23$ versus $233/948 = 0.24$—evidence that the AV node does not scale (26,80,88).

Although the effect of digitalis on ventricular rate can be blocked by atropine, as already shown by Mackenzie (8), this does not necessarily prove that digitalis acts through the vagal nerve, as at that time already asserted by Sir Thomas Lewis (91). The histograms (Fig. 1) show that digitalis increases the FRP of the AV junction and that it increases the number of long RR intervals due to its (direct or indirect) effect on the atrial myocardium. Whether or not digitalis also affects other electrophysiological properties of the AV junction cannot be stated with certainty. It may act both ways, but at the therapeutic level digitalis probably does not affect refractoriness or conduction in the His-Purkinje system (92).

ATRIAL FIBRILLATION IN THE WOLFF-PARKINSON-WHITE PATIENT

Although beyond the scope of this chapter, in the light of our gatekeeper theory a single remark may be devoted to atrial fibrillation in patients with WPW. These patients have an aberrant connection between atrial and ventricular myocardium without AV junctional electrophysiological properties, which short-circuits the protective function of the AV node. In the presence of atrial fibrillation a high ventricular rate or even ventricular fibrillation may be the result of this (93). A short refractory period and low apparent threshold will allow many more atrial impulses to reach the ventricles than in the absence of such a bypass short circuit (94).

The difference between the effect of atrial fibrillation on the ventricular rates in patients with WPW and without WPW must reside in the difference of electrophysiological properties between the Kent bundle(s) and the AV junction. The Kent bundles probably conduct most of the atrial impulses, while the AV node probably acts as an entrained pacemaker. Both systems (normal and aberrant) are confronted with the same atrial electrical activity, although in a different spatial setting. The AV node consists of cells with specific electrophysiological properties and is embedded in, and therefore electrotonically susceptible to, the surrounding atrial myocardium. The Kent bundle(s) directly connect(s) the atrial and ventricular myocardium and have basically the same electrophysiological properties as myocardium. The analysis of the ventricular rhythm in patients with WPW and atrial fibrillation deserves further attention.

THE ROLE OF THE ATRIOVENTRICULAR NODE DURING ATRIAL FIBRILLATION

We have seen that the classical theory of concealed conduction in the AV node during atrial fibrillation is challenged by:

1. the occurrence of a compensatory pause following properly timed ventricular extrasystoles and a shift of the postextrasystolic histogram to the right (79);

2. the occurrence of complete anterograde block during RV pacing at pacing intervals of approximately twice the length of the shortest spontaneous RR previous to RV pacing (78);
3. the constancy of the CV of the ventricular rhythm at different ventricular rates (80,88).

Several investigators have studied the behavior of the AV node during sinus rhythm as well as during atrial fibrillation with mathematical or electronic modeling (52). These studies showed that during sinus rhythm the electrophysiological properties of the AV node can be explained on the basis of an entrained biological oscillator. We may add to this that the AV node demonstrates its pacemaker properties during atrial arrest. Moreover, the AV node shows pacemaker activity during RV pacing and following ventricular extrasystoles. We therefore postulate that in atrial fibrillation the AV node behaves as a pacemaker electrotonically modulated or entrained by the fibrillating atrial myocardium.

This conclusion is supported by the comparison of AV nodal electrical behavior and SA nodal electrical behavior during atrial fibrillation. Functionally and morphologically there is a close resemblance between the mammalian SA and AV nodes (43,95). Kirchhof et al. (96) showed that during induced atrial fibrillation the intracellular recordings from the sinus node area point to local SA conduction block and dissociated electrical activity.

The same investigators (97) also found evidence that the pacemaker activity of the AV node is electrotonically depressed, thus modulated by surrounding fibrillating atrial myocardium. Outward conduction of impulses from the center of the SA node toward the atrium is practically impossible, mainly because the surrounding fibrillating atrial myocardium is continuously refractory. The AV node, however, albeit also surrounded by fibrillating atrial myocardium, has an outlet and is directly connected to the His bundle, so impulses originating in the AV node, their intervals modulated by the electrical activity of atrial myocardium, can reach the His-Purkinje system.

Assuming the AV node is a pacemaker electrotonically modulated or entrained by the surrounding fibrillating atrial myocardium, it should be realized that we do not know how this electrotonic modulation is affected. Jalife (98) demonstrated striking similarities between the characteristics of the sucrose gap model and those of an AV node. For instance, nonconducted impulses originating from a proximal segment can delay or advance the approach to threshold of a subsequent impulse (53). This may result in an irregular and chaotic-like response in rhythmically driven, nonoscillatory cardiac conducting tissue. Our observations agree well with the idea that the distal side of a weakly coupled junctional area may behave as the "rhythm determining element" without the need for a manifest pacemaker within the AV node. However, the pacemaker function of the AV node manifest during atrial arrest and possible entrainment by the atrial excitation during sinus rhythm seem to favor the pacemaker hypothesis over the sucrose gap theory.

From the available evidence we thus hypothesize that during atrial fibrillation, atrial impulses of sufficient strength and of random but proper timing cause an AV nodal pacemaker to fire in a random fashion (26,78). Local atrial impulses impart to cells within the AV node a random rhythm that ultimately reaches the ventricles. Threshold and refractory period of the His-Purkinje system, together with the random production in the AV node of impulses of sufficient strength to overcome the threshold, suffice to explain the ventricular rate and rhythm during atrial fibrillation.

THE GATEKEEPER REVISITED

When we now return to the gatekeeper metaphor, our hypothesis is that the gatekeeper allows only those atrial impulses to enter the gate that fulfill certain qualifications of form, strength, or direction. These impulses impart, by whatever means, an impulse-forming source behind the gate to send out new impulses through the His bundles to the ventricles. The AV node, like the SA node, is surrounded by fibrillating atrial myocardium; the atrial impulses do not arrive at the gate from somewhere else but are continuously created locally. In all probability during atrial fibrillation the AV node behaves in the same fashion as the SA node (95). The atrial impulses need certain qualities to affect the AV node and occur at random intervals. This assertion is supported by the observation that an overall high rate atrial electrical activity, e.g., caused by digitalis treatment, creates fewer suitable impulses and therefore a slower ventricular rhythm; a slow rate atrial electrical activity, e.g., caused by quinidine treatment, creates more suitable impulses and therefore a faster ventricular rhythm. The gatekeeper's behavior may change under the influence of autonomic nervous interference or drug action. However, these influences will affect the electrical activity of the atrial myocardium as well.

FINAL REMARKS

In the foreword of his book *The Emperor's New Mind* (99), Roger Penrose gives a classification of theories. Theories may be superb, useful, tentative, or misguided. Our theory on AV nodal function during atrial fibrillation does not go beyond tentative, and we certainly hope it will not misguide our readers. The current available evidence convinced us that the classical theory of concealed conduction in the AV node cannot stand the test of the real-life situation. But not only concealed conduction, the fairly simple and attractive model of electrotonic modulation of phase 4 of an AV nodal pacemaker equivalent does not explain all observations, e.g., the absence of scaling in atrial fibrillation, either. So we can only guess how an AV nodal pacemaker is electrotonically affected by the fibrillating atria.

Until now, our present theory that the AV node behaves as a pacemaker during atrial fibrillation has not been experimentally confirmed nor has it been disproved. Together with the multiple wavelet theory (18), it offers a credible explanation for all electrocardiographic phenomena related to or occurring during atrial fibrillation. It also offers a basis for the understanding of most drug action, autonomic nervous control in relation to ventricular rate and rhythm in atrial fibrillation. It reduces the small differences between the ventricular rates in dogs, humans, and horses during atrial fibrillation to the well-known limited difference in electrophysiological behavior of the respective AV junctions and the probable, similar behavior of the fibrillating atria. We have good reason to believe that our theory on AV nodal pacemaker function may also be valid in the absence of atrial fibrillation. As said before, the flaw in our theory is that as yet we cannot offer a credible mechanism of how the atrial electrical activity affects the function of the AV node. We are working on a model that we hope will fill in the holes in our theory. During sinus rhythm and other forms of organized atrial electrical activity, entrainment of an AV nodal pacemaker (51) can explain the mismatch between PR interval and heart size and the varying PR intervals under varying conditions.

CONCLUSION

During atrial fibrillation the AV node does not conduct, but behaves as a (nonprotected) electrotonically modulated or entrained pacemaker. Ventricular rate and rhythm are dictated by

1. the atrial electrical activity itself,
2. its effect on the AV nodal pacemaker,
3. the inherent properties of the AV nodal pacemaker,
4. the refractory period and threshold of the His-Purkinje system.

ACKNOWLEDGMENT

Supported by the Wijnand M. Pon Foundation, Leusden, The Netherlands.

REFERENCES

1. Kannel WB, Abbot RD, Savage DD, McNamara PM. Epidemiologic features of chronic atrial fibrillation. The Framingham Study. *N Engl J Med* 1982;302:1018–1022.
2. Selzer A. Atrial fibrillation revisited. *N Engl J Med* 1982;306:1044–1045.
3. Godtfredsen J. *Atrial fibrillation. Etiology, course and prognosis. A follow-up study of 1212 cases.* Thesis. University of Copenhagen, 1975.
4. Hering HE. Analyse des Pulsus irregularis perpetuus. *Prager Med Wochenschr* 1903;28:377–381.
5. Meijler FL. The pulse in atrial fibrillation. *Br Heart J* 1986;56:1–3.
6. Lewis, T. *The mechanism of the heart beat.* London: Shaw & Sons, 1911;194–215.
7. Lewis T. Irregularity of the heart's action in horses and its relationship to fibrillation of the auricles in experiment and to complete irregularity of the human heart. *Heart* 1911–1912;3:161–171.
8. Mackenzie J. *Diseases of the heart,* 3rd ed. London: Oxford, 1914;211–236.
9. Wenckebach KF, Winterberg H. *Die Unregelmässige Herztätigkeit.* Leipzig: Wilhelm Engelmann, 1927;441–467.
10. Brill IC. Auricular fibrillation: the present status with a review of the literature. *Ann Intern Med* 1937;10:1487–1502.
11. Einthoven W, Korteweg AJ. On the variability of the size of the pulse in cases of auricular fibrillation. *Heart* 1915;6:107–120.
12. Bohn FK, Patterson DF, Pyler RL. Atrial fibrillation in dogs. *Br Vet J* 1971;127:485–496.
13. Deem DA, Fregin GF. Atrial fibrillation in horses: a review of 106 clinical cases, with consideration of prevalence, clinical signs, and prognosis. *J Am Vet Med Assoc* 1982;180:261–265.
14. Braunstein JR, Franke EK. Autocorrelation of ventricular response in atrial fibrillation. *Circ Res* 1961;9:300–304.
15. Horan LG, Kistler JC. Study of ventricular response in atrial fibrillation. *Circ Res* 1961;9:305–311.
16. Hoopen M ten. Ventricular response in atrial fibrillation. A model based on retarded excitation. *Circ Res* 1966;19:911–918.
17. Moe GK, Abildskov JA. Atrial fibrillation as a self-sustaining arrhythmia independent of focal discharge. *Am Heart J* 1959;58:59–70.
18. Moe GK. On the multiple wavelet hypothesis of atrial fibrillation. *Arch Int Pharmacodyn* 1962;140:183–188.
19. Allessie MA, Lammers WJEP, Bonke FIM, Holten J. Experimental evaluation of Moe's multiple wavelet hypothesis of atrial fibrillation. In: Zipes DP, Jalife J, eds. *Cardiac electrophysiology and arrhythmias.* Orlando: Grune & Stratton, 1985;265–275.
20. Mazgalev T, Dreifus LS, Bianchi J, Michelson EL. Atrioventricular nodal conduction during atrial fibrillation in rabbit heart. *Am J Physiol* 1982;243:H754–H760.
21. Moore EN. Observations on concealed conduction in atrial fibrillation. *Circ Res* 1967;21:201–208.
22. Robles de Medina EO, Bernard R, Coumel P, et al. WHO-ISFC Task Force. Definition of terms related to cardiac rhythm. *Am Heart J* 1978;95:796–806.
23. Giraud GI, Latour H, Puech P. La fibrillation auriculaire. Analyse électrocardiographique endocavitaire. *Arch Mal Coeur* 1956;49:419–440.

24. Puech P, Grolleau R, Rebuffat G. Intra-atrial mapping of atrial fibrillation in man. In: Kulbertus HE, Olsson SB, Schlepper M, eds. *Atrial fibrillation.* Mölndal: Astra Cardiovasc, 1982;94–108.
25. Meijler FL, Van der Tweel I, Herbschleb JN, Hauer RNW, Robles de Medina EO. Role of atrial fibrillation and AV conduction (including Wolff-Parkinson-White syndrome) in sudden death. *J Am Coll Cardiol* 1985;5:B17–B22.
26. Bootsma BK, Hoelen AJ, Strackee J, Meijler FL. Analysis of the R-R intervals in patients with atrial fibrillation at rest and during exercise. *Circulation* 1970;41:783–794.
27. Billette J, Roberge FA, Nadeau RA. Roles of the AV junction in determining the ventricular response to atrial fibrillation. *Can J Physiol Pharmacol* 1975;53:575–585.
28. Meijler FL, Van der Tweel I, Herbschleb JN, Heethaar RM, Borst C. Lessons from comparative studies of atrial fibrillation in dog, man and horse. In: Zipes DP, Jalife J, eds. *Cardiac arrhythmias.* New York: Grune & Stratton 1985;489–493.
29. Meijler FL, Strackee J. Dr. Gordon Moe and the analysis of sustained irregularity of the pulse. *J Cardiovasc Electrophysiol* 1990;1:349–353.
30. Langendorf R. Concealed A-V conduction: the effect of blocked impulses on the formation and conduction of subsequent impulses. *Am Heart J* 1948;35:542–552.
31. Fisch C. *Electrocardiography of arrhythmias.* Philadelphia: Lea & Febiger, 1990;1.
32. Hoffman PF, Paes de Calvalho A, De Mello WC, Cranefield PF. Electrical activity of single fibers of the atrioventricular node. *Circ Res* 1959;7:11–18.
33. Hoffman BF, Cranefield PF. *Electrophysiology of the heart.* New York: McGraw-Hill, 1960;156–162.
34. Langendorf R, Pick A, Katz LN. Ventricular response in atrial fibrillation: role of concealed conduction in the A-V junction. *Circulation* 1965;32:69–75.
35. Meijler FL, Janse MJ. Morphology and electrophysiology of the mammalian atrioventricular node. *Physiol Rev* 1988;68:608–647.
36. Dreifus LS, Mazgalev T. "Atrial paralysis." Does it explain the irregular ventricular rate during fibrillation? *J Am Coll Cardiol* 1988;11:546–547.
37. Meijler FL. An "account" of digitalis and atrial fibrillation. *J Am Coll Cardiol* 1985;5:A60–A68.
38. Goldman MJ. Quinidine treatment of auricular fibrillation. *Am J Med Sci* 1951;186:382–391.
39. Gibson D, Sowton E. The use of beta-adrenergic receptor blocking drugs in dysrhythmias. *Prog Cardiovasc Sci* 1969;12:16–39.
40. Schamroth L. The philosophy of calcium-ion antagonists. In: Zanchetti A, Krikler DM, eds. *Calcium antagonism in cardiovascular therapy.* Amsterdam: Excerpta Medica, 1985;5–10.
41. Grant RP. The mechanism of A-V arrhythmias with an electrotonic analogue of the human A-V node. *Am J Med* 1956;20:334–344.
42. Katholi CR, Urthaler F, Macy J, James TN. A mathematical model of automaticity in the sinus node and AV junction based on weakly coupled relaxation oscillators. *Comp Biomed Res* 1977;10:529–543.
43. Lewis T. *The mechanism and graphic registration of the heart beat.* London: Shaw & Sons, 1925;377.
44. Van der Pol B, Van der Mark J. The heartbeat considered as a relaxation oscillation, and an electrical model of the heart. *Philos Mag* 1928;6:763–775, *Arch Neerl Physiol* 1929;14:418–443.
45. Van der Tweel LH, Meijler FL, Van Capelle FJL. Synchronisation of the heart. *J Appl Physiol* 1973;34:283–287.
46. Van der Tweel I, Herbschleb JN, Borst C, Meijler FL. Deterministic model of the canine atrioventricular node as a periodically perturbed, biological oscillator. *J Appl Cardiol* 1986;1:157–173.
47. Brugada P, Wellens HJJ. Entrainment as an electrophysiologic phenomenon. *J Am Coll Cardiol* 1984;3:451–454.
48. Segers M, Lequime J, Denolin H. Synchronization of auricular and ventricular beats during complete heart block. *Am Heart J* 1947;33:685–691.
49. Jalife J, Michaels DC. Phase-dependent interactions of cardiac pacemakers on mechanisms of control and synchronization in the heart. In: Zipes DP, Jalife J, eds. *Cardiac electrophysiology and cardiac arrhythmias.* New York: Grune & Stratton, 1985;109–119.
50. Winfree AT. *When time breaks down. The three dimensional dynamics of electrochemical waves and cardiac arrhythmias.* Princeton, NJ: Princeton Univerity Press, 1987;292.
51. Meijler FL, Fisch C. Does the atrioventricular node conduct? *Br Heart J* 1989;61:309–315.
52. Cohen RJ, Berger RD, Dushane ThE. A quantitative model for the ventricular response during atrial fibrillation. *IEEE Trans Biomed Eng* 1983;30:769–780.
53. Antzelevitch C, Moe GK. Electrotonic inhibition and summation of impulse conduction in mammalian Purkinje fibers. *Am J Physiol* 1983;245:H42–H53.
54. Waller AD. Cardiology and cardiopathology. *Br Med J* 1913;2:375–376.
55. Clark AJ. Conduction in the heart of mammals. In: *Comparative physiology of the heart.* Cambridge, England: Cambridge University Press, 1927;49–51.

56. Meijler FL. Atrioventricular conduction versus heart size from mouse to whale. *J Am Coll Cardiol* 1985;5:363–365.

57. Sommer JR, Johnson EA. Ultrastructure of cardiac muscle. In: Berne RM, Sperelakis N, Geiger SR, eds. *Handbook of physiology. The cardiovascular system. I. The heart.* Bethesda, MD: American Physiological Society, 1979;113–186.

58. James TN. Structure and function of the AV junction. *Jpn Circ J* 1983;47:1–47.

59. Jack JJB, Noble D, Tsien RW. *Electric current flow in excitable cells.* Oxford: Clarendon Press, 1975;292–296.

60. De Mello WC. Passive electrical properties of the atrioventricular node. *Pflugers Arch* 1977;371:135–139.

61. Durrer D, Janse MJ, Lie KI, Van Capelle FJL. Human cardiac electrophysiology. In: Dickinson CJ, Marks J, eds. *Developments in cardiovascular medicine.* Lancaster: MTP Press, 1978;53–75.

62. Pressler ML. Membrane properties of the cardiac conduction system: comparative aspects. *Proc R Neth Acad Sci* 1990;93:477–487.

63. King RL, Jenks JL, White PD. The electrocardiogram of a Beluga whale. *Circulation* 1953;8:397–393.

64. White PD, King RL, Jenks J. The relation of heart size to the time intervals of the heart beat with particular reference to the elephant and the whale. *N Engl J Med* 1953;248:69–70.

65. Kawamura K. Size of the atrio-ventricular node in mammals. *Proc R Neth Acad Sci* 1990;93:431–435.

66. Meijler FL. The mismatch between size and function of the heart. *Proc R Neth Acad Sci* 1990;93:463–467.

67. Meijler FL. An off beat whale hunt. *Br Med J* 1989;299:1563–1565.

68. Weinberg SL. A whale of an electrocardiogram. *Dayton Med* 1990;46:116–118.

69. Buchanan JW. Spontaneous arrhythmias and conduction disturbances in domestic animals. *Ann NY Acad Sci* 1965;127:224–238.

70. Meijler FL, Heethaar RM, Harms FMA, et al. Comparative atrioventricular conduction and its consequences for atrial fibrillation in man. In: Kulbertus HE, Olsson SB, Schlepper M, eds. *Atrial fibrillation.* Mölndal: Astra Cardiovasc, 1982;72–80.

71. Meijler FL, Kroneman J, Van der Tweel I, Herbschleb JN, Heethaar RM, Borst C. Nonrandom ventricular rhythm in horses with atrial fibrillation and its significance for patients. *J Am Coll Cardiol* 1984;4:316–323.

72. Wellens HJJ. Wolff-Parkinson-White syndrome. Part I. Diagnosis: arrhythmias and identification of the high risk patient. *Mod Concepts Cardiovasc Dis* 1983;52:53–56.

73. Dreifus LS, Haiat R, Watanabe Y, Arriage J, Reitman N. Ventricular fibrillation. A possible mechanism of sudden death in patients with Wolff-Parkinson-White syndrome. *Circulation* 1971;43:520–527.

74. Boineau JP, Moore EN. Evidence for propagation of activation across an accessory atrioventricular connection in types A and B pre-excitation. *Circulation* 1970;41:375–397.

75. Wellens HJJ, Durrer D. Wolff-Parkinson-White syndrome and atrial fibrillation. Relation between refractory period of acccessory pathway and ventricular rate during atrial fibrillation. *Am J Cardiol* 1974;34:777–782.

76. Deleted at proofs.

77. James TN. Automaticity in the atrioventricular junction. In: Rosen MR, Janse MJ, Wit AL, eds. *Cardiac electrophysiology: a textbook.* Mount Kisco, NY: Futura, 1990.

78. Wittkampf FHM, De Jongste MJL, Lie KI, Meijler FL. Effect of right ventricular pacing on ventricular rhythm during atrial fibrillation. *J Am Coll Cardiol* 1988;11:539–545.

79. Wittkampf FHM, De Jongste MJL, Meijler FL. Atrioventricular nodal response to retrograde activation in atrial fibrillation. *J Cardiovasc Electrophysiol* 1990;1:437–447.

80. Wittkampf FHM, Robles de Medina EO, Strackee J, Meijler FL. Scaling in atrial fibrillation? In: Wittkampf FHM, ed. *Atrioventricular nodal transmission in atrial fibrillation.* Thesis, State University Utrecht, The Netherlands, 1991;89–104.

81. Langendorf R, Pick A. Artificial pacing of the human heart: its contribution to the understanding of the arrhythmias. *Am J Cardiol* 1971;26:516–525.

82. Pritchett LC, Smith WM, Klein SJ, Hammill SC, Gallagher JJ. The "compensatory pause" of atrial fibrillation. *Circulation* 1980;62:1021–1025.

83. Scherf D, Schott A. *Extrasystoles and allied arrhythmias,* 2nd ed. Chicago: William Heinemann, 1973;76–78.

84. Moore EN, Spear JF. Experimental studies on the facilitation of AV conduction by ectopic beats in dogs and rabbits. *Circ Res* 1971;29:29–39.

85. Lehmann MH, Mahmud R, Denker S, Soni J, Akhtar M. Retrograde concealed conduction in the atrioventricular node: differential manifestations related to level of intranodal penetration. *Circulation* 1984;70:392–401.

86. Wittkampf FHM, De Jongste MJL, Meijler FL. Competitive anterograde and retrograde atrio-

ventricular junctional activation in atrial fibrillation. *J Cardiovasc Electrophysiol* 1990;1:448–456.

87. Fisch C. *Electrocardiography of arrhythmias*. Philadelphia: Lea & Febiger, 1990;427–428.
88. Kirsch JA, Sahakian AV, Baerman JM, Swiryn S. Ventricular response to atrial fibrillation: role of atrioventricular conduction pathways. *J Am Coll Cardiol* 1988;12:1265–1272.
89. Schmidt-Nielsen K. *Scaling. Why is animal size so important?* Cambridge, England: Cambridge University Press, 1984;126–130.
90. Armitage P, Berry G. *Statistical methods in medical research,* 2nd ed. Oxford: Blackwell, 1987;90.
91. McMichael J. Sir James Mackenzie and atrial fibrillation—a new perspective. *J R Coll Gen Pract* 1981;31:402–406.
92. Hoffman BF, Singer DH. Effects of digitalis on electrical activity of cardiac fibers. *Prog Cardiovasc Dis* 1964;7:226–260.
93. Wellens HJJ, Bär FW, Ross D, Vanagt EJ. Sudden death in the Wolff-Parkinson-White syndrome. In: Kulbertus HE, Wellens HJJ, eds. *Sudden death.* The Hague: Martinus Nijhoff, 1980;392–399.
94. Wellens HJJ, Durrer D. Effect of digitalis on atrioventricular conduction and circus-movement tachycardias in patients with Wolff-Parkinson-White syndrome. *Circulation* 1973;47:1229–1233.
95. James TN. Anatomy of the sinus node. AV node and os cordis of the beef heart. *Anat Rec* 1965;153:361–372.
96. Kirchhof CJHJ, Allessie MA, Bonke FIM. The sinus node and atrial fibrillation. *Ann NY Acad Sci* 1990;591:166–177.
97. Kirchhof CJHJ, Bonke FIM, Allessie MA. Evidence for the presence of electrotonic depression of pacemakers in the rabbit atrioventricular node. The effects of uncoupling from the surrounding myocardium. *Basic Res Cardiol* 1988;83:190–201.
98. Jalife J. The sucrose gap preparation as a model of AV nodal transmission: are dual pathways necessary for reciprocation and AV nodal "echoes"? *PACE* 1983;6:1106–1122.
99. Penrose R. *The emperor's new mind*. New York/Oxford: Oxford University Press, 1989.
100. Meijler FL, Van der Tweel I. Comparative study of atrial fibrillation and AV conduction in mammals. *Heart Vessels* 1987;(suppl 2):24–31.

Atrial Fibrillation: Mechanisms and Management, edited by
R. H. Falk and P. J. Podrid.
Raven Press, Ltd., New York © 1992.

5

Epidemiology of Atrial Fibrillation

*William B. Kannel and †Philip A. Wolf

*Department of Medicine, University Hospital, *†Section of Preventive Medicine and
Epidemiology, Evans Memorial Department of Clinical Research, †Department of
Neurology, Boston University School of Medicine, Boston, Massachusetts 02118*

Atrial fibrillation (AF) is now recognized as the most common cardiac disorder leading to systemic emboli. In the past, chronic AF without valvular heart disease was considered relatively innocuous, but more recent evidence indicates that it is associated with a high risk of thromboembolic events, particularly stroke. Because, once established, AF is difficult to revert to sinus rhythm; prevention of its occurrence and anticoagulation are needed to cope with the problem.

This chapter deals with the factors predisposing to AF and its prognostic outlook. It is based on epidemiologic data derived chiefly from the Framingham study. This study has routinely obtained ECGs on the entire cohort at 2-year intervals over the past 40 years allowing a complete and unbiased detection of all chronic AF that has evolved. In addition transient AF has been detected from hospital records on subjects admitted to the only hospital in town. Cardiovascular risk factors and cardiovascular status have also been routinely assessed biennially and thus examined in relation to subsequent development of AF. In this way it is possible to provide undistorted insights into the prevalence, incidence, precursors, and prognosis of AF in the general population.

INCIDENCE AND PREVALENCE

Next to premature atrial and ventricular systoles, AF is alleged to be the most frequently occurring cardiac rhythm disturbance. It is much more common than the other atrial tachyarrhythmias. The prevalence of AF is reported to be 2 to 3 per 1,000 at age 25 to 35 years, 30 to 40 per 1,000 at age 55 to 64 years, and 50 to 90 per 1,000 at age 62 to 90 years. It is estimated that about 1 to 1.5 million Americans may have chronic nonvalvular AF (1).

The Framingham study provides more representative data on the occurrence of AF in the general population because it is largely free of selection bias. In that study, the occurrence, precursors, and prognosis of AF have been examined in a 22- to 30-year follow-up of a cohort of 5,209 men and women aged 30 to 62 years at entry (2–7). After 30 years, 376 of the participants had developed AF. The incidence of AF was observed to increase progressively with age with a modest male predominance (Fig. 1). Overall, in this adult cohort the chance of developing AF over two decades was 2%. Although not well documented, AF is believed to begin with brief, unde-

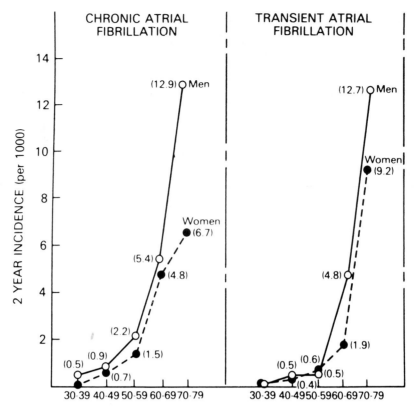

FIG. 1. Two-year incidence of chronic and transient atrial fibrillation by age and sex from the Framingham study. (From ref. 4, with permission.)

tected transient bouts that evolve into more persistent and refractory episodes, eventually becoming a persistent rhythm disturbance. Once achieving this chronic stage, it seldom spontaneously reverts to sinus rhythm.

ECG CHARACTERISTICS

AF is characterized by a rapid, totally irregular beating of the atria provoking an irregular response of the ventricles. The atrial rate varies between 350 and 550 beats per minute with a ventricular response ranging between 60 and 160 beats per minute. Definite P-waves are replaced by continuous undulating waves of varying amplitude, contour, and spacing (f-waves). Sometimes these are barely perceptible. AF may be transient and may even appear and disappear within minutes on a single ECG examination. This often evolves into a chronic persistent AF that no longer spontaneously reverts to normal. It often alternates with atrial flutter.

The ECG precursors are not well understood. Transient AF and atrial flutter are likely antecedents of chronic AF. Unproven precursors include left ventricular hypertrophy, intra-atrial conduction delay, atrial premature beats, and atrial tachycardia. In the Framingham study ECG criteria for left ventricular hypertrophy (LVH) carry a two- to threefold risk of developing AF and nonspecific repolarization abnormalities a 1.7-fold risk (Table 1).

TABLE 1. *Cardiovascular risk factors in cases with atrial fibrillation (AF) compared to matched controls in the Framingham study*

Risk factor	Men (%)			Women (%)		
	Cases	Controls	Risk ratio	Cases	Controls	Risk ratio
Smoking	55.1	61.6	0.8	38.8	30.2	1.5
Hypertension	59.2	44.5	1.9	61.2	49.4	1.8
Diabetes	10.2	4.5	2.3	10.2[a]	3.7	3.0
LVH	30.6[a]	12.2	3.0	28.6[a]	14.7	2.4
Nonspecific abnormality on ECG	36.7	27.8	1.6	38.8	28.2	1.8

[a]$p<0.05$ compared to control valve.

For men only, the presence of left ventricular hypertrophy (LVH) on a 12-lead ECG was statistically associated with development of AF. For women, both LVH and diabetes were associated.

ETIOLOGY

AF is usually a consequence of established heart disease. In the past it was most commonly a consequence of rheumatic heart disease with mitral stenosis. Today AF usually occurs without valvular disease in persons with hypertension and coronary heart disease, particularly in the setting of cardiac failure. AF also occurs in association with mitral valve calcification and prolapse, hypertensive cardiovascular disease with LVH, an enlarged left atrium, cardiomyopathy, and, acutely, following myocardial infarction and cardiac surgery.

AF may also result from such extracardiac conditions as hyperthyroidism, acute alcohol intoxication, cholinergic drug use, surgery, or diagnostic procedures. Occasionally, no contributing factors can be identified, a condition characterized as "lone AF."

Cardiovascular disease increases the risk of AF three- to fivefold (Table 2). However, the attributable risk is greater in those without primary cardiovascular disease

TABLE 2. *Risk of development of atrial fibrillation (AF) by cardiovascular (CV) disease status in 2,326 men and 2,866 women after 24 years of follow-up in the Framingham study*[a]

Predisposing cardiovascular disease	Chronic AF		Transient AF	
	Men	Women	Men	Women
Coronary heart disease	2.2[b]	0.5[c]	2.1[b]	4.5[b]
Hypertension CV disease	4.7[b]	4.0[b]	4.4[b]	4.6[b]
Cardiac failure	8.5[b]	13.7[b]	8.2[b]	20.4[b]
Rheumatic heart disease	9.9[b]	27.5[b]	7.6[b]	24.3[b]
Any cardiovascular disease	3.2[b]	4.8[b]	4.4[b]	5.4[b]

[a]Two-year age-adjusted risk ratio.

[b]$p<0.05$.

[c]Not significant.

All patients with coronary heart disease, defined as prior infarction and/or angina, are included regardless of coexistence of other risk factors such as hypertension. Hypertensive cardiovascular disease is defined as hypertension with either evidence of left ventricular hypertrophy by ECG, cardiomegaly on x-ray, or cardiac failure.

See ref. 4.

TABLE 3. *Attributable risk for developing atrial fibrillation in populations with various cardiovascular diseases during 24 years of follow-up in the Framingham study—26-year follow-up*

CV disease	Percentage of attributable risk	
	Men	Women
Stroke	3	—
CHD	8	3
CHF	5	8
HCVD	13	15
RHD	8	28
Any CV disease	25	31
Other conditions[a]	75	69

[a]Includes lone AF, diabetes, and ECG abnormalities without overt CV disease hypertension.
Attributable risk is a function of the prevalence of a precursor and the strength of the association between the precursor and AF.
AF, atrial fibrillation; CHF, congestive heart failure; CV, cardiovascular; HCVD, hypertensive cardiovascular disease; RHD, rheumatic heart disease. Definitions as in Table 2.

due to the higher prevalence of these predisposing conditions. Thus, in aggregate, hypertension, diabetes, LVH, and nonspecific repolarization are responsible for 70% to 75% of AF in the general population (Table 3). Among those with cardiovascular disease, most AF in women is attributable to hypertensive cardiovascular disease (15%) and rheumatic heart disease (28%). In men, hypertensive cardiovascular disease accounts for 13% and rheumatic heart disease 8%. Mitral annular calcification is associated with a twofold increased prevalence of AF (8–12).

PREDISPOSING FACTORS

The incidence of AF increases when cardiovascular disease occurs. Coronary heart disease, which is responsible for 8% of the AF in men, doubles the risk of developing chronic AF (Table 4), but no increased risk was demonstrated in women. Rheumatic heart disease escalates the AF occurrence in both sexes: eightfold in men and 27-fold in women. Hypertensive cardiovascular disease, responsible for about 14% of AF, increases AF risk about fourfold. Among the cardiac conditions, congestive heart failure rivals rheumatic heart disease, imposing a substantial AF risk, particularly in women.

TABLE 4. *Risk of atrial fibrillation by clinical manifestation of coronary heart disease*

	Chronic AF age-adjusted risk ratio		Transient AF age-adjusted risk ratio	
	Men	Women	Men	Women
Coronary attacks	1.8	2.1	3.5[a]	8.7[a]
Angina pectoris	2.1[a]	0.3	2.1	1.8[a]
Any coronary heart disease	2.2[a]	0.5	2.1[a]	4.5[a]

[a]$P<0.05$.
Coronary attack = myocardial infarction. Angina pectoris excludes patients with prior infarction.

Among the other predisposing factors, diabetes and ECG-LVH were associated with the highest (two- to threefold) risk ratios (Table 1). Cigarette smoking was not a risk factor for AF in men. In women, there was a 50% excess risk observed (not statistically significant). Hypertension appears to almost double the risk in both sexes.

Coronary Disease

AF is a fairly common rhythm disturbance in coronary heart disease. It may occur in 20% of acute myocardial infarctions, usually transient, during the first 3 days in the coronary care unit (13–18). Some have postulated pericarditis as the mechanism, causing irritation of the sinoatrial (SA) node and atrium, but the evidence is inconsistent and unconvincing (13,16,19,20,24). Increased right atrial pressure associated with more extensive myocardial infarction seems the more likely mechanism. Also, transient ischemia of the atrial myocardium cannot be excluded. The prognostic significance of AF during an acute myocardial infarction remains controversial, some studies finding it dangerous (13–16), some not (17–21). The long-term survival of hospitalized myocardial infarctions with AF is likewise uncertain (16,22,23). Coronary heart disease doubled the risk of developing AF in men in the Framingham study. It was more strongly related to development of transient AF in women (Table 4). In men angina was as strong a cause of AF as a coronary attack. In women, angina was a weak risk factor for AF, and when it did occur, it was apt to be transient (Table 4). Coronary heart disease appears to promote AF even excluding coexistent hypertensive cardiovascular disease and cardiac failure.

Valvular Atrial Fibrillation

In the past rheumatic heart disease was the major cause of AF, which often caused systemic emboli. As the incidence of rheumatic heart disease declined, so did the prevalence of AF attributable to rheumatic heart disease. However, valvular heart disease continues to be a common cause of AF and systemic embolism. Mitral valve disease, whether manifested as mitral stenosis or mitral insufficiency, is particularly likely to produce AF. Only when AF is present is there a significant increased risk, on the order of three- to fourfold, of systemic embolism associated with deformed mitral valves. Persons with other forms of valvular heart disease also have some increased risk of AF.

Mitral annular calcification has been implicated as a valvular abnormality associated with AF and with an increased incidence of stroke. Aronow et al. (9) reported that left atrial enlargement was 2.4 times more prevalent and AF 1.9 times more prevalent in patients with mitral annular calcification than in those without this condition (9). Others have also found a higher prevalence of AF in patients with mitral annular calcification (9–11,24).

PROGNOSIS

Chronic AF in the presence of rheumatic valvular disease clearly increases stroke risk; in the absence of valvular disease, chronic AF is definitely not innocuous (Fig. 2). Recent evidence indicates that it is a dangerous hallmark for disease outcome

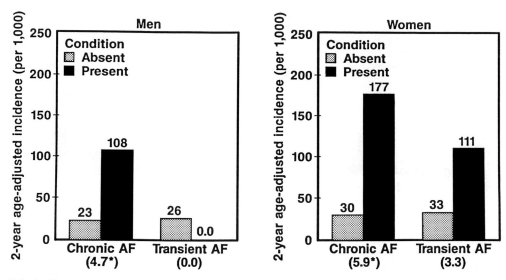

FIG. 2. Two-year age-adjusted incidence of stroke in a population with coronary heart disease, with (condition present) and without (condition absent) atrial fibrillation. Although atrial fibrillation was a risk marker for stroke in this population, all stroke patients also had predisposing or coexisting hypertensive or rheumatic heart disease or congestive heart failure. (Modified from ref. 4.)

and death, and AF has been found to be associated with a doubled cardiovascular mortality and death due to all causes (Table 5).

AF has been identified as the rhythm disturbance responsible for more than 85% of systemic thromboembolism from the heart (25). Furthermore, the brain was the target in more than two-thirds of all clinical embolic events in several postmortem series of fibrillators (26,27). Since AF often develops in the presence of cardiac impairments such as coronary heart disease, cardiac failure, and hypertension, it is argued that the strokes that occur are thrombotic and these cardiac contributors are

TABLE 5. *Mortality among 49 men and 49 women who developed atrial fibrillation (AF)
during a 22-year follow-up period in the Framingham study*

Mortality	Men, % (N)			Women, % (N)		
	Cases	Controls	Risk ratio	Cases	Controls	Risk ratio
Total deaths	59.2[a] (29)	34.3 (84)	1.7	44.9[a] (22)	25.3 (62)	1.8
Deaths from cardiovascular causes	42.9[a] (21)	21.2 (52)	2.0	40.8[a] (20)	15.1 (37)	2.7
Average time to death (years)	5.9[a]	7.7	—	6.6	6.7	—

[a]Significant difference between values for cases and those for controls among all subjects 38 to 78 years old at death ($P < 0.05$).
    Five control subjects, free of atrial fibrillation (AF), were matched with each AF subject and constitute the control group.
    Modified from ref. 2.

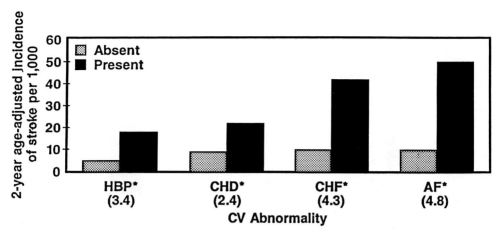

FIG. 3. The Framingham study: 34-year follow-up. Incidence of stroke in men and women, age 50–89, by cardiovascular abnormality. Atrial fibrillation (AF) was responsible for 14.7% of all strokes and was associated with a 4.8 fold increased risk of stroke. HBP, high blood pressure; CHD, coronary heart disease; CHF, congestive heart failure. *, significant excess of stroke, $p < 0.001$. (Modified from ref. 4.)

largely responsible for their occurrence (28). To address this question, the mechanism of stroke was determined in a recent comprehensive clinical study of 154 consecutive anterior circulation stroke patients with AF. They were evaluated for alternative causes of stroke, other than AF, by means of carotid angiography or noninvasive carotid testing and exclusion of lacunar infarction by computed tomographic (CT) scan (29). In 76% of these cases, no alternate stroke mechanism, other than cerebral embolus from AF, was found.

The Framingham data also indicate that AF exerts a significant impact on risk of stroke (Fig. 3). This effect is independent of the often associated cardiovascular abnormalities (3). Furthermore, while the other cardiovascular contributors have a decreasing influence with advancing age, the impact of AF increases into the ninth decade of life (3). In another prospective study, this one in Denmark, AF was also found to be an independent risk factor for stroke (30). Recent reports of a significant reduction in the incidence of stroke in randomized clinical trials by warfarin anticoagulation (31–33) and by aspirin (32) suggest these drugs may be safely used and are indicated in persons with AF.

SEVERITY OF STROKE IN ATRIAL FIBRILLATION

The embolus that causes cerebral infarction when the source is the heart, particularly in persons with AF, is of a relatively large size and often results in occlusion of a major cerebral artery (34). Withholding treatment until symptoms of cerebral ischemia develop is clearly not adequate since the initial stroke usually occurs without warning or a transient ischemic attack and often results in significant disability or death. The ensuing infarct is often large and results in a severe or fatal stroke. In one series of hospitalized patients with stroke associated with AF, 71% died or had a severe permanent neurologic deficit from the initial embolic stroke (35). Epidemiologic investigations have provided a more precise estimate of the importance of this

TABLE 6. *Stroke incidence associated with AF (men and women combined): Framingham study—30-year follow-up*

Age	Stroke rate per 1,000		Percentage of strokes with AF
	Without AF	With AF	
30–49	0.8	0.0	0.0
50–59	4.1	55.0	6.7
60–69	9.0	42.5	8.1
70–79	18.0	97.5	20.3
80–89	28.7	142.9	36.2
Total	6.2	76.0	14.7

AF, atrial fibrillation.

arrhythmia as a precursor of stroke (5,36). The age-specific relative risk of stroke in the presence of AF is rather uniform from age 50 to 89. However, since the prevalence of AF is so much greater in the elderly, this fivefold increase in risk makes nonvalvular AF the most powerful precursor of strokes in the elderly; the proportion of strokes associated with AF increases from about 7% at ages 50 to 59 years to 36% at ages 80 to 89 years (Table 6). Even AF in the absence of cardiac disease ("lone AF") increases the stroke risk fourfold (7). In the recent clinical trial, the Boston Area Anticoagulation Trial in Atrial Fibrillation (BAATAF), more than half of the patients enrolled did not have underlying heart disease (33). Preliminary analysis did not disclose any lower risk of stroke in these subjects with "lone AF." Furthermore, stroke prevention with low-dose warfarin was no less effective in them.

Following a stroke, AF increases the risk of recurrence more than twofold; a third of these new strokes occur within 6 months after the first event (6) (Fig. 4). In AF

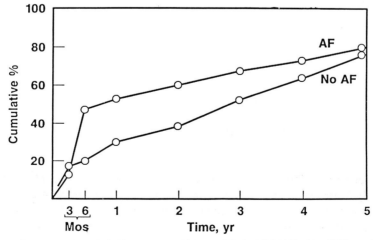

FIG. 4. Time of recurrence of stroke in 15 subjects with atrial fibrillation (AF) and 84 patients without atrial fibrillation (No AF) who had a first stroke during a 30-year follow-up period in the Framingham heart study. During this period a total of 501 strokes occurred in 5,184 patients. In the AF group, 47% of stroke recurrences occurred in the first 6 months. (Data from ref. 6.)

the risk of peripheral embolism is also increased, occurring at about a rate of 2% per year, compared to a 4% to 6% per year rate for stroke. In addition to clinically evident strokes, AF has been found to be associated with asymptomatic or "silent" strokes. As many as 35% to 37% of patients with nonrheumatic AF without a history of a stroke have been found to have cerebral infarcts on CT scan. This amounts to approximately a threefold increased rate of silent strokes seen on acute CT scan at the time of initial stroke. AF is clearly a major threat to the brain.

PREVENTIVE IMPLICATIONS

AF is a common condition in advanced age that warrants serious concern. Contrary to past clinical impressions, chronic AF is associated with a worse prognosis than transient AF. However, neither can be safely ignored. Also, although AF in association with cardiac disease, particularly with rheumatic mitral stenosis, is more dangerous, "lone AF" cannot be prudently overlooked. Strokes and recurrences of stroke are the most devastating consequence of the arrhythmia, which often occur soon after the onset of chronic AF.

Control of hypertension and diabetes and their cardiovascular sequelae of hypertensive cardiovascular disease, coronary disease, and cardiac failure are required in order to reduce AF incidence. Prevention of myocardial damage and atrial dilatation in persons with cardiac disease are required if AF is to be avoided.

Data from recently completed randomized clinical trials in AF provide strong evidence that warfarin, and perhaps aspirin, prevents stroke in patients with nonrheumatic AF (31–33). Although risk of stroke is increased in persons with AF, stroke does not occur in everyone with this arrhythmia, and some are undoubtedly more susceptible than others. One of the secondary goals of the clinical trials was to define a high-risk subgroup on the basis of demographic, clinical, or echocardiographic characteristics. Of the variables evaluated in the BAATAF study, mitral valve calcification was the sole characteristic that was significantly more prevalent in AF subjects who developed stroke.

Secondary Prevention of Stroke in Atrial Fibrillation

Stroke in persons with AF is particularly likely to recur; the recurrence rate in the first year after the initial stroke varies between 13% and 32% (37). Furthermore, recurrence is particularly high in the week following the initial event and has been estimated to be approximately 1% per day for the first 10 days. The need for prevention of recurrent embolic stroke by immediately instituting heparin anticoagulation is widely accepted. This urgency must be tempered by the approximately 4% to 8% risk of spontaneous hemorrhagic transformation of the infarct. Recent cooperative multicenter accumulation of cases of stroke resulting from cardiogenic embolism have greatly improved our understanding of the natural history of embolic infarction (38). Spontaneous hemorrhagic transformation of embolic stroke varies in degree from microscopic diapedesis of red blood cells through damaged capillary walls to accumulations of more than 30 cm^3 of gross hematoma with mass effect. The gross hemorrhagic transformation seemed to be more likely in large infarcts. However, if heparin anticoagulants are administered at the time of hemorrhagic transformation, the resulting hematoma may indeed be lethal. As a result, it has been suggested that if no evidence of hemorrhage is seen on CT performed 24 to 48 hr after stroke, heparin anticoagulation should be instituted. Chronic warfarin is then indicated since risk of recurrence persists at a level rate for at least 3 to 5 years (6,39).

SUMMARY

The occurrence, precursors, and prognosis of AF is examined in the Framingham cohort based on 22 to 30 years of follow-up of 5,209 men and women aged 30 to 62 years on entry. After 30 years 376 men and women developed chronic or transient AF, the incidence increasing progressively with age with no significant difference in the sexes. Overall, there was a 2% chance of developing AF over two decades in the adult cohort.

Although the *relative* risk of developing AF was greatest in those with overt, clinically manifest cardiac disease (four- to fivefold), the *attributable* risk was greatest for those without overt cardiovascular disease owing to the higher prevalence of predisposing conditions such as hypertension, diabetes, LVH, and nonspecific ECG repolarization abnormalities. Some 70% of AF evolving in the general population arose from these conditions prior to onset of overt cardiac disease. Among these, diabetes and ECG-LVH were associated with the highest risk ratios (two- to threefold). Among the cardiac conditions predisposing cardiac failure and rheumatic heart disease imposed the greatest AF risk, particularly in women. Coronary heart disease doubled the risk of AF in men and quadrupled the risk in women, but only 3% to 8% of AF in women and men, respectively, was attributable to overt coronary heart disease. Hypertensive cardiovascular disease was responsible for 13% to 15%.

In the past chronic AF without valvular disease was considered relatively innocuous. Recent evidence indicates that it doubles both cardiovascular and all cause mortality. AF is the most powerful stroke precursor in the elderly, increasing risk fivefold even when not accompanied by rheumatic heart disease. The proportion of strokes associated with AF increases from 6.7% at ages 50 to 59 years to 36.2% at ages 80 to 89 years. Even "lone AF," which tended to occur in association with ventricular conduction disturbances and repolarization ECG abnormalities, increased risk of stroke fourfold. Stroke recurrences are more common when AF is present, and most will occur within 6 months. After adjustment for concomitant coronary disease, cardiac failure, blood pressure, and age, AF imposes an independent stroke risk of 2.7-fold. It increases the stroke risk of persons with coronary heart disease fivefold.

Protection against cerebral embolism is urgently needed in patients with chronic AF; recent successful randomized trials have shown warfarin, and perhaps aspirin, to be safe and effective for stroke prevention.

REFERENCES

1. Halpern JL, Hart RG. Atrial fibrillation and stroke: new ideas, persisting dilemmas. *Stroke* 1988;19:937–941.
2. Kannel WB, Abbott RD, Savage DD, McNamara PM. Epidemiologic features of atrial fibrillation. The Framingham study. *N Engl J Med* 1982;306:1018–1022.
3. Wolf PA, Abbott RD, Kannel WB. Atrial fibrillation: a major contributor to stroke in the elderly. *Arch Intern Med* 1987;147:1561–1564.

4. Kannel WB, Abbott RD, Savage DD, et al. Coronary heart disease and atrial fibrillation: the Framingham study. *Am Heart J* 1983;106:389–396.
5. Wolf PA, Dawber TR, Thomas HE, Kannel WB. Epidemiologic assessment of chronic atrial fibrillation and risk of stroke. The Framingham study. *Neurology* 1978;28:973–977.
6. Wolf PA, Kannel WB, McGee DL, et al. Duration of atrial fibrillation and imminence of stroke: the Framingham study. *Stroke* 1983;14:664–667.
7. Brand FN, Abbott BD, Kannel WB, et al. Characteristics and prognosis of lone atrial fibrillation: 30 year follow-up in the Framingham study. *JAMA* 1985;254:3445–3453.
8. Falkerson PK, Beauer BM, Anseon JC, Graber HC. Calcification of the mitral annulus: etiology, clinical associations, complications and therapy. *Am J Med* 1979;66:967–977.
9. Aronow WS, Schmoetz KS, Koenigsberg M. Correlation of atrial fibrillation with presence or absence of mitral annular calcium in 604 persons older than 60 years. *Am J Cardiol* 1987;59:1213–1214.
10. Savage DD, Garrison RJ, Castelli WP, et al. Prevalence of saturated (annular) calcium and its correlates in a general population-based sample: the Framingham study. *Am J Cardiol* 1983;57:1375–1378.
11. Noir CK, Thomas W, Ryschan K, Cook C, Hec TT, Sketch MH Sr. Longterm follow-up of patients with echocardiographically detected mitral annular calcium and comparison with age and sex: control subjects. *Am J Cardiol* 1989;63:465–470.
12. Aronow WS, Koenigsberg M, Kronzan I, Gutstein H. Association of mitral annular calcium with new thromboembolic stroke and cardiac events at 39 month follow-up in elderly patients. *Am J Cardiol* 1990;66:1511–1515.
13. Cristal N, Szwarcberg J, Gueron M. Supraventricular arrhythmias in acute myocardial infarction—prognostic importance of clinical setting; mechanism of production. *Ann Intern Med* 1975;82:35–39.
14. Helmes C, Lundman T, Mogersan L, et al. Atrial fibrillation in acute myocardial infarction. *Acta Med Scand* 1973;193:39–44.
15. Klass M, Haywood LJ. Atrial fibrillation associated with acute myocardial infarction: a study of 34 cases. *Am Heart J* 1970;79:752–760.
16. Luria MH, Knoke JD, Wachs JS, et al. Survival after recovery from acute myocardial infarction: two and five year prognostic indices. *Am J Med* 1979;67:7–14.
17. Fluch D, Olsar E, Pentecost BL, et al. Natural history and clinical significance of arrhythmias after acute myocardial infarction. *Br Heart J* 1967;29:170–189.
18. Jewitt DE, Balcon R, Raffery EB, et al. Incidence and management of supraventricular arrhythmias after acute myocardial infarction. *Lancet* 1967;2:734–738.
19. Julian D, Valentine P, Miller G. Disturbance of rate, rhythm, and conduction in acute myocardial infarction. *Am J Med* 1964;37:915–927.
20. Meltzen L, Kitchell J. The incidence of arrhythmia associated with acute myocardial infarction. *Prog Cardiovasc Dis* 1960;9:50–58.
21. Stock E, Goble A. Assessment of arrhythmias in myocardial infarction. *Br Med J* 1967;2:719–723.
22. Kitchin AA, Pocock SJ. Prognosis of patients with acute myocardial infarction admitted to a coronary care unit. II. Survival after discharge. *Br Heart J* 1977;39:1167–1171.
23. Pardeans J, Lesaffre E, Williams JL, et al. Multivariate analysis for the assessment of prognostic factors and risk categories after recovery from acute myocardial infarction: the Belgian situation. *Am J Epidemiol* 1985;122:805–819.
24. Korn D, DeSanctis RW, Sell S. Massive calcification of the mitral annulus: a clinicopathologic study of 14 cases. *N Engl J Med* 1962;267:900–909.
25. Abbott WM, Maloney RD, McCabe CC, Lee CE, Wirthlin LS. Arterial embolism: a 44 year perspective. *Am J Surg* 1982;1243:460–464.
26. Aberg H. Atrial fibrillation. 1. A study of atrial thrombosis and systemic embolism in a necropsy material. *Acta Med Scand* 1969;185:373–379.
27. Hinton RC, Kistler JP, Fallon JT, Friedlich AL, Fisher CM. Influence of etiology of atrial fibrillation on incidence of systemic embolism. *Am J Cardiol* 1977;40:509–513.
28. Chesebro JH, Fuster V, Halperin JL. Editorial: atrial fibrillation—risk marker for stroke. *N Engl J Med* 1990;323:1556–1558.
29. Bogousslavsky J, Van Melle G, Regli F, Kappenberger L. Pathogenesis of anterior circulation stroke in patients with nonvalvular atrial fibrillation: the Lausanne stroke registry. *Neurology* 1990;40:1046–1050.
30. Boysen G, Nyboe J, Appleyard M, et al. Stroke incidence and risk factors for stroke in Copenhagen, Denmark. *Stroke* 1988;19:1345–1353.
31. Petersen P, Boysen G, Godtfredsen J, Andersen B. Placebo-controlled, randomised trial of warfarin and aspirin for prevention of thromboembolic complications in chronic atrial fibrillation: the Copenhagen AFASAK study. *Lancet* 1989;1:175–179.
32. Stroke Prevention in Atrial Fibrillation Study Group Investigators. Preliminary report of the stroke prevention in atrial fibrillation study. *N Engl J Med* 1990;322:863–868.

33. The Boston Area Anticoagulation Trial for Atrial Fibrillation Investigators. The effect of low-dose warfarin on the risk of stroke in patients with nonrheumatic atrial fibrillation. *N Engl J Med* 1990;323:1505–1511.
34. Yamanouchi H, Tomonaga M, Shimada H, Matsushita S, Kuramoto K, Toyokura Y. Nonvalvular atrial fibrillation as a cause of fatal massive cerebral infarction in the elderly. *Stroke* 1989;20:1653–1656.
35. Fisher CM. Reducing risks of cerebral embolism. *Geriatrics* 1979;34:59–66.
36. Friedman GD, Loveland DB, Ehrlich SP Jr. Relationship of stroke to other cardiovascular disease. *Circulation* 1968;38:533–541.
37. Sherman DG, Hart RG, Easton JD. The secondary prevention of stroke in patients with atrial fibrillation. *Arch Neurol* 1986;43:68–70.
38. Cardiac Embolism Task Force. Immediate anticoagulation of embolic stroke: a randomized trial. *Stroke* 1983;14:668–676.
39. Sage JI, Van Uitert RL. Risk of recurrent stroke in patients with atrial fibrillation and non-valvular heart disease. *Stroke* 1983;14:537–540.

Atrial Fibrillation: Mechanisms and Management, edited by
R. H. Falk and P. J. Podrid.
Raven Press, Ltd., New York © 1992.

6

Atrial Fibrillation in the Absence of Overt Cardiac Disease

Richard A. Leather and Charles R. Kerr

*Division of Cardiology, Department of Medicine, University of British Columbia,
Vancouver, British Columbia, Canada V6T 2B5*

The majority of the cases of atrial fibrillation in the adult population are related to a cardiovascular abnormality. The existence of atrial fibrillation in the absence of overt cardiovascular disease has been recognized since the early 1900s. Although most reports agree that it comprises only 2% to 6% of all cases of atrial fibrillation (1–5), proportions as high as 31% have been cited (6,7). Variations in the estimated frequency likely reflect the diagnostic criteria used in the study population (8).

Because of its relative infrequency compared to atrial fibrillation with overt cardiac disease, atrial fibrillation in the absence of cardiac disease has been incompletely studied and information about its true etiology, course, and prognosis is still lacking. The purpose of the chapter is to review this clinical entity particularly with respect to etiology, prevalence, significance, and management.

POTENTIAL ETIOLOGIES OF IDIOPATHIC ATRIAL FIBRILLATION

Occult Structural Cardiac Disease

Complete history and physical examination are essential to rule out organic heart disease, particularly rheumatic heart disease, coronary artery disease, cardiomyopathy, and hypertension. Even with careful and complete history and physical examination, advanced cardiac abnormalities may be overlooked. Noninvasive assessment with electrocardiogram, chest radiography, and echocardiogram to determine heart chamber dimensions, wall thickness, and motion as well as valvular morphology and function may be useful (9). These investigations, however, may not reveal cardiac abnormalities due to the limits of resolution of currently available diagnostic methods. It has been postulated that idiopathic atrial fibrillation is secondary to a diffuse fibrodegenerative disease involving the heart in general but particularly the sinus node, atrioventricular node, and atrial muscle. This is suggested by the greater incidence of atrial fibrillation in elderly patients, particularly those with organic heart disease. Pathologic studies in patients with sinus node dysfunction support this, and it is suspected that the diffuse changes are secondary to previous single or multiple exposures to various toxins, infectious agents, or inflammatory disease. If these changes were to result in slowing of conduction velocity, shortening of atrial refractoriness, or a combination of both, a more hospitable substrate for sustaining atrial fibrillation could exist. However, in postmortem studies in patients with atrial fibrillation (without specific reference to associated sinus node disease), there has been a notable absence of abnormalities (3,10–13). Despite these negative postmortem results, the presence of micro scars and infiltrates in a proportion of patients with atrial fibrillation without a clear etiology remains speculative since changes in the myocardium at the microscopic or electrophysiologic level would escape clinical detection.

Occult Primary Electrical Abnormalities

The presence of a concealed accessory pathway should be considered in individuals, particularly young, otherwise healthy patients, with no clear cause for atrial fibrillation. Approximately 20% of patients with Wolff-Parkinson-White syndrome develop spontaneous atrial fibrillation (14–17). Patients with concealed accessory pathways may also develop atrial fibrillation, but, in the absence of preexcitation, if reciprocating tachycardia has not been documented, there would be no reason to suspect the presence of an accessory pathway. The association of atrial fibrillation with Wolff-Parkinson-White syndrome has been well documented, and the elimination of paroxysmal atrial fibrillation after surgical ablation of the accessory pathway occurs in most patients (16,18–20). There are several factors that may predispose to development of atrial fibrillation in these individuals, including extrastimuli, substrate, and mechanical factors. An appropriate trigger is required to initiate atrial fibrillation. In most patients these are closely coupled extrastimuli occurring in the vulnerable zone of the atrial action potential (14). Most spontaneous ventricular premature beats will result in subsequent atrial activation due to retrograde activation of the atrium over the accessory pathway. In addition, appropriately timed atrial premature beats may conduct over the atrioventricular node and produce an echo beat from the ventricle conducting retrogradely to the atrium via the accessory pathway creating a situation whereby the atrium is exposed to two sequential atrial extrastimuli. Campbell (17) suggested that multiple colliding inputs from the accessory pathway, sinus node, and atrial catheter explain susceptibility to atrial fibrillation. Further, Jackman et al. (21,22) by carefully observing local electrograms, reported a number of cases of atrial fibrillation that originate in the region of the accessory pathway. These may represent local reentry within the accessory pathway fibers themselves.

Although there are ample potential triggers to initiate atrial fibrillation in patients with accessory pathways, a critical mass of atrial tissue with appropriate electrophysiologic properties is necessary to sustain atrial fibrillation. Evidence to suggest that this substrate exists is circumstantial. Extrastimuli delivered in electrophysiologic study in patients without accessory pathways infrequently result in atrial fibrillation. The association of abnormal atrial myocardium near the junction of the atrium with the accessory pathway may be important. One would not expect, however, that simply destroying the accessory pathway fibers locally with surgery or a catheter, which usually eliminates atrial fibrillation, would result in any change in the atrial substrate responsible for atrial fibrillation maintenance. In addition, in electrophysiologic study, although some atrial fibrillation seems to originate near the atrium-accessory pathway junction or within the accessory pathway itself, in many other instances the site of initiation is well removed from the atrioventricular annulus (18).

Reciprocating tachycardia induced in the electrophysiology laboratory has been noted to degenerate spontaneously to atrial fibrillation in approximately 15% of cases (19,20,23,24) and is often precipitated by a premature atrial beat during tachycardia (16,17). Excitation-contraction feedback has been suggested as a possible mechanism (19,24–26). It is well recognized that as reciprocating tachycardia develops, the pressure and volume within the atrium increase. This mechanical change is reflected electrophysiologically by a decrease in the atrial effective refractory period and an increase in intra-atrial conduction time. These modifications provide the appropriate electrophysiologic substrate to allow atrial fibrillation to develop and sustain. The influence of the autonomic nervous system on the substrate is unknown but presumably maximal fluctuations in vagal and sympathetic tone occur at the onset of reciprocating tachycardia and will influence both refractoriness and conduction (27).

Unfortunately, to establish the proportion of patients with atrial fibrillation without overt cardiac disease who have concealed accessory pathways would require mapping retrograde conduction during ventricular pacing in a large, consecutive series of patients with idiopathic atrial fibrillation. These studies would be difficult and incomplete due to the inherent invasive nature of the test.

Noncardiac Triggers of Atrial Fibrillation

A vast assortment of noncardiac metabolic and physiologic derangements have been reported to cause atrial fibrillation. In most, such as the pleuropulmonary diseases, atrial fibrillation is simply an acute complication and would usually not be the presenting problem. The arrhythmia will usually resolve even without specific management, and one would not expect recurrent paroxysmal or chronic atrial fibrillation to result. On occasion, toxins or medications might be responsible but may not be suspected. There are case reports of atrial fibrillation due to bronchial inhalants (28,29) as well as reports of atrial fibrillation occurring with antihistamines and other cold remedies, local anesthetics, and coffee (30). The influence of extreme fatigue or emotional stress may be additive (30,31). Atrial fibrillation can occur secondary to various infections affecting the cardiovascular and pulmonary system (diphtheria, typhoid, pneumonia, empyema), toxic exposures, noxious gases, anesthetic agents, metabolic abnormalities such as hypokalemia, hypocalcemia, hypomagnesemia, and hypoglycemia (32,33), hypothermia, and hypoxia (1,34).

Two other potential noncardiac causes, alcohol and hyperthyroidism, deserve special attention because of their prevalence in the population and because of the possibility of controlling atrial fibrillation with their appropriate management.

Alcohol and Atrial Fibrillation

It has long been suspected that alcohol plays an etiologic role in atrial fibrillation not only in patients with organic heart disease but also in those without overt cardiac disease (3,5,30,35). Since occasional use of alcohol is common and events such as paroxysmal atrial fibrillation are relatively uncommon, it is difficult to firmly establish a direct relationship. Although not universal, a number of studies strongly suggest a link (36). Ettinger et al. (37) reported observations on 24 patients with a history of heavy alcohol use preceding presentation with arrhythmias. No patient had overt cardiac disease. Twelve of the 24 patients experienced paroxysmal atrial fibrillation and six experienced atrial flutter. They noted that the majority of admissions to hospital with atrial arrhythmias occurred over weekends or holidays when alcohol intake was more marked and that with long-term abstinence arrhythmias appeared to resolve. They coined the term "holiday heart." Atrial fibrillation was thought to be precipitated by acute effects of alcohol on atrial refractoriness and conduction as well as the cumulative effects of chronic use creating preclinical cardiac dysfunction. These findings were substantiated by others (38,39). Engel and Luck (39) assessed 14 men, 11 of whom were habitual alcohol abusers, and four of whom had a past history of atrial fibrillation and flutter when drinking alcohol. Atrial refractory periods and conduction properties before and after 60 to 120 ml of whiskey were measured. Five of the 10 patients without inducible atrial fibrillation in the basal state had atrial fibrillation after whiskey. There was no significant change in atrial refractory periods or in dispersion of refractoriness. This likely reflected the effect of a relatively low dose as changes in atrial refractory period have been noted in animals with larger doses of alcohol (40). In another study alcohol was noted to prolong intraatrial conduction (41).

Chronic cardiac sequelae of long-term alcohol use are well described and include both myocardial dysfunction and arrhythmias (37,42,43). Histologically, patchy inflammatory lesions are noted in the hearts of both humans and animals (33,44).

An acute alcohol binge at times of emotional stress in individuals without a history of previous alcohol use and without cardiac disease has been implicated as a cause of paroxysmal atrial fibrillation (30,31,45–47). Thornton (31) suggested that a history of acute, unusual alcohol intake in a patient presenting with atrial fibrillation with nothing by history or examination to indicate organic heart disease should reassure the physician that elaborate and invasive testing is not warranted. He appropriately pointed out that an occult underlying metabolic or structural cause for atrial fibrillation exacerbated by alcohol could not be ruled out.

The acute electrophysiologic effects in these individuals may be secondary to catecholamine surges during withdrawal, to electrolyte fluxes, or to direct toxic effects of alcohol on the myocardium. These changes may persist for some time since presentation with atrial fibrillation the day after an alcohol binge when blood alcohol levels are low or normal has been frequently observed.

Several case control studies have attempted to correlate paroxysmal atrial fibrillation with alcohol use. Rich et al. (48) retrospectively reported that 62% of 64 patients with idiopathic paroxysmal atrial fibrillation versus 33% of 64 randomly selected age- and sex-matched hospital controls were heavy users of alcohol as indicated by analysis of medical records. In a Finnish study, Koskinen et al. (46), also using a case controlled design, reported on 98 consecutive young and middle aged patients with recurrent paroxysmal atrial fibrillation presenting to the emergency room. History of alcohol use was determined by a screening questionnaire for alcohol abuse. They used two control groups, 98 randomly selected age- and sex-matched patients presenting to the emergency room with acute illnesses, and 50 randomly selected individuals from the local community. The matched control group excluded patients presenting with alcohol-related problems. Mean alcohol consumption was significantly greater for patients who had paroxysmal atrial fibrillation than among the matched control groups. In a subgroup analysis this association held for men but not for women, although this may simply be due to the relatively small number of women (23) versus men (75) in the study. These data were in general agreement with their findings in a previous study of patients with new onset atrial fibrillation (45) as well as findings of others (49).

Thus, there is accumulating anecdotal and epidemiologic evidence that alcohol plays an etiologic role in atrial fibrillation in patients with and without organic heart disease. Whether atrial fibrillation will recur in these individuals in the absence of alcohol use is unclear and has not been prospectively addressed.

Hyperthyroidism in Atrial Fibrillation

Hyperthyroidism has been recognized clinically as a cause for atrial fibrillation even before the development of sophisticated radioimmunoassays of thyroid function. The incidence of atrial fibrillation in patients with overt hyperthyroidism is approximately 10% to 20% (50,51), occurring much more frequently in the elderly and rarely in individuals under age 40 (52,53). This age difference may be partially related to the greater prevalence of associated illness in the elderly. Camm et al. (54) noted that atrial fibrillation was present in 11% of ambulatory individuals with hyperthyroidism over age 75. The incidence in the elderly hospital population is similar (55,56). In the elderly, hyperthyroidism may be masked (apathetic hyperthyroidism) and, therefore, not suspected if the usual clinical criteria for hyperthyroidism are used (57,58). The potential difficulties in recognizing hyperthyroidism are further complicated by controversies regarding true gold standards. Therefore, although it is relatively easy to estimate the incidence of atrial fibrillation in patients with a diagnosis of hyperthyroidism, the converse is not true.

With the development of radioimmunoassays, hyperthyroidism has been diagnosed by measuring total T4, total T3, and basal thyroid-stimulating hormone (TSH). Since 99.96% of T4 and 99.5% of T3 is bound to plasma proteins, levels of binding proteins, primarily thyroid-binding globulin (TBG), will influence measured and free thyroid hormone levels (59). A significant number of physiologic and disease states and medications will alter TBG levels. With the availability recently of free T4 and T3 levels, this problem can be avoided.

In patients with thyroid adenomas, the free T4 levels may be normal if the tumor secretes only T3, and therefore both T3 and T4 levels should be measured (60). High levels of thyroid hormone feed back at the level of the hypothalamus to suppress TSH. Initially assays for TSH were not reliable in the low ranges, but with new superselective TSH assays, hyperthyroidism can be diagnosed by significant suppression of TSH levels to less than 0.2 μU/ml. In fact, a level of TSH above 0.2 μU/ml virtually rules out hyperthyroidism (61,62). The previously used thyrotropin-releasing hormone (TRH) stimulation test may have led to overdiagnosis of hyperthyroidism in some studies (51,61–69).

The incidence of overt and occult hyperthyroidism in patients presenting with atrial fibrillation has been addressed (51,63,64,66,69–72). When patients with atrial fibrillation of any cause are analyzed, hyperthyroidism appears to be a rare etiology responsible for only 2% to 3% of cases (67,69,70) even when sensitive tests for hyperthyroidism are used. For example, Fagerberg et al. (69) prospectively evaluated 110 consecutive ambulatory patients with atrial fibrillation and found that, using free T3 and T4 determinations, only three patients had hyperthyroidism, and in two of these patients the diagnosis was not clinically evident. All studies are limited by the relatively small number of patients with idiopathic atrial fibrillation. Forfar et al. (51) assessed 75 consecutive patients with sustained, idiopathic atrial fibrillation (although 23 patients had some underlying cardiac disease). They found that 10 (13%) had hyperthyroidism, eight of 52 patients with true idiopathic atrial fibrillation, and two of 23 with organic heart disease. However, the diagnosis of hyperthyroidism was made using the TRH stimulation test. Total T3 and T4 levels and thyroid scans were normal in all but two and three patients, respectively. No studies have used the newer assays of TSH as the gold standard for assessing thyroid status.

The identification of hyperthyroidism as a precipitant for atrial fibrillation is important since there is evidence that, with antithyroid management, conversion and long-term maintenance of sinus rhythm can be expected in at least 60% of patients (51,53,64). The conversion rate appears highest when hypothyroidism or the euthyroid state is induced promptly (53). When atrial fibrillation has persisted for longer periods, conversion to sinus rhythm is more difficult (73). This may be related to changes in atrial morphology induced by atrial fibrillation (74).

In summary, hyperthyroidism is a rare cause of atrial fibrillation. It may account for a significant percentage of patients with truly idiopathic atrial fibrillation, but this has not yet been evaluated in a prospective controlled fashion with large enough numbers of patients. Hyperthyroidism may not be evident clinically, particularly in the elderly, and, therefore, biochemical screening is imperative in the patient with idiopathic atrial fibrillation since prompt treatment may result in restoration of sinus rhythm. With the availability of more sophisticated assays, a normal free T3 and T4 or superselective TSH should rule out hyperthyroidism.

PREVALENCE OF IDIOPATHIC ATRIAL FIBRILLATION

The exact prevalence and incidence of atrial fibrillation, including idiopathic atrial fibrillation, in the general population are difficult to determine. Atrial fibrillation may be intermittent and, particularly in the elderly and in those with a controlled ventricular rate, may be asymptomatic. Many studies have attempted to determine both the prevalence and incidence but suffer from limitation of patient numbers and the bias inherent in studying a selected population. It is difficult to compare the various studies directly due to inhomogeneity in patient demographics, recruitment site (community, clinic, hospital), and presence or absence of associated cardiovascular and other medical illnesses. There is also much inhomogeneity in study design. Some authors report on the prevalence of atrial fibrillation by using screening electrocardiograms (30,75,76). Others, such as the Framingham study, report the incidence of atrial fibrillation occurring in a general population over a long follow-up (6,36,77), while still others are descriptive reports on series of patients with atrial fibrillation (1–5,7,12,13,78,79). Determining the true proportion of atrial fibrillation patients who are idiopathic is restricted not only by limitations of clinical examination and currently available diagnostic techniques, but also by the relative lack of representative epidemiologic data.

Atrial fibrillation occurring in the absence of overt organic heart disease was recognized as early as the turn of this century (80,81). Further reports of atrial fibrillation without evidence of heart disease followed in the 1930s (4,5,7,12,82) and 1940s (1,3). Most patients were young males and reports included cases of both paroxysmal and chronic atrial fibrillation, of which 5% to 10% were idiopathic. The entity had been variously described as benign, functional, idiopathic, senile, of unknown etiology, and atrial fibrillation without heart disease. Evans and Swann (78) in 1954 coined the term "lone atrial fibrillation." They described 20 elderly male patients with chronic atrial fibrillation in whom there was no evidence of cardiac disease by history, clinical examination, electrocardiogram, phonocardiogram, and cardioscopy and stressed that symptoms were mild and the prognosis was excellent.

Although not unusual in the young adult, idiopathic atrial fibrillation is more common in the elderly. By screening routine yearly electrocardiograms, Hiss and Lamb (76) found atrial fibrillation in only 5 of 122,043 healthy flying personnel aged 16 to 60. They noted that by history the incidence of paroxysmal atrial fibrillation was undoubtedly higher. Lamb and Pollard (30), in a similar manner, found only 60 cases of atrial fibrillation in over 250,000 flying personnel aged 22 to 49 years. A British study reported on electrocardiographic findings in 18,403 middle aged civil servants (75). They found an age-related prevalence of atrial fibrillation with 0.16% between ages 40 and 49 years, 0.37% between ages 50 and 59 years, and 1.13% of individuals between ages 60 and 64 years. Campbell (50) found higher prevalences (2%–5%) of atrial fibrillation in elderly fit Scotsmen.

From the Framingham study comes some of the most compelling data (6,36). In a general community, 2,325 men and 2,866 women aged 30 to 62 years, none with history of atrial fibrillation, were followed biennially for 22 years. Forty-nine men and 49 women developed chronic atrial fibrillation during the follow-up. The incidence increased with advancing age. In 18 men and 12 women (31% of the atrial fibrillation group), no cause for atrial fibrillation could initially be found; however, during the course of the study cardiovascular disease was detected in all but five of these individuals. Therefore, depending on the strictness of definition the etiology of atrial fibrillation was idiopathic in between 5% and 31% of these community-based individuals. The potentially higher proportion of patients with idiopathic atrial fibrillation likely represents a healthier, generally younger set of patients.

Thirty-year follow-up of the Framingham cohort (36) revealed that 193 of 2,336 men and 183 of 2,873 women developed atrial fibrillation. Mean age was 70.6 years. Of those developing atrial fibrillation, 32 men (16.6%) and 11 women (6%), or 0.8% of the total population, had idiopathic atrial fibrillation. For men, but not women, there was a greater proportion of individuals with idiopathic atrial fibrillation in the older age groups compared with the younger. Although coronary artery disease, congestive heart failure, hypertensive heart disease, and rheumatic heart disease were not present in this group of patients with idiopathic atrial fibrillation, 16.7% and 26.1% had preexisting nonspecific abnormalities or intraventricular conduction delay, respectively, on electrocardiogram.

A total of 3,623 patients with atrial fibrillation from Olmsted County, Minnesota, were seen at the Mayo Clinic over a 30-year period (77). Retrospective analysis of their medical records identified 97 (2.7%) patients with idiopathic atrial fibrillation. Only 9% were chronic, but by a mean 8-year follow-up, 12 of 68 patients with recurrent paroxysmal atrial fibrillation had progressed to chronic atrial fibrillation. Recently, Davidson et al. (2) noted 33 of 704 consecutive patients with atrial fibrillation presenting to the emergency room over an 8-year period had idiopathic atrial fibrillation. Only two of these 33 cases were chronic.

Therefore, studies have shown that idiopathic atrial fibrillation makes up 2% to 31% of all cases of atrial fibrillation. It is more frequent in the nonhospitalized, elderly male and less frequent in the general hospital population, in which an underlying etiology is more likely. Idiopathic atrial fibrillation is unusual in the young, healthy population. Definitions can become blurred since with follow-up many patients with idiopathic atrial fibrillation will develop cardiovascular disease. Whether this is simply natural progression of a common entity or whether occult cardiovascular disease was already present and predisposed to development of atrial fibrillation is unclear.

PROGNOSIS OF IDIOPATHIC ATRIAL FIBRILLATION

The influence of idiopathic atrial fibrillation on morbidity (primarily stroke and other cardiovascular complications) and mortality is still poorly defined because of the low incidence of idiopathic atrial fibrillation. Many of the original papers on idiopathic atrial fibrillation remarked on its low mortality (1,3,5,78), and more recently (30,75,77), in young individuals, its benign prognosis has been reemphasized. In the prevalence study by Rose et al. (75), the 5-year mortality for 70 patients with atrial fibrillation (of whom 43% had no evidence of cardiovascular disease) was only 4.8%. Ninety-seven consecutive patients under the age of 60 at the time of diagnosis of idiopathic atrial fibrillation were followed for a mean of 15 years and 19 patients died (77). Mortality increased significantly after 20 years of atrial fibrillation but by this time mean age at death was 73 years. At diagnosis 80% of cases were paroxysmal. Thromboembolic events were low, averaging 0.55 per 100 patient years and occurred approximately equally among the paroxysmal and chronic atrial fibrillation groups. The benign prognosis in this moderately sized general population study was at variance with the data from the Framingham study (6,36,83,84). Kannel et al. (6) noted nearly twice the annual total mortality in all cases with chronic atrial fibrillation compared with controls (5% vs 2.8%). In the subgroup of 30 patients with idiopathic atrial fibrillation, yearly mortality was still increased at 3.8%. Brand et al. (36) was able to obtain long-term follow-up on 30 of the 43 patients from Framingham with idiopathic atrial fibrillation. Eight of 30 (28%) presented with stroke at a mean of 8.5 years from beginning of follow-up. Compared with the 51 of 988 controls (6.8%) who developed stroke, this was a four- to fivefold increase in risk of stroke, suggesting chronic idiopathic atrial fibrillation is not benign.

Although the Framingham data seem to conflict with that of Kopecky et al. (77), important differences existed in the patient characteristics. Kopecky et al. reported on young patients (mean age 44 years) with predominantly paroxysmal atrial fibrillation (80%). Patients in the Framingham study, however, were older (mean age 70 years) and all had chronic atrial fibrillation. In addition 32% had hypertension and 40% who developed atrial fibrillation subsequently developed other cardiovascular disease, suggesting that some patients in the Framingham cohort were not truly idiopathic (6,36,83,84).

Further evidence suggesting a poor prognosis for patients with idiopathic atrial fibrillation comes from questionnaires gathered from several hundred insurance companies (85). One hundred twenty-six cases of chronic and 1,645 cases of paroxysmal atrial fibrillation were identified. Two-thirds of the patients were under age 50, and of this younger group 50% with chronic and 72% with paroxysmal atrial fibrillation were called idiopathic. Mean follow-up of 3.3 years revealed an almost eightfold increase in mortality in the chronic idiopathic atrial fibrillation group versus controls as determined using standard insurance tables. Mortality in the paroxysmal atrial fibrillation group was not significantly different from controls. Since cardiovascular disease was ruled out only retrospectively by insurance questionnaires, the incidence of cardiovascular disease in both the chronic and paroxysmal atrial fibrillation groups was probably substantially higher than estimated.

The influence of patient age, chronicity of atrial fibrillation, and associated cardiovascular disease on prognosis has recently been reviewed (86). Although data are still limited, the prognosis in patients with idiopathic atrial fibrillation, as defined by absence of overt cardiovascular disease by history, examination, electrocardiogram, and chest radiograph, appears to be excellent in the young, nonhospitalized patients with paroxysmal atrial fibrillation. Prognosis in the elderly patient with chronic atrial fibrillation, however, particularly if hospitalized at diagnosis, is far from benign. These patients have increased risk of stroke and mortality. Whether the risks are intermediate in younger patients with chronic atrial fibrillation or older patients with paroxysmal atrial fibrillation is uncertain and awaits further population-based studies.

MANAGEMENT

The management strategies for atrial fibrillation in the absence of cardiac disease are fourfold: to control rate, identify precipitating factors, consider conversion to sinus rhythm, and maintain sinus rhythm. Special concerns include complications of antiarrhythmic drugs, stroke risk, and complications of anticoagulant therapy.

Control of Rate

Rapid ventricular response to atrial fibrillation cannot be allowed to persist and conventionally is controlled using digoxin, beta-blockers, or calcium channel antagonists. Prompt cardioversion is indicated for hemodynamic deterioration, but this is seldom necessary in this group of patients with ostensibly normal hearts. Atrial fibrillation with a controlled ventricular response in the absence of drug therapy is occasionally seen. Although not all would include these patients in the group with idiopathic atrial fibrillation, these patients have abnormal atrioventricular node function and usually have some element of sinus node and atrial disease predisposing them to atrial fibrillation (87,88).

Identification of Precipitating Factors

The identification of precipitating factors is essential. Full history and physical examination, electrocardiogram, and chest radiograph to rule out cardiovascular disease, acute illnesses such as pericarditis, pulmonary emboli, and infections, metabolic abnormalities, toxic exposures (particularly to alcohol), new medications, and hyperthyroidism are important. These should be supplemented by laboratory investigations including electrolytes and free T3 and T4 or a superselective TSH. Particularly in younger patients with new or paroxysmal atrial fibrillation an echocardiogram is indicated. In the absence of cardiovascular disease the presence of an acute precipitant makes one more optimistic that treating the cause will prevent further recurrences of atrial fibrillation. The possibility of an underlying abnormal atrial substrate rendered more susceptible to atrial fibrillation by the acute precipitant cannot be ruled out. Therefore, in a subset of these patients atrial fibrillation may recur either with or without further precipitating insults. Alcohol abuse acutely or chronically may be more common than is generally appreciated. There is evidence that abstinence from alcohol can decrease or eliminate atrial fibrillation recurrences (31,37). Although hyperthyroidism is not likely a common cause for idiopathic atrial fibrillation, in many patients with hyperthyroidism treatment with antithyroid medication leads to a resumption and maintenance of sinus rhythm (51,53,64). The possibility of conversion decreases the longer atrial fibrillation has persisted (53,73), thus stressing the importance of early detection and treatment. In the elderly patient with idiopathic atrial fibrillation, apathetic hyperthyroidism must be considered in the differential diagnosis (50).

Conversion of Atrial Fibrillation to Sinus Rhythm

Conversion to sinus rhythm is much less likely if atrial fibrillation has persisted for longer than 1 year. Attempts probably should be made to convert most patients with atrial fibrillation of unknown duration. Certainly in those individuals with atrial fibrillation of short duration, cardioversion should be attempted. Conversion may be pharmacologic or electrical. Type 1A, 1C, or 3 antiarrhythmic drugs are commonly used and conversion of recent onset idiopathic atrial fibrillation may approach 94% (2). There have been no randomized, prospective studies comparing anticoagulants in the few weeks before and after medical or electrical cardioversion of atrial fibrillation, but from retrospective studies in all types of atrial fibrillation most would agree that full anticoagulation in idiopathic atrial fibrillation is warranted prior to attempted restoration of sinus rhythm (89–92).

Maintenance of Sinus Rhythm

The question of long-term antiarrhythmic medication often arises. In individuals with frequent recurrences of rapid and symptomatic atrial fibrillation prophylactic therapy is clearly indicated. In those with less frequent or asymptomatic bouts with controlled ventricular rates, the major concern becomes the risk of thromboembolic events. The benefits of therapy must be balanced by the known adverse effects of antiarrhythmic medications. Although the newer antiarrhythmic drugs have lower noncardiac side effect profiles, proarrhythmia may occur in as many as 10% of patients treated with type 1C medications (93–96). Proarrhythmia manifests either as a new arrhythmia or as acceleration of ventricular response to atrial fibrillation or flutter. The proarrhythmic effect of these drugs in patients without organic heart disease is uncertain.

Frequently restoration and maintenance of sinus rhythm is not possible or only attainable with high-dose single or combination antiarrhythmic drugs. In these circumstances chronic slowing and smoothing of rhythm is desirable. This can usually be achieved by medication. However, frequently the rate cannot be adequately slowed, particularly during exercise, or the patient remains symptomatic in spite of medication. In these cases, atrioventricular nodal ablation is becoming increasingly popular. The use of radiofrequency energy makes this a particularly safe and well-tolerated procedure (97,98). Subsequent placement of a ventricular (in chronic atrial fibrillation) or dual-chamber (in paroxysmal recurrent atrial fibrillation) pacemaker provides a smooth rhythm that responds to physiologic demand.

Risk of Stroke

The risk of stroke in patients with idiopathic atrial fibrillation has been discussed. Appropriate management to prevent embolism depends on the risk of embolism in the untreated state, but clearly maintenance of sinus rhythm is the best method of prevention.

In a nonrandomized retrospective study from the Montreal Heart Institute, 15% of 254 patients with atrial fibrillation had idiopathic atrial fibrillation (99). Most of the patients had cardiac disease, with mitral valve disease being the most common. Average age was 54 years. The average follow-up was 3.3 years. For nonanticoagulated patients with paroxysmal or chronic atrial fibrillation unrelated to mitral valve disease, the risk of thromboembolism was 5.91 per 100 patient years. With anticoagulation the incidence of thromboembolic events was only 0.70 per 100 patient years. There were two thromboembolic events (both extracerebral) in the 37 patients with idiopathic atrial fibrillation, one each in the anticoagulated and nonanticoagulated groups. In this group of fairly young patients, the stroke risk without anticoagulation was substantially greater (approximately 10 times) than the Kopecky et al. group (77) of patients at 0.55 per 100 patient years. The Olmsted County patients, however, were even younger than the Montreal Heart Institute patients, and all had idiopathic atrial fibrillation (compared with the 50% of nonmitral valve patients in the Montreal Heart group with cardiomyopathy, coronary artery disease, or hypertension). Only 8% and 1%, respectively, were being treated with warfarin or aspirin.

There have been three randomized prospective studies evaluating the efficacy of anticoagulant therapy in prevention of embolism in atrial fibrillation. In a Danish study 1,007 patients with nonrheumatic chronic atrial fibrillation were randomized to open-label warfarin ($n = 335$), aspirin 75 mg daily ($n = 336$), or placebo ($n = 336$) and followed for 2 years (100). Thromboembolic complications in the aspirin and placebo groups were virtually identical (20 and 21 events, respectively), while only five events occurred in the warfarin-treated group. Yearly incidence of thromboembolism of 2% in the warfarin group and 5.5% in the aspirin and placebo groups corresponded to a risk reduction of more than 60%. These patients were elderly (median age 74.2 years) with chronic atrial fibrillation and most did not have idiopathic atrial fibrillation. Whether the benefit of anticoagulants in this group of patients applies to individuals with idiopathic atrial fibrillation and/or younger patients with paroxysmal and chronic atrial fibrillation is unclear.

Preliminary results of the second study (101) in which 34% of the patients had paroxysmal atrial fibrillation showed an 81% reduction in embolic events with both warfarin and aspirin at a dose of 325 mg daily (1.6% yearly) compared with control (8.3% yearly). Younger patients appeared to respond better to aspirin than older patients. There were no strokes occurring in the group of patients under age 55 with idiopathic atrial fibrillation compared with an approximately 5% risk of stroke in patients with lone atrial fibrillation over age 65.

The most recently reported Boston Area Anticoagulation Trial for Atrial Fibrillation (BAATAF) randomized 420 patients with nonrheumatic atrial fibrillation to low-dose warfarin (prothrombin time 1.2–1.5 times control) versus placebo in an unblinded fashion (102). Follow-up averaged 2.2 years. Most patients were elderly (85% over 60 years of age) with chronic atrial fibrillation (83% vs 17% with paroxysmal atrial fibrillation) and more than 50% had organic heart disease. The trial was terminated early when a highly significant 80% reduction in stroke (from 3.0% to 0.41% yearly) in the warfarin-treated group was noted. Aspirin was used in 46% of the control patients, which might explain their lower stroke risk compared with an 8.3% yearly risk in a similar but seemingly healthier control population not treated with aspirin or warfarin in the previous trial (101).

Although the BAATAF results seem to confirm those of the previous two trials, the patient population was elderly with a significant preponderance of organic heart disease. In all trials, stroke risk was less in younger patients and in those with no evidence of other cardiac disease.

Atrial fibrillation is likely a risk factor for stroke, as indicated by the epidemiologic data. The low absolute stroke risk in individuals with idiopathic atrial fibrillation would indicate that left atrial stasis leading to mural thrombus formation and subsequent thromboembolism is only one aspect of stroke risk. The etiology of stroke, particularly in individuals with other cardiovascular disease, is multifactorial, involving a combination of fibrin formation and platelet activation. The relative importance of these various factors will influence the benefits of warfarin and aspirin (103). In none of these trials was a control group without atrial fibrillation used. A similar stroke risk reduction with aspirin or warfarin in patients with sinus rhythm might have indicated that atrial fibrillation is more a high-risk marker for embolic events rather than being primarily responsible.

Anticoagulant therapy with warfarin in the older patient with chronic atrial fibrillation in the presence of valvular or nonvalvular cardiac disease has been shown to reduce stroke risk. The absolute risk of stroke in the younger patient with idiopathic paroxysmal atrial fibrillation, although greater than that in a healthy young individual, is small and aspirin therapy at a dose of 325 mg daily is likely adequate. In the younger patient with chronic atrial fibrillation or the older patient with paroxysmal atrial fibrillation, stroke risk is likely intermediate and in the absence of contraindications and until results of ongoing trials are available, anticoagulation should be instituted.

SUMMARY

Atrial fibrillation is a common arrhythmia occurring in 0.4% to 5% of the adult population. The incidence increases with advancing age. Approximately 5% of atrial fibrillation is idiopathic. After acute treatment one must identify and treat any precipitating factors and suspect and rule out the presence of occult cardiac disease, hyperthyroidism, and alcohol. The prognosis is largely related to the risk of thromboembolism. Embolic risk increases with advancing age, chronicity of atrial fibrillation, and associated illnesses. This risk will be significantly reduced if sinus rhythm can be maintained. The relative benefit of anticoagulation with warfarin or aspirin needs to be clarified but it is likely that anticoagulation is warranted in the absence of contraindications for the older patient with careful titration of warfarin to keep the INR between 2.0 and 3.0 to lessen the risk of bleeding complications. Younger patients with idiopathic atrial fibrillation may benefit from aspirin therapy of 325 mg daily. However, since atrial fibrillation and, thus, stroke risk will be present for many years, the relative benefits of warfarin versus aspirin remain to be determined by further trials.

REFERENCES

1. Hanson HH, Rutledge DI. Auricular fibrillation in normal hearts. *N Engl J Med* 1949;240:947–953.
2. Davidson E, Weinberger I, Rotenberg Z, Fuchs J, Agmon J. Atrial fibrillation: cause and time of onset. *Arch Intern Med* 1989;149:457–459.
3. Phillips E, Levine SA. Auricular fibrillation without other evidence of heart disease. *Am J Med* 1949;7:478–489.
4. Mohler HK, Lintgen C. Auricular fibrillation and analysis of 220 cases. *Pa Med J* 1931;35:68–74.
5. Friedlander RD, Levine SA. Auricular fibrillation and flutter without evidence of organic heart disease. *N Engl J Med* 1934;211:624–629.
6. Kannel WB, Abbott RD, Savage DD, McNamara PM. Epidemiologic features of chronic atrial fibrillation. *N Engl J Med* 1982;306:1018–1022.
7. Parkinson J, Campbell M. Paroxysmal auricular fibrillation: record of 200 patients. *Q J Med* 1930;23:67–100.
8. Selzer A. Atrial fibrillation revisited. *N Engl J Med* 1982;306:1044–1045.
9. Grand A, Fichter C, Ferry M, Fichter P, Pernot F. Value of echocardiography in aged patients with presumed idiopathic auricular fibrillation. *Ann Cardiol Angeiol (Paris)* 1990;39:7–12.
10. Yater WM. Pathologic changes in auricular fibrillation and in allied arrhythmias. *Arch Intern Med* 1929;43:808–834.
11. Frothingham C. The auricles in cases of auricular fibrillation. *Arch Intern Med* 1925;36:437.
12. Fowler M, Baidridge CW. Auricular fibrillation as only manifestation of heart disease. *Am Heart J* 1930;6:183–191.
13. Orgain ES, Wolff L, White PD. Uncomplicated auricular fibrillation and auricular flutter: frequent occurrence and good prognosis in patients without other evidence of cardiac disease. *Arch Intern Med* 1936;57:493–513.
14. Bennett MA, Pentecost BL. The pattern of onset and spontaneous cessation of atrial fibrillation in man. *Circulation* 1970;41:981–988.
15. Bauernfeind RA, Swiryn SP, Wyndham CR, Palilio E, Rosen KM. Telephonic documentation of paroxysmal atrioventricular reentrant tachycardia in preexcitation with recurrent paroxysmal atrial fibrillation. *Chest* 1980;78:771–773.
16. Sung RJ, Castellanos A, Mallon SM, Bloom MG, Gelband H, Myerburg RJ. Mechanism of spontaneous alternation between reciprocating tachycardia and atrial fibrillation/flutter in the Wolff-Parkinson-White syndrome. *Circulation* 1977;56:409–416.
17. Campbell RWF, Smith RA, Gallagher JJ, Prichett ELC, Wallace AG. Atrial fibrillation in the preexcitation syndrome. *Am J Cardiol* 1977;40:514–520.
18. Sharma AD, Klein GJ, Guiraudon GM, Milstein S. Atrial fibrillation in patients with Wolff-Parkinson-White syndrome: incidence after surgical ablation of the accessory pathway. *Circulation* 1985;72:161–169.
19. Shen EN, Sung RJ. Initiation of atrial fibrillation by spontaneous ventricular premature beats in concealed Wolff-Parkinson-White syndrome. *Am Heart J* 1982;103:911–912.
20. Morady F, Sledge C, Shen E, Sung RJ, Gonzalez R, Scheinman MM. Electrophysiologic testing in the management of patients with the Wolff-Parkinson-White syndrome and atrial fibrillation. *Am J Cardiol* 1983;51:1623–1628.
21. Jackman W, Yeung-Lai-Wah JA, Friday K, Khan A, Sakural M, Lazzara R. Tachycardias originating in accessory pathway networks mimicking atrial flutter and fibrillation (abstract). *J Am Coll Cardiol* 1986;7:6A.
22. Jackman W, Friday K, Yeung-Lai-Wah JA, Aliot E, Lazzara R. Accessory pathways: branching networks and tachycardia (abstract). *Circulation* 1985;72(suppl III):270.
23. Fujimura O, Klein GJ, Yee R, Sharma AD. Mode of onset of atrial fibrillation in the Wolff-Parkinson-White syndrome: how important is the accessory pathway. *J Am Coll Cardiol* 1990;15:1082–1086.
24. Kaseda S, Zipes DP. Contraction-excitation feedback in the atria: a cause of changes in refractoriness. *J Am Coll Cardiol* 1988;11:1327–1336.
25. Klein LS, Miles WM, Zipes DP. Effect of atrioventricular interval during pacing or reciprocating tachycardia on atrial size, pressure and refractory period. Contraction-excitation feedback in human atrium. *Circulation* 1990;82:60–68.

26. Lab MJ. Contraction-excitation feedback in myocardium. *Circ Res* 1982;50:757–766.
27. Leitch JW, Klein GJ, Yee R, Murdock C, Teo WS. Neurally mediated syncope and atrial fibrillation. *N Engl J Med* 1991;324:495–496.
28. Ridker PM, Gibson CM, Lopez R. Atrial fibrillation induced by breath spray (letter). *N Engl J Med* 1989;320:124.
29. Breeden CC, Safirstein BH. Spacer induced atrial fibrillation. *N Engl J Med* 1990;87:113–114.
30. Lamb LE, Pollard LW. Atrial fibrillation in flying personnel. Report of 60 cases. *Circulation* 1964;29:694–701.
31. Thornton JR. Atrial fibrillation in healthy non alcohol people after an alcohol binge. *Lancet* 1984;2:1013–1014.
32. Chugh SN, Jaggal KL, Ram S, Singhal HR, Mahajan SK. Hypomagnesemic atrial fibrillation in a case of aluminium phosphide poisoning (letter). *J Assoc Physicians India* 1989;37: 548–549.
33. Yinnon AM, Rosenmann D, Zion MM. Hypoglycemia: a rare case of atrial fibrillation. *Isr J Med Sci* 1989;25:346–347.
34. Bashour TT, Gualberto A, Ryan C. Atrioventricular block in accidental hypothermia: a case report. *Angiology* 1989;40:63–66.
35. Singer K, Lundberg WB. Ventricular arrhythmias associated with the ingestion of alcohol. *Ann Intern Med* 1972;77:247–248.
36. Brand FN, Abbott RD, Kannel WB, Wolf PA. Characteristics and prognosis of lone atrial fibrillation. Thirty year follow-up in the Framingham study. *JAMA* 1985;254:3449–3453.
37. Ettinger PO, Wu CF, De La Cruz C, Weisse AB, Ahmed SS, Regan TJ. Arrhythmias and the holiday heart: alcohol associated cardiac rhythm disorders. *Am Heart J* 1978;95:555–562.
38. Greenspon AJ, Stang JM, Lewis RP, Schaal SF. Provocation of ventricular tachycardia after consumption of alcohol. *N Engl J Med* 1979;301:1049-1050.
39. Engle TR, Luck JC. Effect of whiskey on atrial vulnerability and holiday heart. *J Am Coll Cardiol* 1983;1:816–818.
40. Gimeno AL, Gimeno MD, Webb JL. Effects of ethanol on cellular membrane potentials and contractility of isolated atrium. *Am J Physiol* 1962;203:194–196.
41. Gould L, Reddy CV, Becker W, Oh KC, Kim SG. Electrophysiologic properties of alcohol in man. *J Electrocardiol* 1978;11:219–226.
42. Brigden W, Robinson J. Alcoholic heart disease. *Br Med J* 1964;2:1283–1289.
43. Burch GE, Colcolough HL, Harb JM, Tsui CY. The effects of ingestion of ethyl alcohol, wine and beer on the myocardium of mice. *Am J Cardiol* 1971;27:522–528.
44. Hibbs RG, Ferrans VJ, Black WC, Weilbaecher DG, Walsh JJ, Burch GE. Alcoholic cardiomyopathy. An electron microscopic study. *Am Heart J* 1965;69:766–779.
45. Koskinen P, Kupari M, Leinonen H. Role of alcohol in recurrence of atrial fibrillation in persons less than 65 years of age. *Am J Cardiol* 1990;66:954–958.
46. Koskinen P, Kupari M, Leinonen H, Luomanmaki K. Alcohol and new onset atrial fibrillation: a case control study of a current series. *Br Heart J* 1987;57:468–473.
47. Lowenstein AJ, Gabow PA, Cramer J, Oliva PB, Ratner K. The role of alcohol in new onset atrial fibrillation. *Arch Intern Med* 1983;143:1882–1885.
48. Rich EC, Siebold C, Campion B. Alcohol related acute atrial fibrillation: a case control study and review of 40 patients. *Arch Intern Med* 1985;145:830–833.
49. Cohen EJ, Klatsky AL, Armstrong MA. Alcohol use and supraventricular arrhythmia. *Am J Cardiol* 1988;62:971–973.
50. Campbell M. The paroxysmal atrial tachycardia. *Lancet* 1947;2:641–647.
51. Forfar JC, Miller HC, Toft AD. Occult thyrotoxicosis: a correctable cause of idiopathic atrial fibrillation. *Am J Cardiol* 1979;44:9–12.
52. Bartels EC. Hyperthyroidism in patients over 65. *Geriatrics* 1965;20:459–462.
53. Scott GR, Forfar JC, Toft AD. Graves disease in atrial fibrillation: the case for even higher doses of therapeutic iodine-131. *Br Med J* 1984;289:399–400.
54. Camm AJ, Evans KE, Ward DE, Martin A. The rhythm of the heart in active elderly subjects. *Am Heart J* 1980;99:598–603.
55. Wosika PH, Feldman E, Chesrow EJ, Myers GB. Unipolar precordial and limb lead electrocardiograms in the aged. *Geriatrics* 1950;5:131–141.
56. Mihalick MJ, Fisch C. Electrocardiographic findings in the aged. *Am Heart J* 1974;87:117–128.
57. Thomas FB, Mazzferri EL, Skillman TK. Apathetic thyrotoxicosis: a distinctive clinical and laboratory entity. *Ann Intern Med* 1970;72:679–685.
58. Campbell AJ. Thyroid disorders in the elderly: difficulties in diagnosis and treatment. *Drugs* 1986;31:455–461.
59. Olsen T, Laurberg P, Week J. Low serum tri-idiothyronine and high serum reverse tri-idiothyroinine: an effect of disease not old age. *J Clin Endocrinol Metab* 1981;53:764–771.
60. Marsden P, Facer P, Acosta M, McKerron CG. Serum tri-iodothyronine in solitary autonomic nodules of the thyroid. *Clin Endocrinol* 1975;4:327–330.

61. Burrow G, Oppenheimer J, Volpe R. In: *Thyroid function and disease*. Philadelphia: WB Saunders, 1989;124–139.
62. Sulimani RA. Diagnostic algorithm for atrial fibrillation caused by occult hyperthyroidism. *Geriatrics* 1989;44:61–69.
63. Forfar JC, Toft AD. Thyrotoxic atrial fibrillation: an underdiagnosed condition. *Br Med J* 1982;285:909–910.
64. Forfar JC, Feek CM, Miller HC, Toft AD. Atrial fibrillation and isolated suppression of the pituitary thyroid axis: response to specific antithyroid therapy. *Int J Cardiol* 1981;1:43–48.
65. Platzer R, Wimpfheimer C, Burgi H. Use of a single TSH after oral thyrotropin releasing hormone: an economical and highly sensitive thyroid screening test. *Acta Endocrinol* 1982;100:369–372.
66. Rohmer V, Hocq F, Galland F, et al. Occult thyrotoxicosis revealed by atrial arrhythmia. *Presse Med* 1984;13:145–148.
67. Davies AB, Williams I, John R, Hall R, Scanlon MF. Diagnostic value of thyrotropin releasing hormone tests in elderly patients with atrial fibrillation. *Br Med J* 1985;291:773–776.
68. Daly JG, Greenwood RM, Helmsworth RL. Thyrotoxic atrial fibrillation (letter). *Br Med J* 1982;285:1574.
69. Fagerberg B, Lindstedt G, Stromblad SO, et al. Thyrotoxic atrial fibrillation: an under diagnosed or over diagnosed condition? *Clin Chem* 1990;36:620–627.
70. Presti CF, Hart RG. Thyrotoxicosis, atrial fibrillation and embolism revisited. *Am Heart J* 1989;117:976–977.
71. Bortin MM, Silvers S, Yohalem SB. Diagnosis of masked hyperthyroidism in cardiac patients with auricular fibrillation. *Am J Med* 1951;11:40–43.
72. Cobbler JL, Williams ME, Greenland P. Thyrotoxicosis in institutionalized elderly patients with atrial fibrillation. *Arch Intern Med* 1984;144:1758–1760.
73. Nakazawa HK, Sakurai K, Hamada M, Momotani N, Ito K. Management of atrial fibrillation in a post thyrotoxic state. *Am J Med* 1982;72:903–906.
74. Iwasaki T, Naka M, Hiramatsu K, et al. Echocardiographic studies on the relationship between atrial fibrillation and atrial enlargement in patients with hyperthyroidism of Graves disease. *Cardiology* 1989;76:10–17.
75. Rose G, Baxter PJ, Reid DD, McCartney P. Prevalence and prognosis of electrocardiographic findings in middle aged men. *Br Heart J* 1978;40:636–643.
76. Hiss RG, Lamb LE. Electrocardiographic findings in 122,043 individuals. *Circulation* 1962; 25:947–962.
77. Kopecky SL, Gersh BJ, McGoon MD, et al. The natural history of lone atrial fibrillation. A population base study over 3 decades. *N Engl J Med* 1987;317:669–674.
78. Evans W, Swann P. Lone auricular fibrillation. *Br Heart J* 1954;16:189–194.
79. Godtfredsen J. *Atrial fibrillation. Etiology, course and prognosis. A follow-up study of 1212 cases.* Copenhagen: Munksgaard, 1975.
80. Mackenzie J. Digitalis. *Heart* 1911;2:273–386.
81. Gossage AM, Hicks JAB. On auricular fibrillation *Q J Med* 1913;6:435–440.
82. Brill IC. Auricular fibrillation with congestive failure and no other evidence of organic heart disease. *Am Heart J* 1937;13:175–182.
83. Wolf PA, Kannel WB, McGee DL, Meeks SL, Bharucha NE, McNamara PM. Duration of atrial fibrillation and imminence of stroke: the Framingham study. *Stroke* 1983;14:664–667.
84. Wolf PA, Dawber TR, Thomas HE Jr, Kannel WB. Epidemiologic assessment of chronic atrial fibrillation and risk of stroke: the Framingham study. *Neurology* 1978;28:973–977.
85. Gajewski J, Singer RB. Mortality in an insured population with atrial fibrillation. *JAMA* 1981;245:1540–1544.
86. Petersen P, Godtfredsen J. Atrial fibrillation—a review of course and prognosis. *Acta Med Scand* 1984;216:5–9.
87. Kerr CR, Chung DC. Atrial fibrillation: fact, controversy and future. *Clin Prog Electrophysiol Pacing* 1985;3:319–337.
88. Ferrer MI. *Sick sinus syndrome*. New York: Futura, 1974.
89. Bjerklund C, Orning OM. An evaluation of DC shock treatment of atrial arrhythmias: immediate results and complications in 437 patients, with longterm results in the first 290 of these. *Acta Med Scand* 1968;184:481–491.
90. Bjerklund C, Orning OM. The efficacy of anticoagulant therapy in preventing embolism related to DC electrical conversion of atrial fibrillation. *Am J Cardiol* 1969;23:208–215.
91. Weinberg DM, Mancini GJB. Anticoagulation for conversion of atrial fibrillation. *Am J Cardiol* 1989;63:745–746.
92. Mancini GBJ, Goldberger AL. Cardioversion of atrial fibrillation: consideration of embolization, anticoagulation, prophylactic pacemaker and longterm success. *Am Heart J* 1982;104:617–621.
93. Feld GK, Chen PS, Nicod P, Fleck RP, Mezer D. Possible atrial proarrhythmic effects of class Ic antiarrhythmic drugs. *Am J Cardiol* 1990;66:378–383.

94. Marcus FI. The hazards of using type 1c antiarrhythmic drugs for the treatment of paroxysmal atrial fibrillation. *Am J Cardiol* 1990;66:366–367.
95. Falk RH. Flecainide induced ventricular tachycardia and fibrillation in patients treated for atrial fibrillation. *Ann Intern Med* 1989;111:107–111.
96. Murdock CJ, Kyles AE, Yeung-Lai-Wah JA, Qi A, Vorderbrugge S, Kerr CR. Atrial flutter in patients treated for atrial fibrillation with propafenone. *Am J Cardiol* 1990;66:755–757.
97. Langbert JJ, Chin MC, Rosenqvist M, et al. Catheter ablation of the atrioventricular junction with radiofrequency energy. *Circulation* 1989;80:1527–1535.
98. Yeung-Lai-Wah JA, Kerr CR, Murdock CJ, Bonet J. Low energy radiofrequency current for AV nodal ablation (abstract). *J Am Coll Cardiol* 1990;15:20A.
99. Roy D, Marchand E, Gagne P, Chabot M, Cartier R. Usefulness of anticoagulation therapy in the prevention of embolic complications of atrial fibrillation. *Am Heart J* 1986;112:1039–1043.
100. Peterson P, Godtfredsen J, Boysen G, Andersen ED, Andersen B. Placebo-controlled, randomized trial of warfarin and aspirin for prevention of thromboembolic complications in chronic atrial fibrillation. *Lancet* 1989;1:175–179.
101. Stroke Prevention in Atrial Fibrillation Study Group Investigators. Preliminary report of the stroke prevention in atrial fibrillation study. *N Engl J Med* 1990;322:863–868.
102. The Boston Area Anticoagulation Trial for Atrial Fibrillation Investigators. The effect of low dose warfarin on the risk of stroke in patients with nonrheumatic atrial fibrillation. *N Engl J Med* 1990;323:1505–1511.
103. Chesebro JH, Fuster V, Halpern JL. Atrial fibrillation—risk marker for stroke. *N Engl J Med* 1990;323:1556–1558.

Atrial Fibrillation: Mechanisms and Management, edited by
R. H. Falk and P. J. Podrid.
Raven Press, Ltd., New York © 1992.

7

Neural Aspects of Paroxysmal Atrial Fibrillation

Philippe Coumel

Department of Cardiology, Hôpital Lariboisière, 75010 Paris, France

Atrial fibrillation (AF), a common arrhythmia, is a convenient model for investigating the relationship between rhythm disturbances and the autonomic nervous system. Experimental data in animal models are abundant, and the clinical correlates of the arrhythmia can be easily studied in humans. In humans, the mode of onset of fibrillation can be observed repeatedly without serious hemodynamic consequences, and, because of the relatively benign nature of the arrhythmia, therapeutic failures or mistakes are tolerable. A reliable image of the vagosympathetic balance is provided by analysis of the rate and behavior of the prevailing sinus rhythm, which can be analyzed both by cycle-to-cycle dynamic variations and by observations of longer heart rate trends. Since experimental models of AF probably share many features with the arrhythmia observed in humans, conclusions derived from laboratory data can be helpful in understanding mechanisms of spontaneous paroxysmal AF.

CONSIDERATIONS FROM EXPERIMENTAL STUDIES

The conditions necessary to produce AF include a critical mass of tissue (1,2), a relatively short atrial refractory period, and heterogeneity of refractoriness (3,4). While in diseased atria, the associated depression of conduction plays a major role, in the experimental, undiseased animal model of AF, arrhythmia sustenance is closely related to refractory period shortening and nonuniformity, and AF terminates as soon as provoking maneuvers are discontinued. Many agents have an effect on atrial tissue. For example, isoproterenol produces shortening of the action potential and a slow response in potassium depolarized fibers. The membrane effects of muscarinic agonists are more complex (5), and their action is dependent on the underlying milieu. Thus, acetylcholine seems to play a protective role when the profibrillatory milieu is produced by isoproterenol or glucagon (agents that increase cyclic AMP levels in myocardial fibers), but not when it is produced by dibutyryl cyclic AMP, ouabain, or electrical stimulation (6).

Vagosympathetic interactions are complex, and, although at the atrial level both limbs of the autonomic nervous system shorten the action potential (7), they do not modify the intra-atrial conduction in the same way. Vagosympathetic interactions may occur in at least two sites: the first at nerve endings where cholinergic control of neuronal release of norepinephrine is thought to be mediated by presynaptic muscarinic receptors located in the membranes of postganglionic sympathetic terminals and the second at the target organ's membrane receptor. The autonomic nervous system produces effects on intra-atrial conduction, but its effect on producing inhomogeneity of atrial conduction is a crucial factor in the provocation of arrhythmia. The mechanism of production of this inhomogeneity is not exactly clear, but evidence suggests that it may result either from the nonuniformity of the anatomic distribution of nerve endings (4) or from a temporal inhomogeneity of stimulation.

Sympathetic and parasympathetic terminals lie in close proximity to one another and both are close to the target cells. However, they do not have an identical distribution. Stimulation of the sympathetic system may affect vagal function and vice versa. For example, acetylcholine released from vagal nerve endings diminishes norepinephrine release from neighboring sympathetic nerve endings (8). The functional responses to cholinergic stimulation occur within a few milliseconds, while those to adrenergic stimulation require seconds for target activation (9). This temporal difference has important clinical implications for heart rate variability as discussed below.

Other factors, extrinsic to the autonomic nervous system, can play a role in arrhythmogenesis. Thus, in diseased atria the nonuniform state of the diseased cells may independently precipitate AF. Digitalis therapy illustrates the complexity of a single factor: its effect depends not only on the dose used, but also on the state of the atrial cell and on the catecholamine storage. Hordof et al. (10) showed that in normal human atrial cells, low doses of ouabain (like acetylcholine) induce an increase in maximal diastolic potential, action potential amplitude, and upstroke velocity of phase-0 depolarization, as well as a decrease in the action potential duration and automaticity. These effects are blocked by atropine. However, large doses of ouabain result in an opposite effect on maximal diastolic potential, action potential amplitude, and upstroke velocity and provoke a further decrease in the action potential duration and an increase in phase-4 depolarization and spontaneous rate, and cause delayed afterdepolarizations. In addition, the direct effects of ouabain are more rapidly obtained in diseased than in normal cells. A further factor to consider is that chronic digoxin therapy in the neurally intact heart has significant vagally mediated effects. Thus, the complexity of pharmacological actions of digoxin and other drugs can explain both the favorable and deleterious effects that may be observed in patients with atrial arrhythmias (11).

AF starts with a period of rapid ectopic activity that may be caused by reentry, discharge of an automatic focus, or afterpotentials. In the setting of an enhanced catecholamine state, the two latter mechanisms may be responsible for triggering AF, but they probably do not play a role in vagally mediated AF. Vagal stimulation has long been known to aid in the provocation of experimental AF (12,13). Such stimulation causes hyperpolarization in atrial fibers, an effect that does not favor either pacemaker activity (14) or delayed afterdepolarizations (15). Since the refractory period of atrial fibers subject to strong vagal activity may actually be shorter than the duration of the P wave, the time required to excite the whole chamber can be greater than the refractory period of individual fibers, allowing for the development of reentry. Thus, vagally mediated AF appears to be precipitated by a reentrant mechanism. This hypothesis is strengthened by the observation that typical atrial flutter, which is clearly a reentrant arrhythmia, can be provoked by vagal stimulation. In addition, vagally induced sinus node reentry can be demonstrated in experimental preparations (16). It is recognized that rapid stimulation as well as pauses or bradycardia may favor reentry circuits, by either modification of conduction speed and refractoriness, or by the development of enhanced afterpotentials (15). Thus, the intrinsic sinus rate is, in some patients, an important precursor for the development of paroxysmal AF (17).

Although the above mechanisms can be demonstrated in experimental preparations, it is not possible to clearly define the mechanisms of AF induction in humans even when precise invasive investigation is performed. However, pharmacological interventions in humans that affect the autonomic nervous system confirm observations made in animal models, as illustrated in Figs. 1–3. Figure 1 illustrates a patient with a history of paroxysmal AF who presented with numerous atrial premature beats demonstrating the behavior of enhanced automaticity (i.e., variable morphology and coupling intervals and nonsustained repetitive activity). Isoproterenol dramatically increased these manifestations and provoked short runs of AF. Figure 2 demonstrates the effect of a bolus of adenosine in another patient—an intervention that reproduces strong vagal stimulation. A sudden atrial tachycardia with a very high rate (500/min) is provoked, reflecting the dramatic shortening of the refractory period. Figure 3 also shows the destabilizing effect of adenosine in a stable atrial tachycardia: the local electrical activity becomes much faster and irregular at the same time as the vagal effect on atrioventricular conduction is most apparent.

CLINICAL CONSIDERATIONS

Few authors have studied the precursors of spontaneously occurring AF (18,19). While some features, in some patients, indicate the role of an increased sympathetic drive, other features suggest that the vagus nerve may play a central role. In studying patients with frequent paroxysmal attacks of AF, we found that not only do disturbances of the autonomic nervous system clearly play a role but that two opposite mechanisms can be identified (vagal and sympathetic), which often interact (20–22).

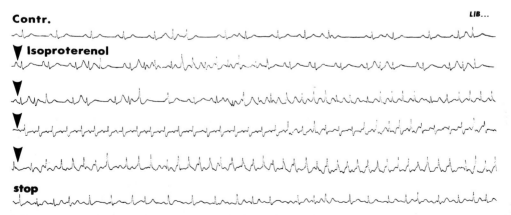

FIG. 1. Provocation of atrial fibrillation (AF) by isoproterenol. In a patient with a history of paroxysmal AF and frequent atrial premature beats, isoproterenol infusion rapidly increases the frequency of potential automatic foci and provokes AF.

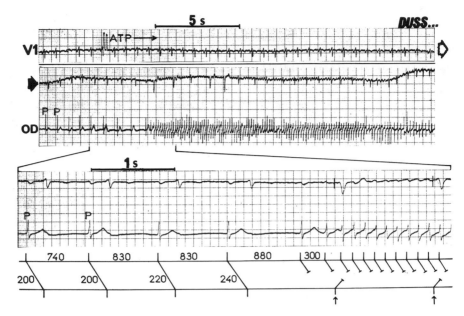

FIG. 2. Induction of atrial fibrillation (AF) by adenosine. *Top traces:* Continuous lead V1 with associated right atrial (OD) recordings after the injection of adenosine triphosphate (ATP). Note the slowing of sinus rate immediately preceding the onset of AF, indicating the vagal effect of the drug. *Bottom traces:* Expanded view of onset of AF, with ladder diagram (numbers in milliseconds). The last two beats are ventricular escape beats.

The patterns of pure vagal and adrenergic paroxysmal AF are rather easy to distinguish provided one closely examines the clinical history and pays attention to the heart rate changes occurring in the period preceding the onset of the arrhythmia. Unfortunately, the separation of the two modes of initiation of AF in an individual patient may be less clear-cut, particularly in subjects with very frequent paroxysms. In such cases, a complex interplay between vagal and sympathetic influences presides over the onset of AF. Sinus node behavior is used as an indication of the state of the autonomic nervous system, but it may not reliably reflect the status of autonomic activity at other levels in the heart. Thus, the effects of the autonomic nervous system on the sinoatrial node may be discrepant with simultaneous effects on the atrium, atrioventricular node, and ventricle (23). However, even though some discrepancies in response have been demonstrated, one may assume that atrial tissues undergo equivalent influences from the autonomic nervous system in terms of timing, and, despite its limitations, monitoring the heart rate remains the easiest way to obtain important, albeit indirect, information about the variation in autonomic tone.

Examination of the mean heart rate cannot provide an exact, complete, and precise image of the vagosympathetic balance throughout the atria since humoral adrenergic stimulation will also have an effect. While humoral adrenergic activity can, in part, be assessed by plasma catecholamine measurement, the neurogenic vagal and sympathetic drives can be only explored in terms of heart rate variability. Classical physiologic studies have demonstrated that the respiratory variations of the RR cycles form oscillations over a few seconds, whereas longer oscillations (more than 10–15 sec) form the classical Mayer waves resulting from sympathetic modulation

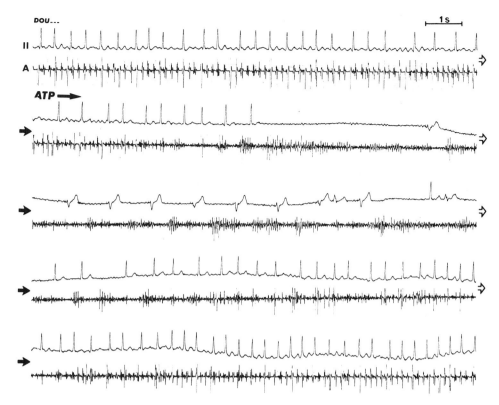

FIG. 3. Effect of adenosine on atrial flutter (continuous surface and intra-atrial recording). In a patient with a known vagal atrial arrhythmia but stable atrial flutter at the time of examination, adenosine destabilizes the flutter into fibrillation. The pattern of fibrillation in the atrium precisely coincides in time with the impairment of the atrioventricular conduction due to the vagal effect of adenosine triphosphate.

(Fig. 4). Several techniques have been proposed to approach this variability. The power spectral analysis using fast Fourier transformation is a classical one and can be used in the frequency domain to isolate high- and low-frequency peaks corresponding to the shorter and longer oscillations. We chose to develop an approach that is better adapted to studying heart rate variability in the time domain, based on the evaluation of the number and the amplitude of the RR cycle oscillations of a preselected "wavelength" (24). Its modalities and application will be described below in individual cases.

Atrial Flutter and Fibrillation of Vagal Origin

Our vast experience with these patients has confirmed our original observation of the syndrome (21). Vagally mediated AF occurs more frequently in men than women with a ratio of about 4:1. The age at which the first symptoms appear is classically between 40 and 50 years, with a range of 25 to 60 years. The clinical history may range from 2 to 10 years, but cases with paroxysms for 15 to 20 years have been seen. A remarkable pattern of the syndrome is the lack of tendency toward permanent AF.

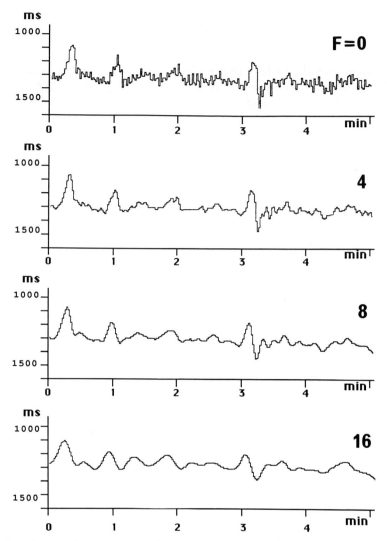

FIG. 4. Various types of heart rate oscillations. Short, respiration-induced heart rate oscillations in sinus rhythm are the result of vagal influences on the sinus node automaticity. They are clearly visible on the beat-by-beat tachograms directly derived from the Holter tracings (*top trace*). A filtering process (F) by averaging the RR intervals over 4, 8, 16 cycles (*bottom three traces*) artificially suppresses these short-term oscillations of the heart rate, thus exposing longer and longer oscillations due to sympathetic influences of neurogenic and humoral origin.

In all cases the arrhythmia is idiopathic and thus can be classified as a form of lone AF. The number of the attacks varies from patient to patient, and it may take from 2 to 15 years for infrequent episodes to develop into daily attacks. The most common pattern is that of weekly episodes, lasting from a few minutes to several hours. The essential feature is the occurrence of the AF at night, often ending in the morning. Rest, the postprandial state (particularly after dinner), and alcohol are also precipitating factors. Neither physical exertion nor emotional stress triggers the arrhythmia. On the contrary, on feeling the sensation of an impending arrhythmia (frequent atrial extrasystoles), many patients observe that they could prevent it by exercising. However, the relaxed period that *follows* effort or emotional stress frequently coincides with the onset of AF.

Figure 5 illustrates the history of a patient who systematically noted the hour of onset of his symptoms over a period of 16 years. During this period (1963–1979) he had a total of 1,128 attacks and three peaks are clearly visible. The first one (at 7 A.M.) corresponds with the attacks having started at night, usually terminating shortly after awakening. The two others correspond with lunch and dinner, which the patient took very regularly at noon and 7 P.M. The number of attacks decreased in the afternoon, but the most important feature is that only very few started during the morning activity.

Vagally induced atrial arrhythmia typically consists of a mixed picture of atrial flutter and fibrillation. The deterioration of typical atrial flutter into AF is a rather common feature. This again suggests a vagal mechanism as it is associated with an acceleration of the intrinsic flutter rate due to the vagally induced shortening of the atrial refractory period (Fig. 6) (25). A typical feature of these patients is to have the reverse pattern, i.e., AF converting into typical flutter, but the apparently different features on the surface ECG may correspond, in endocavitary tracings, to slight rate changes of a rapid and regular atrial activity. The arrhythmia is typically preceded

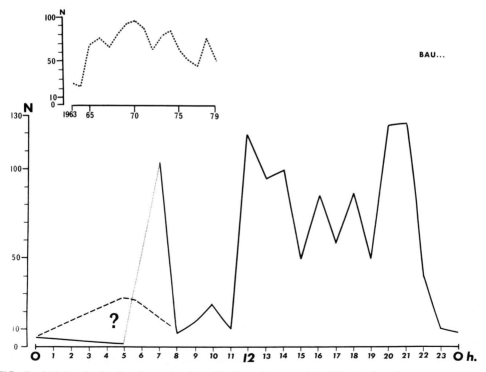

FIG. 5. Atrial arrhythmia of vagal origin. Timing of onset of 1,128 attacks of paroxysmal atrial flutter and fibrillation over 17 years in the same patient. The *upper panel* shows the number (N) of attacks per year from 1963 to 1979. The *lower panel* displays their timing during the 24-hr period, with three peaks: before 7 A.M. (i.e., during sleep), between noon and 2 P.M., and between 7 and 10 P.M.

by a progressive, mild bradycardia (55–60/min), reflecting the predominance of the vagal drive, and the onset of AF is often immediately preceded by a further lengthening of the sinus cycle (Fig. 6). Vagal maneuvers or administration of vagotonic drugs may artificially reproduce this process. We have never observed sinus node dysfunction in these patients, even after years of progression of the disease. Thus, the syndrome of vagal atrial arrhythmia should be clearly distinguished from the bradycardia-tachycardia syndrome or from the sick sinus syndrome, even though atrial pacing may have a favorable effect in both disorders.

Heart Rate Variability Analysis

Our experience with the evaluation of heart rate variability has allowed us to further document the vagal mechanism of paroxysmal AF. Heart rate variability is analyzed from a 24-hr Holter monitor interfaced with minicomputer utilizing a specially designed program. The duration of sequences to be analyzed can be preset to any required length, and the computer analyzes each RR interval, seeking trends of heart rate acceleration or deceleration in the preceding or subsequent beats. Artifact or atrial premature beats are excluded by setting an upper limit for changes in RR in-

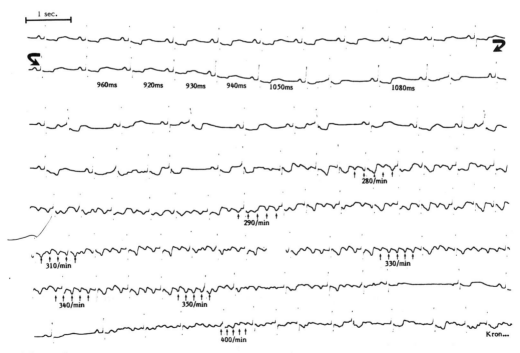

FIG. 6. Onset of atrial flutter, degenerating into atrial fibrillation (AF). Isolated atrial premature beats are preceded by longer and longer sinus cycle lengths due to an increased vagal drive. Atrial flutter initially begins with an atrial rate of 280 beats/min, but the continuing vagal influence is responsible for its acceleration to 350 to 400 beats/min with subsequent transformation into AF (*bottom two tracings*).

tervals, and insignificant changes are indicated by a gradient of less than 40 msec (the term "gradient" refers to the difference between the longest and shortest cycle in a given oscillation). The product of the gradient (in milliseconds) and the number of oscillations per minute can be expressed in milliseconds per minute and provides a global quantification of the heart rate variability. Figure 7A and B displays the pattern of a 1-hr period in terms of heart rate variability. In Fig. 7A, segments numbered 1 to 6 represent 2- to 3-min periods displayed on a beat-by-beat basis so that the variations in the short oscillations can be demonstrated. In panel 1 (between 23.30 and 23.35 hr), the rate is less than 60 beats per minute, but the number of short oscillations is limited. In contrast, panel 6 (00.18 hr) shows a striking difference: although the mean heart rate is clearly higher than 60 beats per minute, the number and amplitude of oscillations are at their maximum during this period, which terminates with the onset of AF. This acute vagal drive actually starts in the preceding 3 min, as represented in panel 5. The initial period of panel 5 is characterized by a sudden acceleration of heart rate lasting 2 min. Because of the absence of "long" oscillations within this acceleration, it is interpreted as an adrenergic discharge of humoral origin. The last 3 min of short oscillations probably represent the vagal response to this humoral stimulus and precipitates AF. Such a phenomenon is, in fact, very frequent. In the lower panel of Fig. 7B, the whole 1-hr period is represented diagrammatically in terms of the product of gradient and oscillation duration for every 2½-min period. The sharp increase in the short oscillations is well illustrated just before the onset of AF. The peak of vagal activity responsible for the AF is very transient and reaches a value of 500 msec/min, which was four to five times the usual value for this patient.

Adrenergic Atrial Tachyarrhythmias

Not all patients suffering from paroxysmal attacks of AF have a history compatible with classical vagally provoked arrhythmia. In such cases analysis of Holter recordings may show an opposite heart rate trend suggesting that the arrhythmia depends on sympathetic tone rather than on the vagal drive. Adrenergically induced arrhythmias are much less frequently observed than those produced by vagal mechanisms, and they may occasionally be associated with disorders such as hyperthyroidism, pheochromocytoma, or primary myocardial disease. The palpitations occur primarily or exclusively during the day, particularly in the morning, during exercise, or with emotional stress, and are frequently accompanied by polyuria. The ECG findings may consist of typical AF, but frequently, at least in the early manifestations of the disease, it consists of runs of atrial tachycardia alternating with sinus rhythm, without any episodes of classical atrial flutter. Typically, the onset of arrhythmia occurs at a specific heart rate, which is gradually attained and can be well documented by the rate trend analysis of the Holter recording. The increasing sinus rate to a value of about 90 beats per minute in these patients contrasts strikingly with the decreasing sinus rate down to 55 to 60 beats per minute in patients with vagal arrhythmias. Usually, the arrhythmia can be reproduced by administering beta-adrenergic agonists (Fig. 1).

The most obvious evidence of adrenergic stimulation in this arrhythmia is the typical pattern of AF occurring after a rapid sinus acceleration, e.g., during exercise

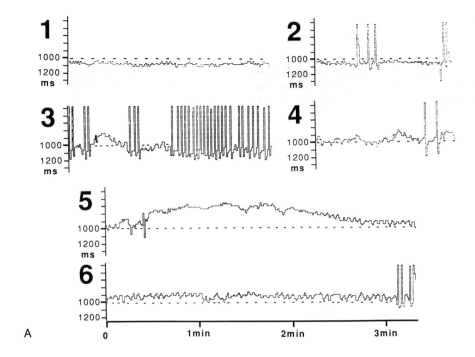

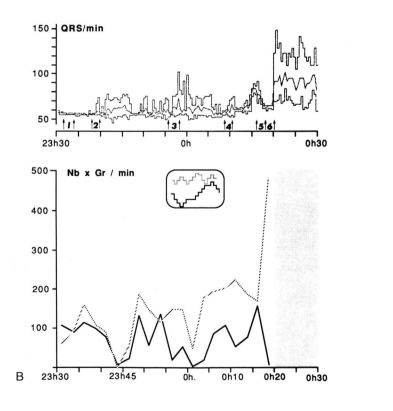

(20,22). However, we deliberately chose not to show the typical pattern, but rather we illustrate a case that was difficult to analyze (Fig. 8A). In this patient there were no apparent circumstances surrounding arrhythmia occurrence except its predominant onset in the morning, a feature that practically excluded vagally mediated AF. The trends visible in Fig. 8A show that the AF occurring at 12:30 P.M.. is preceded by a dramatic sinus acceleration. The heart rate variability analysis further confirms the predominance of long, sympathetically mediated oscillations, and Fig. 8B confirms this pattern. No respiration-related oscillations are visible, suggesting humoral mechanisms. Eventually hyperthyroidism was diagnosed in this patient, the initial manifestation of which had been the paroxysmal AF in the absence of other clinical manifestations.

Mixed Picture of Vagal and Adrenergic Atrial Fibrillation

Figure 9 shows that the distinction between the two mechanisms is not always clear-cut and that autonomic imbalance is probably more important than vagal or sympathetic drive alone. The tracings were recorded from a 34-year-old athletic patient whose history was typical of vagal AF. As the paroxysms were rather infrequent, it was initially impossible to record either their onset or the several hours of sinus rhythm preceding the arrhythmia. Since in our experience of mixed arrhythmia it is rather common to observe that the more strenuous the daytime physical activity, the more likely the attack will occur at night, we applied a Holter recording the day that the patient participated in a 20-km walk (Fig. 9, rhythm a). At the end of the competition, the predominant vagal effect on the atrioventricular node following the intense exercise was apparent since there were several blocked P waves, despite a persistent sinus tachycardia (rhythm b). AF started in the evening of the same day (rhythm c), and it was briefly preceded by a sinus rate that was relatively slow in comparison to the previous rapid sinus rate.

FIG. 7. A: Cycle-by-cycle analysis of heart rate variation. Panels 1 to 6 represent 2-min beat-by-beat tachograms, the heart rate variability of which is quantified in terms of maximal, minimal, and mean heart rates (**B**). There are characteristic patterns to the oscillations. In panel 1 the mean heart rate is slow and regular, without large beat-to-beat variations. Atrial premature beats are present in panels 2 and 3: their presence explains the pattern of the maximal and minimal heart rate trends in the upper diagram of **B** (segments 2 and 3) and prevents the oscillations from being quantified. Panel 4 shows a few large oscillations and panel 5 shows a prolonged acceleration probably related to an adrenergic stimulation of humoral origin. It is immediately followed in panel 6 by a strong vagal reaction responsible for characteristic numerous and ample short oscillations that terminate with the onset of atrial fibrillation (AF). For further details see text. **B:** Heart rate variability analysis of the last hour preceding AF. The *upper panel* shows the maximal, minimal, and mean heart rate trends for a 1-hr period. Segments 1 to 6 correspond to the beat-to-beat tachograms illustrated in A. In the *lower panel,* the "product" (number of oscillations per minute × amplitude) has been determined for each 2½-min period of the 1-hr recording. The *broken* and *solid lines* represent the product of the shorter (vagal) and longer (adrenergic) oscillations, respectively. The inset is simply a schematic representation of the time course of short and long oscillations and is not derived from this patient's data. The dramatic increase in short, vagally dependent oscillations is clearly visible in the period immediately preceding the arrhythmia. For further details see text. Nb, number; Gr, gradient of heart rate oscillations.

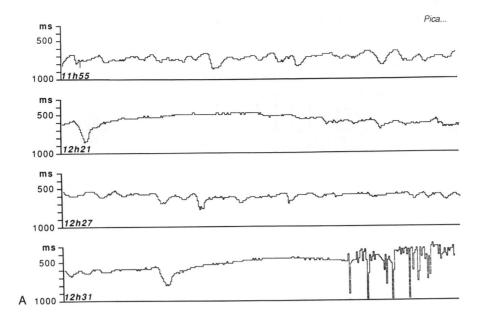

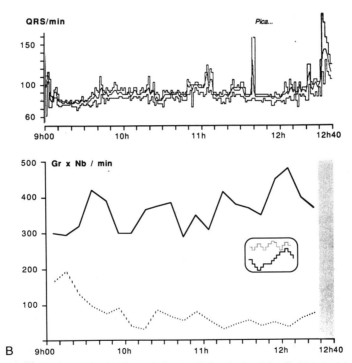

FIG. 8. **A:** Adrenergic atrial fibrillation. Samples of beat-to-beat tachograms of about 3 min each in the hour preceding the onset of AF show the absence of short-term heart rate oscillations reflecting the vagal influences. The sympathetic modulation of neurogenic origin in the form of long oscillations over 10 to 20 beats is clearly visible. From time to time, they are overwhelmed by long accelerations resulting from humoral influences. They finally culminate with the onset of AF. **B:** Heart rate variability and adrenergic paroxysmal atrial fibrillation (AF) (same patient). Heart rate oscillations of shorter and longer wavelengths have been quantified in the same way as in Fig. 7B. The pattern, however, is totally different from the patient illustrated in Fig. 7 with an almost invisible vagal activity and a clearly exaggerated adrenergic activity finally responsible for the paroxysmal attack of AF. Abbreviations as in Fig. 7.

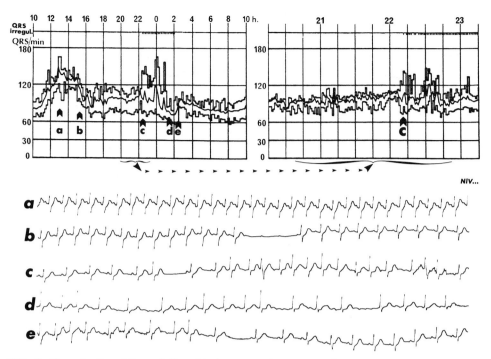

FIG. 9. Complexity of the relationship between the autonomic nervous system balance and atrial fibrillation (AF). **Top:** Computerized analysis of Holter recordings during 24 (on the left) and 3 hr (on the right) (note different scales). The irregular ventricular response is detected by the computer and indicated by the small vertical bars in the upper part of the diagram between 22 and 2 h. **Bottom:** Tracings a–e correspond to the letters on the diagrams above. They show the sinus tachycardia during the prolonged exercise (a), the strong vagal reaction with several dropped P waves when the effort is discontinued (b), the onset (c) of AF shortly after 10 P.M. preceded on a short-term basis by the slowed sinus rate, the continuation of the arrhythmia (d), and its termination (e).

THERAPEUTIC CONSIDERATIONS

Not surprisingly, beta-blocking drugs are unsuccessful in treating most cases of paroxysmal AF. Patients with vagal AF may have the number of their attacks increased by either beta-blockers or digoxin, and they may tolerate these drugs very poorly when in sinus rhythm. In only a very few anecdotal cases have patients benefited from beta-blockers: such patients tend to be those with a mixed picture of vagosympathetic imbalance (like the case just described) in whom the nocturnal attacks were clearly preceded by an intense physical activity during the day and a subsequent "vagal rebound" mechanism. In these cases the beneficial effect of beta-blockers is most often seen with small doses of relatively weak compounds, preferably one having some intrinsic adrenergic activity such as a single morning dose of 100 or 200 mg of acebutolol. In contrast, patients with adrenergic-dependent AF need a stronger degree of beta-blockade: in our experience the long-acting agent nadolol appears far more effective than the other beta-blockers (22). However, a curious escape phenomenon is observed in about two-thirds of cases. After spectacular efficacy during the initial 3 to 6 weeks, attacks of AF recur with a less typical pattern of diurnal, exertional, or emotional palpitations. In such cases it becomes necessary to add other antiarrhythmics, which may have previously been ineffective when used alone, such as type 1A or 1C drugs.

Type 1A drugs like disopyramide or quinidine have a well-known vagolytic effect that may, at least in part, be the explanation of their activity in the treatment of paroxysmal AF. As far as type 1C drugs are concerned, it is our experience that flecainide and propafenone have a clearly different effect on paroxysmal AF. Flecainide is much more active than propafenone every time a vagal mechanism is involved, possibly because it may have some vagolytic action in addition to its direct antiarrhythmic effect (26). The case illustrated in Fig. 10 is suggestive of such an action. Interestingly, we have noted the development of hypertension in about 10% of patients treated with flecainide—an observation we believe is related to unopposed sympathetic tone in susceptible subjects. In contrast to flecainide, the beta-inhibitory action of propafenone is deleterious in vagal AF but is often effective when adrenergic-precipitating factors are present (27). The effects of amiodarone are more complex. Amiodarone has a mild beta-inhibitory effect but is active in vagally induced AF. This is possibly due to a direct atrial effect that prevents the dramatic shortening of the action potential induced by vagal stimulation. In contrast, propafenone does not manifest this electrophysiologic property. In some cases, the beta-inhibitory and/or negative chronotropic effects of amiodarone are prominent and may produce a significant sinus bradycardia, which aggravates the tendency for AF to occur. In such a situation the implantation of an atrial pacemaker in combination with amiodarone may alleviate the paroxysms of AF.

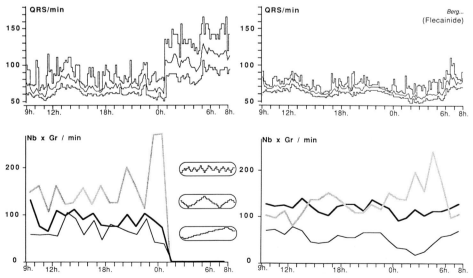

FIG. 10. Antiarrhythmic and vagolytic action of flecainide. **Left:** The vagal mechanism of atrial fibrillation in this patient is shown: the attack that occurs at night is preceded by 2 hr of a large predominance of short, vagally mediated heart rate oscillation (*shaded lines*) over the longer ones. **Right:** The same patient treated with flecainide. The balance of the heart rate oscillations (hence probably of the autonomic nervous system itself) has been changed, with a much less marked evidence of vagal tone and an increased sympathetic activity.

We first reported the favorable effect of atrial pacing in the prevention of resistant paroxysmal AF several years ago (28), and subsequent experience has confirmed our original observations. Again, we stress that these patients do not have evidence of sick sinus syndrome or post-tachycardia sinus arrest. Rather, atrial pacing is performed to maintain the atrium at a critical rate above which arrhythmia control is easier. Figure 11 demonstrates the results of atrial pacing in a patient who previously had paroxysmal AF that could be reproducibly produced by adenosine. Following pacing adenosine had no proarrhythmic effect.

SUMMARY AND CONCLUSION

Experimental AF in animals has long been produced by manipulation of the autonomic nervous system and our observations indicate that in a subgroup of patients autonomic factors play a critical role. In our experience, vagal arrhythmias are far more frequent than adrenergic AF in undiseased hearts, and remarkably, we have never observed evidence of vagally induced arrhythmias in diseased atria. However, our failure to observe this phenomenon in diseased atria does not mean that it will not occasionally occur. Some patients with paroxysmal AF may be difficult to classify, and Holter recordings often show that the adrenergic stimulation may be the best way to provoke the "rebound" vagal reaction that can precipitate AF.

There is no evidence that the autonomic nervous system is fundamentally abnormal in patients with autonomically triggered AF, although vagal arrhythmias are predominantly observed in people displaying vagal hypertonicity (such as athletes and

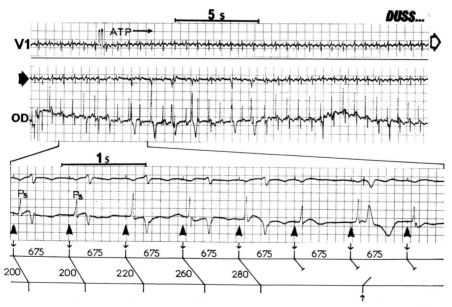

FIG. 11. Preventive effect of atrial pacing in vagal arrhythmia. In the patient illustrated in Fig. 2 in whom atrial fibrillation was consistently induced by adenosine triphosphate (ATP), atrial pacing of 89/min prevents the arrhythmia, although the evidence of the vagal effect is still clear from its effect on the atrioventricular conduction. (Note blocked paced beats in lower tracing.)

patients with digestive problems) and adrenergic arrhythmias most commonly occur in circumstances associated with a hyperadrenergic state. In favor of the concept that the disorder is primarily an electrical abnormality of the atrium that is exposed by autonomic stimuli is the observation that, on long-term follow-up, sustained "lone" AF may occur. This suggests that the preceding paroxysms of AF were triggered by autonomic mechanisms but required an abnormal electrophysiologic substrate.

Studying the relationship between the vagosympathetic balance and atrial tachyarrhythmias necessitates a complex analysis of heart rate variability. This tool is very promising and observations of variability can predict the clinical outcome of therapeutic intervention. Careful analysis of heart rate variability in a patient with paroxysmal AF may not only aid in the appropriate use and prevent the misuse of beta-blockers but also can indicate which patients may benefit from atrial pacing. The necessity for atrial pacing in some resistant cases of paroxysmal AF does not lessen the importance of the autonomic nervous system as a triggering factor but merely underscores the complexity of these patients and the need to carefully individualize their treatment.

REFERENCES

1. Moe GK, Rheinboldt WC, Abildskov JA. A mathematical model of atrial fibrillation. *Am Heart J* 1964;67:200–207.
2. West TC, Landa JF. Minimal mass required for induction of a sustained arrhythmia in isolated atrial segments. *Am J Physiol* 1962;202:232–236.
3. Allessi R, Nusynowitz M, Abildskov JA, Moe GK. Nonuniform distribution of vagal effects on the atrial refractory period. *Am J Physiol* 1958;194:406–410.
4. Ninomyia I. Direct evidence of nonuniform distribution of vagal effects on dog atria. *Circ Res* 1966;19:576–583.
5. Hewett KW. Membrane effects of muscarinic agonists. In: Rosen MR, Janse MJ, Wit AL, eds. *Cardiac electrophysiology*. Mount Kisco, NY: Futura, 1990;877–888.
6. Watanabe AM, Bailey JC, Lathrop D, Besch HR Jr. Acetylcholine antagonism of the cellular electrophysiologic effects of isoproterenol. In: Schartz PJ, Brown AM, Malliani A, Zanchetti A, eds. *Neural mechanisms in cardiac arrhythmias*. New York: Raven Press, 1978;349–358.
7. Hutter OF, Trautwein W. Vagal and sympathetic effects on the pacemaker fibers in the sinus venosus of the heart. *J Gen Physiol* 1956;39:715–732.
8. Levy MN. Autonomic interactions in cardiac control. In: Coumel P, Garfein OB, eds. *Electrocardiography: past and future*. 1990;209–221.
9. Randall WC. Sympathetic modulation of normal cardiac rhythm. In: Rosen MR, Janse MJ, Wit AL, eds. *Cardiac electrophysiology*. Mount Kisco, NY: Futura 1990;889–901.
10. Hordof AJ, Spotnitz A, Mary-Rabine L, Edie RN, Rosen MR. The cellular electrophysiologic effects of digitalis on human atrial fibers. *Circulation* 1978;57:223–229.
11. Allessie MA, Bonke FIM, Lammers WJEP. The effects of carbamylcholine, adrenaline, ouabain, quinidine and verapamil on circus movement tachycardia in isolated segments of rabbit atrial myocardium. In: Kulbertus H, ed. *Reentrant arrhythmias*. Lancaster: MTPress, 1977;63.
12. Lewis T, Drury AN, Bulger HA. Observations upon flutter and fibrillation. Part VII: the effect of vagal stimulation. *Heart* 1921;8:141–169.
13. Nahum LH, Hoff HE. Production of auricular fibrillation by application of acetyl-beta-methylcholine chloride to localized region of the auricular surface. *Am J Physiol* 1940;129:428–436.
14. Loeb JM, Moran JM. Autonomic interactions among subsidiary foci. *Am J Cardiol* 1981;48:690–697.
15. Cranefield PF. *The conduction of the cardiac impulse*. Mount Kisco, NY: Futura, 1975.
16. Spear JF, Moore EN. Patterns of atrial responses following vagally induced reentry in the isolated sinus node of the rabbit. In: Schwartz PJ, Brown AM, Malliani A, Zanchetti A, eds. *Neural mechanisms in cardiac arrhythmias*. New York: Raven Press, 1978;167–178.
17. Nadeau RA, Roberge FA, Billette J. Role of the sinus node in the mechanism of cholinergic atrial fibrillation. *Circ Res* 1970;27:129–138.
18. Killip T, Gault JH. Mode of onset of atrial fibrillation in man. *Am Heart J* 1965;70:172–179.

19. Bennett MA, Pentecost BL. The pattern of onset and spontaneous cessation of atrial fibrillation in man. *Circulation* 1970;41:981–988.

20. Coumel P. Atrial fibrillation. In: Surawicz B, Pratap Reddy C, Prystowsky EN, eds. *Tachycardias*. Boston: Martinus Nijhoff, 1984;231–244.

21. Coumel P, Attuel P, Lavallée JP, Flammang D, Leclercq JF, Slama R. Syndrome d'arythmie auriculaire d'origine vagale. *Arch Mal Coeur* 1978;71:645–656.

22. Coumel P, Escoubet B, Attuel P. Beta-blocking therapy in atrial and ventricular tachyarrhythmias: experience with nadolol. *Am Heart J* 1984;108:1098–1108.

23. Inoue H, Zipes DP. Effects of simultaneous vagal and sympathetic stimulation on spontaneous sinus cycle length, atrial and ventricular refractoriness and atrioventricular nodal conduction. In: Brugada P, Wellens HJJ, eds. *Cardiac arrhythmias: where to go from here?* Mount Kisco, NY: Futura, 1987;209–218.

24. Coumel P, Hermida JS, Leenhardt A, et al. Heart rate variability in myocardial hypertrophy and heart failure, and the effects of beta-blocking therapy. A non-spectral analysis of heart rate oscillations. *Eur Heart J* 1991;12:612–622.

25. Allessie MA, Lammers WJEP, Rensma PL, Bonke FIM. Flutter and fibrillation in experimental models: what has been learned that can be applied to humans? In: Brugada P, Wellens HJJ, eds. *Cardiac arrhythmias: where to go from here?* Mount Kisco, NY: Futura, 1987;67–82.

26. Alboni P, Paparella N, Cappato R, Candini GC. Direct and autonomically mediated effects of oral flecainide. *Am J Cardiol* 1988;61:759–763.

27. Coumel P, Leclercq JF, Assayag P. European experience with the antiarrhythmic efficacy of propafenone for supraventricular and ventricular arrhythmias. *Am J Cardiol* 1984;54:D60–D66.

28. Coumel P, Friocourt P, Mugica J, Attuel P, Leclercq JF. Long-term prevention of vagal arrhythmias by atrial pacing at 90/mn. Experience with 6 cases. *PACE* 1983;6:552–560.

Atrial Fibrillation: Mechanisms and Management, edited by
R. H. Falk and P. J. Podrid.
Raven Press, Ltd., New York © 1992.

8

Atrial Fibrillation Following Cardiac Surgery

*Michael S. Lauer and †Kim A. Eagle

*Section of Cardiology, Lahey Clinic Medical Center, Burlington, Massachusetts 01805;
†Cardiac Unit, Massachusetts General Hospital, Boston, Massachusetts 02114*

Atrial fibrillation is one of the most common postoperative complications of cardiac surgery, including both valvular (1–4) and coronary artery bypass surgery (CABG) (1,6–23). Atrial fibrillation after CABG (6) has been studied more extensively than after other types of cardiac surgery. This chapter will address the epidemiology, pathogenesis, diagnosis, treatment, prevention, and complications of atrial fibrillation following cardiac surgery with particular attention to post-CABG atrial fibrillation.

EPIDEMIOLOGY

Studies of patients undergoing CABG have shown that postoperative atrial fibrillation has an incidence of 5% to 40% (1,8–23). An early prospective review of post-CABG arrhythmias was reported from the Texas Heart Institute in 1974 (6). The most common arrhythmias following CABG were ventricular premature beats with a small proportion of patients having ventricular tachycardia and ventricular fibrillation; ventricular arrhythmias of some type occurred in 21 of 78 (35%) patients. Seven patients (10%) experienced atrial fibrillation or atrial flutter, lasting between 1 hr and 4 days. More recent and larger studies by Taylor and colleagues (24) and Fuller and colleagues (25) reported 19% and 28.4% incidences of post-CABG atrial fibrillation, respectively. Thus, atrial fibrillation is a common post-CABG arrhythmia.

The incidence and nature of atrial arrhythmias after noncoronary bypass cardiac surgery have been less well studied (see elsewhere in this volume). However, it is clear that atrial fibrillation is quite common after valvular surgery (1–4) and likely is similar in terms of pathogenesis, clinical consequences, and management. At least one study (1) suggests that valvular surgery increases the risk for postoperative atrial fibrillation. Also, mitral valve operations may be associated with more refractory postoperative arrhythmias (3).

While most observers agree that atrial tachyarrhythmias are frequently associated with CABG, there is less consensus as to the clinical correlates or risk factors of these arrhythmias. Fuller and colleagues (25) studied 1,666 consecutive patients undergoing CABG and evaluated the relationship of atrial fibrillation to a number of preoperative, intraoperative, and postoperative variables in a multivariate logistic regression analysis. The preoperative variables examined included age, gender, medications, diabetes, hypertension, previous myocardial infarction, and left ventriculography; intraoperative variables included aortic cross-clamp time, volume of cardioplegic solution, acid-base balance during bypass, number of grafts, endarterectomy, sequential grafts, use of defibrillator, and ventricular pacing; postoperative variables included hemorrhage, myocardial infarction, infection, embolism, stroke, death, CK-MB levels, bundle branch block, ventricular arrhythmias, and beta-blocker therapy. The variable that had the strongest independent association with postoperative atrial fibrillation was age ($P = 0.0001$), with atrial fibrillation far more likely in older patients. The only other variables that had an independent association with postoperative atrial fibrillation were male sex ($P = 0.02$), and postoperative beta-blocker therapy ($P = 0.001$), with beta-blockers having a protective effect.

Other studies have also evaluated possible clinical correlates of post-CABG atrial fibrillation. Roffman and Feldman (9) found that patients with supraventricular arrhythmias tended to be older than those without (61 vs 55 years; $P < 0.001$), had more bypass grafts (4.0 vs 3.3; $P < 0.01$), and longer aortic cross-clamp times (68.4 vs 59.0 min; $P < 0.01$). The last two were likely interrelated. Loop (1987, *personal communication*) has also noted a relationship with age; in his series atrial fibrillation occurred in 17.6% of patients younger than 65 years, 33.5% of those 65 to 74, and 46.3% of those older than 75. Douglas and colleagues (4), in reviewing 135 patients undergoing surgery for aortic stenosis with or without CABG, also noted a clear association between postoperative atrial fibrillation and age; atrial fibrillation occurred in 61% of patients older than 70 years as compared to 38% of patients younger than 70 ($P < 0.004$).

Several clinical studies have examined the role of beta-blockers and digoxin in the pathogenesis of post-CABG atrial arrhythmias. As beta-blockers are frequently used in the treatment of coronary artery disease, many patients have received chronic beta-blockade before surgery (8,26). A number of centers had advocated routinely discontinuing beta-blockade before surgery for fear of deleterious intra- and postoperative hemodynamic effects (8,27,28). In fact, such withdrawal may play a major role in the pathogenesis of a number of adverse perioperative cardiac events (8,28,29) including atrial arrhythmias. Thus, White and colleagues (10) and Salazar and colleagues (11) both noted a two- to fivefold increased incidence of atrial arrhythmias in patients in whom beta-blockers were discontinued when compared to those who continued to receive beta-blocking drugs preoperatively and postoperatively. Reasons for this observation may include increased postoperative adrenergic tone (27), as reflected by increased 24-hr urine epinephrine and norepinephrine excretion, along with the effects of beta-blocker withdrawal on beta-adrenergic receptor density (30–32).

The role of chronic digoxin administration is less clear. Rose and colleagues (15) and Morrison and Killip (33) failed to find any correlation between digoxin levels and atrial arrhythmias.

Other groups (1,8,9,15,34) have also studied a number of possible clinical correlates of post-CABG atrial fibrillation; none, however, appeared to correlate well with the occurrence of atrial fibrillation. These included gender, hypertension, previous myocardial infarction, unstable angina, poor left ventricular function, extent of coronary artery disease, serum electrolyte levels (including calcium and magnesium), lipid profiles, arterial blood gas values, heart size by chest x-ray, and postoperative right and left atrial pressures.

In summary, atrial fibrillation is a common arrhythmia after CABG. With the probable exceptions of advanced age and beta-blocker use, a number of reviews considering a large number of clinical correlates have failed to demonstrate clearly reproducible preoperative, intraoperative, and postoperative correlates of postoperative atrial fibrillation. This may be because potentially independent causes of arrhythmias are operating simultaneously. In addition, sample sizes in several of the studies are too small to allow meaningful evaluation of a large number of independent and interrelated arrhythmogenic factors (35,36).

PATHOGENESIS

Atrial fibrillation is generally considered to be the result of multiple small atrial reentrant circuits that cause numerous circulating excitation wavefronts; this is known as the multiple wavelet hypothesis (37). Electrophysiologic studies of canine atrial fibrillation indicate that the initiation and perpetuation of atrial fibrillation depend, at least in part, on increasing atrial size and decreasing atrial refractory period (37). Thus, a large atrial size and a small reentry circuit probably enhance vulnerability to atrial tachyarrhythmia.

The pathophysiology of postoperative atrial tachyarrhythmias has been investigated in both humans and dogs. Boyden and Hoffman (38) studied the effects of surgically induced right atrial enlargement on atrial electrophysiology. One group of mongrel dogs underwent atriotomy with septal tricuspid leaflet excision and partial pulmonary artery constriction. To control for the effects of atriotomy and electrode placement, another group of dogs underwent sham procedures. In the former, atrial enlargement was successfully achieved without a marked effect on right atrial pressure. These dogs were more susceptible to induced atrial tachyarrhythmias, primarily atrial flutter. Histologic changes noted in the dilated atria included myofibril hypertrophy and interstitial fibrosis. Of particular interest, cellular transmembrane potential characteristics were unaffected. Consistent with the noted increased susceptibility to atrial tachycardias after atrial enlargement, it has been observed that patients with chronic left atrial enlargement are unlikely to achieve successful long-term conversion from atrial fibrillation or flutter to sinus rhythm (39–42). Bush and colleagues (43) studied the electrophysiologic properties of right atrial biopsy material in patients undergoing surgery for aortic stenosis. Atrial fibrillation occurrence correlated well with abnormal phase-four depolarizations, conduction velocities, and transmembrane action potentials among patients aged 40 years or older. Other factors that possibly may be related to postoperative atrial fibrillation include atrial infarction, left atrial hypertension, local surgical trauma such as occurring from cannulation of the atria, pericarditis, and age-dependent atrial atrophic changes (7).

Buxton and Josephson investigated the role of P wave duration as a predictor of postoperative atrial arrhythmias (44). They studied 99 patients undergoing CABG; all of the patients were in sinus rhythm preoperatively. Total P wave duration was determined from simultaneous recording of three standard leads. Twenty-nine patients (30%) experienced postoperative atrial fibrillation or flutter. Of note, the mean total P wave duration of patients with atrial flutter or fibrillation was 160 msec compared to only 126 msec for those patients without arrhythmia ($P<0.001$). The presence of an intra-atrial conduction defect, as reflected by a prolonged total P wave duration, was a sensitive (sensitivity$=83\%$), but not very specific (specificity = 43%), predictor of postoperative atrial tachyarrhythmia. Thus, the presence of an underlying atrial conduction defect may predispose some patients to post-CABG arrhythmia.

Electrocardiographic studies of postoperative atrial fibrillation have revealed it to be an electrophysiologically heterogeneous arrhythmia. Wells and colleagues (45) followed bipolar atrial electrograms in 34 postoperative patients. They noted four distinct atrial electrocardiographic patterns. Type I atrial fibrillation was characterized by discrete atrial complexes with an isoelectric baseline. In Type II atrial fibrillation, discrete complexes were interspersed within a perturbed nonisoelectric baseline. Type III atrial fibrillation has completely chaotic patterns. Finally, Type IV was characterized by a combination of Type III with either Type I or II. Of note, in 22 patients atrial electrograms were recorded more than once; 50% of these 22 showed pattern variability. Thus, the electrophysiologic properties of postoperative atrial fibrillation do not appear to be homogeneous. The clinical significance of these different electrical patterns of atrial fibrillation is unclear.

CLINICAL DIAGNOSIS AND MANAGEMENT

Diagnosis

The diagnosis of post-CABG atrial fibrillation is often easily made from the ECG. However, in certain instances, atrial electrograms may be useful to confirm the diagnosis (46–49). Waldo and colleagues (47) used high right epicardial atrial wires in 57 patients undergoing cardiac surgery and found them to be useful for diagnosing and/or confirming a wide variety of arrhythmias including atrial fibrillation, atrial flutter, atrial tachycardia, atrioventricular junctional tachycardia with or without aberrancy, atrioventricular dissociation, and ventricular tachycardia.

Treatment

Treatment of post-CABG atrial fibrillation differs little from treatment of this arrhythmia in other circumstances (46). Behrendt and Austen (7) refrain from treating the arrhythmia unless the ventricular rate is unacceptably fast. Rate can be reduced with digoxin (0.25 mg doses every 3 to 4 hr up to 1.0 to 1.5 mg), propranolol (1 mg every 5 min up to 0.1 mg/kg total) or other beta-blocking agents, or verapamil (5–10 mg doses every 1 to 4 hr as needed), preferably given intravenously (46). Rate control with digoxin may be difficult owing to high postoperative sympathetic tone. One study of the ultrashort-acting beta-blocking agent esmolol (50) found it to be effective for rate control in most patients, but there were frequent side effects including hypotension (10 of 15 patients), gastrointestinal disturbances, and somnolence. In patients without a prior history of atrial fibrillation, spontaneous conversion to sinus rhythm will almost always eventually occur.

Whether digoxin actually aids in conversion from atrial fibrillation to sinus rhythm is controversial. Weiner and colleagues (51) prospectively studied 45 nonsurgical patients with acute atrial fibrillation and noted a very high conversion rate with rapid digitalization. The authors did not study a control (nondigitalized) group, however. Falk and colleagues (52) showed no digitalis-conversion effect in a prospective, randomized, placebo-controlled trial of 36 patients with acute atrial fibrillation. Furthermore, in canine models (53) digoxin has not been shown to reduce atrial fibrillation threshold.

Finally, some authors (46) advocate the use of quinidine, procainamide, or electrical cardioversion. In at least one recent series (35) electrical cardioversion was never required. Waldo and colleagues (46) think that direct cardioversion is not indicated in the early postoperative period, as recurrence of arrhythmia is likely and eventual spontaneous and sustained conversion to sinus rhythm is likely. However, in occasional patients who suffer serious hemodynamic deterioration as a result of the atrial fibrillation, urgent cardioversion may be necessary. We generally use quinidine, or other similar antiarrhythmic drugs, for the suppression of the arrhythmia in the rare instances in which it is stubbornly recurrent.

Aside from quinidine and procainamide, other groups have considered the use of amiodarone, sotalol, and disopyramide. A recent trial (3) randomized patients with postoperative atrial fibrillation or flutter for more than 2 hr to either intravenous amiodarone bolus (5 mg/kg over 20 min) or oral quinidine (400 mg immediately and 400 mg in 4 hr) with crossover at 8 hr if the arrhythmia persisted. The quinidine strategy resulted in a higher rate reversion to sinus rhythm (64% vs 41%; $P = 0.04$), but there were more side effects caused by quinidine including torsades de pointes ventricular tachycardia, severe nausea and vomiting, hypotension, and enhancement of atrioventricular node conduction. Another trial found that both sotalol, a beta-blocker with Type III antiarrhythmic activity, and a combination of disopyramide and digoxin were equally effective in converting postbypass atrial fibrillation or flutter to sinus or junctional rhythm, but sotalol tended to work faster (54).

Prophylaxis

The prevention of postoperative supraventricular arrhythmias (including atrial fibrillation) with digitalis or beta-blockers has been analyzed in a number of nonrandomized studies during the 1960s and 1970s (55–61). We will review only recent controlled studies. A summary of these and doses of drugs used can be found in Tables 1 and 2.

Preoperative Digitalis

Nonrandomized Trials

Chee and colleagues (1) studied 182 patients undergoing a variety of cardiac procedures. One group received 0.75 mg of digoxin orally in divided doses on the day before surgery; a second group received no digoxin, while a third group, previously taking digoxin, had it discontinued 48 hr preoperatively. Supraventricular arrhythmias, including atrial fibrillation and flutter, occurred in 72% of patients not receiving digoxin but in only 5% of those who had received digoxin preoperatively. The authors noted a relationship between postoperative supraventricular tachyarrhythmias and valvular surgery or ECG evidence of myocardial infarction. They therefore recommended preoperative digitalization for patients undergoing cardiac valve replacement and those with ECG evidence of prior myocardial infarction. However, the nonrandomized nature of this study and the failure to stratify for the use of beta-blockade are major limitations.

TABLE 1. *Digoxin prophylaxis trials*

Author	Preoperative or postoperative	Regimen for different groups	Design	SVT (AF) occurrence (%)
Chee et al.	Preoperative	(1) 0.75 mg p.o. 1 day (2) No drug (3) Discontinued 48 hr preoperatively	Nonrandomized	(1) 5 (2) 72 } $P<0.01$ } $P<0.01$ (3) 95
Johnson et al.	Preoperative	(1) 1.0 mg p.o. load 2 to 3 days preoperatively (2) Control	Randomized	(1) 5 (6) } $P<0.01$ (2) 26 (11)
Tyras et al.	Preoperative	(1) 1.0 mg p.o. load 1 day preoperatively (2) 1.5 mg p.o. load 1 day preoperatively (3) Control		(1) 31.6 } (2) 21.7 } $P<0.05$ } $P<0.05$ (3) 11.4
Csicsko et al.	Postoperative	(1) 1.0 mg i.v. load 4 to 12 hr postoperatively (2) Control		(1) 2.2 (1.5) } $P<0.01$ (2) 15.7 (5.9)
Weiner et al.	Postoperative	(1) 1.0 mg i.v. load 6 to 24 hr postoperatively (2) Control		(1) 15 (10) } NS (2) 16 (10)

All prospective controlled. All received maintenance therapy. The *P* values refer to SVT unless otherwise indicated.
Abbreviations: NS, not seen; SVT, supraventricular tachycardia; AF, atrial fibrillation.
From ref. 5, with permission.

TABLE 2. *Beta-blocker prophylaxis trials*

Author	Regimen for different groups	Design[a]	SVT (AF) occurrence[b]
Matangi et al.	(1) Propranolol 5 mg orally q.i.d. (2) Control (all received preoperative beta-blocker)	Randomized	(1) 9.8% (8%) (2) 23% (15%) } $P<0.02$
White et al.	(1) Timolol 0.5 mg i.v. 3 to 7 hr postoperatively, then timolol 10 mg orally b.i.d. (2) Control (placebo)	Randomized	(1) 84 episodes (2) 581 episodes } $P<0.05$
Daudon et al.	(1) Acebutolol 200 mg orally b.i.d. starting 36 hr postoperatively (2) Control	Randomized	(1) 0% (2) 40% (34%) } $P<0.001$

All gave beta-blocker postoperatively.
[a]All prospective, controlled.
[b]See text.
From ref. 5, with permission.

Randomized Trials

Johnson and colleagues (21) randomized 120 patients undergoing CABG (no valvular or aneurysmal surgery) to control or digoxin loading 2 to 3 days before surgery. Supraventricular tachyarrhythmias occurred in 26% of control patients but in only 5% of digitalized patients. The incidence of atrial fibrillation in particular was significantly reduced from 11% to 6% ($P<0.01$). Six control patients underwent electrical cardioversion compared to only one digitalized patient. By omitting digitalis on the morning of surgery, no cases of digitalis toxicity occurred. The authors concluded that prophylactic preoperative digitalis was safe and effective. Another study by Parker and colleagues (22) yielded similar results.

Tyras and colleagues (23) evaluated the effects of prophylactic digitalization given 24 hr preoperatively. Patients assigned to the digoxin group received either 1 or 1.5 mg loading doses. In contrast to the results of other studies (21,22) treated patients had a significantly higher incidence of supraventricular tachyarrhythmias than control patients. This was noted in both the 1 and 1.5 mg groups. Of note, pre- and postoperative digoxin levels were "subtherapeutic" or "barely therapeutic" in all digitalized patients. Other groups (21,22) did not record digoxin levels in their studies.

Postoperative Digitalis

Nonrandomized Trials

Csicsko and colleagues (62) evaluated the effects of immediate (under 4 hr) postoperative digitalization in patients undergoing CABG. Supraventricular tachycardia occurred in 13% of untreated patients but in only 2% of treated patients. The incidence of atrial fibrillation was also significantly reduced from 5.9% to 1.5%. There were no differences in the rates of ventricular arrhythmias, perioperative myocardial infarction, or hospital mortality.

Randomized Trials

A small prospective trial by Weiner and colleagues (63) showed a 15% incidence of supraventricular arrhythmias in both control and treated patients. The latter received first a digoxin load and maintenance therapy thereafter. Atrial fibrillation occurred in 10% of patients regardless of digoxin use. Most patients in both groups were receiving beta-blockers preoperatively and continued to receive them in reduced dosages postoperatively.

Postoperative Beta-Blockade

Randomized Trials

While digoxin has had mixed success in preventing postoperative atrial fibrillation, studies of beta-blockers have found them to be almost uniformly beneficial (8,10,13, 14,16,18,20,34,63). Four representative studies will be reviewed.

Mantangi and colleagues (13) studied 164 patients undergoing CABG and without histories of asthma, previous tachyarrhythmias, preoperative beta-blockade, congestive heart failure, inotropic support, atrioventricular block, or sick sinus syndrome. Patients were randomly assigned to control or treatment groups; the latter received low-dose propranolol (5 mg orally every 6 hr). The incidence of both supraventricular and ventricular arrhythmias was markedly reduced in the propranolol group. Patients who had supraventricular tachycardias were initially treated with digoxin. Quinidine, disopyramide, and/or electrical cardioversion were added as necessary. Of note, only one of the 82 treated patients required additional antiarrhythmic therapy compared to 13 of 82 control patients. Three control patients required elective cardioversion. Major hemodynamic complications did not occur in the treatment group. Thus, the authors concluded that very low doses of beta-blockade could safely prevent a wide variety of supraventricular tachyarrhythmias including atrial fibrillation.

White and colleagues (10) evaluated the efficacy of timolol in 21 patients for prevention of supraventricular tachyarrhythmias after CABG; their trial was also prospective, controlled, and randomized. Instead of recording the number of patients experiencing or not experiencing arrhythmias, they noted episodes of arrhythmia as ascertained by 8 consecutive days of ECG recording. Severe arrhythmias were defined as those lasting more than 5 min and/or at rates greater than 200 beats per minute. Mild episodes lasted less than 30 sec or at rates less than 150 beats per minute. Timolol successfully and dramatically reduced the number of all and mild episodes of atrial fibrillation. Severe arrhythmias also occurred less often but statistical significance was not achieved. Adverse effects of timolol were minimal.

Daudon and colleagues (64) performed a randomized, controlled trial of acebutolol in CABG patients. The incidence of postoperative atrial fibrillation or flutter was reduced from 40% to 0% in the acebutolol group. Adverse effects of acebutolol were also minimal.

There has been at least one study that directly evaluated the efficacies of digoxin and propranolol in a head-to-head fashion. In a prospective, randomized trial, Rubin and colleagues (34) followed 150 patients who were randomized to three groups: group I received no drug; group 2 received intravenous digoxin 0.5 mg on the first postoperative day followed by 0.25 mg daily by mouth for the next 6 weeks; group

3 received propranolol 20 mg every 6 hr for 6 weeks beginning on the first postoperative day. Patients with previous atrial fibrillation, bronchospasm, brittle diabetes, bradycardia, high-degree atrioventricular block, or ejection fractions of less than 50% were excluded. Of note, 27 patients were excluded from data analysis, including 19 for "protocol deviations." Sustained atrial fibrillation, defined as arrhythmias lasting more than 30 sec, occurred in 15 of 40 (37.5%) of control patients, 15 of 46 (32.6%) of digoxin patients ($P = NS$), but in only six of 37 (16.2%) of propranolol patients ($P = 0.03$). After 26 ± 7 months of follow-up, there were no differences in cardiovascular or cerebrovascular mortality or morbidity among the patients who had atrial fibrillation as compared to those who did not have atrial fibrillation.

Thus, postoperative beta-blockade appears to successfully prevent most episodes of atrial fibrillation and may reduce the need for various other treatment modalities.

Other Strategies

Combined Prophylaxis

Roffman and Feldman (9), in a nonrandomized, controlled study, compared postoperative administration of digoxin plus propranolol and digoxin alone to a control group. Both controls and patients given digoxin only had a 22% incidence of supraventricular arrhythmias compared to only 2.1% in the digoxin plus propranolol group. Thus, it appears that the beta-blocker played the major role in preventing postoperative arrhythmias. Mills and colleagues (17) also showed a beneficial effect of digoxin plus propranolol for both supraventricular and ventricular arrhythmias but did not study either agent alone among their patients.

Verapamil

Davison and colleagues (12) evaluated postoperative oral verapamil for the prevention of post-CABG atrial fibrillation. While atrial fibrillation, when it occurred, was significantly slower (115 vs 156 beats per minute) in the treatment group, the overall incidence of the arrhythmia was not significantly reduced. Furthermore, the incidence of hypotension was significantly higher in the treated patients.

Magnesium

Katholi and colleagues (65) recently reported the preliminary results of a double-blinded randomized trial of magnesium chloride replacement after CABG. One hundred and twenty-eight patients were randomized to either $MgCl_2$ (48 mEq i.v. followed by 15 mEq p.o. daily) or placebo. "Responders" were defined as patients whose magnesium levels increased to 2.0 mEq/liter or more after magnesium replacement. The incidence of postoperative atrial fibrillation was significantly reduced (7% vs 14%; $P < 0.05$) compared to placebo in responders but was not affected in nonresponders. The authors concluded that $MgCl_2$ replacement can be effective as prophylaxis of post-CABG atrial fibrillation, but only when the magnesium level is increased to 2.0 mEq/liter or more.

Current Practices

In order to identify the most common approach to the treatment and prevention of post-CABG atrial fibrillation, we surveyed chiefs of cardiac surgery in the United

TABLE 3. *Post-CABG atrial fibrillation: current practices*

Is post-CABG atrial fibrillation a significant problem at your hospital?	Yes	58 (80%)
	No	14 (20%)
What is your estimated incidence of atrial fibrillation at your hospital?	Range	5%–50%
	Mean	20%
	Median	25%
What method of supraventricular arrhythmia prophylaxis do you use?	Preop digoxin	5 (7%)
(Several centers use more than one method.)	Postop digoxin	20 (27%)
	Preop beta-blocker	9 (12%)
	Postop beta-blocker	33 (44%)
	None	27 (36%)
	Verapamil	2 (3%)
How is method of prophylaxis determined?	Department policy	33%
	Physician choice	67%

Based on survey of 75 US chiefs of cardiothoracic surgery.
From ref. 5, with permission.

States regarding their current practices relating to post-CABG arrhythmias. Eighty percent considered post-CABG atrial fibrillation to be a significant problem; some thought it to be frequent but not serious (D. Roe, 1987, *personal communication*). Reported incidences of atrial fibrillation ranged from 5% to 50% with a median of 20%. A wide diversity of prophylactic practices was noted. One-third stated that they did not use any routine prophylactic modality. Slightly less than one-half use postoperative beta-blockade, while a small fraction use preoperative or postoperative digitalis glycosides. These data are listed in Table 3. At Massachusetts General Hospital there has been a gradual shift from routine postoperative prophylaxis with i.v. followed by oral digoxin (with postoperative beta-blockade reserved for those patients who were on beta-blockers before CABG) to a more widespread use of preoperative and postoperative beta-adrenergic blocker treatment. Postoperative beta-blockade is quite uniformly given to those patients who were on these drugs in advance of surgery.

PROGNOSIS AND COMPLICATIONS

Post-CABG atrial fibrillation usually occurs 24 to 60 hr after surgery (12–14,20). In a recent large Australian review, the peak incidence occurred 2 days after the operation; a small proportion (4.7%) developed atrial tachyarrhythmia the day of the operation, while very few (0.4%) experienced atrial fibrillation after more than 9 days. The arrhythmia is usually benign without significant long-term sequelae (7,46). Nevertheless, complications may occur, and in a small proportion of patients these may result in adverse clinical consequences. Potential complications include embolic phenomena, especially cerebrovascular accidents, hemodynamic compromise, sustained atrial fibrillation, and increased length of hospital stay.

Atrial Thrombus Formation and Systemic Emboli

Stroke is an infrequent, yet serious, consequence of CABG (66). A 10-year retrospective review of 3,279 cases at Johns Hopkins University (67) revealed an increasing incidence of stroke from 0.57% in 1979 to 2.4% in 1983. Using case-control analysis, a number of preoperative and intraoperative risk factors for stroke were identified; these included increasing age, preexisting cerebrovascular disease, severe atherosclerosis of the ascending aorta, protracted cardiopulmonary bypass time, and severe perioperative hypotension. No analysis of association between stroke and postoperative arrhythmia was carried out.

Embolic stroke is a well-known complication of both chronic and paroxysmal atrial fibrillation, even in the absence of rheumatic or valvular heart disease (68,69). Pertinent to the problem of post-CABG atrial fibrillation is the risk of paroxysmal arrhythmia. A retrospective Danish study (70) of 426 patients found a lower incidence of cerebrovascular events in patients with paroxysmal atrial fibrillation than in patients with chronic atrial fibrillation. Nonetheless, systemic arterial emboli occurred in 18.5% of these patients, and 58% of emboli were to the cerebral vessels. Nearly one-third of these events occurred near the onset—that is, less than 1 month and often within days—of the arrhythmia. Data from the Framingham study have shown similar results (71).

A recent report by Taylor and colleagues (24) provides more compelling evidence for an association between postoperative stroke and atrial fibrillation in patients undergoing CABG. They prospectively evaluated 453 consecutive patients undergoing CABG for neurologic complications—stroke or transient ischemic attacks (TIA). Stroke or TIA occurred in 10 patients (2.2%). Postoperative atrial fibrillation occurred in six of these 10 patients (60%) compared to its occurrence in 80 of 443 patients (18%) who did not have stroke or TIA ($P<0.005$). Other clinical correlates of post-CABG stroke or TIA included a prior history of stroke or TIA and the presence of a carotid bruit. Using stepwise logistic regression, both a history of stroke or TIA and postoperative atrial fibrillation were identified as independent predictors of post-CABG neurologic events, even after accounting for age and clinical evidence of carotid disease. These findings are further supported by a recent case-control study done at Massachusetts General Hospital (72). In this study, 54 patients with postoperative stroke or TIA were compared to 54 randomly chosen control patients among 5,915 consecutive patients who had CABG from 1970 to 1984. Postoperative atrial fibrillation occurred in 29 cases (54%), but in only 15 controls (28%); the odds ratio for stroke with postoperative atrial fibrillation was 3.0 (95% confidence interval 1.4–6.7).

While these and other data do not conclusively show a cause-effect relationship between brief paroxysms of atrial fibrillation and clinically significant systemic emboli, they do heighten the concern that such an association exists.

Hemodynamic Deterioration

An important potential complication of post-CABG atrial fibrillation is hemodynamic deterioration—either hypotension, congestive heart failure, or both—as a consequence of the arrhythmia. How well atrial fibrillation is tolerated depends on three major factors: (a) the ventricular rate; (b) the status of the patient's underlying ventricular function; and (c) the duration of the arrhythmia. In addition, the loss of atrial systole may contribute to hemodynamic deterioration. The relative importance of atrial contraction in augmenting cardiac output remains controversial. Most studies that have examined this issue involved patients with abnormal hearts (73–79). Furthermore, results of such studies are often obscured by the effects of rapid heart rates and irregular rhythms as well as mitral regurgitation (80). Two studies using healthy canine models with artificially induced atrial fibrillation showed a 15% to 30% decrease in cardiac output and stroke volume (80,81) when compared to sinus rhythm. In the otherwise healthy heart, the loss of atrial systole may not be clinically deleterious. In the diseased, noncompliant heart, however, the loss of atrial systole when combined with tachycardia and a reduced diastolic filling time and increased myocardial oxygen consumption may have deleterious clinical effects. This may be especially true in patients with diseased atrioventricular valves, ischemic heart disease, acute myocardial infarction or ischemia, and dilated or hypertrophic cardiomyopathy (73,74). Thus, one study demonstrated a 20% increase in cardiac output after cardioversion in eight patients with chronic atrial fibrillation and known coronary artery disease (75); other studies, however, have revealed conflicting results (76,77,79).

In the post-CABG patient, atrial fibrillation does not commonly result in hypotension severe enough to require use of sympathomimetic pressors or other therapy, although few data address this point specifically. Davison and colleagues (12), in a controlled trial of verapamil for the prevention of post-CABG atrial fibrillation, observed 34 occurrences of atrial fibrillation among 200 patients. Twenty-three of these patients were in the control group. Within this group, only one clinically significant episode of hypotension occurred. Rubin and colleagues (34) followed 123 patients postoperatively; 36 developed atrial fibrillation. Two of these patients, as compared to four of the 87 patients without atrial fibrillation, experienced syncope ($P = $ NS). No patients required direct-current cardioversion.

Thus, while hemodynamic decompensation from post-CABG atrial fibrillation is a concern, its occurrence in clinical practice appears to be unusual. There are several likely reasons for this. First, episodes of post-CABG atrial fibrillation are usually of short duration. Second, the bypass procedure itself reduces the ischemic jeopardy imposed by the arrhythmia. Finally, patients with very poor left ventricular function are not commonly subjected to CABG. Nonetheless, in occasional patients atrial fibrillation can precipitate serious hemodynamic deterioration. For these individuals the urgent termination of the arrhythmia and its further prevention are of paramount importance.

Prolonged Atrial Fibrillation

In one recent European study (82) 19 of 100 (19%) of consecutive patients undergoing CABG developed atrial fibrillation; one-quarter of these patients were still in atrial fibrillation at time of hospital discharge. Most studies of patients previously free of atrial tachyarrhythmias (1,8–13,16–18,20–23,62,64) suggest this arrhythmia rarely persists for longer than a few days, even though it is often recurrent when it develops. Thus, chronic atrial fibrillation developing *de novo* post-CABG appears to be unusual.

Resource Utilization and Potential for Iatrogenesis

Angelini and colleagues (6) noted that seven of 78 patients undergoing surgery for coronary heart disease developed postoperative atrial fibrillation. These arrhythmias lasted between 1 hr and 4 days. Of interest, the length of hospital stay was significantly increased for patients with atrial fibrillation; length of stay increased from 9.9 to 11.4 days. Similarly Rubin and colleagues (34), in a study of 123 patients, noted that atrial fibrillation occurrence was associated with a 2-day increase in length of stay (14.4 ± 6 vs 12.4 ± 4 days; $P<0.02$). It is not clear whether the association between atrial fibrillation and increased length of stay is causal or confounded by other factors. Also, to our knowledge, the relationship between atrial arrhythmia occurrence and the need for more intensive and expensive care, i.e., longer intensive care unit stays, has not been documented.

As post-CABG atrial fibrillation sometimes requires treatment (46), there exists the potential for adverse consequences secondary to antiarrhythmic drugs, including digoxin, beta-blockers, verapamil, quinidine, and others. These agents alone or in various combinations can cause gastrointestinal and central nervous system toxicity, hypotension, atrioventricular block, and increased predisposition to ventricular arrhythmias (15,83,84). To our knowledge, the incidence of such events in treated post-CABG patients with atrial fibrillation is unknown, but presumably small.

POSTOPERATIVE ATRIAL FIBRILLATION AFTER VALVULAR SURGERY

As previously mentioned, atrial fibrillation after valvular surgery has been less well studied than atrial fibrillation after CABG. In a prospective study of 50 consecutive patients undergoing cardiac valve replacement, Smith and colleagues (85) found that atrial fibrillation was the most common postoperative arrhythmia, occurring in 21 of 66 arrhythmic episodes (32%). One interesting finding of this study was that supraventricular arrhythmias were more common after mitral valve replacements than after aortic valve replacements (73% vs 43%; $P<0.05$). In a study of 70 patients undergoing cardiac surgery by one surgeon over a 2-month period, atrial fibrillation occurred in nine of 15 patients (60%) undergoing valve surgery, whereas it occurred in only 19 of 50 patients (38%) undergoing CABG ($\chi^2 = 1.42$; $P = NS$) (2).

Another study also suggests that valvular surgery is associated with an increased risk of postoperative atrial fibrillation.

Douglas and colleagues (4) evaluated clinical correlates of postoperative atrial fibrillation in 135 consecutive patients undergoing valve replacement for aortic stenosis. The strongest independent predictor of postoperative atrial fibrillation was age; atrial fibrillation occurred in 61% of patients greater than 69 years of age. In younger patients (less than 70 years of age) the presence of significant mitral valve disease and pulmonary hypertension were significant risk factors for postoperative atrial fibrillation.

An additional issue in valvular heart disease patients is whether it is worthwhile to attempt to restore sinus rhythm after mitral valve replacement or repair in patients with chronic atrial fibrillation preoperatively. Flugelman and colleagues (86) studied 40 patients with pure mitral stenosis and chronic atrial fibrillation who underwent mitral valve replacement or commissurotomy. Cardioversion with direct current shock and quinidine or disopyramide was performed in all patients less than 6 months after the procedure. Twenty-four patients (60%) remained in sinus rhythm for more than 3 months after cardioversion and were therefore considered successes. Using univariate analysis, the authors noted that patients who were successes were younger (38 vs 47 years; $P<0.05$), had symptoms for a shorter period of time (3.0 vs 6.4 years; $P<0.02$), and by echocardiography had a smaller preoperative left atrial size (4.9 vs 5.5 cm; $P<0.03$). After subjecting their data to multivariate regression analysis, the authors concluded that for patients with preoperative left atrial sizes of greater than 5.2 cm and symptoms for more than 3 years, the likelihood of successful cardioversion was too low to justify any attempt.

CONCLUSIONS

Atrial fibrillation is a frequent complication of CABG and other types of cardiac surgery, occurring in 5% to 40% of patients, and is especially common in elderly patients (25,87). Despite a wealth of data, its specific pathogenesis or precipitants are incompletely understood. Although it occurs commonly, it is most often a benign, self-limited arrhythmia with adverse effects primarily limited to possible increases in length of hospital stay, need for antiarrhythmic therapies, and postoperative stroke (88; F. Loop, 1987, *personal communication*). Treatment primarily consists of rate control using digitalis glycosides, beta-adrenergic blocking agents, or verapamil. In some cases there may be a need for additional antiarrhythmic agents, such as quinidine; electrical cardioversion may be required in the rare patient suffering serious hemodynamic instability from atrial fibrillation. A number of researchers have investigated the issue of prophylaxis of post-CABG atrial fibrillation; low-dose beta-adrenergic blocking drugs appear to be the safest and most effective drugs for this purpose.

REFERENCES

1. Chee TP, Prakash NS, Dresser KB, et al. Postoperative supraventricular arrhythmias and the role of prophylactic digoxin in cardiac surgery. *Am Heart J* 1982;104:974–977.
2. Michelson EL, Morganroth J, MacVaugh H III. Postoperative arrhythmias after coronary artery and cardiac valvular surgery detected by long-term electrocardiographic monitoring. *Am Heart J* 1979;97:442–448.
3. McAlister HF, Luke RA, Whitlock RM, Smith WM. Intravenous amiodarone bolus versus oral quinidine for atrial flutter and fibrillation after cardiac operations. *J Thorac Cardiovasc Surg* 1990;99:911–918.
4. Douglas P, Hirshfeld JW Jr, Edmunds H. Clinical correlates of postoperative atrial fibrillation. *Circulation* 1984;70(suppl II):II-165.
5. Lauer MS, Eagle KA, Buckley MJ, DeSanctis RW. Atrial fibrillation following coronary artery bypass surgery. *Prog Cardiovasc Dis* 1989;31:367–378.
6. Angelini P, Feldman MJ, Lutschanowski R, et al. Cardiac arrhythmias during and after heart surgery; diagnosis and management. *Prog Cardiovasc Dis* 1974;16:469–495.
7. Behrendt DM, Austen WG. *Patient care in cardiac surgery.* Boston: Little, Brown, 1985.
8. Silverman NA, Wright R, Levitsky S. Efficacy of low-dose propranolol in preventing postoperative supraventricular tachyarrhythmias: a prospective, randomized study. *Ann Surg* 1982;196:194–197.
9. Roffman JA, Feldman A. Digoxin and propranolol in the prophylaxis of supraventricular tachydysrhythmias after coronary artery bypass surgery. *Ann Thorac Surg* 1981;31:496–501.
10. White HD, Antman GM, Glynn MA, et al. Efficacy and safety of timolol for prevention of supraventricular tachyarrhythmias after coronary artery bypass surgery. *Circulation* 1984;70:479–484.
11. Salazar C, Frishman W, Friedman S, et al. Beta-blockade therapy for supraventricular tachyarrhythmias after coronary surgery: a propranolol withdrawal syndrome? *Angiology* 1979;30:816–819.
12. Davison R, Hertz R, Kaplan K, et al. Prophylaxis of supraventricular tachyarrhythmia after coronary bypass surgery with oral verapamil: a randomized, double-blinded trial. *Ann Thorac Surg* 1985;39:336–339.
13. Mantangi MF, Neutze JM, Graham IC, et al. Arrhythmia prophylaxis after aorta-coronary bypass: the effect of minidose propranolol. *J Thorac Cardiovasc Surg* 1985;89:439–443.
14. Stephenson LW, MacVaugh H, Tomasello DN, et al. Propranolol for prevention of postoperative cardiac arrhythmias: a randomized study. *Ann Thorac Surg* 1980;29:113–116.

15. Rose MR, Glassman E, Spencer FC. Arrhythmias following cardiac surgery: relation to serum digoxin levels. *Am Heart J* 1975;89:288–294.
16. Vecht RJ, Nicolaides EP, Ikweuke JK, et al. Incidence and prevention of supraventricular tachyarrhythmias after coronary bypass surgery. *Int J Cardiol* 1986;13:124–134.
17. Mills SA, Poole GV Jr, Breyer RH, et al. Digoxin and propranolol in the prophylaxis of dysrhythmias after coronary artery bypass grafting. *Circulation* 1983;68(suppl II):II-222–II-225.
18. Ivey MF, Ivey TD, Bailey WW, et al. Influence of propranolol on supraventricular tachycardia early after coronary artery revascularization: a randomized trial. *J Thorac Cardiovasc Surg* 1983;85:214–218.
19. Abel R, Gelder HM, Pores IH, et al. Continued propranolol administration following coronary bypass surgery: anti-arrhythmic effects. *Arch Surg* 1983;118:727–731.
20. Mohr R, Smolinsky A, Goor DA. Prevention of supraventricular tachyarrhythmia with low-dose propranolol after coronary bypass. *J Thorac Cardiovasc Surg* 1981;81:840–845.
21. Johnson LW, Dickstein RA, Freuhan CT, et al. Prophylactic digitalization for coronary artery bypass surgery. *Circulation* 1976;53:819–822.
22. Parker FB Jr, Greiner-Hayes C, Bowe EL, et al. Supraventricular arrhythmias following coronary artery bypass: the effect of preoperative digitalis. *J Thorac Cardiovasc Surg* 1983;86:594–600.
23. Tyras DH, Stothert JC Jr, Kaiser GC, et al. Supraventricular tachyarrhythmias after myocardial revascularization: a randomized trial of prophylactic digitalization. *J Thorac Cardiovasc Surg* 1979;77:310–314.
24. Taylor GJ, Malik SA, Colliver JA, et al. Usefulness of atrial fibrillation as a predictor of stroke after isolated coronary artery bypass grafting. *Am J Cardiol* 1987;60:905–907.
25. Fuller JA, Adams GC, Buxton B. Atrial fibrillation after coronary artery bypass grafting: is it a disorder of the elderly? *J Thorac Cardiovasc Surg* 1989;97:821–825.
26. Vilgoen JR, Estataneous FG, Kellner GA. Propranolol and cardiac surgery. *J Thorac Cardiovasc Surg* 1972;64:826–830.
27. Boudalas H, Snyder GL, Lewis RP, et al. Safety and rationale for continuation of propranolol therapy during coronary bypass operation. *Ann Thorac Surg* 1978;26:222–229.
28. Jones EL, Kaplan JA, Dorney ER, et al. Propranolol therapy in patients undergoing myocardial revascularization. *Am J Cardiol* 1976;38:696–700.
29. Leftkowitz RJ, Caron MG, Stiles GL. Mechanisms of membrane receptor regulation. Biochemical, physiological, and clinical insights derived from studies of the adrenergic receptors. *N Engl J Med* 1984;310:1570–1579.
30. Miller RR, Olson HG, Amsterdam EA, et al. Propranolol-wtihdrawal rebound phenomenon. Exacerbation of coronary events after abrupt cessation of anti-anginal therapy. *N Engl J Med* 1975;293:416–418.
31. Aarons RD, Nies AS, Gal J, et al. Elevation of beta-adrenergic receptor density in human lymphocytes after propranolol administration. *J Clin Invest* 1980;65:949–957.
32. Boudalas H, Lewis RP, Kates RE, et al. Hypersensitivity to adrenergic stimulation after propranolol withdrawal in normal subjects. *Ann Intern Med* 1977;87:433–436.
33. Morrison J, Killip T. Serum digitalis and arrhythmia in patients undergoing cardiopulmonary bypass. *Circulation* 1973;47:341–352.
34. Rubin DA, Nieminski KE, Reed GE, Herman MV. Predictors, prevention, and long-term prognosis of atrial fibrillation after coronary artery bypass graft operations. *J Thorac Cardiovasc Surg* 1987;94:331–335.
35. Pocock SJ. *Clinical trials: a practical approach.* New York: Wiley, 1983.
36. Freiman JA, Chalmers TC, Smith H Jr. The importance of beta, the type II error, and sample size in the design and interpretation of the randomized control trial: survey of 71 "negative" trials. *N Engl J Med* 1978;297:690–694.
37. Waldo AL. Mechanisms of atrial fibrillation, atrial flutter, and ectopic atrial tachycardia: a brief review. *Circulation* 1987;75(suppl III):III-37–III-40.
38. Boyden PA, Hoffman BF. The effects on atrial physiology and structure of surgically induced right atrial enlargement in dogs. *Circ Res* 1981;49:1319–1331.
39. Benditt DG, Benson DW Jr, Dunningan A, et al. Atrial flutter, atrial fibrillation, and other primary atrial tachycardias. *Med Clin North Am* 1984;68:895–918.
40. Mancini GBJ, Goldberger AL. Cardioversion of atrial fibrillation: consideration of embolization, anticoagulation, prophylactic pacemaker, and long term success. *Am Heart J* 1982;104:617–621.
41. Henry WL, Morganroth J, Perlman AS, et al. Relation between echocardiographically determined left atrial size and atrial fibrillation. *Circulation* 1976;53:273–279.
42. Ewy GA, Ulfers L, Hager WD, et al. Response of atrial fibrillation to therapy: role of etiology and left atrial diameter. *J Electrocardiol* 1980;13:119–123.
43. Bush HL, Gelband H, Hoffman BF, et al. Electrophysiologic basis for supraventricular arrhythmias following surgical procedures for aortic stenosis. *Arch Surg* 1971;103:620–625.
44. Buxton AE, Josephson ME. The role of P wave duration as a predictor of postoperative atrial arrhythmias. *Chest* 1981;80:68–73.

45. Wells JL Jr, Karp RB, Kouchoukos NT, et al. Characterization of atrial fibrillation in man: studies following open heart surgery. *PACE* 1978;1:426–438.
46. Waldo AL, Henthorn RW, Epstein AE, et al. Diagnosis and treatment of arrhythmias during and following open heart surgery. *Med Clin North Am* 1984;68:1153–11570.
47. Waldo AL, MacLeen WA, Cooper TB, et al. Use of temporarily placed epicardial atrial wire electrodes for the diagnosis and treatment of arrhythmias following open heart surgery. *J Thorac Cardiovasc Surg* 1978;76:500–505.
48. Waldo AL, Henthorn RW, Plumb VJ. Temporary epicardial wire electrodes in the diagnosis and treatment of arrhythmias after open heart surgery. *Am J Surg* 1984;148:275–283.
49. Waldo AL, MacLeen WA, Karp R, et al. Continuous rapid atrial pacing to control recurrent or sustained supraventricular tachycardias following open heart surgery. *Circulation* 1976;54:245–250.
50. Schwartz M, Michelson EL, Savin HS, MacVaugh H III. Esmolol: safety and efficacy in postoperative cardiothoracic patients with supraventricular tachyarrhythmias. *Chest* 1988;93:705–711.
51. Weiner P, Bessan MM, Jacchovsky J, et al. Clinical course of acute atrial fibrillation treated with rapid digitalization. *Am Heart J* 1983;105:223–227.
52. Falk RH, Knowlton AA, Bernard SA, et al. Digoxin for converting recent-onset atrial fibrillation to sinus rhythm: a randomized, double-blinded trial. *Ann Intern Med* 1987;106:503–506.
53. Gold RL, Bren GB, Katz RJ, et al. Independent and interactive effect of digoxin and quinidine on the atrial fibrillation threshold in dogs. *J Am Coll Cardiol* 1985;6:119–123.
54. Campbell TJ, Gavaghan TP, Morgan JJ. Intravenous sotalol for the treatment of atrial fibrillation and flutter after cardiopulmonary bypass: comparison with disopyramide and digoxin in a randomized trial. *Br Heart J* 1985;54:86–90.
55. Berman SO. The prophylactic use of digitalis before thoracotomy. *Ann Thorac Surg* 1972;14:359–367.
56. Berman SO. Digitalis and thoracic surgery. *J Thorac Cardiovasc Surg* 1965;6:873–881.
57. Shields TW, Ujiki GT. Digitalization for prevention of arrhythmias following pulmonary surgery. *Surg Gynecol Obstet* 1968;126:743–746.
58. Juler GL, Stemmer EA, Connolly JE. Complications of prophylactic digitalization in thoracic surgical patients. *J Thorac Cardiovasc Surg* 1969;58:352–360.
59. Willman VL, Cooper T, Hanlan CR. Prophylactic and therapeutic use of digitalis in open-heart operations. *Arch Surg* 1959;80:168–171.
60. Gianelly G, Griffin JR, Harrison DC. Propranolol in the treatment and prevention of paroxysmal arrhythmias with propranolol therapy. *Ann Intern Med* 1967;66:667–676.
61. Gettes LS, Surawicz B. Long term prevention of paroxysmal arrhythmias with propranolol therapy. *Am J Med Sci* 1967;254:257–265.
62. Csicsko JF, Schatzlein MH, King RD. Immediate post-operative digitalization in the prophylaxis of supraventricular arrhythmias following coronary artery bypass. *J Thorac Cardiovasc Surg* 1981;81:419–422.
63. Weiner B, Rheinlader HF, Decker EL, et al. Digoxin prophylaxis following coronary artery bypass surgery. *Clin Pharm* 1986;5:55–58.
64. Daudon P, Corcos T, Gardjbakah I, et al. Prevention of atrial fibrillation or flutter by acebutolol after coronary bypass grafting. *Am J Cardiol* 1986;58:933–936.
65. Katholi RE, Taylor GJ, Woods WT Jr, et al. Magnesium chloride replacement after bypass surgery to prevent atrial fibrillation: a double blind, randomized trial. *Circulation* 1990;82(suppl III):III-58.
66. Gardner TJ, Horneffer PJ, Manolio TA, et al. Stroke following coronary artery bypass grafting: a ten year study. *Ann Thorac Surg* 1985;50:574–581.
67. Bojar RM, Najafi H, DeLaria GA, et al. Neurologic complications of coronary revascularization. *Ann Thorac Surg* 1983;36:427–432.
68. Kelley BE, Berger JR, Alter M, et al. Cerebral ischemia and atrial fibrillation: a prospective study. *Neurology* 1984;34:1285–1291.
69. Sago JL, Uitert RLV. Risk of current stroke in patients with atrial fibrillation and non-valvular heart disease. *Stroke* 1983;14:537–540.
70. Peterson P, Godtfredson J. Embolic complications in paroxysmal atrial fibrillation. *Stroke* 1986;17:622–626.
71. Wolf PA, Kannel WB, McGee DL, et al. Duration of atrial fibrillation and imminence of stroke: the Framingham study. *Stroke* 1983;14:664–667.
72. Reed GL, Singer DE, Picard EH, et al. Stroke following coronary-artery bypass surgery: a case-control estimate of the risk from carotid bruits. *N Engl J Med* 1988;319:246–250.
73. Moran BJ, Bonow RO, Cannon RO III, et al. Hypertrophic cardiomyopathy: interrelations of clinical manifestations, pathophysiology, and therapy (second of two parts). *N Engl J Med* 1987;316:844–852.
74. Chamberlain DA, Leinbach RC, Vassaux CE, et al. Sequential atrioventricular pacing in heart block complicating myocardial infarction. *N Engl J Med* 1970;282:577–582.

75. Khaja F, Parker JO. Hemodynamic effects of cardioversion in chronic atrial fibrillation. *Arch Intern Med* 1972;129:433–440.
76. Braunwald E. Symposium on cardiac arrhythmias: introduction: with comments on the hemodynamic significance of atrial systole. *Am J Med* 1964;37:665–669.
77. Benchimol A, Ellis JG, Dimund EG, et al. Hemodynamic consequences of atrial and ventricular arrhythmias in men. *Am Heart J* 1965;70:775–788.
78. Oberman A, Harrell RR, Russell RO. Surgical versus medical treatment in disease of the left main coronary artery. *Lancet* 1976;2:591–594.
79. Orlando JF, Herick R, Aronow W, et al. Hemodynamics and echocardiograms before and after cardioversion of atrial fibrillation to normal sinus rhythm. *Chest* 1979;76:521–526.
80. Naito M, David D, Michelson EL, et al. The hemodynamic consequences of cardiac arrhythmias: evaluation of the relative roles of abnormal atrioventricular sequencing, irregularity of ventricular rhythm and atrial fibrillation in a canine model. *Am Heart J* 1983;106:284–291.
81. Friedman HS, Scozza J, McGuinn R, et al. The effects of atrial fibrillation on myocardial blood flow and energetics. *Proc Soc Exp Biol Med* 1985;180:1–8.
82. Yousif H, Davies G, Oakley CM. Peri-operative supraventricular arrhythmias in coronary bypass surgery. *Int J Cardiol* 1990;26:313–318.
83. Zipes DP. Specific arrhythmias: diagnosis and treatment. In: Braunwald E, ed. *Heart disease: a textbook of cardiovascular medicine,* 3rd ed. Philadelphia: WB Saunders, 1987;658–716.
84. Smith WM, Gallagher JJ. "Les torsades de pointes"; an unusual ventricular arrhythmia. *Ann Intern Med* 1980;93:578–584.
85. Smith R, Grossman W, Johnson L, et al. Arrhythmias following cardiac valve replacement. *Circulation* 1972;45:1018–1023.
86. Flugelman MY, Hasin Y, Katznelson N, et al. Restoration and maintenance of sinus rhythm after mitral valve surgery for mitral stenosis. *Am J Cardiol* 1984;54:617–619.
87. Hochberg MS, Levine FH, Daggett WM, et al. Isolated coronary artery bypass grafting in patients seventy years of age and older. *J Thorac Cardiovasc Surg* 1982;84:219–223.
88. Turnipseed WD, Berkoff HA, Belzer FO. Postoperative stroke in cardiac and peripheral vascular disease. *Ann Surg* 1980;192:365–368.

Atrial Fibrillation: Mechanisms and Management, edited by
R. H. Falk and P. J. Podrid.
Raven Press, Ltd., New York © 1992.

9

Exercise Hemodynamics of Atrial Fibrillation

J. Edwin Atwood

*Cardiology Division, Department of Medicine, Stanford University,
Stanford, California 94305; Palo Alto Veterans Administration Hospital,
Palo Alto, California 94304*

HISTORICAL PERSPECTIVE

Ever since the turn of the century, when Sir James Mackenzie first described new cardiac auscultatory findings, specifically a loss of the presystolic accentuation of the mitral rumble along with an irregular rhythm, and Sir Thomas Lewis produced atrial fibrillation in dogs, there has been an increasing interest in atrial fibrillation (1). Controversy has always been present concerning the treatment of atrial fibrillation and its rate control, as evidenced by the interchange of Lewis and Mackenzie describing the uncertain effects of digitalis on atrial fibrillation (2). After these two pioneers pooled their observations and described various features of auricular fibrillation (now termed atrial fibrillation), physicians have attempted to scientifically observe the hemodynamic effect of rest and exercise on heart rate and cardiac output during atrial fibrillation, either in animal models or in humans.

In 1916 Gesell (3–6) first documented, in the river terrapin, an increased ventricular output with auricular systole. Invasive human studies during the 1950s and 1960s primarily evaluated the hemodynamic effects of atrial fibrillation pre- and postcardioversion; however, these invasive studies involved patients with acute and chronic atrial fibrillation with variable disease etiologies; rheumatic, coronary artery disease, hypertensive, and idiopathic (lone) atrial fibrillation (7–20). Additional studies investigated the role of atrial contribution to cardiac output at rest and exercise in patients with complete heartblock and pacemakers (21–28). While these invasive studies were being completed, American and Scandinavian researchers began to evaluate patients with atrial fibrillation both during rest and exercise, while on placebo versus digoxin therapy (29–34). In the late 1970s and 80s, American and European researchers evaluated pharmacologic rate control in atrial fibrillation during rest and exercise (34–49). Digoxin was used in single drug therapy and in conjunction with either a beta-adrenergic blocker or calcium channel-blocker. Most exercise studies involving pharmacologic agents, performed during this time period evaluated patients with heterogeneous causes for atrial fibrillation, e.g., the Scandinavian studies enrolled patients primarily with rheumatic valvular heart disease who were clinically more ill at baseline evaluation. For the most part, these studies used treadmill or bicycle time to estimate levels of oxygen uptake when evaluating functional capacity, since direct measurements using the Douglas bag method were cumbersome and time-consuming.

When gas exchange analysis, which measures functional capacity in terms of actual oxygen uptake (VO_2) and CO_2 production (VCO_2), became an easy, viable, reproducible method to measure VO_2 on a breath-by-breath basis, exercise studies shifted from the previous inaccurate estimated VO_2 to actual measured gas exchange. By utilizing gas exchange analysis these studies evaluating pharmacologic therapy for rate control (29,49) or electrocardioversion (50,51) have allowed for improved comparison of true measured functional data despite varying methodologies such as varying exercise protocols, different subject populations, and multiple study designs.

This chapter will review the development of our current understanding of the hemodynamics of atrial fibrillation with emphasis on the role of exercise testing with gas exchange analysis. Specifically, the role of atrial contraction in contributing to cardiac output, the effect of heart rate and atrioventricular synchrony, and the effect of cardioversion of atrial fibrillation to sinus rhythm will be discussed. Exercise testing methodology will be described and the effect of exercise in patients with atrial fibrillation will be reviewed with respect to four parameters of exercise, i.e., heart rate, functional capacity, blood pressure response, and the ECG.

THE ATRIAL CONTRIBUTION TO CARDIAC OUTPUT

Sir Thomas Lewis (1) first noted the effect of atrial contribution when he described the reduction in aortic pressure and cardiac output during induced atrial fibrillation in dogs, but he attributed this to increased heart rate. In a series of animal experiments from 1910 to 1916, Gesell (3–6) demonstrated the atrial systolic contribution to cardiac output and the importance of the timing of atrial systole in increasing cardiac output. Other early animal studies by Wiggers and Katz (52) and Jochim (53) confirmed his findings. Braunwald and Frahm (7) described, in humans, the relationship of atrial systole to mean left atrial pressure and left ventricular end diastolic pressure in both normal subjects and 26 patients with abnormal left ventricular function. They emphasized that "left atrial and left ventricular contraction are functions of the pressures in these chambers," thereby supporting Starling's law. Further human studies have underscored the contributory "booster pump function" of the atria in several diseases, particularly in coronary artery disease after infarction. Thus, Rahimtoola et al. (54) demonstrated a greater contribution of atrial systole to left ventricular end diastolic volume, stroke volume, and cardiac output in patients 3 to 6 weeks after a myocardial infarction. He also noted that there was less of a contribution in patients with increased end diastolic volume. Greenberg et al. (55) also noted less of an atrial contribution to cardiac output with higher pulmonary artery wedge pressures.

Patients with complete heart block offer a unique opportunity to study the effect of heart rate and of atrial systole and synchrony on cardiac output at rest and during exercise. Samet et al. (21), in 1965, studied 20 patients with complete heart block and noted an increase in the rate of rise of systemic arterial pressure and peak pressures when there was a "normal temporal relation between the P and QRS." Karlof (22), in 1975, demonstrated in 12 patients with complete heart block the importance of atrial systole to resting cardiac output, which increased by 18% when patients were paced at similar atrial and ventricular heart rates. He also noted that during exercise, cardiac output increased in patients undergoing ventricular pacing at a fixed rate, despite the absence of either atrial synchrony or increase in heart rate, thus indicating a contribution from increased myocardial contractility. In another group of patients, he increased the ventricular pacing rate during exercise to match that of atrial synchronized ventricular pacing and noted only a meager 8% increase in cardiac output during exercise when atrial synchronized pacing was present versus pacing at a similar fixed rate in the ventricle. After calculating the cardiac output of 12 patients during rest and exercise from radionuclide studies, Ausubel et al. (25) confirmed this work and concluded that heart rate and not atrial systole increased cardiac output, noting a small additional increment (less than 5%) of atrial synchrony during exercise. Of interest, Ausubel et al. demonstrated no increase in resting cardiac output with atrial synchronized pacing. Numerous other studies have demonstrated improved functional capacity and increased exercise time when atrial synchronized pacing was employed (23–27,56,57). Benditt et al. (28), in a very complete study, demonstrated in 12 patients that activity-initiated ventricular pacing when compared to fixed-rate ventricular pacing significantly increased heart rate (128 vs 90 bpm), prolonged exercise duration (10.2 vs 7.7 min), and increased VO$_2$ both at maximal effort (1,617 vs 1,325 ml O$_2$/min) and at the anaerobic threshold. In summary, both exercise functional studies and invasive studies demonstrate the important contribution of both appropriately timed atrial systolic contraction and increasing heart rate to cardiac output, but which factor contributes more to improved cardiac output at a given level of activity is not well defined.

In general cardiac output measured by invasive means increases in patients who have been converted from atrial fibrillation to normal sinus rhythm (9–20). These acute hemodynamic studies are listed in Table 1. The loss of atrial booster pump function as a consequence of atrial fibrillation remains the most likely mechanism for reduction in cardiac output, but other potential causes have been suggested, such

TABLE 1. *Catheterization cardiac output data on conversion of atrial fibrillation to normal sinus rhythm*

Authors (ref.)	Year	No. of patients	Change with rest (%)	Change with exercise (%)
Hansen et al. (9)	1952	14	27[a]	30[a]
Graettinger et al. (10)	1964	17 converted	10[a]	7.4[a]
Kahn et al. (11)	1964	10	22[a]	27[a]
Benchimol et al. (12)	1965	8	6.6	8.3[a]
Morris et al. (13)	1965	11	16[a]	18[a,c]
Reale (14)	1965	12	7[b]	—
Killip & Baer (15)	1966	10 (MVD)	30[a]	22[a]
		5 (AVD)	38[a]	15
		4 (LAF)	8[a]	6.6
Rowlands et al. (16)	1966	12	11[b]	—
Resnekov (17)	1967	15	2	16[a]
Kaplan et al. (18)	1968	16	15[a]	—
Shapiro & Klein (19)	1968	11	12	14.8[a]
Khaja & Parker (20)	1972	13	9.2[b]	—

[a]Significant.
[b]Possibly significant.
[c]Five patients only.
MVD, mitral valve disease; AVD, aortic valve disease; LAF, lone atrial fibrillation.

as deranged mitral and tricuspid valve closure, wasted ventricular energy during episodes of inadequate ventricular contraction, and a reduction in diastolic filling time resulting in reduced coronary flow. These hemodynamic studies are complicated by the fact that they were performed in patients with various types of heart disease, with varying degrees of left ventricular function, and with atrial fibrillation of varying duration. These differences may be responsible for differing conclusions. Thus, Graettinger et al. (10) noted a significantly greater atrial contribution to cardiac output only in patients whose heart rate decreased when in sinus rhythm, while Killip and Baer (15) concluded that a significant contribution to cardiac output after cardioversion occurred in subjects with mitral and aortic valvular disease, but not in patients with idiopathic atrial fibrillation. Nevertheless, despite various qualifiers, there was a general consensus that atrial contraction adds both to resting and exertional cardiac output.

EFFECT OF EXERCISE IN PATIENTS WITH ATRIAL FIBRILLATION

Exercise testing is a useful noninvasive method for evaluating the cardiovascular response in a variety of populations ranging from normal to the severely ill cardiomyopathy patient with congestive heart failure. As noted in Table 2, studies to evaluate the response of patients with atrial fibrillation to exercise were performed as early as 1968. These studies noted specific differences in the response to exercise in atrial fibrillation when compared to subjects in normal sinus rhythm. A common finding was an inordinately rapid heart rate response to atrial fibrillation during the initial stage of exercise, which is unlike the linear heart rate response to increasing work levels found in patients in normal sinus rhythm whose rate is dependent on the autonomic/catecholaminergic effect on the sinoatrial node. Early studies also tended to demonstrate a reduced functional capacity when estimating energy expenditure at maximal treadmill or bicycle work. The systolic blood pressure response was found to remain within ranges of those found in subjects in normal sinus rhythm.

Estimation of functional capacity from exercise duration has several potential inaccuracies that may seriously flaw conclusions of exercise studies. In order to avoid these pitfalls, we routinely perform gas exchange analysis during exercise. The pitfalls of standard exercise testing and the technique of gas exchange analysis with particular reference to atrial fibrillation will now be reviewed in detail.

Exercise Testing Methodology

Exercise testing is an excellent method to evaluate a patient's heart rate response, blood pressure response, electrocardiographic response, and maximal functional capacity. However, most studies utilizing exercise as a method for stressing patients in atrial fibrillation to evaluate the therapeutic efficacy of pharmacologic agents such as digoxin, beta-blockers, and calcium channel-blockers, are not comparable because of the numerous methodologic variations including a variety of protocols using either treadmill exercise (Bruce, modified Bruce, or modified Balke-Ware protocols) or bicycle exercise, different patient populations, and unclear endpoints (47). General conclusions can therefore be made, but comparisons may be made only with reservation.

TABLE 2. *Previous studies of exercise testing in patients with atrial fibrillation*

	Investigator (ref.)												
	Hornsten & Bruce (29)	Aberg et al. (30)	Aberg et al. (31)	Aberg et al. (32)	Khalsa & Olsson (35)	Davidson & Hagan (36)	Lang et al. (41)	Molajo et al. (40)	DiBianco et al. (38)	Roth et al. (42)	Steinberg et al. (44)	Atwood et al. (47)	Lundstrom & Ryden (49)
Year	1968	1972	1972	1977	1979	1979	1983	1984	1984	1986	1987	1988	1990
No. of patients	65	179	24	15	11	11	20	10	20	12	14	50	13
Mean age (year)	48	47	45	45	56	55	59	52	60	48	66	65	65
Exercise protocol	Bruce	Bike	Bike	Bike	Bike	Bruce	Bike	Bruce	Mod. Bruce	Mod. Bruce	Mod. Bruce	Mod. B-W	Bike
Mean max HR heart rate (bpm)	176	134	157	138	142	176	169	162	175	170	163	176	179
Estimated METs	7	3.5	3.5	4	5.9	6.5	3.5	5	7	—	7	7.5	6.5
Estimated max VO$_2$ (ml/kg/min)	25	12	12	13	21	23	12	18	25	—	—	26	22.3
Resting blood pressure	132/76	—	—	—	—	143/—	132/82	125/—	131/84	118/77	136/83	138/85	150/—
Exercise blood pressure	160/76	—	—	—	—	165/—	166/42	157/—	*166/91	151/88	*160/80	175/83	193/—

[a]Submaximal exercise.
—, not reported; Mod. Bruce, modified Bruce; B-W, Balke-Ware.

Maximal functional capacity or exercise capacity is that level of exertion or VO_2 at which point the participant is subjectively unable to continue exercising and is measured or estimated in ml O_2/kg/min or described in terms of number of METs (a unit of basal energy expenditure equal to 3.5 ml O_2/kg/min). Functional capacity is extremely difficult to estimate accurately from a workload level of treadmill speed and grade in individual subjects. Variables that influence functional capacity include genetic endowment, age, sex, health status of the individual, presence of disease such as cardiomyopathy or coronary artery disease, activity status of the individual, familiarity with exercise testing, hanging on to or grasping handrails, willingness to push to a maximal level of exercise, and commonly in serial exercise studies the so-called learning or habituation effect (60). Several studies have demonstrated that on serial exercise testing despite no significant change in measured maximal VO_2, a significant increase in treadmill exercise time may occur (63–68). To eliminate the habituation or learning effect, it has been suggested for reproducibility that peak measured VO_2 be within 10% on consecutive studies. In one study employing exercise time, 21 of 30 patients required four or more tests (eight required six or more tests) before three consecutive tests were within 60 sec of each other (65). Froelicher et al. (67) studied more than 1,000 asymptomatic men and demonstrated a range of more than 20 ml O_2 kg/min (approximately 6 METs) in measured VO_2 at a given fixed workload of exercise, thereby lending further evidence for the variability and/or potential error in estimating energy expenditure from workload or exercise time. This variability or potential inaccuracy is of particular relevance in studies involving a therapeutic comparison in which a 10% to 20% change may be considered significant.

Because exercise testing with gas exchange analysis directly measures VO_2/consumption, it is the most accurate method to assess subject performance or evaluate specific therapy. Breath-by-breath gas exchange analysis of O_2, CO_2, and air flow has replaced the cumbersome method of the 1-min Douglas bag collection. Measuring expiratory gas during exercise has many advantages, viz., the results are more accurate and reproducible than simple estimation of VO_2 from exercise duration and intensity; it is less affected by serial testing; oxygen kinetics can be measured; submaximal measurements of oxygen consumption may be measured—in particular the anaerobic threshold (a point at which minute ventilation (VE) and VCO_2 production increase out of proportion to VO_2). In addition other elements of exercise capacity besides VO_2 can be measured such as VCO_2, VE, the respiratory exchange ratio (RER), which is simply a ratio of VCO_2/VO_2, and calculations of ventilatory dead space and tidal volume (58–60).

When performing an exercise test to evaluate functional capacity, certain methodologic considerations must be made in addition to the routine heart rate, blood pressure, and ECG monitoring. Treadmill exercise rather than erect bicycle ergometry is more commonly used because higher levels of VO_2 and heart rate are attained with treadmill exercise, although higher systolic pressures are noted at maximal levels of bicycle exercise (71,72). The type of protocol used is also very important and should be individualized to the subject. Older, less conditioned patients may require a less rigorous protocol than the Bruce protocol, which at Stage I (estimated to be approximately 5 to 6 METs) may prove to be 70% to 80% of the subjects maximal exercise capacity. The modified Balke-Ware protocol with an initial treadmill speed of 2.0 mph and 0% grade and a maximal treadmill speed of 3.0 mph offers a superior alternative. Buchfuhrer et al. (72) have demonstrated that an exercise duration of approximately 10 min is optimal for data collection. Longer duration tests may measure endurance more than maximal exercise capacity. Recent data suggest that rather than 2- or 3-min stages for each incremental workload, a ramp protocol utilizing a progressively increasing work rate without defined stages or "increments" may offer more accuracy and be better suited for pharmacologic studies (60).

During exercise testing with gas exchange analysis subjects have a mouthpiece and noseclip in place and use hand signals to communicate on a chart with the Borg scale of rate of perceived exertion (77). Each minute throughout the exercise test, the subject rates his/her perceived exertion on a scale of 6 to 20 (very very hard). We use a rating of perceived exertion of 18 to 20 as an indicator of maximal effort. Maximal exercise has been determined by various other methods such as symptoms or rate of perceived exertion, maximal predicted heart rate, a RER of 1.1 or greater, and a plateau in VO_2 despite an increase in workload. These latter two measurements require exercise testing with gas exchange analysis. The measurement of a VO_2 plateau employs an arbitrary assignment of a sampling time interval, but this "plateau" may be present in as few as 7% of subjects (73,74). The RER and predicted heart rate at maximal effort vary extensively from patient to patient. At maximal effort the standard deviation in heart rate may reach as high as ±15 bpm (80). Interestingly, while studying nine patients in atrial fibrillation during three different therapeutic regimens of placebo, high-dose beta-adrenergic blocker, and medium-dose calcium channel-blocker, we noted that VE was more closely related to perceived exertion than heart rate or VO_2 (61).

Blood pressure and heart rate and gas exchange values of VO_2, VCO_2, RER, and VE are obtained not only at maximal exercise but also at submaximal levels. Submaximal levels are variably defined and might include a common workload that all subjects have attained, workloads either at a matched double product (heart rate multiplied by systolic pressure) or when 1 mm of ST-segment depression occurs on the ECG (particularly useful in angina studies), and/or the gas exchange anaerobic threshold. The anaerobic threshold is a reproducible point at which there is a nonlinear increase in VE and VCO_2 in contrast to the linear increase in VO_2. Although initially thought to be the noninvasive delineation of lactate accumulation, the mechanism for gas exchange anaerobic threshold has come under intense scrutiny and remains controversial (61,75,76). Nevertheless, it has remained a reproducible submaximal level of exertion useful in pharmacologic studies and for predicting fitness.

The reproducibility of exercise testing with gas exchange analysis has been well demonstrated in patients in normal sinus rhythm (63). As mentioned previously, the importance of multiple exercise tests and sequential exercise testing is underscored by the fact that patients who are inexperienced with treadmill testing may have an increase in total treadmill exercise time without an actual increase in measured maximal VO_2 since repeated testing can result in improved neuromuscular coordination, which may decrease VO_2. At submaximal workloads, both VO_2 and heart rate may likewise decrease, consistent with the "learning effect" and increased work efficiency with serial testing. The effect of repeated exercise testing on performance time may be greater with treadmill testing than bicycle testing, owing to the greater learning effect on gait with the former modality. Thus, Aberg and associates (32) demonstrated little or no significant differences in submaximal or maximal heart rate responses to sequential bicycle exercise testing in patients in atrial fibrillation. Although not significant, they did note a 6% lower heart rate on the second test, at submaximal workloads. In contrast, in our own study of patients with atrial fibrillation, we found that at submaximal levels of exercise on a follow-up test, there was a reduction in heart rate and VO_2, whereas maximal VO_2 remained relatively unchanged (78). This was consistent with a learning or habituation effect. In addition to the improvement in neuromuscular coordination on serial exercise testing, there is also the effect of autonomic/catecholaminergic activity, which may have marked effect on the atrioventricular node in patients in atrial fibrillation. With reduced anxiety on serial tests the rate may fall because of diminished catecholamine effect on the atrioventricular node. On the other hand, patients in normal sinus rhythm, whose rate is entirely dependent on the sinoatrial node, may have a less dramatic heart rate reduction.

Heart Rate Response

Accurate measurement of heart rate during exercise testing and rest in patients with atrial fibrillation may be difficult because the irregular rate causes high variability (79). We noted that in atrial fibrillation a 1-sec sample had a 33-beat range of inaccuracy, whereas a 20-sec sample yielded an average error of 2.4 beats when compared to a 60-sec count (Fig. 1). A 6-sec calculation of heart rate led to an average of a 5.5-bpm error. In comparison, 1- and 2-sec sampling intervals of patients in sinus rhythm led to an error of 3.9 and 3.2 bpm, and longer intervals ranging up to 20 sec led to an approximate error of 1 to 2 bpm average. We concluded that accurate efficient estimates of heart rate during atrial fibrillation at rest and during exercise are obtained if intervals of greater than or equal to 6 sec are used and that, ideally, an average of two 6-sec measurements during a 1-min strip would improve the precision (79).

Heart rate response during treadmill exercise is generally higher in patients with atrial fibrillation (Table 2) than heart rates predicted for patients in sinus rhythm (58,80). The marked variability of heart rate response in subjects with atrial fibrillation is evidenced by such large standard deviations as 30 bpm. Our laboratory noted a higher heart rate response in patients with lone atrial fibrillation than in those with atrial fibrillation with known heart disease (189 ± 32 vs 166 ± 24 bpm) (47). Bicycle exercise is generally associated with lower heart rate response for patients in sinus rhythm and as noted in Table 2, in studies by Aberg et al. (30–32) and Khalsa and Olsson (35), mean maximal heart rate response in patients with atrial fibrillation undergoing bicycle exercise was 20 to 40 bpm lower than those on treadmill exercise. The low heart rate response in these studies may also have been due to the population tested by these two investigators, which tended to be sicker, as evidenced by the markedly lower functional capacity.

Most of the exercise studies involved the use of digoxin, which some authors suggest may decrease submaximal heart rates and may even reduce maximal heart rate response. Hornsten and Bruce (29) noted a higher heart rate response and higher functional capacity in their population of patients with rheumatic valvular disease on a digitalis preparation, when compared to a similar group in sinus rhythm, thereby suggesting that his patients had a lesser degree of disease. The other studies in Table 2 were selected from studies evaluating the therapeutic efficacy of various medical regimens when compared to digoxin. They too demonstrate higher heart rate responses than one would expect for a similar age-matched population in sinus rhythm.

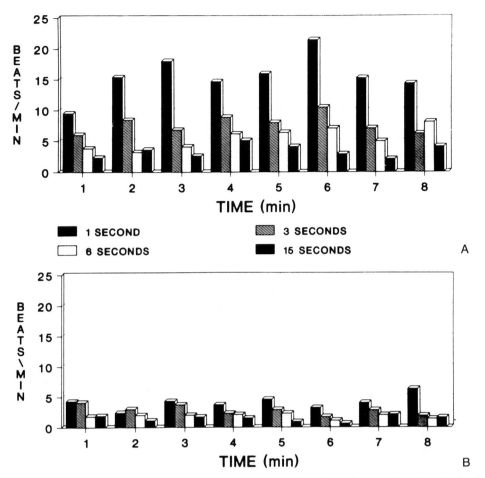

FIG. 1. A: Mean differences between heart rate obtained and true heart rate using 1-, 3-, 6-, and 15-sec sampling intervals among patients with atrial fibrillation. **B:** Mean differences between heart rate obtained and true heart rate using 1-, 3-, 6-, and 15-sec sampling intervals among subjects in normal sinus rhythm. (From ref. 79, with permission.)

In reviewing these and other studies, it becomes clear that heart rate in patients with atrial fibrillation, as in patients in sinus rhythm, is directly related to total body oxygen demand or stage of exercise. Most studies used a Bruce protocol in an older aged population whose maximal exercise capacity was relatively diminished because of either age and/or intrinsic heart disease. However, by using lower workloads in our population of 50 subjects, we demonstrated a linear response in our subject population when comparing heart rate to VO_2 (Fig. 2) (47). Hence, a workload of 70% maximal exertion would have a heart rate of approximately 70% of the maximal heart rate. This suggests that, contrary to the generally accepted belief, the heart rate response to exercise in many patients with atrial fibrillation may not be pathologically rapid but may partially represent a functional response to the underlying heart disease.

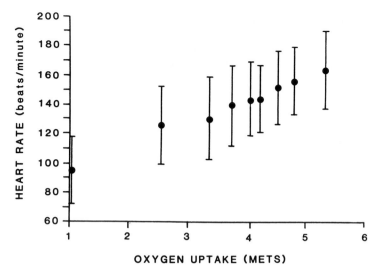

FIG. 2. Relation between maximal heart rate and VO_2 for all 50 patients with atrial fibrillation during progressive exercise (0–8 min). Heart rate and VO_2 were significantly correlated ($r = 0.54$, $p < 0.001$) despite a large variance in heart rate (SD ± 28 bpm), and they covaried significantly over time ($F = 27.1$, $p < 0.001$). Group membership (lone vs atrial fibrillation with heart disease) did not affect these relations. METs = multiples of oxygen consumption at rest. (From ref. 51, with permission.)

When comparing patients with lone atrial fibrillation to those with intrinsic heart disease, we noted similar resting heart rates but significantly lower maximal heart rate responses in the subjects with intrinsic heart disease (166 ± 24 vs 189 ± 32 bpm). Possible explanations for this finding might include (a) a greater degree of atrioventricular node disease in patients with intrinsic heart disease; (b) a blunted catecholamine rise in the diseased population, and/or (c) a greater degree of anterograde concealed conduction in patients with intrinsic atrial fibrillation related to finer, more frequent fibrillatory waves. The higher heart rate response in atrial fibrillation patients than expected for their age in comparison to that predicted for subjects in sinus rhythm has many possible explanations. Teleologically, it would be satisfying to conjecture that higher maximal heart rates serve as a compensatory mechanism for the loss of "atrial kick" to cardiac output. However, it is more likely that the enhanced atrioventricular node response to catecholamines during exercise with atrial fibrillation allows for greater heart rate response than does a similar catecholamine stimulation of the sinoatrial node during sinus rhythm.

After conversion from atrial fibrillation to sinus rhythm the maximal heart rate response to exercise falls to below that anticipated in a similar age-matched population without a history of arrhythmia (50,51). In the Lipkin et al. (50) study, mean maximal heart rate fell from 168 ± 7 while in atrial fibrillation, to 135 ± 6 bpm in normal sinus rhythm 1 day after cardioversion. This is lower than the anticipated maximal sinus rate for a healthy age-matched population and probably represents chronotropic incompetence related to the underlying cardiac disease. The maximal heart rate response to exercise after cardioversion did not increase after 1 month when subjects were retested. Our group of patients also demonstrated this chronotropic incompetence after an even longer period postcardioversion (51).

In summary, in subjects in atrial fibrillation: (a) heart rate response is highly variable; (b) heart rates are significantly higher than expected in age-matched patients in sinus rhythm; (c) significantly higher heart rates occur in subjects with lone atrial fibrillation than in those patients with atrial fibrillation and known heart disease; and (d) heart rate response relates linearly to or parallels oxygen consumption (i.e., 70% of maximal VO_2 is associated with approximately 70% of the maximal heart rate); (e) maximal exercise heart rate response after cardioversion to sinus rhythm is markedly reduced compared to atrial fibrillation and also is often lower than that expected for an age-matched normal population.

Functional Capacity

As noted in Table 2, functional capacity varies in patients with atrial fibrillation. The Scandinavian studies of Aberg et al. and Khalsa and Olsson demonstrate a much lower functional capacity than that in other studies. In reviewing these studies, the population tended to be more severely ill with valvular heart disease and other intrinsic heart disease, which is consistent with the idea that intrinsic heart disease is associated with reduced maximal exercise capacity. In addition, they used bicycle exercise, which is associated with a lower maximal VO_2 than treadmill exercise. Interestingly, in the study by Hornsten and Bruce (29) although their population had predominantly rheumatic valvular heart disease, their subjects had a relatively high estimated functional capacity. DiBianco's group (38) had 11 patients with idiopathic atrial fibrillation, although six had associated hypertension. Both these studies have high estimated MET levels and suggest a fitter population.

In order to determine whether reduction in functional capacity is primarily due to intrinsic heart disease or to atrial fibrillation, we studied 50 patients in chronic atrial fibrillation (47). Twenty-one had lone atrial fibrillation, and 29 had intrinsic heart disease (including eight with regurgitant valvular heart disease, eight with dilated cardiomyopathy, seven with a history of congestive heart failure, three with ischemic heart disease, two with moderate lung disease, and one with sick sinus syndrome). There was a significantly higher exercise capacity in the lone atrial fibrillation group compared to those with associated heart disease (mean VO_2 of 22.7 vs 19.1 ml O_2/kg/min; $p<0.05$). The maximal VO_2 and the estimated functional capacity of the lone atrial fibrillation group equaled values typical of an age-matched group of normal men in sinus rhythm. Likewise, the functional capacity in those with intrinsic heart disease was approximately 20% less than that expected for a similar age group. We concluded that exercise capacity in patients with atrial fibrillation was limited by intrinsic heart disease and not the rhythm of atrial fibrillation.

Blood Pressure Response

Because of the variability in the diastolic filling period, the determination of the onset of systolic blood pressure in patients with atrial fibrillation is difficult to assess, poorly reproducible, and has not been well described in the literature. This is particularly true at rest when, after long RR intervals, Korotkoff's sounds may be heard more distinctly, either at a higher or lower level than those with shorter RR intervals. Interestingly enough, in exercise as the heart rate increases, the variability in blood pressure seems to diminish *(personal finding)*, but this has not been verified in the literature.

Both from review of the literature and by personal experience, systolic blood pressure increases, diastolic pressure remains the same or diminishes, and mean arterial pressure increases, as expected in any normal subject in normal sinus rhythm during exercise (see Table 2) (47). A normal increase in systolic blood pressure from rest to exercise in men should be at least 60 ± 25 mm Hg and in women 40 ± 20 mm Hg with an increment of approximately 6 mm Hg/MET (58). In our large study describing the hemodynamic response of 50 patients in atrial fibrillation (47), a stepwise regression analysis done for the 50 patients demonstrated that systolic blood pressure (an excellent correlate of ventricular function) was the best predictor of maximal exercise capacity, accounting for 19% of the variance. Maximal heart rate was the only other significant predictor and accounted for only 8% of the variance. Of 21 patients with lone atrial fibrillation, the systolic blood pressure response was 15 mm Hg higher than those 29 patients with atrial fibrillation and known heart disease ($p<0.05$), thereby implying better cardiac function. There was also no significant difference in diastolic pressure at any stage of exercise in either population.

In summary, (a) the blood pressure responses in patients with atrial fibrillation parallel those in subjects in sinus rhythm, i.e., systolic pressure increases, mean arterial pressure increases, and diastolic blood pressure remains unchanged; (b) systolic blood pressure seems to be the best predictor of exercise capacity in patients with atrial fibrillation; (c) the systolic blood pressure response in patients with lone atrial fibrillation is significantly greater than those in patients with atrial fibrillation and known heart disease.

Electrocardiogram

The ECG primarily serves to make the diagnosis of atrial fibrillation by documenting an undulating baseline, lack of defined atrial activity or a chaotic atrial rhythm, and a variable RR interval. Accurate efficient measurement of heart rate during exercise testing is difficult because of the irregular rate causing high variability. We found that either an average of two 6-sec sampling measurements during a 1-min strip or one 6-sec sample were the most efficient intervals to produce an accurate heart rate without counting QRS complexes for 1 min (73).

Arrhythmia diagnosis during exercise testing is difficult, especially distinguishing premature ventricular complexes from aberrant conduction. At higher exercise workloads, differentiating between aberrant ventricular conduction, ventricular tachycardia, and a rate-dependent bundle-branch block may be extremely challenging. ST-segment changes are also difficult to assess, because most subjects in atrial fibrillation are receiving digoxin and that may produce ST-segment shifts unrelated to coronary artery disease. Hence, interpretation of the ECG changes during exercise testing should be done with caution.

USE OF GAS EXCHANGE ANALYSIS TO EVALUATE THERAPY IN ATRIAL FIBRILLATION

As mentioned previously, exercise testing with gas exchange analysis is the most accurate method of measuring actual functional capacity or VO_2 at various levels of

TABLE 3. *Exercise response to therapy in patients with atrial fibrillation*

	Heart rate	Blood pressure	Maximal exercise capacity
Digoxin	↓	NC	SI ↑
Digoxin and beta-blockers	↓ ↓ ↓	↓ ↓	↓
Digoxin and calcium channel-blockers	↓ ↓	NC	NC or ↑
Cardioversion	↓ ↓ ↓	↑	↑ ↑

↓, mild decrease; ↓ ↓, moderate decrease; ↓ ↓ ↓, marked decrease; NC, no change; ↑, increase; SI ↑, slight increase; ↑ ↑, moderate increase.

exercise. Hence, it is particularly useful in evaluating the efficacy of a specific therapy such as cardioversion to sinus rhythm or pharmacologic attenuation of heart rate response by such agents as digoxin, calcium channel-blockers, and beta-adrenergic blockers (see Table 3).

Evaluation of Pharmacologic Therapy

In the past, most studies evaluating the effectiveness of therapy employed exercise time rather than measured VO_2, as has been done more recently. Only one study employing gas exchange analysis has evaluated the effectiveness of digoxin for controlling the heart rate response to exercise in patients in atrial fibrillation. Beasley et al. (45) measured heart rate response at a measured workload level of exertion of 20 ml O_2/kg/min in 12 subjects with chronic atrial fibrillation. While on placebo, the resting heart rate was 108 bpm, increasing to 192 bpm at a workload to 20 ml O_2/kg/min. On low-dose (serum levels 0.8 µg/liter) digoxin, and high-dose (serum levels of 1.8 µg/liter) digoxin, resting heart rate fell to 93 and 83 bpm, respectively, and at a workload of 20 ml O_2/kg/min, heart rate fell to 182 and 164 bpm, respectively. In earlier studies not utilizing gas exchange analysis Aberg et al. (31) demonstrated a mild reduction in exercise heart rate response at higher doses of digoxin. Still another study reported that digoxin at levels of 1.3 to 2.6 nmol/liter was only as effective as verapamil 40 mg t.i.d. (81).

Six studies using beta-blockers in conjunction with digoxin all demonstrated a definite reduction in exercise heart rate (37–40,46,82), although the effect on exercise duration was variable. Nadolol was shown to decrease exercise time, which was in contrast to Corwin, a beta-1 adrenoreceptor partial agonist, which increased exercise time by an average of 42 sec (38,40). Practolol, timolol, and propranolol all reduced heart rates at submaximal levels of exercise, but each of these three studies contained patients who deteriorated clinically, suggesting that there might be a significant negative inotropic effect from beta-blockers (37,39,82). Using exercise with gas exchange analysis, we evaluated celiprolol, a beta-1 selective adrenergic blocker, to test whether reducing heart rate and increasing diastolic filling time would possibly improve functional capacity in patients in atrial fibrillation (46). A definite reduction in heart rate response occurred at all levels of exercise, but there was a clear-cut reduction in maximal exercise capacity, with a 16% reduction in measured VO_2 at maximal effort (21.0 ml O_2/kg/min for placebo vs 17.6 ml O_2/kg/min for those on celiprolol). We also noted a significant reduction in systolic pressure at all levels of exertion. Although speculative, the mechanism for the reduction in VO_2 is most likely due to the negative inotropic effect of the beta-adrenergic blockade, which is possibly manifest as the blunted blood pressure response. However, the possibility that an inadequate heart rate response was a source for this reduction in VO_2 could not be excluded. The effect of beta-blockers on maximal VO_2 in patients with normal sinus rhythm is controversial, and these agents have been reported as decreasing or demonstrating no change in maximal VO_2. This may be due to several causes, including different types of adrenergic blockers used, timing of the test, duration of medication, dosage level, exercise protocol used, and patient population (83).

To date only two studies (48,49) have used gas exchange analysis to evaluate the therapy of calcium channel-blockers in patients in atrial fibrillation, although many exercise studies have been performed (41–45,48,49,84–87). Lang and his group (41) demonstrated that verapamil increased exercise capacity on a multistage bicycle ergometry exercise test. Using an elaborate reporting form of exercise units, they noted an increase from 522 to 806 work units when subjects were placed on verapamil therapy. Gas exchange analysis was not performed on this population. Lewis and colleagues (81), although not reporting actual maximal exercise capacity, found that exercise tolerance was similar in both verapamil- and digoxin-treated patients. Roth and colleagues (42), using a fixed maximal level of treadmill exercise in 12 patients, demonstrated that the addition of diltiazem to digoxin significantly reduced the heart rate response more so than when digoxin or diltiazem was given alone. They concluded that a moderate dose of diltiazem with digoxin (diltiazem 240 mg/day) was a safe and effective dose. In a population of nine patients using exercise testing with gas exchange analysis, we demonstrated that diltiazem 60 mg, four times daily, along with digoxin, significantly reduced heart rate response at all levels of exercise (48). In contrast to the findings during celiprolol therapy (46), there was no significant change in exercise capacity or systolic blood pressure at all levels of exercise. More recently, Lundstrom and colleagues (49), using bicycle ergometric testing, along with gas exchange analysis, demonstrated a significant reduction in heart rate at rest and at all levels of exercise, using either diltiazem 270 mg/day, or verapamil 240 mg/day. In their group of 18 patients, at maximal exercise they noticed no significant change in systolic blood pressure, and with measured VO_2, they noted that subjects on diltiazem had a small but significant increase in maximal functional capacity when compared to placebo (23.7 vs 22.3 ml O_2/kg/min). Verapamil produced a slight increase to 22.9 O_2/kg/min, but this was not statistically significant. There was no significant difference between diltiazem and verapamil in terms of improving maximal exercise capacity.

In summary, the pharmacologic therapy for atrial fibrillation is variable (see Table 3). Digoxin does reduce heart rate at rest, but only mildly in response to exercise. There are no studies that define in a clear-cut manner that digoxin may improve functional capacity. Beta-adrenergic blockers, when added to digoxin, significantly reduce the heart rate response at all levels of exercise, may reduce systolic blood pressure response, and may reduce VO_2 at maximal exercise. Calcium channel-blockers, when given in conjunction with digoxin, reduce heart rate response to exercise at all levels, do not change systolic blood pressure response at maximal exercise, and have been demonstrated to increase or have no change in VO_2 at maximal levels of exertion.

Electrocardioversion

In theory, functional capacity should improve when patients are converted to normal sinus rhythm from atrial fibrillation because of the contribution of the "atrial

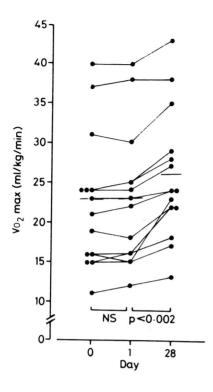

FIG. 3. Change in symptom-limited maximal oxygen consumption (VO_2 max) before and on days 1 and 28 after direct current cardioversion of atrial fibrillation to sinus rhythm. (From ref. 50, with permission.)

kick" to cardiac output. Only two published studies using exercise testing with gas exchange analysis have evaluated this hypothesis (50,51). Lipkin et al. (50) studied 14 individuals in chronic atrial fibrillation using exercise testing with gas exchange analysis, the day prior to cardioversion, 1 day after cardioversion, and 28 days after cardioversion. All patients prior to cardioversion had undergone exercise testing until there was a less than 5% change in VO_2 on two consecutive tests, thereby eliminating the "learning effect." Lipkin et al. demonstrated that there was no significant increase in VO_2, either at the anaerobic threshold or at peak exercise, on the day after cardioversion. However, 28 days after cardioversion and in sinus rhythm, the anaerobic threshold had significantly increased from 17 to 20 ml O_2/kg/min, and maximal exercise capacity had increased from 23 to 26 ml O_2/kg/min (Fig. 3). Doppler echocardiography was performed in 12 of the 14 patients. In all patients, the height of the A-wave and the A-to-E ratio had significantly increased from day 1 to day 28, suggesting delayed improvement in atrial contractility, a finding consistent with several other studies (87–92). They concluded that restoration of sinus rhythm improved exercise capacity, which was in part due to a slow improvement in atrial contractility after cardioversion. No change in maximal heart rate response occurred after being in sinus rhythm for 1 month.

Lipkin et al. noted an average increase of approximately 1 MET of exercise and also noted that most improvement seemed to occur in patients with the most reduced functional capacity, primarily in patients with valvular heart disease or coronary artery disease. In three patients with idiopathic dilated cardiomyopathy, the improvement was 1, 2, and 3 ml O_2/kg/min. In a study of 11 male patients in our laboratory, we noted that the maximal VO_2 was higher after cardioversion, but it was in patients who had normal left ventricular function that we seemed to note the largest increase in functional capacity (51). Because of the small numbers, we could not determine statistical significance. In addition, our patients were not studied at a fixed day after cardioversion, but rather a mean of 39 days following cardioversion. As anticipated, in both the Lipkin et al. study and our study, heart rate was markedly reduced at all levels of exercise following cardioversion. This has also been noted in hemodynamic studies in which the heart rate reduction was as great as 30 bpm during exercise.

In summary, cardioversion results in: (a) an increase in cardiac output, both at rest and during exercise; (b) an improved VO_2 at maximal exercise, but only after atrial function has had a chance to recover (i.e., at least 28 days after cardioversion); (c) a reduction in heart rate response during exercise after cardioversion.

ACKNOWLEDGMENTS

The author wishes to thank Maureen Kelly for her excellent secretarial assistance and typing of this manuscript. I would also like to thank Dr. Vic Froelicher, who was an excellent advisor during all of these studies. Most of all, I would like to thank my research group of John Myers, Michael Sullivan, Susan Forbes, Susan Quaglietti, and Erin Bushell, who have contributed enormously to my knowledge and understanding of atrial fibrillation.

REFERENCES

1. Lewis T. Fibrillation of the auricles; its effects upon the circulation. *J Exp Med* 1912;16:395.
2. Meijler FL. Atrial fibrillation: a new look at an old arrhythmia. *J Am Coll Cardiol* 1983;2:391–393.
3. Gesell RA. Cardiodynamics in the heart block as affected by auricular systole, auricular fibrillation and stimulation of the vagus nerve. *Am J Physiol* 1916;40:267.
4. Gesell RA. Initial length-initial tension and tone of auricular muscle in relation to myo and cardiodynamics. *Am J Physiol* 1916;39:239.
5. Gesell RA. The effects of change in auricular tone and amplitude of auricular systole on ventricular output. *Am J Physiol* 1915;38:404.
6. Gesell RA. Auricular systole and its relation to ventricular output. *Am J Physiol* 1911;29:32.
7. Braunwald E, Frahm CJ. Studies on Starling's law of the heart: IV. Observations on the hemodynamic functions of the left atrium in man. *Circulation* 1961;24:633–641.
8. Braunwald E. Symposium on cardiac arrhythmias: introduction with comments on the hemodynamic significance of atrial systole. *Am J Med* 1964;37:665–669.
9. Hansen WR, McClendon RO, Kinsman JM. Auricular fibrillation. Hemodynamic studies before and after conversion with quinidine. *Am Heart J* 1952;44:499.
10. Graettinger JS, Carleton RA, Muenster JJ. Circulatory consequences of changes in cardiac rhythm produced in patients by transthoracic direct-current shock. *J Clin Invest* 1964;43:2290–2302.
11. Kahn DR, Wilson WS, Weber W, Sloan H. Hemodynamic studies before and after cardioversion. *J Thorac Cardiovasc Surg* 1964;48:898–905.
12. Benchimol A, Lowe HM, Akre P. Cardiovascular response to exercise during atrial fibrillation and after conversion to sinus rhythm. *Am J Cardiol* 1965;16:31–41.
13. Morris JJ, Entman M, North WC, Kong Y, McIntosh H. The changes in cardiac output with reversion of atrial fibrillation to sinus rhythm. *Circulation* 1965;31:670–678.
14. Reale A. Acute effects of countershock conversion of atrial fibrillation upon right and left heart hemodynamics. *Circulation* 1965;32:214–223.
15. Killip T, Baer RA. Hemodynamic effects after reversion from atrial fibrillation to sinus rhythm by precordial shock. *J Clin Invest* 1966;45:658–671.
16. Rowlands DJ, Logan WFWE, Howitt G. Atrial function after cardioversion. *Am Heart J* 1967;74:149–160.
17. Resnekov L. Hemodynamic studies before and after electrical conversion of atrial fibrillation and flutter to sinus rhythm. *Br Heart J* 1967;29:700–708.

18. Kaplan MA, Gray RE, Iseri LT, Williams RL. Metabolic and hemodynamic responses to exercise during atrial fibrillation and sinus rhythm. *Am J Cardiol* 1968;22:543–549.

19. Shapiro W, Klein G. Alterations in cardiac function immediately following electrical conversion of atrial fibrillation to normal sinus rhythm. *Circulation* 1968;38:1074–1084.

20. Khaja F, Parker JO. Hemodynamic effects of cardioversion in chronic atrial fibrillation. *Arch Intern Med* 1972;129:433–440.

21. Samet P, Bernstein W, Levine S. Significance of the atrial contribution to ventricular filling. *Am J Cardiol* 1965;15:195–202.

22. Karlof I. Haemodynamic effect of atrial triggered versus fixed rate pacing at rest and during exercise in complete heart block. *Acta Med Scand* 1975;197:195.

23. Kruse I, Arnman K, Conradson TB, Ryden L. A comparison of the acute and long-term hemodynamic effects of ventricular inhibited and atrial synchronous ventricular inhibited pacing. *Circulation* 1982;65:846–855.

24. Kruse I, Ryden L. Comparison of physical work capacity and systolic time intervals with ventricular inhibited and atrial synchronous ventricular inhibited pacing. *Br Heart J* 1981;46:129.

25. Ausubel K, Steingart RM, Shimshi M, Klementowicz P, Furman S. Maintenance of exercise stroke volume during ventricular versus atrial synchronous pacing: role of contractility. *Circulation* 1985;72:1037.

26. Fananapazir L, Bennett DH, Monks P. Atrial synchronized ventricular pacing: contribution of the chronotropic response to improved exercise performance. *PACE* 1983;6:601.

27. Fananapazir L, Srinivas V, Bennett DH. Comparison of resting hemodynamic indices and exercise performance during atrial synchronized and asynchronous ventricular pacing. *PACE* 1983;6:202.

28. Benditt DG, Mianulli M, Fetter J, et al. Single-chamber cardiac pacing with activity-initiated chronotropic response: evaluation by cardiopulmonary exercise testing. *Circulation* 1987;75:184–191.

29. Hornsten TR, Bruce RA. Effects of atrial fibrillation on exercise performance in patients with cardiac disease. *Circulation* 1968;37:543–548.

30. Aberg H, Strom G, Werner I. Heart rate during exercise in patients with atrial fibrillation. *Acta Med Scand* 1972;191:315–320.

31. Aberg H, Strom G, Werner I. The effect of digitalis on the heart rate during exercise in patients with atrial fibrillation. *Acta Med Scand* 1972;191:441–445.

32. Aberg H, Strom G, Werner I. On the reproducibility of exercise tests in patients with atrial fibrillation. *Uppsala J Med Sci* 1977;82:27–30.

33. Redfors A. Digoxin dosage and ventricular rate at rest and exercise in patients with atrial fibrillation. *Acta Med Scand* 1971;190:321–333.

34. Redfors A. Plasma digoxin concentration—its relation to digoxin dosage and clinical effects in patients with atrial fibrillation. *Br Heart J* 1972;34:383–391.

35. Khalsa A, Olsson B. Verapamil-induced ventricular regularity in atrial fibrillation. *Acta Med Scand* 1979;205:509–515.

36. Davidson D, Hagan A. Role of exercise stress testing in assessing digoxin dosage in chronic atrial fibrillation. *Cardiovasc Med* 1979;4:671–678.

37. David D, DiSegni E, Klein HO, Kaplinsky E. Inefficacy of digitalis in the control of heart rate in patients with chronic atrial fibrillation: beneficial effect of an added beta-adrenergic blocking agent. *Am J Cardiol* 1979;44:1378–1382.

38. DiBianco R, Morganroth J, Frietag JA, et al. Effects of nadolol on the spontaneous and exercise-provoked heart rate of patients with chronic atrial fibrillation receiving stable dosages of digoxin. *Am Heart J* 1984;108:1121–1127.

39. Brown RW, Goble AJ. Effect of propranolol on exercise tolerance in patients with atrial fibrillation. *Br Med J* 1969;2:279–280.

40. Molajo AO, Coupe MO, Bennett DH. Effect of corwin (ICI 118587) on resting and exercise heart rate and exercise tolerance in digitalized patients with chronic atrial fibrillation. *Br Heart J* 1984;52:392–395.

41. Lang R, Klein H, Segni E, et al. Verapamil improves exercise capacity in chronic atrial fibrillation: double-blind crossover study. *Am Heart J* 1983;105:820–824.

42. Roth A, Harrison E, Mitani G, et al. Efficacy and safety of medium- and high-dose diltiazem alone and in combination with digoxin for control of heart rate at rest and during exercise in patients with chronic atrial fibrillation. *Circulation* 1986;73:316–324.

43. Klein HO, Pauzner H, DiSegni E, David D, Kaplinsky E. The beneficial effects of verapamil in chronic atrial fibrillation. *Arch Intern Med* 1979;139:747.

44. Steinberg JS, Katz RJ, Bren GB, Buff LA, Varghese PF. Efficacy of oral diltiazem to control ventricular response in chronic atrial fibrillation at rest and during exercise. *J Am Coll Cardiol* 1987;9:405–411.

45. Beasley R, Smith DA, McHaffie DJ. Exercise heart rates at different serum digoxin concentrations in patients with atrial fibrillation. *Br Med J* 1985;290:9–11.

46. Atwood JE, Sullivan M, Forbes S, et al. Effect of beta-adrenergic blockade on exercise performance in patients with chronic atrial fibrillation. *J Am Coll Cardiol* 1987;10:314–320.
47. Atwood JE, Myers J, Sullivan M, et al. Maximal exercise testing and gas exchange in patients with chronic atrial fibrillation. *J Am Coll Cardiol* 1988;11:508–513.
48. Atwood JE, Myers JN, Sullivan MJ, Forbes SM, Pewen WF, Froelicher VF. Diltiazem and exercise performance in patients with chronic atrial fibrillation. *Chest* 1988;93:20–25.
49. Lundstrom T, Ryden L. Ventricular rate control and exercise performance in chronic atrial fibrillation: effects of diltiazem and verapamil. *J Am Coll Cardiol* 1990;16:86–90.
50. Lipkin DP, Frenneaux M, Stewart R, Joshi J, Lowe T, McKenna WJ. Delayed improvement in exercise capacity after cardioversion of atrial fibrillation to sinus rhythm. *Br Heart J* 1988;59:572–577.
51. Atwood JE, Myers J, Sullivan M, et al. The effect of cardioversion on maximal exercise capacity in patients with chronic atrial fibrillation. *Am Heart J* 1989;118:913–918.
52. Wiggers CJ, Katz LN. The contours of ventricular volume curves under different conditions. *Am J Physiol* 122:58:439.
53. Jochim K. The contribution of the auricles to ventricular filling in complete heart block. *Am J Physiol* 1938;122:639.
54. Rahimtoola SH, Ehsain A, Sinno MZ, Loeb HS, Rosen KN, Gunnar RM. Left atrial transport function in myocardial infarction: importance of its booster pump function. *Am J Med* 1975;59:686–694.
55. Greenberg B, Chatterjee K, Parmley WW, Werner JA, Holly AN. The influence of left ventricular filling pressure on atrial contribution to cardiac output. *Am Heart J* 1980;98:742–751.
56. Tyers GFO. Current status of sensor-modulated rate-adaptive cardiac pacing. *J Am Coll Cardiol* 1990;15:412–418.
57. Levine PA, Mace RC. *Pacing therapy: a guide to cardiac pacing for optimum hemodynamic benefit*. New York: Futura, 1983.
58. Froelicher VF, Marcondes GD. *Manual of exercise testing*. Chicago: Year Book Medical, 1989.
59. Jones N, Campbell E. *Clinical exercise testing*. Philadelphia: WB Saunders, 1982;152–155.
60. Myers J, Froelicher VF. Optimizing the exercise test for pharmacologic investigations. *Circulation* 1990;82:1839–1846.
61. Myers J, Atwood JE, Sullivan M, et al. Perceived exertion and gas exchange after calcium and b-blockade in atrial fibrillation. *J Appl Physiol* 1987;63:97–104.
62. American College of Sports Medicine. *Guidelines for graded exercise testing and exercise prescription*. St. Louis: CV Mosby, 1986.
63. Sullivan M, Genter F, Savvides M, Roberts M, Myers J, Froelicher VF. The reproducibility of hemodynamic, electrocardiographic, and gas exchange data during treadmill exercise in patients with stable angina pectoris. *Chest* 1984;86:375–382.
64. Elborn JS, Stanford CF, Nichols DP. Reproducibility of cardiopulmonary parameters during exercise in patients with chronic cardiac failure. The need for a preliminary test. *Eur Heart J* 1990;11:75–81.
65. Pinsky DJ, Ahern D, Wilson PB, Kukin ML, Packer M. How many exercise tests are needed to minimize the placebo effect of serial exercise testing in patients with chronic heart failure? *Circulation* 1989;80(suppl II):II-426.
66. Sullivan M, McKirnan MD. Errors in predicting functional capacity for postmyocardial infarction patients using a modified Bruce protocol. *Am Heart J* 1984;107:486–491.
67. Froelicher VF, Lancaster MC. The prediction of maximal oxygen consumption from a continuous exercise treadmill protocol. *Am Heart J* 1974;87:445–450.
68. Roberts JM, Sullivan M, Froelicher VF, Genter F, Myers J. Predicting oxygen uptake from treadmill testing in normal subjects and coronary artery disease patients. *Am Heart J* 1984;108:1454–1460.
69. Asana K. Relationships of anaerobic threshold and onset of blood lactate accumulation with endurance performance. *Eur J Appl Physiol* 1983;52:51–56.
70. Matsumura N, Nishijima H, Hashimoto F, Minami M, Yasuda H. Determination of anaerobic threshold for assessment of functional state in patients with chronic heart failure. *Circulation* 1983;68:360–367.
71. Hermanasen L, Saltin B. Oxygen uptake during maximal treadmill and bicycle exercise. *J Appl Physiol* 1969;26:31–37.
72. Buchfuhrer MJ, Hansen JE, Robinson TE, Sue DY, Wasserman K, Shipp BJ. Optimizing the exercise protocol for cardiopulmonary assessment. *J Appl Physiol* 1983;55:1558–1564.
73. Myers J, Walsh D, Sullivan M, Froelicher VF. Effect of sampling on variability and plateau in oxygen uptake. *J Appl Physiol* 1990;68:404–410.
74. Noakes TD. Implications of exercise testing for prediction of athletic performance: a contemporary perspective. *Med Sci Sports Exerc* 1988;20:319–330.
75. Brooks GA. Anaerobic threshold: review of the concept and directions for future research. *Med Sci Sports Exerc* 1985;17:22–31.

76. Davis JA. Anaerobic threshold: review of the concept and directions for future research. *Med Sci Sports Exerc* 1985;17:6–18.
77. Borg G. Perceived exertion as an indicator of somatic stress. *Scand J Rehab Med* 1970;2:92–98.
78. Kraemer MD, Sullivan M, Atwood JE, Forbes S, Myers J, Froelicher V. Reproducibility of treadmill exercise data in patients with atrial fibrillation. *Cardiology* 1989;76:234–242.
79. Atwood JE, Myers J, Sandhu S, et al. Optimal sampling interval to estimate heart rate at rest and during exercise in atrial fibrillation. *Am J Cardiol* 1989;63:45–48.
80. Hammond K, Froelicher VF. Normal and abnormal heart rate responses to exercise. *Prog Cardiovasc Dis* 1985;28:271–296.
81. Lewis R, Lakhani M, Moreland TA, McDevitt DG. A comparison of verapamil and digoxin in the treatment of atrial fibrillation. *Eur Heart J* 1987;8:148–153.
82. Yahalom J, Klein H, Kaplinsky E. Beta-adrenergic blockade as adjunctive oral therapy in patients with chronic atrial fibrillation. *Chest* 1977;71:582–596.
83. Wilmore JH, Freund BJ, Joyner MJ, et al. Acute response to sub-maximal and maximal exercise consequent to beta-adrenergic blockade: implications for the prescription of exercise. *Am J Cardiol* 1985;55:135D–141D.
84. Panidis IP, Morganroth J, Baessler C. Effectiveness and safety of oral verapamil in control exercise-induced tachycardia in patients with atrial fibrillation receiving digitalis. *Am J Cardiol* 1983;52:1197–1201.
85. Schwartz JB, Keefe D, Kates RE, Kirstein E, Harrison DC. Acute and chronic pharmacodynamic interaction of verapamil and digoxin in atrial fibrillation. *Circulation* 1982;65:1163–1170.
86. Theisen K, Haufe M, Peters J, Theisen F, Jahrmarker H. Effect of the calcium antagonist diltiazem on atrioventricular conduction in chronic atrial fibrillation. *Am J Cardiol* 1985;55:98–102.
87. Orlando JR, Van Herick R, Aronow WS, Olson HG. Hemodynamics and echocardiograms before and after cardioversion of atrial fibrillation to normal sinus rhythm. *Chest* 1979;76:521–526.
88. DeMaria AN, Lies JE, King JF, Miller RR, Amesterdam EA, Mason DT. Echographic assessment of atrial transport, mitral movement, and ventricular performance following electroversion of supraventricular arrhythmias. *Circulation* 1975;51:273–282.
89. Dethy M, Chassat C, Roy D, Mercier L-A. Doppler echocardiographic predictors of recurrence of atrial fibrillation after cardioversion. *Am J Cardiol* 1988;62:723–726.
90. Manning WJ, Leeman DE, Gotch PJ, Come PC. Pulsed Doppler evaluation of atrial mechanical function after electrical cardioversion of atrial fibrillation. *J Am Coll Cardiol* 1989;13:617–623.
91. Ieri A, Zipoli A, Bartoli P, Marmugi P, Morelli G. Improvement of the cardiac function after electrical cardioversion of atrial fibrillation. *G Ital Cardiol* 1982;12:91–95.
92. Ikram H, Nixon PGF, Arcan T. Left atrial function after electrical conversion to sinus rhythm. *Br Heart J* 1986;30:80–83.

Atrial Fibrillation: Mechanisms and Management, edited by R. H. Falk and P. J. Podrid. Raven Press, Ltd., New York © 1992.

10

Echocardiography in Atrial Fibrillation

Charles Pollick

Echocardiography Laboratory, Vancouver General Hospital, Vancouver, British Columbia, Canada V5Z 1M9; Department of Medicine, University of British Columbia, Vancouver, British Columbia, Canada V5S 1G4

Echocardiography lends itself to the investigation and management of atrial fibrillation for many reasons. From the anatomic standpoint, echocardiography permits the accurate determination of atrial size, which plays a major role in the instigation of atrial fibrillation. Physiologically, by performing pulsed and color-flow Doppler studies, the hemodynamics of atrial contraction and atrial flow patterns can be assessed, both of which have implications for the development of atrial fibrillation and the propagation of complications of hemodynamic instability and atrial thrombus. Pathologically, by using transthoracic and transesophageal echocardiography, a whole host of potential valvular and cardiomyopathic causes of atrial fibrillation can be diagnosed as well as the consequences of atrial fibrillation, which include left atrial cavity and left atrial appendage spontaneous contrast and thrombus.

In this chapter I begin with a section on atrial function that highlights some basic articles that by derivation have implications for our understanding and assessment of atrial fibrillation. The next section examines the contentious issue of which comes first, the enlarged left atrium or atrial fibrillation. The third section details selected reports that deal with the echocardiographic determination of success and maintenance of cardioversion. I then summarize the current interest in the ability of echocardiography, particularly by the transesophageal route, to display left atrial and left atrial appendage spontaneous contrast and thrombus, both of which have implications for the development of systemic emboli. Finally, I discuss the issue of whether all patients with atrial fibrillation should undergo echocardiography.

ASSESSMENT OF ATRIAL FUNCTION BY ECHOCARDIOGRAPHY

Atrial Size

Left Atrium

The benchmark of the echocardiographic assessment of atrial fibrillation is maximal, end-systolic left atrial size, readily determined by M-mode and two-dimensional echocardiography. This measurement has implications for understanding the etiology and pathophysiology of atrial fibrillation and, possibly, determining the appropriateness of cardioversion.

Controversy surrounds (a) the most appropriate single echocardiographic dimension to represent left atrial size, (b) the method of echocardiographic measurement, and (c) the upper normal echocardiographic range.

a. In the early M-mode echocardiographic literature, left atrial dimension (representing the anteroposterior dimension of the left atrium at the aortic root level) was found to correlate significantly with left atrial angiographic area (1). Wade et al. (2), however, found that this standard dimension correlates poorly with left atrial volume as determined by two-dimensional echocardiography, thereby questioning the use of this single measurement to represent left atrial size.

b. In the original M-mode echocardiographic literature the left atrium was measured using a "leading edge" convention, from the anterior border of the echo originating from the posterior left atrial wall to the anterior edge of the posterior aortic wall (1). In a survey of members of the American Society of Echocardiography (3), only 34% used this method versus 64% who used the "inner edge" convention in which the left atrium is measured from the anterior border of the posterior left atrial wall to the posterior border of the posterior aortic root. The American Society of Echocardiography, however, recommended, for the sake of reproducibility, that M-mode left atrial dimension should be measured using the "leading edge" convention (3). The thickness of the posterior aortic wall may range from 1 to 3 mm. In children, this difference in convention may significantly affect left atrial size, which may only be a few millimeters, but in adults the difference only represents 2% to 5%, which is within observer variability (4).

c. Feigenbaum (5) reported M-mode echocardiographic values of normal range of left atrial size from 19 to 40 mm ("inner edge" convention). Two-dimensional echocardiographic measurement of left atrial size was reported by Triulzi et al. (6) as 23 to 38 mm ("inner edge" convention) and by Schnittger et al. (7) as 27 to 45 mm ("leading edge" convention). As left atrial size correlates with body surface area, it seems logical to index the measured dimension for appropriate interpatient comparisons (5).

In our laboratory, we report left atrial dimension taken from the parasternal long-axis, two-dimensional image at end-systole, using an inner edge convention, and use 40 mm as the upper normal dimension. We rarely will report left atrial size in the apical four-chamber view (length or width) if the parasternal long-axis measurement does not appear to accurately reflect true left atrial size.

Right Atrium

Right atrial size cannot be adequately assessed by M-mode echocardiography but is optimally assessed by two-dimensional echocardiography from the apical four-chamber view. Other than defining normal values for right atrial size (6,7), there do not appear to have been any studies correlating right atrial size with predictors of atrial fibrillation.

Atrial Wall Motion

The echocardiographic patterns of atrial wall motion during atrial arrhythmias can be helpful in diagnosis. An appreciation of atrial wall motion during sinus rhythm provides information on atrial function that may clarify mechanisms of atrial arrhythmias.

Sinus Rhythm

Left atrial wall motion may be deduced by assessment of the posterior aorta. Using this method, Strunk et al. (8) reported that left atrial size diminishes in three defined periods within the cardiac cycle: by more than 40% in the first third of diastole; in mid-diastole there is a phase of diastasis represented by a flat motion of the posterior aortic root; in the final third of the cardiac cycle with atrial systole the left atrium diminishes further. The timing of atrial contraction was studied by Egeblad and Rasmussen (9) in 25 patients in sinus rhythm. They reported that right atrial contraction preceded left atrial contraction by 42 ± 31 msec. M-mode assessment of left atrial function by transthoracic echocardiography depends on normal aortic anatomy and would be distorted by an aortic aneurysm.

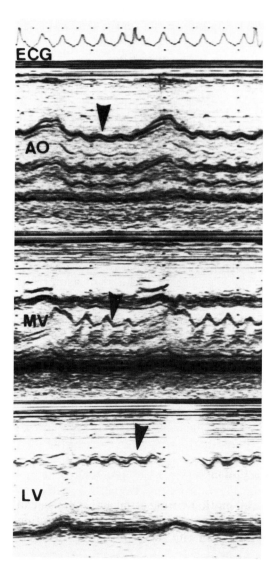

FIG. 1. M-mode echocardiogram of a patient in atrial flutter. *Top:* Aortic root (AO); *arrow* points to flutter of anterior aortic root. *Middle:* Mitral valve (MV); *arrow* points to flutter of anterior mitral leaflet. *Lower:* Left ventricle (LV); *arrow* points to flutter of interventricular septum.

M-mode echocardiography of the atrium using transesophageal echocardiography permits assessment of atrial size throughout the cardiac cycle from the atrial septum to the outer edge of the atrium, for both atria, thereby excluding the aorta from measurement. Toma et al. (10) have shown that this method correlates significantly with left atrial volume determined by angiography and may be the preferred method of assessing changes in atrial size during the cardiac cycle.

Arrhythmias

The normal pattern of atrial wall motion is altered in patients with arrhythmias. Motion of the aortic root, posterior left atrial wall, interatrial septum, posterior right atrial wall, mitral valve, and interventricular septum (Fig. 1) by precordial and subcostal echocardiography may clarify the nature of an arrhythmia (11–15). Abrupt inward motions of these structures are considered to reflect atrial mechanical systole. By this methodology, atrial tachycardia, atrial flutter, atrial fibrillation, ventricular tachycardia, and undefined tachyarrhythmias can be diagnosed; this is of particular value when the standard 12-lead ECG does not provide the correct diagnosis. Differences in extent of cardiac movement between atrial fibrillation and atrial flutter can sometimes be seen, but this is not invariable; some patients with fibrillation may have as much or more movement of the mitral valve or surrounding cardiac structures as patients with flutter. Echocardiography is the most practical method of diagnosing fetal arrhythmias. Steinfeld et al. (16) reconstructed the fetal ECG from M-mode echocardiography by matching atrial and ventricular wall contractions with assumed P-waves and QRS complexes. In 57 pregnancies referred specifically because of an irregular fetal heartbeat, they diagnosed ventricular premature beats (21 cases), atrial premature contractions (12 cases), complete heart block (4 cases), sinus or junctional bradycardia (8 cases), atrial bigeminy with 2:1 block (1 case), and atrial flutter (4 cases).

Atrial Hemodynamics

Because high atrial pressure may cause atrial fibrillation, it is useful to review echocardiographic methodologies of assessing atrial hemodynamics.

Left Atrial Pressure

Several methods of predicting left ventricular diastolic pressure and pulmonary wedge pressure (and thereby left atrial pressure), from echo/Doppler techniques, have been reported. By the use of combined echo measurements and systolic time intervals, Askenaze et al. (17) derived a formula that correlated well with the invasive measurement of pulmonary wedge pressure ($r = 0.91$). Kuecherer et al. (18) estimated left atrial pressure by transesophageal assessment of pulmonary venous flow. The systolic component of the pulmonary venous inflow Doppler velocity profile decreased linearly with increasing mean left atrial pressure ($r = -0.81$; $p < 0.0001$). A shift from systolic to early diastolic forward flow predominance was associated with a high mean left atrial pressure (>15 mm Hg). A "systolic fraction" (pulmonary venous systolic velocity-time integral as fraction of the sum of systolic and early diastolic velocity-time integral) less than 55% was 91% sensitive and 87% specific for mean left atrial pressure greater than 15 mm Hg. The systolic fraction of flow provided a clinically useful approximation of pulmonary wedge pressure within ± 6 mm Hg, although the authors indicate that borderline raised wedge pressure may not be recognized.

Some information about left atrial pressure and function may be derived from the mitral inflow velocity profile. The ratio of early diastolic (M^1 or E) to late diastolic filling velocity (M^2 or A) due to atrial contraction is decreased with impaired left ventricular relaxation, and the deceleration time of early diastolic filling (M^1 or E) is decreased with increased left ventricular chamber stiffness [19]. These abnormalities are usually a reflection of increased left ventricular diastolic pressure and thereby left atrial pressure. These signs, however, lack sensitivity and specificity, as demonstrated by Klein et al. [20], who reported pseudonormalization of the mitral inflow pattern in patients with cardiac amyloidosis, giving the mistaken impression of normal left ventricular diastolic filling and pressure.

It seems logical to suppose that a large A-wave may categorize a patient with higher than normal risk of developing atrial fibrillation. It may also indicate that if that patient does develop atrial fibrillation, then it may be poorly tolerated as the patient is dependent on a strong atrial contraction to maintain stroke volume. Tischler et al. [21] studied 87 consecutive patients with new-onset atrial fibrillation by pulsed Doppler interrogation of mitral inflow velocity when the patients were subsequently in sinus rhythm. They found that a large A-wave predicted clinical instability. In particular they reported that atrial fraction (atrial velocity integral/total diastolic velocity integral) greater than 40% could predict the development of angina, congestive heart failure, syncope, or hypotension during atrial fibrillation with a sensitivity of 80% and specificity of 72%.

Right Atrial Pressure

Indirect assessment of right atrial pressure can be obtained by assessment of inferior vena cava size and response to respiration. Simonson and Schiller [22] reported that minimal inferior vena cava diameter was directly related to mean right atrial pressure ($r = 0.56$); minimal/maximal inferior vena cava diameter ratio was inversely related to mean right atrial pressure ($r = 0.57$). These findings may have particular relevance in patients with cor pulmonale, who may develop atrial fibrillation secondary to high right atrial pressure.

Atrial Flow

Normal right atrial flow topography has been studied by Miyatake et al. [23]. Flow from the inferior and superior vena cava merge into a "belt" of flow that courses along the atrial septum. The "belt" of blood then flows through the tricuspid valve and into the right ventricle. Similarly, in our laboratory, we have observed that flow from the pulmonary veins converges along the interatrial septum before entering the mitral valve (Fig. 2). The significance of these belt-like formations has not been established. Nevertheless, they imply more stagnant flow in the outer portions of

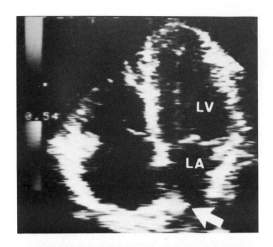

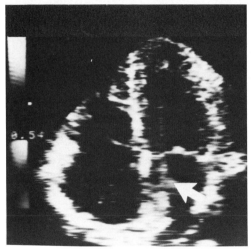

FIG. 2. Two-dimensional echocardiogram with color-flow imaging in a normal subject in four-chamber view in two successive systolic frames (**top, bottom**) displaying flow coursing along the atrial septum in a "belt" of flow from the back of the left atrium (top) to the mitral valve (bottom).

the atrium, which may partially explain why thrombus forms in these parts of the atrium and not along the atrial septum.

Left Atrial Appendage: Structure and Function

While the left atrial appendage is rarely seen by transthoracic echocardiography, it can be well demonstrated by transesophageal echocardiography. In healthy subjects the left atrial appendage demonstrates (Fig. 3) a characteristic pattern of emptying (24). The apex of the triangle-shaped appendage contracts and obliterates (following the ECG P-wave) and produces a characteristic Doppler signal. The base of the left atrial appendage (at its entrance into the body of the left atrium) is relatively noncontractile. The characteristics of left atrial appendage contraction have implications for the development of left atrial appendage thrombus formation, as described later in this chapter.

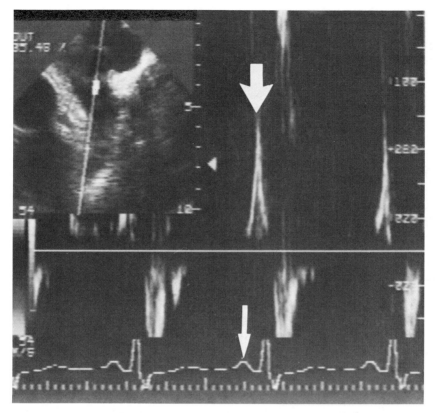

FIG. 3. Pulsed Doppler display of left atrial appendage contraction (*large arrow*) following the ECG P-wave (*small arrow*). Two-dimensional duplex image of sample volume at the neck of the left atrial appendage is displayed at the top left.

LEFT ATRIAL ENLARGEMENT AND ATRIAL FIBRILLATION—CAUSE OR EFFECT?

Left atrial size, in patients with atrial fibrillation, has implications for the success and maintenance of cardioversion to sinus rhythm and for the development of spontaneous contrast and left atrial thrombus formation. The pathophysiology of left atrial dilatation in atrial fibrillation, however, remains speculative and controversial. There is evidence that the left atrium dilates in response to increased left atrial pressure in patients with mitral stenosis (25) and that atrial fibrillation develops because of left atrial enlargement (26). Further atrial enlargement may occur without significant hemodynamic worsening.

Keren et al. (27) studied 155 subjects with mitral stenosis and found no significant hemodynamic differences between patients who were in either sinus rhythm or atrial fibrillation. The left atrium was larger in patients with mitral stenosis and atrial fibrillation (37.6 cm^2) than in patients in sinus rhythm (27.8 cm^2) ($p<0.001$). By multiple regression analysis, they showed that the severity of mitral stenosis accounted for 38%, and atrial fibrillation for 11%, of the change in the size of the left atrium.

Their analysis suggested that the onset of left atrial dilatation in mitral stenosis is the result of an early increase in left atrial pressure. Atrial fibrillation, which develops irrespective of the severity of the mitral stenosis, contributes to a further enlargement of the left atrium. These authors also studied the right atrium and found that atrial fibrillation accounts for 24% and mitral valve area for only 3% of the change in the size of the right atrium. They therefore concluded that atrial fibrillation contributes to left and right atrial enlargement in patients with mitral stenosis.

It is likely that hemodynamic and pathological changes in the left and right atria as well as atrial size per se are contributors to the development of atrial fibrillation. Patients with similarly enlarged atria and comparable hemodynamics have a different prevalence of atrial fibrillation, depending on the underlying pathology. Papazoglou (28) studied 3,679 patients without ischemic heart disease and noted atrial fibrillation in 44% of patients with mitral stenosis, 12% with aortic valve disease, 22% with high blood pressure, 11% with primary myocardial disease, and 4% with congenital cardiac disorders. In a study of congestive cardiomyopathy, only 17% of patients were in atrial fibrillation, despite a mean left atrial size of 51 mm (29).

Petersen et al. (30) studied the relationship between left atrial dimension and duration of atrial fibrillation and found a significant increase in left atrial dimension after 6 months of follow-up in both atrial fibrillation of short and long duration. They studied 36 patients with atrial fibrillation of less than 3 months duration (group 1) and 34 patients with atrial fibrillation of at least 1 year duration (group 2). In group 1, the mean left atrial dimension increased from 43 ± 5 to 49 ± 6 mm ($p < 0.001$). In group 2, left atrial dimension increased from 49 ± 5 to 53 ± 5 mm. They concluded, therefore, that atrial fibrillation contributes to the development of enlargement of the atria. Similar findings were reported by Sanfilipo et al. (31). They studied 15 patients with atrial fibrillation over an average time period of 21 months. Despite normal atrial dimensions at the onset of atrial fibrillation, both left and right atria increased in size (45.2 to 64.1 cm^3, $p < 0.001$; 49.2 to 66.2 cm^3, $p < 0.001$, respectively) despite unchanged left ventricular dimensions.

In conclusion, there is clearly an interplay between left atrial pressure, inflammatory changes in the left atrial musculature, and duration of atrial fibrillation in the determination of left atrial size in patients in atrial fibrillation. Incorrect assumptions about the severity of the underlying disorder may be made if left atrial size is considered only a marker of the underlying hemodynamic abnormality.

ECHO/DOPPLER ASSESSMENT OF PREDICTORS OF SUCCESSFUL AND MAINTAINED CARDIOVERSION OF ATRIAL FIBRILLATION

Initial Success

The assessment of left atrial size by echocardiography is one measure that has been used to predict successful cardioversion from atrial fibrillation to sinus rhythm. Several groups (32–34) have suggested that left atrial dimension greater than or equal to 45 mm is associated with a low likelihood of pharmacological and electrical cardioversion. In these studies, the drugs used were mainly Class 1A antiarrhythmic drugs such as quinidine, disopyramide, and procainamide. Newer drugs such as amiodarone and Class 1C agents such as flecainide and propafenone appear more potent and permit cardioversion of patients with left atrial dimension up to 60 mm

(35). Dittrich et al. (36), however, were unable to discover a relationship between left atrial size and successful electrical cardioversion when left atrial size was measured by the assessment of left atrial area and long-axis dimension by two-dimensional echocardiography.

Maintenance

Echocardiography

As with the echo predictor of left atrial size less than 45 mm predicting successful cardioversion, so this measurement also was found to predict successful maintenance of sinus rhythm in the long term following cardioversion (32–34). Brodsky et al. (35) also reported that, using amiodarone and Class 1C agents, sinus rhythm was maintained in patients with moderate left atrial dilatation (45–60 mm) but not with patients with left atrial dimension greater than 60 mm. Dittrich et al. (36) found that left atrial area and long-axis dimension by two-dimensional echocardiography were significantly larger in patients remaining in sinus rhythm than in those who had reverted to atrial fibrillation at 1 month (28 ± 7 vs 24 ± 5 cm^2 and 65 ± 9 vs 59 ± 8 mm, respectively, both $p<0.05$), but overlap was great (and this may represent a type I statistical error). They concluded that atrial size did not appear to strongly influence the outcome of cardioversion and should not be included as an important variable when considering patients for cardioversion. It should be noted, from their study, that only two of six patients were in sinus rhythm at 6 months with left atrial dimension greater than or equal to 60 mm. Dethy et al. (37) also did not find any correlation between left atrial dimension and eventual outcome of cardioversion. They found that left atrial dimension greater than 45 mm had a positive predictive value of 66%, with a sensitivity of 59% and specificity of 61% for recurrence of atrial fibrillation.

It is my practice to take into account left atrial dimension as one factor in the decision-making process. I would rarely consider electrically cardioverting a patient with a left atrial dimension greater than 55 mm.

Doppler

The Doppler assessment of atrial function from the mitral inflow velocity profile has been used to predict maintenance of sinus rhythm following cardioversion. Dethy et al. (37) reported that the percentage of increase of the A-wave from 4 to 24 hr less than 10% had the highest positive predictive value (80%) for recurrence of atrial fibrillation (sensitivity 71% and specificity 71%). Manning et al. (38) reported that immediately after cardioversion, peak A-wave velocity was significantly higher (0.40 ± 0.21 m/sec) in patients with ultimate reversion to atrial fibrillation than in those who remained in sinus rhythm (0.24 ± 0.16 m/sec; $p<0.05$). In patients in whom sinus rhythm was maintained, however, peak A-wave velocity increased over the period of observation, whereas in six of eight patients with reversion to atrial fibrillation, peak A-wave velocity declined or failed to increase during the period of observation. These differences, however, did not reach statistical significance.

While these results are of interest, they do not suggest a clinical role for Doppler evaluation in this setting. The relative height of the A-wave can be influenced by many factors, e.g., mitral regurgitation, left ventricular compliance, and dehydration, and may not reflect merely atrial function.

Atrial Function Following Cardioversion (Fig. 4)

The return of the ECG P-wave after successful cardioversion does not necessarily imply significant atrial contraction. Sharpiro et al. (39) reported that atrial function, as determined by peak atrial velocity and A/E ratios performed within 24 hr of cardioversion, showed normal atrial function in patients with acute atrial fibrillation of less than 1 week duration. Atrial function was diminished, however, in patients with chronic atrial fibrillation when assessed within 24 hr. They found the patients with chronic atrial fibrillation who maintained sinus rhythm showed an increase in the A/E ratio to control levels at 48 days after conversion. Manning et al. (38) reported that peak A-wave velocity and percentage of atrial contribution to total left ventricular filling did not return to normal until 3 weeks after cardioversion in patients who remained in sinus rhythm. These results suggest that patients should remain on anticoagulants for at least 3 weeks after conversion to sinus rhythm as poor atrial function during this time may continue to predispose the patient to left atrial thrombus formation.

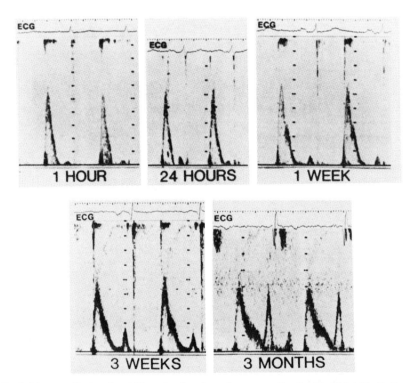

FIG. 4. Serial transmitral pulsed Doppler tracings from a patient with atrial fibrillation, electrically cardioverted to sinus rhythm. There is a progressive increase in the height and area of the A-wave over a 3-month period. Horizontal distances between calibrations represent 1 sec; vertical calibrations indicate 0.2 m/sec velocity. (From ref. 38, with permission.)

ECHOCARDIOGRAPHIC ASSESSMENT OF ATRIAL THROMBI AND INTRACAVITARY BLOOD STASIS

Left Atrial Thrombus

Transthoracic Echocardiography

Pathological studies have demonstrated left atrial thrombus in approximately one-third of patients with mitral stenosis (40). Transthoracic echocardiography has a poor sensitivity for such left atrial thrombus as demonstrated in a study by Scheizer et al. (41) who studied 92 patients with mitral stenosis and found left atrial thrombi in four patients by transthoracic two-dimensional echo but in 12 patients at the time of surgery, for a sensitivity of 33%. Better results were obtained by Shrestha et al. (42) who studied 293 patients with rheumatic mitral stenosis and regurgitation and discovered thrombi in 30 of 51 patients preoperatively. Their sensitivity and specificity were 59% and 99%, respectively, for two-dimensional echocardiography. Bansal et al. (43) correlated transthoracic echo and surgical findings in 148 patients with mitral valve disease and reported sensitivity of 46% and specificity of 99%.

Transesophageal Echocardiography

Improved sensitivity of left atrial thrombus is demonstrated by transesophageal echocardiography (Fig. 5). Aschenberg et al. (44) reported on six of 21 patients with

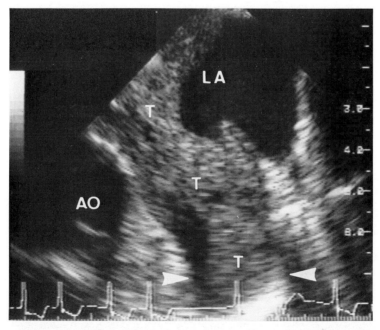

FIG. 5. Transesophageal echocardiogram in a patient with recent-onset atrial fibrillation and stroke. Thrombus in the left atrial appendage is *arrowed*. LA, left atrium; AO, aorta; T, thrombus.

mitral stenosis in whom a left atrial appendage thrombus was diagnosed by trans-esophageal echocardiography when transthoracic echocardiography had failed. The transesophageal findings were confirmed at surgery for mitral valve replacement in all cases. Malone et al. (45) assessed the effect of atrial fibrillation in producing thrombus in 63 patients with mitral valve disease. Group 1 consisted of 11 patients with systemic embolus and group 2 consisted of 52 patients without recent systemic embolus. Left atrial thrombus was detected in four (36%) of group 1 patients and three (6%) of group 2 patients ($p<0.005$). All but one of these thrombi were confined to the left atrial appendage, and none was detected by transthoracic echocardiography.

Combined anatomic and physiologic factors likely account for left atrial appendage thrombus formation. The appendage is a long cul-de-sac with trabeculated ridges from pectinate muscles (the rest of the left atrium is not trabeculated). This anatomic predisposition to stasis is enhanced by the lack of normal appendage contraction in atrial fibrillation (46).

Left Atrial Spontaneous Contrast

Transthoracic Echocardiography

In addition to left atrial thrombus, the presence of blood stasis in the left atrium (Fig. 6) appears to have significant implications with regard to subsequent systemic

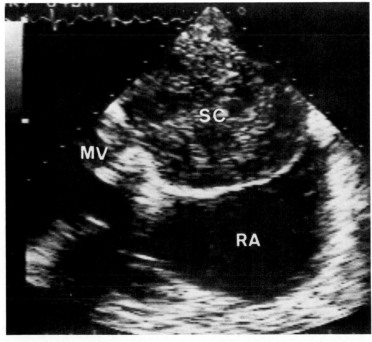

FIG. 6. Transesophageal echocardiogram of left atrial spontaneous contrast in a patient with atrial fibrillation and a bioprosthetic mitral valve. SC, spontaneous contrast; MV, mitral valve; RA, right atrium.

emboli. Garcia-Fernandez et al. (47) reported four patients with characteristics of blood stasis in the left atrium. They reported on a cloud of intra-atrial echoes with a slow circular movement that changed in confirmation and acoustic density. All four patients had aneurysmal dilatation of the left atrium subsequent to long-standing mitral valve disease without a history of peripheral embolism.

Transesophageal Echocardiography

Daniel et al. (48) reported 122 patients studied by echocardiography. Group 1 consisted of 52 patients with mitral stenosis and group 2 consisted of 70 patients with mitral valve replacement. Spontaneous echo contrast was seen in the left atrium in 35 group 1 patients (67.3%) (including seven patients with sinus rhythm) and 26 patients in group 2 (37.1%) (all with atrial fibrillation). Patients with spontaneous echo contrast had a larger left atrium and a greater incidence of both left atrial thrombi and history of arterial embolic episodes than did patients without spontaneous echo contrast. Transthoracic echocardiography allowed the visualization of atrial spontaneous echo contrast in only one of the studied patients. They concluded that left atrial spontaneous echo contrast on echocardiography may help to identify increased thromboembolic risk in patients with mitral stenosis or mitral valve replacement. DeBelder et al. (49) performed transesophageal echocardiography on 80 patients with atrial fibrillation. Of 62 patients with chronic atrial fibrillation, 40% had spontaneous contrast versus 5.6% of 18 patients with paroxysmal atrial fibrillation ($p = 0.01$). Left atrial thrombus was seen in seven patients, six (86%) of whom demonstrated spontaneous contrast ($p = 0.006$). Patients with spontaneous contrast were four times more likely to have suffered a thromboembolic event ($p = 0.009$). They concluded that spontaneous contrast in the left atrium is a useful marker for thromboembolic risk in patients with atrial fibrillation. Red cell aggregation and possibly platelet aggregation are postulated causes of spontaneous contrast (50).

The above studies on left atrial thrombus and contrast clearly demonstrate a pivotal role for transesophageal echocardiography in patients with atrial fibrillation. Prospective studies need to be performed to see whether transesophageal echocardiography should be performed in all patients with atrial fibrillation to determine whether only selected patients require anticoagulation based on echocardiographic findings of left atrial spontaneous contrast, poor left atrial appendage contraction, or left atrial thrombus. Following stroke in a patient with atrial fibrillation, in the absence of another cause of stroke (on clinical grounds or from transthoracic echocardiography), it is my practice to assume that left atrial thrombus is a likely cause of stroke and to recommend anticoagulation (and cardioversion, if appropriate).

Atrial Fibrillation and Stroke: Risk of Left Atrial Enlargement

Controversy surrounds the role of left atrial enlargement as a risk factor in producing stroke in patients with atrial fibrillation. In contrast to earlier studies demonstrating this relationship (51), Wiener et al. (52) retrospectively studied 115 patients with nonrheumatic atrial fibrillation. Left atrial size was not different between 17 patients with (53 ± 10 mm) or 95 patients without emboli (54 ± 9 mm).

ROLE OF ECHOCARDIOGRAPHY IN THE MANAGEMENT OF ATRIAL FIBRILLATION

The role of routine echocardiography in patients with atrial fibrillation is questioned by Kupari et al. (53) who performed echocardiography on 95 patients less than 65 years old with new-onset atrial fibrillation. Echocardiography contributed to diagnosis in six (6.3%) patients. An otherwise unsuspected diagnosis was made in three of 38 patients (8%) classified as having lone atrial fibrillation, but this had no effect on short-term treatment. Two of the three patients had evidence of myocardial infarction, and one had evidence of dilated cardiomyopathy. In one further patient, clinical examination suggested myocardial infarction, whereas echocardiography revealed hypertrophic cardiomyopathy. In two patients with hypertension, ECG suggested left ventricular hypertrophy that was unsubstantiated by echocardiography. They concluded that echocardiography is unnecessary for the initial evaluation and treatment of new-onset atrial fibrillation. Echocardiography, in their opinion, should be considered only to assess the severity of the underlying heart disease and to guide its specific therapy.

In my experience, combined echo/Doppler studies are often of enormous benefit in clarifying the cause of atrial fibrillation. The recognition of the underlying disease has implications regarding the need for appropriate antiarrhythmics. For example, a patient with left ventricular dysfunction is at risk of heart failure with sotalol or disopyramide. In addition, the cardiac diagnosis helps stratify the patient according to the risk of stroke and the need for warfarin (54). High-risk patients include those with prosthetic heart valves and mitral stenosis, medium risk patients are those with heart failure and coronary disease, and low-risk patients include those with lone atrial fibrillation. These diagnoses can be reliably made by history, physical examination, and echo/Doppler examination.

The recently published guidelines for the clinical application of echocardiography reported by the combined American College of Cardiology/American Heart Association Task Force (55) has placed atrial fibrillation in Class II of recommendations (conditions for which echocardiography is frequently used, but there is a divergence of opinion with respect to its appropriateness).

SUMMARY

Echocardiographic studies have contributed greatly to our understanding of the diagnosis, mechanism, complications, and therapy of atrial fibrillation. The assessment of left atrial size as a determinant of successful cardioversion, although not as reliable an indicator as was initially thought, continues to be a useful clinical parameter for predicting initial and long-term success. Echo/Doppler assessment permits accurate cardiac diagnosis facilitating the appropriate choice of pharmacological antiarrhythmic therapy, and correctly stratifies the patient for consideration of warfarin. It remains to be seen whether transesophageal echocardiography is indicated in selected cases of atrial fibrillation to further refine management strategies for anticoagulation.

REFERENCES

1. Hirata T, Wolfe SB, Popp RL, Helmen C, Feigenbaum H. Estimation of left atrial size using ultrasound. *Am Heart J* 1969;78:43.

2. Wade MR, Chandraratna PAN, Reid CL, Lin SL, Rahimtoola SH. Accuracy of nondirected and directed M-mode echocardiography as an estimate of left atrial size. *Am J Cardiol* 1987;60:1208–1211.
3. Sahn DJ, DeMaria A, Kisslo J, Weyman A. Recommendations regarding quantitation in M-mode echocardiography: results of a survey of echocardiographic measurements. *Circulation* 1978; 58:1076–1083.
4. Hagan AD, Deely WJ, Sahn DJ, Freidman WF. Echocardiographic criteria for the normal newborn infants. *Circulation* 1973;50:248.
5. Feigenbaum H. *Echocardiography*, 4th ed. Philadelphia: Lea and Febiger, 1983.
6. Triulzi M, Gillam LD, Gentile F, Newell MJB, Weyman AE. Normal adult cross-sectional echocardiographic values: linear dimensions and chamber areas. *Echocardiography* 1984;1:403–426.
7. Schnittger I, Gordon EP, Fitzgerald PJ, Popp RL. Standardized intracardiac measurements of two-dimensional echocardiography. *J Am Coll Cardiol* 1983;2:934–938.
8. Strunk BL, Fitzgerald JW, Lipton M, Popp RL, Barry WH. The posterior aortic wall echocardiogram: its relationship to left atrial volume change. *Circulation* 1976;54:744.
9. Egeblad H, Rasmussen V. Analysis of arrhythmias based on atrial wall motion. *Acta Med Scand* 1986;219:283–289.
10. Toma Y, Matsuda Y, Matsuzaki M, et al. Determination of atrial size by esophageal echocardiography. *Am J Cardiol* 1983;52:278–280.
11. Zoneraich S, Zoneraich O, Rhee JJ. Echocardiographic findings in atrial flutter. *Circulation* 1975;52:455–459.
12. Drinkovic N. Subcostal M-mode echocardiography of the right atrial wall in the diagnosis of cardiac arrhythmia. *Am J Cardiol* 1982;50:1104–1108.
13. Drinkovic N. Subcostal M-mode echocardiography of the right atrial wall for differentiation of supraventricular tachyarrhythmias with aberration from ventricular tachycardia. *Am Heart J* 1984;107:326–331.
14. Tel C, Tanaka H, Kashima T, Nakao S, Tahara M, Kanehisa T. Echocardiographic analysis of interatrial septal motion. *Am J Cardiol* 1979;44:472–477.
15. Wren C, Henter S, Campbell RWF. The use of echocardiography in the assessment of arrhythmias. *Echocardiography* 1986;3:129–141.
16. Steinfeld L, Rappaport HL, Rossbach HC, Martinez E. Diagnosis of fetal arrhythmias using echocardiographic and Doppler techniques. *J Am Coll Cardiol* 1986;8:1425–1433.
17. Askenaze J, Koenigsberg DI, Ribner HS, Plucinski D, Silverman IM, Lesch M. Prospective study comparing different echocardiographic measurements of pulmonary capillary wedge pressure in patients with organic heart disease other than mitral stenosis. *J Am Coll Cardiol* 1983;2: 919–925.
18. Kuecherer HF, Muhiudeen IA, Kusumoto FM, et al. Estimation of mean left atrial pressure from transesophageal pulsed Doppler echocardiography of pulmonary venous flow: an intraoperative transesophageal study. *Circulation* 1990;82:1127–1139.
19. Appleton CP, Hatle LK, Popp RL. Relation of transmitral flow velocity patterns to left ventricular diastolic function: new insights from a combined hemodynamic and Doppler echocardiographic study. *J Am Coll Cardiol* 1988;12:426–440.
20. Klein A, Hatle LK, Burstow DJ, et al. Doppler characterization of left ventricular diastolic function in cardiac amyloidosis. *J Am Coll Cardiol* 1988;13:1017–1026.
21. Tischler MD, Lee TH, McAndrew KA, Sax PE, Sutton MSJ, Lee RT. Clinical, echocardiographic and Doppler correlates of clinical instability with onset of atrial fibrillation. *Am J Cardiol* 1990;66:721–724.
22. Simonson JG, Schiller NB. Sonospirometry. A new method for non-invasive estimation of mean right atrial pressure based on two-dimensional echographic measurements of the inferior vena cava during measured inspiration. *J Am Coll Cardiol* 1988;11:557–564.
23. Miyatake K, Izumi S, Shimizu A, et al. Right atrial flow topography in healthy subjects studies with real-time two-dimensional Doppler flow imaging technique. *J Am Coll Cardiol* 1986;7:425–431.
24. Sullivan H, Pollick C. Incomplete left atrial appendage ligation that simulates mitral regurgitation. *J Am Soc Echocardiogr* 1990;3:75–77.
25. Selzer A, Cohn KE. Natural history of mitral stenosis: a review. *Circulation* 1972;45:878.
26. Abildskov JA, Millar K, Burgess MJ. Atrial fibrillation. *Am J Cardiol* 1971;28:263.
27. Keren G, Etzion T, Sherez J, et al. Atrial fibrillation and atrial enlargement in patients with mitral stenosis. *Am Heart J* 1987;114:1146.
28. Papazoglou NM. Atrial fibrillation and mitral stenosis. *Circulation* 1974;49:1019.
29. Mann B, Ray R, Goldberger AL, Shabetai R, Green C, Kelly M. Atrial fibrillation in congestive cardiomyopathy: echocardiographic and hemodynamic correlation. *Cathet Cardiovasc Diagn* 1984;7:387.
30. Petersen P, Kastrup J, Brinch K, Godtfredsen J, Boysen G. Relation between left atrial dimension and duration of atrial fibrillation. *Am J Cardiol* 1987;60:382–384.
31. Sanfilippo AJ, Abascal VM, Sheehan M, et al. Atrial enlargement as a consequence of atrial fibrillation, a prospective echocardiographic study. *Circulation* 1990;82:792–797.32.

32. Henry WL, Morganroth J, Pearlman AS, et al. Relation between echocardiographically deter-mined left atrial size and atrial fibrillation. *Circulation* 1976;53:273–279.

33. Ewy G, Ulfers L, Hager WD, Rosenfeld AR, Roeske WR, Goldman S. Response of atrial fibril-lation to therapy: role of etiology and left atrial diameter. *J Electrocardiol* 1980;13:119–124.

34. Flugelman MY, Hasin Y, Katznelson N, Kriwisky M, Shefer A, Gotsman MS. Restoration and maintenance of sinus rhythm after mitral valve surgery for mitral stenosis. *Am J Cardiol* 1984;54:617–619.

35. Brodsky MA, Allen BJ, Capparelli EV, Luckett CR, Morton R, Henry WL. Factors determining maintenance of sinus rhythm after chronic atrial fibrillation with left atrial dilatation. *Am J Car-diol* 1989;63:1065–1068.

36. Dittrich HC, Erickson JS, Schneiderman T, Blacky AR, Savides T, Nicod PH. Echocardiographic and clinical predictors for outcome of elective cardioversion of atrial fibrillation. *Am J Cardiol* 1989;63:193–197.

37. Dethy M, Chassat C, Roy D, Mercier LA. Doppler echocardiographic predictors of recurrence of atrial fibrillation after cardioversion. *Am J Cardiol* 1988;62:723–726.

38. Manning W, Leeman DE, Gotch PJ, Come PC. Pulsed Doppler evaluation of atrial mechanical function after electrical cardioversion of atrial fibrillation. *J Am Coll Cardiol* 1989;13:617–623.

39. Shapiro EP, Effron MB, Lima S, Ouyang P, Siu CO, Bush D. Transient atrial dysfunction after conversion of chronic atrial fibrillation to sinus rhythm. *Am J Cardiol* 1988;62:1202–1207.

40. Lie JT. Atrial fibrillation and left atrial thrombus: an insufferable odd couple. *Am Heart J* 1988;116:1374–1377.

41. Scheizer P, Bardos P, Erbel R, et al. Detection of left atrial thrombi by echocardiography. *Br Heart J* 1981;45:148.

42. Shrestha NK, Moreno FL, Narciso FV, et al. Two-dimensional echocardiographic diagnosis of left atrial thrombus in rheumatic heart disease: a clinicopathologic study. *Circulation* 1983;67:341.

43. Bansal RC, Heywood JT, Applegate PM, Jutzy KR. Detection of left atrial thrombi by two-di-mensional echocardiography and surgical correlation in 148 patients with mitral valve disease. *Am J Cardiol* 1989;64:243–246.

44. Aschenberg W, Schluter M, Kremer P, Schroder E, Siglow V, Bleifeld W. Transesophageal two-dimensional echocardiography for the detection of left atrial appendage thrombus. *J Am Coll Cardiol* 1986;7:163–166.

45. Malone SA, Palac RT, Imus RL, Andrilenas KK, McDonald RW, Giraud GD. Prevalence of left atrial thrombi in symptomatic versus asymptomatic patients with nonvalvular atrial fibrillation. *Circulation* 1989;80:II-1(abstract).

46. Pollick C, Taylor D. Assessment of left atrial appendage function by transesophageal echocardi-ography: implications for the development of thrombus. *Circulation* 1991;84:223–231.

47. Garcia-Fernandez MA, Moreno M, Banuelos F. Two-dimensional echocardiographic identifica-tion of blood stasis in the left atrium. *Am Heart J* 1985;109:600–601.

48. Daniel WG, Nellessen U, Schroder E, et al. Left atrial spontaneous echo contrast in mitral valve disease: an indicator for an increased thromboembolic risk. *J Am Coll Cardiol* 1988;11:1204–1211.

49. de Belder MA, Tourikis L, Leech G, Camm AJ. Spontaneous contrast echos are markers of throm-boembolic risk in patients with atrial fibrillation. *Circulation* 1989;80:II-1(abstract).

50. Mahony C, Evans JM, Spain C. Spontaneous contrast and circulating platelet aggregates. *Circu-lation* 1989;80:II-1(abstract).

51. Caplan LR, D'Cruz I, Hier DB, et al. Atrial size, atrial fibrillation and stroke. *Ann Neurol* 1986;19:158–161.

52. Wiener I, Hafner R, Nicolai M, Lyons H. Clinical and echocardiographic correlates of systemic embolization in nonrheumatic atrial fibrillation. *Am J Cardiol* 1987;59:177.

53. Kupari M, Leinonen H, Koskinen P. Value of routine echocardiography in new-onset atrial fi-brillation. *Int J Cardiol* 1987;16:106–108.

54. Stein B, Halperin JL, Fuster V. Should patients with atrial fibrillation be anticoagulated prior to and chronically following cardioversion? In: Cheitlin MD, ed. *Dilemmas in clinical cardiology*. Philadelphia: FA Davis, 1990;231–247.

55. Ewy G, Appleton CP, DeMaria AN, et al. Guidelines for the clinical application of echocardiog-raphy. A report of the American College of Cardiology American Heart Association Task Force on Assessment of Diagnostic and Therapeutic Cardiovascular Procedures. *Circulation* 1990;82:2323–2345.

Atrial Fibrillation: Mechanisms and Management, edited by
R. H. Falk and P. J. Podrid.
Raven Press, Ltd., New York © 1992.

11

Electrical Cardioversion of Atrial Fibrillation

*Rodney H. Falk and †Philip J. Podrid

*Division of Cardiology, Boston City Hospital, Boston, Massachusetts 02118;
†Arrhythmia Service, University Hospital, Boston, Massachusetts 02118;
†Boston University School of Medicine, Boston, Massachusetts 02118

Electrical cardioversion is a safe and effective method of terminating atrial fibrillation (1). Remarkably little has changed in the technique of cardioversion since its introduction in the early 1960s (2–4), although progress has been made in understanding factors responsible for success, in defining more precisely which patients will benefit from this technique, and in reducing the already low complication rate. In this chapter we briefly review the technique of cardioversion, discuss indications and relative contraindications of cardioversion in patients with atrial fibrillation or flutter, and examine some of the controversies still surrounding the procedure.

TECHNIQUE OF CARDIOVERSION

Premedication the evening before cardioversion with a sedative such as diazepam or a short-acting barbiturate is recommended by some authorities (1) in the belief that anxiety may increase endogenous catecholamine levels and thereby increase the energy requirement for a successful outcome. While evidence for this belief is lacking, it is certainly appropriate to reassure all patients undergoing the procedure and to premedicate those who are particularly anxious.

Prior to the procedure it must be ascertained that serum potassium is within the normal range and that patients receiving warfarin have been adequately anticoagulated for the preceding 2 to 3 weeks. We are particularly careful to maintain serum potassium at or above 4.0 mEq/liter in patients receiving diuretics who are to be prescribed type IA antiarrhythmic agents, as even mild hypokalemia may precipitate torsades de pointes. This may only occur after reversion to sinus rhythm when the heart rate has been reduced (5). If the patient is receiving digoxin, it is appropriate to check the serum level and to hold the drug if the level is above the accepted therapeutic range (see below). In addition to the defibrillator-cardioverter, full resuscitation equipment should be available and a physician skilled in airway management should be present. Lidocaine and atropine are probably the most commonly required drugs for cardioversion-associated arrhythmias and should be rapidly accessible.

A variety of sedative or short-acting anesthetic agents have been used for cardioversion. We generally use either diazepam in 2- to 5-mg increments until adequate sedation is produced, or Brevital given by an anesthesiologist. It has been suggested that the benzodiazepine midazolam may be preferable to diazepam as it has a shorter half-life and produces a greater degree of amnesia (6). Whatever sedation/anesthesia is used, it is crucial to ensure that the patient does not remember the shock, which, when the subject is inadequately sedated, may be extremely painful (7).

Cardioversion involves the delivery of an electrical impulse to the heart, synchronized to the QRS complex to avoid the vulnerable period of the cardiac cycle (8,9). Early defibrillator-cardioverters had an adjustable dial permitting alteration of the delivered impulse in relation to the QRS complex, but present-day devices automatically detect the QRS. Familiarity with the device being used for cardioversion is essential. Most current models of defibrillator-cardioverter will function in the synchronized mode only when the input from the patient is from ECG cables directly interfacing with the device. Some earlier models permitted synchronization in a "quick-look" mode that monitored the ECG through defibrillator paddles placed directly on the chest. Generally, the quality of the ECG tracing derived from paddles is suboptimal and subject to errors of R-wave sensing (Fig. 1). Therefore this mode should not be used for elective cardioversion.

The behavior of the synchronized mode on defibrillators after a shock has been delivered varies. In some models the defibrillator remains in the synchronized mode so that serial shocks can be given. However, if ventricular fibrillation is produced by a synchronized cardioversion shock, it is imperative to defibrillate with a nonsynchronized countershock, and failure to disengage the synchronized mode will prevent the device from firing. Consequently, most current models revert to nonsynchronized mode after each shock, thereby necessitating repeated activation of the "synchronize" button for serial shocks. If the nonsynchronized mode is used, particularly at lower energies, there is a risk of precipitation of ventricular fibrillation (10).

Once the appropriate QRS complex has been selected for synchronization, the tracing is examined to confirm the site of synchronization and the R-wave height is reduced to the minimum necessary for each QRS complex to be sensed. This reduces the risk of T-wave sensing. Gently shaking the ECG cables attached to the patient will indicate whether movement artifact is a potential problem. Shocks may be administered through preapplied self-adhesive defibrillation electrodes or directly through well-gelled defibrillator paddles. Despite early suggestions that anteroposterior paddle/electrode placement resulted in lower energy requirements than anteroapical placement (11), there is probably no clear advantage to either position (12), as discussed below. The major factor to consider in paddle placement is adequate skin contact, with adequate gel to prevent burns. Although some defibrillators label one paddle as "sternum," paddle placement over the sternum or other bony sites

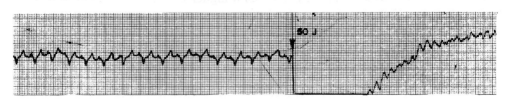

FIG. 1. Attempted cardioversion of atrial flutter. The synchronized mode was incorrectly set resulting in a delivered shock on the T wave, with consequent ventricular fibrillation.

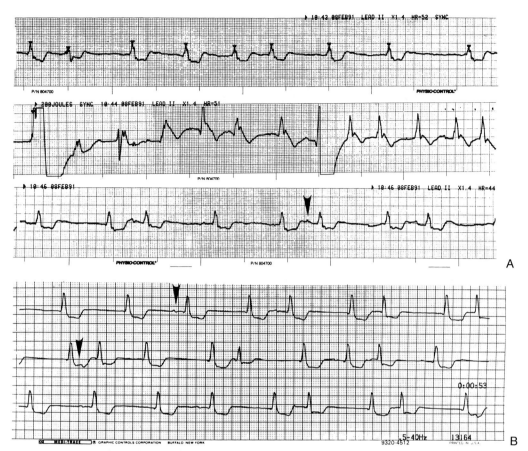

FIG. 2. A: Cardioversion in a patient with atrial fibrillation, slow ventricular response and sinus node disease. *Top:* Precardioversion. *Middle:* Synchronized 200-J shock, followed by irregular rhythm with ST elevation. *Bottom:* 2 min later, ST segments have gone down but rhythm still appears irregular. Careful examination revealed possible P waves (*arrow*). **B:** Rhythm strip with less baseline artifact reveals rhythm to be profound sinus bradycardia with predominant junctional escape rhythm and occasional sinus beats (indicated by *arrows*).

(e.g., scapula) should be avoided as this increases the impedance to current flow. The appropriate anteroapical position is right parasternal and apex (avoiding the nipple as burns are particularly painful). For anteroposterior placement the right or left parasternal position is used in combination with a subscapular electrode. Firm pressure must be applied at the time of shock.

Termination of atrial fibrillation requires a higher energy than either ventricular tachycardia or other supraventricular tachycardias, particular atrial flutter. In the absence of suspected digoxin toxicity, it is reasonable to give an initial shock of 100 J, increasing on successive shocks to the maximal output (usually 320 J of delivered energy). In patients with possible digoxin toxicity in whom cardioversion is urgently required, "titrated cardioversion" (see below) is advisable to avoid precipitating malignant ventricular arrhythmia (13). Careful examination of the ECG after each shock is mandatory to determine whether sinus rhythm has resumed (Fig. 2). An occasional patient may have resumption of sinus rhythm for two or three beats followed by immediate recurrence of arrhythmia—under these circumstances a repeat attempt at cardioversion may be of very little value. In some patients the P-wave voltage following resumption of sinus rhythm may be very low and, if atrial premature beats are present, the postcardioversion rhythm strip may give the appearance of persistent atrial fibrillation, resulting in the application of further, unnecessary shocks.

FACTORS AFFECTING SUCCESSFUL CARDIOVERSION

Electrical termination of atrial fibrillation is successfully accomplished in about 90% of patients, although duration of sinus rhythm varies from a few seconds to permanent resumption. Despite the fact that the energy delivered by the cardioverter is measured in joules (watt seconds), it is the current delivered to the heart (measured in amperes) that determines the success or failure of a given shock (14). The delivered current is a function of the energy selected and the transthoracic impedance, and the latter is affected by a number of factors including higher energy levels, number of shocks, distance between the electrodes, and firm electrode pressure (15–20). Most of these phenomena (with the exception of the use of adequately gelled, low-impedance electrodes and good skin contact) have minimal clinical significance in elective cardioversion, although recent, preliminary information indicates that, while high-energy shocks uniformly terminate atrial fibrillation, lower energy shocks will be successful only if transthoracic impedance is low (21).

Effect of Paddle Position

In the early experience of cardioversion, Lown et al. (11) suggested that anteroposterior paddle placement resulted in a lower energy requirement for successful cardioversion of atrial fibrillation. This was based on the theory that a greater amount of myocardium was affected with the anteroposterior position. Additionally this positioning of the paddles eliminated the problem of the two anterior paddles being too close, since if there is excessive gel, the current may flow across the chest rather than through cardiac tissue. Other authors failed to confirm this observation (22). Kerber et al. (12) suggested that electrode area, rather than position, was responsible for efficacy of cardioversion and performed a randomized trial to test this hypothesis. Over a 2-year period four sets of paddles were used, in 6-month blocks. Two were anterolateral (standard or larger anterior paddle) and two were anteroposterior (standard anterior with large posterior or large anterior and large posterior). Transthoracic resistance was significantly decreased as cumulative paddle area increased. However, no difference could be demonstrated in transthoracic resistance between patients cardioverted with 100 J and those requiring higher energies, and a similar proportion of patients required more than 100 J for conversion in each paddle group.

Digoxin Therapy

Early animal experiments indicated that serious ventricular arrhythmias may occur if a direct current (DC) shock is administered to digoxin-toxic animals (23). The higher the energy of the administered shock, the more likely significant arrhythmias

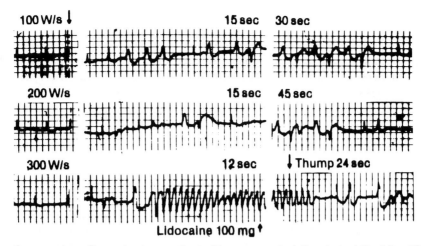

FIG. 3. Attempted cardioversion in a patient with unsuspected digoxin toxicity. After 100 Wsec, ventricular tachycardia followed by biventricular tachycardia occurs (*top*). *Middle:* A shock of 200 Wsec produced similar arrhythmia. *Bottom:* 300-Wsec shock results in ventricular flutter terminated by lidocaine and thump. (Tracings courtesy of Dr. Michael D. Klein.)

are to occur. A similar experience occurs in humans (24) (Fig. 3) and led to recommendations that digoxin be held for 2 to 3 days prior to cardioversion (11). With the easy availability of serum digoxin levels and the recognition of factors likely to provoke digoxin toxicity (such as hypokalemia or the concurrent use of quinidine), the risk of digoxin toxicity is markedly reduced. In digitalized but nontoxic animals (24) and in patients in whom digoxin toxicity is not clinically suspected, cardioversion has been demonstrated to be safe (25,26), and thus digoxin is no longer routinely withheld prior to cardioversion. Occasionally, a patient will be encountered in whom urgent cardioversion is required despite the presence of digoxin toxicity or in whom possible toxicity is suspected despite "therapeutic" levels (e.g., atrial fibrillation with regularization of the ventricular response). Under such a circumstance, it is wise to start with a low-energy shock, for example, 20 J. Although this would not be anticipated to terminate the arrhythmia, digoxin-toxic rhythm, such as ventricular bigeminy, may be provoked (Fig. 3). If this occurs, then digoxin toxicity is likely and the attempted cardioversion should be abandoned unless very urgent, in which case lidocaine should be administered prior to further shocks (1).

CONDUCTION SYSTEM DISEASE

The most common arrhythmia following cardioversion of atrial fibrillation is the appearance of multiple atrial premature beats (27). Usually those last only for a few minutes, but if they persist longer, they may be a harbinger of an early recurrence of atrial fibrillation. A slow ventricular response to atrial fibrillation in the absence of digoxin therapy is suggestive of conduction system disease affecting the atrioventricular node. Such patients often have coexisting sinus node disease and, following cardioversion, may manifest periods of sinus arrest with a slow junctional or atrial escape rhythm that gradually gives way to sinus bradycardia (Fig. 2). Less commonly, a prolonged asystolic period may occur followed by a ventricular escape rhythm or a wandering atrial pacemaker. This may be a particular problem if the patient is receiving a beta-blocker for rate control since these agents depress nodal activity. In view of these potentially unstable rhythms, untreated atrial fibrillation with a slow ventricular response in the absence of medication is considered a contraindication to cardioversion. If cardioversion is deemed necessary in these patients, it may be prudent to perform the procedure with a temporary wire in place or, more conveniently, with external pacing electrodes available for immediate use (28). If external pacing is considered, we always establish a pacing threshold after the sedation/anesthesia has been administered, immediately prior to cardioversion.

Effects of Antiarrhythmic Agents on Energy Requirements

Many patients undergoing cardioversion are prescribed atrial antiarrhythmic agents for the maintenance of sinus rhythm following the procedure. Although quinidine and disopyramide are commonly chosen drugs, class IC agents have been used successfully for the maintenance of sinus rhythm (29). Flecainide has been shown to increase the energy requirements for cardioversion in a small group of subjects (30). A similar effect of flecainide has been found on transvenous pacing thresholds (31). Encainide, also a class IC drug, may increase energy requirements for ventricular defibrillation (32), but its effect on cardioversion threshold for atrial fibrillation has not been studied. Despite these observations of measured cardioversion thresholds, there is little evidence that these or other antiarrhythmic agents have any clinically significant effect on the eventual successful electrical termination of atrial fibrillation, since the increase in energy requirements generally falls below the upper energy limit of the cardioversion device. Nevertheless, if cardioversion of atrial fibrillation is unsuccessful in a patient receiving a IC agent, consideration should be given to changing the drug and repeating the procedure after an interval of a few days.

POSTCARDIOVERSION ST SEGMENT ELEVATION AND MYOCARDIAL DAMAGE

Early in the experience of cardioversion it was noted that transient ST segment elevation occasionally occurred (33) (Fig. 4). Although initially thought to represent myocardial ischemia, such elevations are transient and not associated with myocardial creatine phosphokinase (CPK) release or any other features of necrosis (34,35). The prevalence of postcardioversion ST elevation has been estimated to be 20% (35), and one study suggested that this finding is more common in subjects with previous pericardiotomy (36). The mechanism is unclear, but the major importance lies in the recognition that this is a benign phenomenon and it should not be considered a reason for discontinuing sequential cardioversion shocks if a patient remains in atrial fibrillation.

While ST segment elevation is rarely an indicator of myocardial damage, early studies of cardioversion reported that transthoracic electrical shocks can cause morphologic changes consistent with damage to the myocardium. This was most often recognized when alternating current energy was used for reversion (37–39). Although such damage is less when DC shock is employed, repeated cardioversion in animals may cause myocardial membrane changes resulting in areas of necrosis associated with the release of tissue enzymes and potassium (39). The extent of tissue necrosis is directly related to the cumulative energy delivered to the myocardium (40,41).

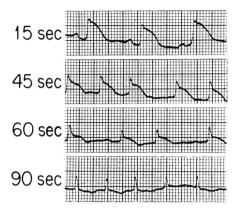

FIG. 4. Postcardioversion ST segment elevation in a subject receiving 320 Wsec for cardioversion of atrial fibrillation. No evidence of myocardial damage was detected. (From ref. 34, with permission.)

There is little significant damage when low energies are used, but progressively more occurs as the delivered energy level is increased, although there is a wide margin of safety (42). In animals receiving multiple high-energy shocks, the extent of myocardial damage and creatine kinase depletion was reduced by pretreatment with verapamil but not propranolol, suggesting a role of calcium accumulation in shock-induced cardiac necrosis (42).

Although early studies in humans suggested that CPK release (43) after cardioversion may be related to myocardial damage, analysis of MB isoenzymes indicate that myocardial necrosis is rarely present, even after multiple shocks. Van Gelder et al. (36) measured CPK-MB isoenzymes in 26 randomly selected subjects undergoing elective cardioversion for atrial arrhythmia, six of whom had postcardioversion ST segment elevation. Total CPK was markedly elevated 24 hr after cardioversion with a minimal elevation in the total MB band. This was considered to represent MB leak from skeletal muscle rather than from the heart. In a similar study, Metcalfe and co-workers (44) assessed total CPK-MB isoenzymes in 25 patients undergoing elective cardioversion. They also performed [99m]technetium stannous pyrophosphate scanning before, and 36 hr after, the procedure. The total CPK release was related to the cumulative energy used, but neither isoenzyme measurement nor pyrophosphate scanning revealed evidence of myocardial damage. These studies indicate that elective cardioversion, in the cumulative ranges of energy most commonly used, causes no overt cardiac damage in humans.

CARDIOVERSION OF ATRIAL FLUTTER TO FIBRILLATION

Atrial flutter is a more organized rhythm than atrial fibrillation, it responds poorly to antiarrhythmic therapy, and cardioversion is often required. Energy requirements for the termination of atrial flutter tend to be lower than for atrial fibrillation, but the flutter may be converted to fibrillation by the DC shock. Lown et al. (45) noted that lower energy shocks (<20 J) for atrial flutter were more likely to produce atrial fibrillation than higher energies. This may be related to failure to fully depolarize the whole atrium with lower energy shocks, thereby allowing the initiation of the multiple reentry circuits necessary for atrial fibrillation. Support for this hypothesis is found in animal experiments of ventricular defibrillation in which it has been demonstrated that a critical mass of tissue requires depolarization for successful arrhythmia termination (46). In the comparative study of Kerber et al. (12), four of 28 subjects (14.3%) with atrial flutter who received an initial shock of 20 to 40 J with anterolateral paddles developed atrial fibrillation, compared to 11 of 28 (42.3%) in whom anteroposterior paddle placement was used. This difference was statistically significant. Although the reason for this is unclear, it may be related to different levels of current reaching the atrium as a result of different directional vectors of current flow.

ANTICOAGULATION AND CARDIOVERSION

The issue of anticoagulation and cardioversion is dealt with in detail in Petersen's chapter in this book and will be discussed only briefly here. The current recommendation of anticoagulation for 2 to 3 weeks prior to and 2 to 3 weeks following cardioversion is to allow time for adherence of any preexisting atrial thrombus before the procedure and to allow for resumption of mechanical atrial activity afterward. The estimated incidence of thromboembolism varies, but in a large, nonrandomized series, published in 1969, which included 437 patients (572 attempted cardioversions), embolism occurred in 5.3% of nonanticoagulated patients compared to 0.8% in those receiving anticoagulation (47). In nonanticoagulated patients with chronic nonvalvular atrial fibrillation, the embolic risk is 3.5% to 8% per annum and appears to be continuously present while atrial fibrillation persists (48–50).

It has been suggested that in patients with no clinical heart disease, atrial fibrillation of less than 3 to 4 days duration does not require anticoagulation prior to defibrillation (1). However, many patients cannot define precisely the onset of their arrhythmia; some conditions may be associated with a clustering of thromboembolism around the onset of atrial fibrillation, and occasionally patients are seen with paroxysmal atrial fibrillation of very short duration who nevertheless develop thromboembolic events. It therefore appears prudent to consider a period of anticoagulation in all patients presenting with atrial fibrillation, even of very recent onset, taking into account duration of arrhythmia in determining the risk-benefit ratio. It is the policy of the authors to immediately anticoagulate, with heparin, all patients presenting with new-onset atrial fibrillation (in the absence of contraindications) while a decision is made regarding further therapy. In the subgroup of patients with arrhythmia clearly documented to be of only a few days duration who do not spontaneously revert to sinus rhythm, this policy permits a more leisurely approach to decision making concerning the optimal time in the patient with recent onset arrhythmia. Certain patients are probably best served by 2 to 3 weeks of anticoagulation prior to cardioversion regardless of arrhythmia duration, owing to a high risk of atrial thromboembolism. These include patients with valvular heart disease and those with dilated or hypertrophic cardiomyopathy. Other patients, with 4 days or less of atrial fibrillation, can be evaluated on a individual basis.

ATRIAL FIBRILLATION DURATION AND ENERGY REQUIREMENT

It has been observed that the energy required for conversion of atrial fibrillation is related to the duration of the arrhythmia (45). In the early experience with cardioversion, it was noted that patients with atrial fibrillation present for less than 3 months were easily cardioverted, with an average energy requirement of 100 J. When the duration of the arrhythmia was more than 6 months, the average energy requirement increased to 150 J. The amplitude of the fibrillatory waves was related to the duration of atrial fibrillation and was also found to be a factor in determining the energy requirements. When the fibrillatory waves are coarse, more than 2 mm in height, atrial fibrillation is usually of a shorter duration and the average energy requirement was 92 J. When the amplitude was 1.0 to 2.0 mm, the average energy requirement was slightly higher at 118 J. An amplitude of less than 1 mm suggested that atrial fibrillation had been present for a longer duration and the average energy requirement for reversion was 140 J.

One exception to these observations is the patient with lone atrial fibrillation, i.e., atrial fibrillation in the absence of any structural cardiac disease and a normal left atrium (1). Often, these patients have no definable provoking factor for their arrhythmia. In such situations, the amplitude of the fibrillatory waves is low, usually less than 1.0 mm, even when the arrhythmia is recent in onset. Nevertheless, this low amplitude does correlate with an increased energy requirement for termination and often 150 to 200 J are required.

ANTIARRHYTHMIC DRUGS BEFORE AND AFTER CARDIOVERSION

A large number of clinical trials of atrial antiarrhythmic agents have demonstrated that the administration of antiarrhythmic therapy increases the likelihood of remaining in sinus rhythm after electrical cardioversion. However, the use of antiarrhythmic agents is associated with a potential for side effects. Although the majority of side effects are tolerable or resolve with discontinuation of therapy, concern over unpredictable proarrhythmic effects of many agents has led some authors to advise an initial cardioversion in the absence of antiarrhythmic drugs (51).

Lundstrom and Ryden (51) reported their experience of DC cardioversion of atrial fibrillation between 1980 and 1982. The initial cardioversion was performed on no antiarrhythmic therapy, and if the patient reverted to atrial fibrillation, a second cardioversion was generally performed using either disopyramide or quinidine prophylaxis. Ninety-five patients underwent their first cardioversion with no antiarrhythmic therapy other than digoxin. By 3 months only 30% were still in sinus rhythm and at 1 year 23% remained in sinus rhythm. The data on the recurrence rate after the second conversion are not clearly documented but are said to be "more successful." The relatively low rate of maintenance of sinus rhythm at 1 year on no therapy is similar to that reported in control groups of studies of individual medicines and less than that reported for patients receiving antiarrhythmic drugs (29,52).

In view of the poor long-term results of cardioversion without maintenance antiarrhythmic therapy, we favor cardioversion after administering adequate doses of an antiarrhythmic agent. This is started after adequate anticoagulation is achieved and shortly before a scheduled cardioversion. The advantages of this approach are several: Approximately 10% to 20% of patients may have restoration of sinus rhythm due to the antiarrhythmic agent. Immediately following DC cardioversion, when atrial premature beats are frequent, the presence of an antiarrhythmic agent may prevent very early recurrence of atrial fibrillation. In addition, starting the agent before cardioversion (as opposed to immediately after) will help to identify patients who have side effects due to the drug (such as quinidine-induced diarrhea) and permit institution of alternative therapy. If all drugs produce side effects, consideration should be given to maintaining atrial fibrillation as the rhythm of choice.

We generally prescribe quinidine sulfate 200 to 300 mg four times daily for 24 hr prior to cardioversion, including the morning of the procedure. Meticulous attention must be paid to potassium levels, and a reduction in digoxin dosage from the pre-quinidine dose is recommended. An alternative first-line agent, which may be better tolerated, is disopyramide 100 to 200 mg three times daily. However, this agent is contraindicated in poorly controlled heart failure and may result in urinary retention, particularly in older males with prostatic hypertrophy, due to its anticholinergic effect. These two drugs, as well as a relatively large number of alternatives are discussed in detail elsewhere in this volume.

Return of full atrial mechanical activity as documented by Doppler echocardiography may take 4 to 6 weeks (53,54), and it is prudent to continue antiarrhythmic drugs for at least this period. After this, antiarrhythmic therapy could be stopped in selected patients, while continuing therapy long-term in others. Patients in whom long-term antiarrhythmic therapy is advisable include those with multiple previous episodes of atrial fibrillation, those with clinical deterioration when in atrial fibrillation, and those with mitral valve disease. In subjects with a single episode of asymptomatic or minimally symptomatic arrhythmia (particularly when the left atrium is normal in size) or those in whom a precipitating factor was identified and adequately treated, a trial of cardioversion without drug therapy is appropriate. Likewise a decision about long-term anticoagulation must be individualized, and warfarin is usually continued for patients at increased risk of recurrence. They have frequent atrial premature beats, have had multiple episodes of atrial fibrillation, or have structural heart disease, especially valvular involvement. Unfortunately many patients do not fit neatly into these categories, and in many cases, a careful judgment has to be made based on an assessment of the risk-benefit ratio.

The overall 1-year success rate of initial cardioversion in the presence of antiarrhythmic drugs varies depending on the agent used and the population studied but is probably about 50%. The decision to repeat a cardioversion with use of another antiarrhythmic agent after one or more relapses is, again, one to be individualized based on clinical factors.

SPECIAL SITUATIONS

Pregnancy

Pregnant women are prone to develop supraventricular tachycardia (usually due to atrioventricular nodal reentry). In the vast majority of cases this is self-terminating but occasionally needs drug therapy or DC cardioversion. A more serious situation is the development of atrial fibrillation during pregnancy, which, although rare, most frequently occurs in the setting of organic heart disease (e.g., mitral stenosis) and may be associated with severe hemodynamic deterioration. DC cardioversion has been successfully used during pregnancy and does not appear to adversely affect the fetus (55,56). Warfarin anticoagulation is contraindicated early in pregnancy (57), but most pregnant patients developing atrial fibrillation are immediately aware of symptoms and thus cardioversion can be performed early after the onset of the arrhythmia, avoiding the necessity for anticoagulation.

Permanent Pacemakers

Cardioversion in a patient with a permanent pacemaker may occasionally damage the pacing device, particularly if the electrodes/paddles are placed too close to the pacemaker (58). In patients with permanent pacemakers requiring cardioversion, care should be taken to position the paddles at a distance from the pacemaker—the anteroposterior position is probably advisable. This topic is discussed in detail elsewhere in this volume.

Automatic Implantable Cardioverter Defibrillator

Patients with an automatic implantable cardioverter defibrillator (AICD) frequently have poor ventricular function and may thus have an increased risk of atrial fibrillation. If the AICD is responsive only to heart rate, a rapid ventricular rate may trigger the device. Although on rare occasions an AICD shock has inappropriately discharged following the onset of atrial fibrillation and fortuitously terminated the arrhythmia, cardioversion rarely occurs and paroxysmal atrial fibrillation in a patient with an AICD may be a cause of multiple inappropriate shocks (59). Patients with an AICD requiring external cardioversion for a ventricular arrhythmia may require an increased energy as the patches on the heart increase transthoracic impedance (60). It is not clear whether increased energy is required for termination of atrial arrhythmias since the atrium is not covered by the AICD patches. However, if unexplained difficulty is experienced converting atrial fibrillation in a patient with an AICD, a different cardioversion paddle position should be tried.

The addition of an atrial antiarrhythmic agent following cardioversion for atrial fibrillation in a patient with an AICD may affect the ventricular defibrillation threshold or it may increase the cycle length of spontaneous ventricular tachycardia so that the rate falls below the device cutoff. It is therefore highly advisable to reinduce a ventricular arrhythmia in order to test the AICD after the introduction of an agent for control of atrial arrhythmia.

HEMODYNAMICS OF CARDIOVERSION

Subjects with atrial fibrillation may have a deterioration in their clinical condition due to loss of the atrial filling component and/or to a poorly controlled ventricular rate. This concept is discussed in detail by Atwood elsewhere in this volume. While control of a rapid ventricular rate may result in immediate symptomatic improvement (e.g., in patients with mitral stenosis), continued improvement may occur for days or weeks after cardioversion possibly related to the delay in the full return of atrial function (53).

Atrial Natriuretic Peptide

Atrial natriuretic peptide (ANP) has been shown to be elevated during atrial fibrillation and to fall following cardioversion (61). Mookherjee et al. (62) measured ANP in a group of patients with atrial flutter or fibrillation before and after cardioversion. ANP levels were elevated and did not differ between patients with flutter and those with fibrillation. Following cardioversion, ANP levels fell significantly. No correlation was found between an elevated ANP level and left atrial size, arrhythmia duration, ventricular rate or blood pressure, and the presence of persistent postcardioversion congestive heart failure did not affect the fall in ANP. The authors concluded that the atrial arrhythmia in these patients was the major stimulus to ANP release.

INTERNAL TRANSCATHETER CARDIOVERSION

Occasionally, patients are seen in whom cardioversion is deemed beneficial but in whom the technique fails to restore sinus rhythm for even a few beats. In such patients, a new and as yet investigational technique of internal transcatheter cardioversion has been reported to be of benefit (63). Unlike internal cardioversion for other arrhythmias, high energies are required, as low energy shocks (0.5–5.0 J) are ineffective for reversion of atrial fibrillation (64). Experience with this technique is still limited and the patient population highly selected, i.e., those in whom both chemical and electric cardioversion have been unsuccessful and in whom ventricular response rates are poorly controlled despite medication.

The technique involves the placement of an electrode catheter in the distal right atrium where atrial fibrillatory electrograms are recorded. A shock of 200 to 300 J is delivered between this electrode and a regular external paddle electrode placed at the back. In one report of 10 patients, sinus rhythm was initially restored in nine, although two patients had early recurrence of atrial fibrillation and three had late recurrences (8 days to 4 months). Overall, five patients were in sinus rhythm after an 11-month follow-up. The only complication observed clinically was transient atrioventricular nodal conduction abnormalities including complete heart block and bundle branch block. However, pathologic studies in animals have demonstrated small foci of subendocardial necrosis, which can be extensive (65). It should be stressed that this technique merely permits the delivery of high intracardiac energy and is of no benefit to patients in whom standard cardioversion results in conversion to sinus rhythm followed by a rapid recurrence of atrial arrhythmia.

CONCLUSIONS

After 30 years of use, synchronized DC shock remains the preferred choice for the termination of atrial fibrillation in the majority of patients with this arrhythmia. The technique is safe and well tolerated and can be repeatedly used if necessary. Newer antiarrhythmic agents are proving effective in maintaining sinus rhythm, although concerns about their safety remain. While some patients clearly show clinical improvement following cardioversion, others are asymptomatic and the procedure is performed on the assumption that restoration of sinus rhythm will reduce the thromboembolic risks known to be associated with atrial fibrillation. As yet such an assumption is unproven, since the risk-benefit ratio of cardioversion followed by antiarrhythmic therapy for asymptomatic atrial fibrillation remains unclear. A trial to determine the value of cardioversion in asymptomatic atrial fibrillation versus long-term anticoagulation might cross the last frontier of unanswered questions concerning DC cardioversion for this common arrhythmia.

REFERENCES

1. DeSilva RA, Graboys TB, Podrid PJ, Lown B. Cardioversion and defibrillation. *Am Heart J* 1980;100:881–895.
2. Lown B, Amarasingham R, Neuman J. New method for terminating cardiac arrhythmias—use of synchronized capacitor discharge. *JAMA* 1962;182:548–555.
3. Lown B, Neuman J, Amarasingham R, Berkovits BV. Comparison of alternating current with direct current electroshock across the chest. *Am J Cardiol* 1962;10:223–233.
4. Lown B. Electrical reversion of cardiac arrhythmias. *Br Heart J* 1967;29:469–489.
5. Roden DM, Woosley RL, Primm RK. Incidence and clinical features of the quinidine-associated long QT syndrome: implications for patient care. *Am Heart J* 1986;111:1088–1093.
6. Khan AH, Malhotra R. Midazolam as intravenous sedative for electrocardioversion. *Chest* 1989;95:1068–1071.
7. Kowey PR. The calamity of cardioversion of conscious patients. *Am J Cardiol* 1988;61:1106–1107.
8. King BG. The effect of electric shock on heart action with special reference to varying susceptibility in different parts of the cardiac cycle. Doctoral thesis, Columbia University, New York, 1934.
9. Wiggers CJ, Wegria R. Ventricular fibrillation due to single, localized induction and condenser shocks applied during the vulnerable phase of ventricular systole. *Am J Physiol* 1921;128:500–505.
10. Chen PS, Shibata N, Dixon EG, Martin RO, Ideker RE. Comparison of the defibrillation threshold and the upper limit of ventricular vulnerability. *Circulation* 1986;73:1022–1028.
11. Lown B, Kleiger R, Wolff G. The technique of cardioversion. *Am Heart J* 1964;67:282–284.
12. Kerber RE, Jensen SR, Grayzel J, Kennedy J, Hoyt R. Elective cardioversion: influence of paddle-electrode location and size on success rates and energy requirements. *N Engl J Med* 1981;305:658–662.
13. Hagemeijer F, Van Houwe E. Titrated energy cardioversion of patients in atrial fibrillation. *Br Heart J* 1975;37:1303–1307.
14. Geddes LA, Tacker VA, Rosboro JP, Moore AG, Kabler PS. Electrical dose for ventricular defibrillation of small and large animals using precordial electrodes. *J Clin Invest* 1974;53:310–319.
15. Lermann BB, Halperin HR, Tsitlik JE, Brin K, Clark CW, Deale OC. Relationship between canine transthoracic impedance and defibrillation threshold. *J Clin Invest* 1987;80:797–803.
16. Kerber RE, Grayzel J, Hoyt R, Marcus M, Kennedy J. Transthoracic resistance in human defibrillation: influence of body weight, chest size, serial shocks, paddle size and paddle contact pressure. *Circulation* 1981;63:676–682.
17. Sirna SJ, Ferguson DW, Charbonnier F, Kerber RE. Factors affecting transthoracic impedance during electrical cardioversion. *Am J Cardiol* 1988;62:1048–1052.
18. Hoyt R, Grayzel J, Kerber RE. Determinants of intracardiac current in defibrillation. Experimental studies in dogs. *Circulation* 1981;64:818–823.
19. Gedder LA, Tacker WA, Cabler P, et al. The decrease in transthoracic impedance during successive ventricular defibrillation trials. *Med Instrum* 1975;9:179–180.
20. Ewy GA, Hellman DA, McCluny S, Taren D. Influence of ventilation phase on transthoracic impedance and defibrillation effectiveness. *Crit Care Med* 1980;8:164–166.
21. Kerber RE, Kienzle MG, Olshansky B, et al. Impedance-based electrical cardioversion of atrial fibrillation: a new method for optimal energy selection (abstract). *J Am Coll Cardiol* 1991; 17:130A.
22. Resnekov L, McDonald L. Appraisal of electrocardioversion in treatment of cardiac dysrhythmias. *Br Heart J* 1968;30:786–811.
23. Lown B, Kleiger R, Williams BJ. Cardioversion and digitalis drugs: changed threshold to electric shock in digitalized animals. *Circ Res* 1965;17:519–531.
24. Leja FS, Euler DE, Scanlon PJ. Digoxin and the susceptibility of the canine heart to countershock-induced arrhythmia. *Am J Cardiol* 1985;55:1070–1075.
25. Ditchey RV, Karliner JS. Safety of electrical cardioversion in patients without digitalis toxicity. *Ann Intern Med* 1981;95:676–679.
26. Mann DL, Maisel AS, Atwood JE, Engler RL, LeWinter M. Absence of cardioversion-induced ventricular arrhythmias in patients with therapeutic digoxin levels. *J Am Coll Cardiol* 1985;5:882–888.
27. Waldecker B, Brugada P, Zehender M, Stevenson W, Wellens HJJ. Dysrhythmias after direct current cardioversion. *Am J Cardiol* 1986;57:120–123.
28. Sharkey SW, Chaffee V, Kapsner S. Prophylactic external pacing during cardioversion of atrial tachyarrhythmias. *Am J Cardiol* 1985;55:1632–1634.
29. Van Gelder IC, Crijns HJGM, Van Gilst WH, Van Wijk LN, Hamer HPM, Lie KI. Efficacy and safety of flecainide acetate in the maintenance of sinus rhythm after electrical cardioversion of chronic atrial fibrillation or atrial flutter. *Am J Cardiol* 1989;64:1317–1321.

30. Van Gelder IC, Crijns HJGM, Van Gilst WH, DeLangen CDJ, Van Wijk LM, Lie KI. Effects of flecainide on the atrial defibrillation threshold. *Am J Cardiol* 1989;63:112–114.
31. Hellestrand KJ, Burnett PJ, Milne JR, et al. Effect of the antiarrhythmic agent flecainide acetate on acute and chronic pacing thresholds. *PACE* 1983;6:892–899.
32. Fain ES, Dorian P, Davy JJ-M, Kates RE, Winkle RA. Effects of encainide and its metabolites on energy requirements for defibrillation. *Circulation* 1986;73:1334–1341.
33. Tacker VA, Van Vleer JF, Geddes LA. Electrocardiographic and serum enzymic alterations associated with cardiac alteration induced in dogs by single transthoracic damped sinusoidal defibrillation shocks of various strengths. *Am Heart J* 1979;98:185–193.
34. Zelinger AB, Falk RH, Hood WB. Electrical-induced sustained myocardial depolarization as a possible cause for transient ST segment elevation post-DC elective cardioversion. *Am Heart J* 1982;103:1073–1074.
35. Chun PK, Davia JE, Donahue DJ. ST segment elevation with elective cardioversion. *Circulation* 1981;63:220–224.
36. Van Gelder IC, Crijns HJ, Van Der Laarse A, Van Gilst WH, Lie KI. Incidence and clinical significance of ST segment elevation after electrical cardioversion of atrial fibrillation and atrial flutter. *Am Heart J* 1991;121:51–56.
37. Peleska B. Cardiac arrhythmias following condenser discharge and their dependence upon strength of current and phase of cardiac cycle. *Circ Res* 1963;13:21–32.
38. Rivkin LM. The defibrillator and cardiac burns. *J Thorac Cardiovasc Surg* 1963;46:755–764.
39. Smith GT, Beeuwkes R, Tomkiewicz M, Abe T, Lown B. Pathological changes in skin and skeletal muscle following alternating current and capacitor discharge. *Am J Pathol* 1965;47:1–18.
40. Davis JS, Lie JT, Bentinck DC, et al. Cardiac damage due to electrical current and energy. Proceedings of the Cardiac Defibrillation Conference, Purdue University, West Lafayette, IN, 1975;27.
41. Dahl CF, Ewy GA, Warner ED, Thomas ED. Myocardial necrosis from direct current discharge. Effect of paddle electrode size and time interval between discharges. *Circulation* 1974;50:956–961.
42. Patton JN, Allen D, Pantridge JF. The effects of shock energy, propranolol and verapamil on cardiac damage caused by transthoracic countershock. *Circulation* 1984;69:357–368.
43. Ehsani A, Ewy GA, Sobel BE. Effects of electrical countershock on serum creatine phosphokinase (CPK) isoenzyme activity. *Am J Cardiol* 1976;37:12.
44. Metcalfe MJ, Smith F, Jennings K, Patterson N. Does cardioversion of atrial fibrillation result in myocardial damage? *Br Med J* 1988;290:1364.
45. Lown B, Perlroth MG, Bey SK, Abe T. "Cardioversion" of atrial fibrillation. A report on the treatment of 65 episodes in 50 patients. *N Engl J Med* 1963;269:325–331.
46. Zipes DP, Fischer J, King RM, et al. Termination of ventricular fibrillation in dogs by depolarizing a critical mass of myocardium. *Am J Cardiol* 1975;36:37–44.
47. Bjerkelund CJ, Orning OM. The efficacy of anticoagulant therapy in preventing embolism related to DC cardioversion of atrial fibrillation. *Am J Cardiol* 1969;23:208–215.
48. Petersen P, Boysen G, Godtfredsen J, Andersen ED, Andersen B. Placebo-controlled, randomized trial of warfarin and aspirin for prevention of thromboembolic complications in chronic atrial fibrillation. The Copenhagen AFASAK Study. *Lancet* 1989;1:175–179.
49. Stroke prevention in atrial fibrillation study group investigators. Preliminary report of the stroke prevention in atrial fibrillation. *N Engl J Med* 1990;322:863–868.
50. The Boston Area Anticoagulation Trial for Atrial Fibrillation Investigators. The effect of low-dose warfarin on the risk of stroke in patients with non-rheumatic atrial fibrillation. *N Engl J Med* 1990;323:1505–1511.
51. Lundstrom T, Ryden L. Chronic atrial fibrillation. Long term results of direct current conversion. *Acta Med Scand* 1988;223:53–59.
52. Jull-Moller S, Edvardsson N, Rehnqvist-Alzberg N. Sotalol versus quinidine for the maintenance of sinus rhythm after direct current cardioversion of atrial fibrillation. *Circulation* 1990;82:1932–1939.
53. Lipkin DP, Frenneaux M, Stewart R, et al. Delayed improvement in exercise capacity after cardioversion of atrial fibrillation to sinus rhythm. *Br Heart J* 1988;59:572–577.
54. Manning WJ, Leeman DE, Gotch PJ, Come PC. Pulsed Doppler evaluation of atrial mechanical function after electrical cardioversion of atrial fibrillation. *J Am Coll Cardiol* 1989;13:617–623.
55. Schroeder JS, Harrison DC. Repeated cardioversion during pregnancy. *Am J Cardiol* 1971;27:445–446.
56. Cullhead I. Cardioversion during pregnancy. A case report. *Acta Med Scand* 1983;214:169–172.
57. Salazar E, Zajarias A, Gutierrez N, Iturbe I. The problem of cardiac prostheses, anticoagulation and pregnancy. *Circulation* 1984;70(suppl I):169–174.
58. Levine PA, Barold SS, Fletcher RD, Talbot P. Adverse acute and chronic effects of electrical defibrillation and cardioversion on implanted unipolar cardiac pacing systems. *J Am Coll Cardiol* 1983;1:1413–1422.

59. Steinberg JS, Sugalski JS. Cardiac rhythm precipitating automatic implantable cardioverter-defibrillator discharge in outpatients as detected from transtelephonic electrocardiographic recordings. *Am J Cardiol* 1991;67:95–97.
60. Chapman PD, Veseth-Rogers JL, Duquette SE. The implantable defibrillator and the emergency physician. *Ann Emerg Med* 1985;18:579–585.
61. Roy D, Paillard F, Cassidy D, et al. Atrial natriuretic factor during atrial fibrillation and supraventricular tachycardia. *J Am Coll Cardiol* 1987;9:509–514.
62. Mookherjee S, Anderson G, Smulyan H, Vardan S. Atrial natriuretic peptide response to cardioversion of atrial flutter and fibrillation and role of associated heart failure. *Am J Cardiol* 1991;67:377–380.
63. Levy S, Lacombe P, Coenti R, Bru P. High energy transcatheter cardioversion of chronic atrial fibrillation. *J Am Coll Cardiol* 1988;12:514–518.
64. Nathan AW, Bexton RS, Spurrell RA, Camm AJ. Internal transvenous low energy cardioversion for the treatment of cardiac arrhythmias. *Br Heart J* 1984;52:377–384.
65. Dunbar DN, Jobler HG, Fetter J, Gormick GC, Benson DW, Benditt DG. Intracavitary electrode catheter cardioversion of atrial tachyarrhythmias in the dog. *J Am Coll Cardiol* 1986;7:1015–1027.

Atrial Fibrillation: Mechanisms and Management, edited by R. H. Falk and P. J. Podrid. Raven Press, Ltd., New York © 1992.

12

Oral Antiarrhythmic Drugs Used for Atrial Fibrillation: Clinical Pharmacology

Philip J. Podrid

Arrhythmia Service, University Hospital, Boston, Massachusetts 02118; Boston University School of Medicine, Boston, Massachusetts 02118

A number of drugs are useful for prevention of atrial fibrillation (AF), while other agents are useful for control of the ventricular response rate. The local anesthetic or membrane agents are primarily effective for termination and prevention of AF, while those agents that have their major action on the atrioventricular node, including digoxin, beta-adrenergic blockers, calcium channel blockers are important for control of the ventricular response rate in patients with chronic AF (Fig. 1).

CLASSIFICATION OF ANTIARRHYTHMIC AGENTS

The antiarrhythmic drugs have been classified by Vaughan Williams (1) based on their major action on the myocardium (Table 1). Although in widespread use, this classification scheme does not imply that drugs of the same class are identical, but rather that their major action and the electrophysiologic effects they produce on the myocardium are similar. It has become clear that some of the agents have several actions, creating difficulty in classifying them and making such distinctions between these drugs questionable. Moreover, each drug is unique and the beneficial or harmful effects of one do not predict the action of any other agent even if of the same class or subclass.

The class 1 agents are the local anesthetic or membrane active drugs that work primarily by blocking the sodium channel, inhibiting the rapid influx of the sodium ion (2). This pharmacologic action is observed in tissue that generates a fast action potential mediated by sodium ions. This includes atrial and ventricular myocardium as well as the His-Purkinje tissue (3). As a result of the interference with sodium ions, there is a significant reduction in the upstroke velocity or phase 0 of the action potential (i.e., the rate of membrane depolarization) that determines the velocity of impulse conduction through the myocardium (4). This reduction in conduction velocity and the increase in the time necessary for complete membrane depolarization are manifest as QRS widening on the surface ECG. Class 1 agents also prolong the membrane refractory period, thereby reducing myocardial excitability. Last, an abnormally increased rate of spontaneous phase 4 depolarization, as can occur with

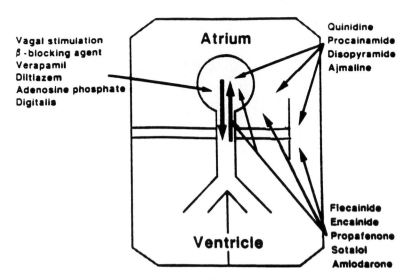

FIG. 1. Site of action of antiarrhythmic drugs. The class 1 and 3 antiarrhythmic agents affect the atrial and ventricular myocardium and accessory pathway as well as the atrioventricular node, while the class 2 and 4 agents and digoxin primarily affect the atrioventricular node.

ischemia or other myocardial disease states, is reduced and therefore abnormal automaticity is suppressed (5).

In addition to direct effects, some of the class 1A agents also have mild vagolytic activity (6). This vagolytic effect is most apparent with quinidine, less so with disopyramide, and the least amount is observed with procainamide. Vagal innervation involves, primarily, the sinus and atrioventricular nodes, and with depression of vagal activity, there are an increase in the rate of impulse generation by the sinus node, a shortening of the refractory period of the atrioventricular node, and an enhancement of impulse conduction through this structure (7). However, when the 1A drugs are used, the direct depressant effect of these drugs on the pacemaker tissue offsets the vagolytic actions, and, as a rule, they do not cause significant changes of the electrophysiologic parameters of these structures (8–10). Vagal innervation is also present in atrial myocardium and stimulation results in an increased conduction velocity and a shortening of the atrial refractory period. Depression of vagal action on atrial tissue by the class 1A drugs may, in part, account for their beneficial role in AF.

Although each of the class 1 membrane active agents has similar actions, there are differences among them in relation to the amount of sodium ion blockade, the magnitude of their effect on the upstroke of phase 0 or membrane depolarization and their effect on action potential duration (phases 2 and 3), i.e., the time for membrane repolarization. This has resulted in a subclassification of the drugs into 1A, 1B, and 1C (11). The class 1A agents (quinidine, procainamide, and disopyramide) have a modest effect on phase 0. Since the upstroke velocity of phase 0 or conduction velocity determines the time for complete membrane depolarization, the QRS is modestly prolonged. In contrast, there is a substantial prolongation of membrane repolarization, manifest on the ECG as QT (or JT) lengthening.

TABLE 1. *Classification of antiarrhythmic drugs*

Class	Action	ECG changes	Agents
1: Membrane stabilizers	Sodium ion inhibition	—	—
1A	Slight reduction in upstroke velocity; prolongation of repolarization	Slight QRS widening; marked QT lengthening	Quinidine, disopyramide, procainamide (amiodarone, recainam)
1B	No change in upstroke velocity; no change or shortening of repolarization	None	Lidocaine, mexiletine, tocainide, ethmozine
1C	Marked slowing of upstroke velocity; no change in repolarization	QRS widening	Encainide, flecainide, propafenone, recainam, indicainide, ethmozine
2: Beta blockers	Block catecholamine action	PR prolongation; slow heart rate; QT shortening	Propranolol, acebutolol, metoprolol, nadolol, timolol, pindolol, atenolol (propafenone, amiodarone)
3	Inhibits potassium fluxes; prolong repolarization	QT prolongation	Amiodarone, sotalol, N-acetyl-procainamide
4: Calcium channel blockers	Calcium channel blockade	PR prolongation	Verapamil, diltiazem (amiodarone)

While the class 1A agents share similar electrophysiologic properties, their effects on atrial tissue and hence their clinical activity against atrial arrhythmias differ. Quinidine and disopyramide exert substantial effects on atrial tissue, while procainamide at clinically used doses exhibits less atrial electrophysiologic activity (12). Consequently, quinidine and disopyramide are more effective against AF and atrial flutter than procainamide.

The class 1B drugs include lidocaine and its oral congeners mexiletine and tocainide. These drugs exert little effect on the rate of phase 0 upstroke or depolarization and do not alter the repolarization time (13,14). Therefore, the QRS and JT intervals are not altered. In general, these agents have no substantial effects on atrial tissue and, as expected, are ineffective against AF or flutter. However, since these agents may have a depressive effect on the accessory pathway tissue in some patients with Wolff-Parkinson-White syndrome, they may slow the ventricular response during AF.

The class 1C drugs (encainide, flecainide, and propafenone) exert a substantial depressive effect on phase 0 upstroke velocity, significantly slowing impulse conduction velocity and therefore prolonging the QRS interval on the ECG. They have little, if any, effect on the time for membrane repolarization, and therefore the JT interval is usually not altered. The class 1C agents exert a potent effect on atrial tissue and are reported to be effective against AF and atrial flutter (15–17). However, data are as yet limited, and unfortunately there are no comparative studies so that it is not certain if there are differences among the 1C agents or between the class 1A and 1C drugs.

The class 2 drugs represent the beta-adrenergic blockers. Although there are many different agents, they all share similar electrophysiologic properties. At clinically used doses, these agents do not exert any significant direct effects on the myocardial membrane, but their actions are mediated principally by blockade of myocardial beta receptors resulting in an antagonism of catecholamine effect on myocardial electrophysiologic properties (18–20). The pharmacologic effects of beta-blocking agents are primarily observed when the sympathetic nervous system is activated or in the presence of an elevated level of circulating catecholamines. Sympathetic stimulation results in an increase in impulse conduction velocity of the membrane, shortening of the membrane refractory period, an increase in its excitability and enhancement of automaticity. The beta-blocking agents prevent these changes in all cardiac tissue. As a rule, the beta-blocking agents do not have significant electrophysiologic action on myocardial tissue in the absence of augmented sympathetic activity and thus are not primary agents for suppression of supraventricular or ventricular arrhythmias except in those cases in which excessive sympathetic stimulation is implicated in arrhythmia genesis or maintenance. In general, the pacemaker tissue of the heart, i.e., the sinus and atrioventricular nodes, is richly innervated by the sympathetic nervous system and is substantially affected by circulating catecholamines (7). The beta blockers therefore have their most obvious clinical effects on these structures. They reduce the rate of sinus node impulse formation, decreasing heart rate at rest and especially during exercise. Since the conduction time through the atrioventricular node and its refractory period are prolonged, these drugs have an important role in controlling ventricular response rate during AF.

The class 3 antiarrhythmic agents (bretylium, *N*-acetyl-procainamide (NAPA), sotalol, and amiodarone) block the potassium channel and interfere with potassium fluxes (21,22). This activity primarily affects membrane repolarization (phases 2 and 3) of the action potential. As a result, there is prolongation of the action potential and refractory periods of all myocardial tissue and a reduction in membrane excitability. On the surface ECG, substantial prolongation of the JT interval is observed. As expected, these agents may be effective for prevention of AF and atrial flutter, although clinically only amiodarone is of established benefit (23).

The class 4 agents are the calcium channel blockers of which the most clinically useful drug for arrhythmia management is verapamil (24). By inhibiting the influx of calcium ions, these drugs primarily act on tissue generating a slow action potential that is mediated by the slow inward movement of calcium ions (25). This includes the sinus and atrioventricular nodes and annular tissue around the mitral and tricuspid valves, the structures capable of exhibiting normal pacemaker activity. A reduction in the inward movement of calcium ions will blunt spontaneous depolarization, the upstroke velocity of phase 0, and the maximum amplitude achieved. This decreases the automaticity of the pacemaker tissue and reduces the rate of impulse conduction within the tissue, particularly important for atrioventricular nodal function. On the surface ECG, these agents produce a slowing of heart rate and prolongation of the PR interval. When AF is present, they reduce the ventricular response.

Although not included as a standard antiarrhythmic agent, digoxin is effective for a wide range of supraventricular arrhythmias, primarily those that involve the atrioventricular node (26). The major direct pharmacologic action of digoxin in the myocardium is to increase intracellular calcium levels by interfering with the sodium potassium ATPase-mediated pump, allowing for an increased exchange between sodium and calcium. The increase in intracellular calcium is the presumed mechanism for its positive inotropic effects (27). The increase in calcium ion influx is responsible for an increase in the frequency and amplitude of delayed afterpotentials (28), a proposed mechanism for certain arrhythmias associated with digoxin toxicity. Digoxin has no other direct electrophysiologic effects on the myocardium, but its major antiarrhythmic action occurs as a result of the enhanced vagal tone produced by this drug. An increase in vagal activity reduces the spontaneous automaticity of pacemaker tissue, slowing the rate of sinus node impulse generation (7,24). Additionally, there is depression of atrioventricular nodal function and prolongation of the refractory period of the node, resulting in a slowing of impulse conduction through this structure, accounting for its useful role in the management of AF and atrial flutter. Although vagal innervation is richest in the sinus and atrioventricular nodes, there is sparse and nonhomogeneous vagal innervation of the atrial and ventricular myocardium. In contrast to the action on pacemaker tissue, an increase in vagal tone increases the conduction velocity and shortens the refractory periods of atrial myocardial tissue. These changes are not uniform within the atrial tissue, a precondition for the development of multiple reentrant circuits, the presumed mechanism for AF. This has major implications in regard to the use of this drug for reversion or prevention of AF.

The most effective agents for termination and prevention of AF are those of classes 1A, 1C, and 3. The drugs of classes 2 and 4 along with digoxin are useful for ventricular rate control as a result of their effect on the electrophysiologic properties of the atrioventricular node (Table 2).

Since there are important clinical differences among these agents, it is important to review their individual pharmacology and side effect profile.

TABLE 2. *Comparative efficacy of antiarrhythmic drugs for atrial fibrillation (AF)*

Drug	AF	AF in WPW
Quinidine	+ +	+ or + +
Procainamide	+	+ +
Disopyramide	+ +	+ or + +
Tocainide	0	0[a]
Mexiletine	0	0[a]
Flecainide	+ + or + + +	+ + +
Encainide	+ +	+ + +
Propafenone	+ +	+ + or + + +
Amiodarone	+ + +	+ + +
Sotalol	+ +	+ + or + + +
Beta blockers	+[b]	−
Verapamil	0[b]	−
Digoxin	0[b]	−

[a]May slow ventricular rate.
[b]Effective for rate slowing only.
0, not effective; −, ineffective, may be harmful; +, occasionally effective; + +, moderately effective; + + +, very effective.

Quinidine

Quinidine is often the first antiarrhythmic drug administered for reversion of AF and is the most frequent agent used for long-term prevention of the arrhythmia. The drug exerts a direct depressant effect on all cardiac tissue and slows impulse conduction (29–31). It also possesses mild anticholinergic activity, considered important because of concerns that this enhanced conduction through the atrioventricular node might result in an acceleration of the ventricular response (6,32). To prevent this, it has been usual clinical practice to administer a drug that blocks atrioventricular nodal conduction, i.e., a beta blocker, calcium channel blocker, or digoxin, prior to administering quinidine. However, rate acceleration is not usually seen. Indeed, His bundle studies have reported no change in the AH interval or atrioventricular nodal conduction during sinus rhythm when quinidine is administered, suggesting that the weak indirect vagolytic action is negated by the direct depressant effect of the drug (6). There have been infrequent cases reported in which quinidine has slowed the atrial rate and resulted in organization of the fibrillatory impulses, observed in the ECG as a slowing and regularization of the fibrillatory waves, resembling atrial flutter. In this situation, there has been slight rate acceleration observed, but it is generally not clinically important. Therefore, in the absence of intermittent atrial flutter, quinidine can be administered as single therapy for AF without the need to block atrioventricular nodal conduction with an additional agent.

Pharmacology (Table 3)

Quinidine is usually administered by the oral route. Although there are preparations that can be given either intramuscularly or intravenously, these are not preferred routes of administration because of associated side effects (33).

Several oral preparations of quinidine are available. Quinidine sulfate is a shorter acting form that is rapidly and completely absorbed from the gastrointestinal tract

TABLE 3. *Quinidine*

Dose	Sulfate 200–400 mg, t.i.d. or q.i.d., oral; gluconate 324 mg t.i.d., oral
Protein binding	70%–90%
Clearance	70%–90% hepatic metabolism; – metabolites have minimal activity; 10%–30% renal
Half-life	5–8 hr
Blood levels	2–5 μg/ml
Drug interactions	Digoxin, barbiturates, phenytoin, rifampin, cimetidine, vasodilators, verapamil
Side effects	Gastrointestinal, hematologic, central nervous system, cardiac

and has a bioavailability of 80% (34). The usual dose is 200 to 300 mg four times per day, although daily doses of up to 2,400 mg have been administered. A slow-release preparation of quinidine sulfate is also available. Quinidine gluconate has a slower rate of absorption and therefore a more prolonged duration of action since blood levels are maintained for a longer period of time (35). The usual dose of quinidine gluconate is 324 mg (one tablet) two or three times per day. This is equivalent to 240 mg of quinidine sulfate. A third preparation is quinidine polygalacturonate, which also is absorbed slowly and has blood levels maintained for a longer time (36). The dose is 275 mg (equivalent to 200 mg of quinidine sulfate) three times daily. Regardless of the preparation, quinidine is 80% to 95% protein bound and has a volume of distribution of 2.0 to 3.5 liters/kg (37). Disease states that affect the level of serum proteins such as cirrhosis or an acute myocardial infarction can affect the concentrations of free quinidine in the plasma by altering the bound fraction. Changes in pH will also alter the binding of quinidine. Protein binding is increased in the presence of alkalosis and reduced with acidosis. Quinidine is 60% to 85% metabolized by the liver to metabolites that are devoid of significant antiarrhythmic activity. The half-life of the drug is 5 to 8 hr and is prolonged when hepatic dysfunction or reduced hepatic blood flow is present (38). The remainder of the drug is excreted unchanged by the kidney. The therapeutic blood level is reported to be 2.5 to 5 μg/ml. In general, blood levels are lower when the long-acting preparations or gluconated formulations are administered.

A number of drug interactions have been reported with quinidine. Digoxin levels rise during quinidine therapy and digoxin toxicity is a potential complication (39). The mechanism is probably multifactorial since quinidine reduces the renal clearance of digoxin and displaces it from skeletal and cardiac muscle binding sites. Drugs that induce hepatic enzymes such as phenobarbital, phenytoin, and rifampin may cause a clinically important increase in the metabolism of quinidine, reducing its half-life (40). The action of warfarin anticoagulants may be enhanced by quinidine (41).

Hemodynamics

Quinidine has several important hemodynamic effects. Although it is a mild negative inotrope (42), the drug also exerts ganglionic-blocking activity, causing vasodilation and a reduction in systemic vascular resistance that may be associated with hypotension (32). As a result of the decrease in afterload, left ventricular function, stroke volume, and cardiac output are maintained and congestive heart failure is infrequently provoked (43,44). However, caution must be used when administering quinidine with other drugs that also lower peripheral vascular resistance and afterload such as calcium channel-blocking drugs, nitrates, vasodilators, and angiotensin-converting enzyme inhibitors. The combined use may occasionally be associated with symptomatic hypotension, and since no further afterload reduction occurs, congestive heart failure may be precipitated in patients with severely depressed ventricular function.

Side Effects

Quinidine is associated with a high incidence of side effects. The most common are those affecting the gastrointestinal tract including nausea, vomiting, abdominal discomfort, and diarrhea (45). Some of these side effects can be prevented or eliminated by administration of quinidine with an aluminum-containing antacid. Not infrequently, an antidiarrheal agent is also required. The gluconated and polygalacturonate formulations may be better tolerated with a lower incidence of gastrointestinal side effects.

Cinchonism is a dose-related constellation of toxic effects including tinnitus, dizziness, nausea, vomiting, headache, palpitations, visual disturbances, confusion, disorientation, memory loss, delirium, or psychosis. Allergic reactions include rash, fever, and granulomatous hepatitis. Immunologically mediated side effects include thrombocytopenia, hemolytic anemia, agranulocytosis, and, rarely, a lupus-like reaction. Ocular involvement is unusual, but there are reports of keratopathy, sicca syndrome, and iritis.

The most serious side effects are cardiac. Congestive heart failure and significant abnormalities of conduction are unusual, while arrhythmia aggravation is relatively common (46). The most frequent reports are of "quinidine syncope," which is most commonly the result of torsades de pointes (47,48). This is associated with significant prolongation of the QT interval (49). Although QT prolongation with quinidine is often dose related and may be a toxic drug effect, QT prolongation with torsades most commonly occurs after a few doses of quinidine when blood levels are low. This represents an idiosyncratic reaction to quinidine and is not predictable. It has been suggested that it may occur in patients with forme fruste of a long QT syndrome who are particularly sensitive to quinidine or other class 1A agents.

Torsades de pointes is a medical emergency that requires immediate therapy. Quinidine should be discontinued and, if high, the serum quinidine levels quickly reduced. This can be accomplished by alkalinization of the blood, which enhances the protein binding of quinidine (50). Since torsades is due to a marked prolongation of the membrane repolarization time and hence the QT interval, interventions that shorten the time for repolarization and decrease the QT interval will reduce or eliminate the arrhythmia. These include rapid or overdrive pacing or the use of isoproterenol. It has also been reported that the intravenous administration of magnesium will terminate torsades (51).

Other forms of arrhythmia aggravation have been reported, including an increase in the frequency of spontaneous ventricular ectopy and the precipitation of a sustained ventricular tachyarrhythmia (46).

Disopyramide

Disopyramide is a class 1A agent that exerts electrophysiologic activity similar to that of quinidine (52). It has direct depressant effects on the electrophysiologic properties of all cardiac tissue as well as indirect vagolytic action, particularly on the atrioventricular node (53,54). However, as with quinidine, these two effects negate each other and atrioventricular nodal function is generally unaltered (8,55).

Pharmacology (Table 4)

Disopyramide is only available for oral use in the United States, and the usual dose is 100 to 200 mg three or four times daily. A long-acting, slow-release preparation is available that can be administered twice per day with adequate maintenance of blood levels (56). The oral drug is rapidly absorbed and has a bioavailability of 83% (57). In Europe, an intravenous preparation of the drug is available where it is in widespread use for the acute termination of AF. The dose administered is generally 1 to 2 mg/kg.

Protein binding of disopyramide is variable and serum concentration dependent (58). The percentage of drug that is protein bound is higher when blood levels are lower. Only 20% of the drug is metabolized by the liver to inactive metabolites, while 80% is excreted unchanged by the kidney (57,59). When renal function is normal, the half-life of the drug is 6 to 8 hr but is significantly prolonged when renal impairment is present (60). The half-life is longer, approximately 12 hr, when the sustained-release preparation is administered (56). The reported therapeutic blood level is 2 to 4 μg/ml. No important drug-drug interactions have been reported with disopyramide.

Hemodynamics

Disopyramide has significant hemodynamic effects. The drug is a potent negative inotrope resulting in a clinically significant decrease in stroke volume and cardiac output (61,62). Disopyramide has no direct effect on peripheral vascular resistance, but as a response to the reduction in cardiac output, there is a reflex vasoconstriction and an increase in peripheral vascular resistance and afterload. This results in an increase in cardiac work, which can further impair left ventricular function, reducing cardiac output.

TABLE 4. *Disopyramide*

Dose	100–200 mg t.i.d. or q.i.d. oral (short-acting); 150–300 mg b.i.d. oral (long-acting)
Protein binding	Variable
Clearance	70% renal unchanged; 15% gastrointestinal unchanged; 15% hepatic (inactive metabolites)
Half-life	5–8 hr
Blood levels	2–5 μg/ml
Drug interactions	Rifampin, phenytoin
Side effects	Cardiac, gastrointestinal, urologic, anticholinergic

Disopyramide can substantially worsen left ventricular function and can precipitate congestive heart failure (63,64). Although this is most commonly observed in patients with a history of congestive heart failure and a significantly reduced left ventricular ejection fraction, heart failure may be precipitated even in those without a prior history (63).

Side Effects

The most frequent side effects caused by disopyramide are the result of its anticholinergic activity (65–67). These effects are dose related and include dry eyes and mouth, constipation, vaginal dryness, urinary retention, and visual disturbances. The sustained-release preparation may cause less frequent and less severe anticholinergic side effects due to the lower serum levels. The coadministration of pyridostigmine may reverse or prevent many of the anticholinergic effects (68).

Other gastrointestinal side effects are nausea, vomiting, and abdominal discomfort, which are less frequent than with quinidine. Neurologic toxicity includes dizziness, fatigue, depression, and psychosis. Hypoglycemia, intrahepatic cholestasis, and skin rash have also been reported.

Cardiac side effects are the most serious and include conduction abnormalities, hypotension, and congestive heart failure (63). There have been reports of electromechanical dissociation, primarily in patients with renal failure in whom disopyramide levels are excessively high (69). Prolongation of the QT interval and torsades de pointes can occur with disopyramide therapy, but it is less common when compared to the incidence reported with quinidine (70,71). Other forms of arrhythmia aggravation have also been reported including an increase in spontaneous arrhythmia or a new sustained tachyarrhythmia (46).

Procainamide

Procainamide is a class 1A agent that has direct effects on cardiac tissue similar to those caused by quinidine and disopyramide (72,73). However, procainamide has less activity on atrial tissue compared to other antiarrhythmic agents and is less effective for termination or prevention of AF compared to the other class 1A drugs (30). Like quinidine and disopyramide, the drug exerts vagolytic activity, especially on the atrioventricular node, although this is not a clinically important effect (73,74).

Pharmacology (Table 5)

Procainamide can be administered orally or intravenously. The usual dose is 100 mg every 3 to 5 min up to a maximum of 1,500 mg, guided by blood pressure and the QRS width (75). In general, the intravenous drug results in slowing of the rate of a supraventricular or ventricular tachycardia, which is an important marker of drug action (76). When given orally, the dose is 500 to 1,000 mg every 4 hr. A sustained-release preparation is available that permits a three or four times per day dosing schedule (77). The oral drug is 75% to 95% bioavailable and only 15% is protein bound (78). It is rapidly metabolized in the liver by acetylation and the major metabolite is NAPA, which has substantial antiarrhythmic activity (79). Its antiarrhythmic

TABLE 5. *Procainamide*

Dose	500–1,000 mg every 4–6 hr oral (short-acting); 750–1,500 mg t.i.d. or q.i.d. oral (long-acting)
Protein binding	15%–25%
Clearance	Hepatic: acetylation to active metabolite (NAPA)
Half-life	1.5–3 hr: procainamide; 6–7 hr: NAPA
Blood levels	4–10 μg/ml NAPA (variable)
Drug interactions	None known
Side effects	Central nervous system, gastrointestinal, cardiac, lupus-like syndrome, hematologic

effects resemble those of class 3 drugs. The metabolic rate of procainamide is genetically determined, and there are fast and slow acetylators (80). Acetylator phenotype can be established by obtaining simultaneous procainamide and NAPA levels 2 hr after a dose. Rapid acetylators have levels of NAPA that are higher than procainamide. The half-life of the oral drug is only 3 hr but is prolonged in the presence of hepatic and renal impairment since a large percentage of the drug and metabolite is excreted by the kidney (81). The reported therapeutic blood levels of procainamide are 4 to 10 μg/ml, but this varies widely because of the active metabolite. Therapeutic levels of NAPA are not well established, but since NAPA and procainamide have different electrophysiologic effects, combining the two levels has no scientific basis or clinical utility.

Similar to the interaction with other drugs, cimetidine reduces renal clearance of procainamide and its metabolite. There are no other drug-drug interactions reported.

Hemodynamics

Like other antiarrhythmic agents, procainamide exerts a mild negative inotropic effect on the myocardium (42,82). Similar to quinidine, the drug exerts ganglionic-blocking activity and may produce peripheral vasodilation resulting in a reduction in systemic vascular resistance or afterload (83). These two actions balance each other and usually cardiac output is maintained. When given by the intravenous route, the effect on peripheral vascular resistance may be more marked and hypotension is relatively common (84,85). Hypotension and congestive heart failure may occur if procainamide is administered to patients with arrhythmia who have severe left ventricular dysfunction already receiving vasodilating agents, as the negative inotropic effect will then predominate.

Side Effects

Toxicity due to procainamide is common (86–88). Gastrointestinal side effects include anorexia, nausea, and vomiting, but these occur less frequently than with quinidine. Neurologic toxicity includes myopathy, tremor, ataxia, depression, thought disorders, and insomnia. Hypersensitivity or allergic reactions include fever, urticaria, agranulocytosis, neutropenia, and nephrotic syndrome. Cardiac toxicity includes conduction abnormalities and congestive heart failure, which are infrequently observed. As with other agents, arrhythmia aggravation occurs with procainamide. Torsades de pointes has been reported, although this is less commonly observed with procainamide in comparison to quinidine (89). An increase in spontaneous arrhythmia or new sustained ventricular tachyarrhythmia has also been reported (46).

The most frequent side effect from procainamide, which generally occurs after several months of therapy, is a lupus-like reaction (90). This is immunologically mediated and is seen most commonly in those who are slow acetylators of the drug, i.e., have high procainamide and low NAPA levels (80). Although antinuclear antibody (ANA) titers are elevated and lupus erythematosus (LE) preparations are positive in more than 80% of patients during long-term therapy, their presence does not always correlate with symptoms of lupus. The lupus-like syndrome is more frequent in those with a LE preparation and ANA titer that become positive within a short time of initiating therapy and rise to high levels rapidly. Manifestations of procainamide-induced lupus include polyarthralgias, arthritis, pleuritis, pneumonitis, pericarditis and myocarditis, fever, hemolytic anemia, and thrombocytopenia. Unlike idiopathic lupus, renal and central nervous system involvement does not occur with the procainamide-induced type.

Encainide

Encainide is classified as a 1C agent and its major electrophysiologic effect is a significant reduction of impulse conduction in all cardiac tissue (91). Since the drug exerts this electrophysiologic action on atrial tissue and the atrioventricular node, it may revert or prevent AF and may slow the ventricular response rate during AF (92).

Pharmacology (Table 6)

Encainide is only available for oral use, and the dose is 25 to 50 mg three or four times daily (93). There is wide individual variation in bioavailability. The drug is metabolized by the liver to at least two metabolites, O-desmethyl encainide (ODE) and 3-methoxy-O-desmethyl encainide (MODE). MODE exerts antiarrhythmic activity equal to and ODE exerts activity greater than that of the parent compound (94). Drug metabolism is genetically determined, and in more than 90% of the population, metabolism is extensive, while the remaining 10% are poor metabolizers (95). Encainide half-life in the extensive metabolizers is 1.5 to 3 hr and 10 hr in the poor metabolizers. The half-lives of the metabolites ODE and MODE are longer than that of encainide, approximately, 6 to 10 hr. At least 3 to 4 days are necessary for the metabolite level to achieve a steady state, and therefore the dose of encainide

TABLE 6. *Encainide*

Dose	25–50 mg t.i.d. or q.i.d. oral
Clearance	Hepatic to active metabolites
Half-life	3 hr parent; 8–10 hr metabolites
Blood levels	Variable
Drug interactions	Cimetidine, beta blockers
Side effects	Central nervous system, cardiac

should be increased only after 3 to 4 days of therapy (96). Blood levels of encainide and its metabolites are highly variable and the defined therapeutic range is wide. Consequently, blood level monitoring is of little clinical use. Since the active metabolites are excreted by the kidneys, the dose of drug must be reduced in the presence of renal insufficiency (97,98). Cimetidine increases the plasma concentrations of encainide. No other drug-drug interactions have been reported.

Hemodynamics

Encainide was initially reported to be a very weak negative inotropic agent, and no clinically significant changes were observed in patients with normal left ventricular function at baseline (99). However, several reports have now documented that encainide can significantly depress left ventricular contractility, primarily when baseline left ventricular function is substantially abnormal and the patient has experienced clinical congestive heart failure. In patients with an underlying cardiomyopathy and congestive heart failure, a single 25-mg dose of encainide produced a significant increase in left ventricular end diastolic pressure and pulmonary wedge pressure, a reduction in cardiac output, and the precipitation of overt congestive heart failure in a number of patients (100). In a large series, congestive heart failure was precipitated in more than 6% of patients, primarily in those with a history of clinical congestive heart failure (101).

Side Effects

The incidence of disturbing or minor side effects from encainide is relatively low. Although many of these are often dose related, some are not related to dose or blood level. The most frequent are neurologic complaints (102,103) including dizziness, lightheadedness, headache, blurred vision, tremor, and paresthesias. Gastrointestinal side effects include nausea, vomiting, constipation, and altered taste. Other infrequent complaints are difficulty in urination, sexual dysfunction, and hyperglycemia. The most frequent serious side effects are cardiac (104). As indicated, congestive heart failure has been reported. Conduction abnormalities are not infrequent and include sinus node dysfunction, atrioventricular nodal conduction disturbances, and slowing of His-Purkinje conduction with the development of intraventricular block (104). While such conduction abnormalities may be apparent at rest and with low heart rates, they are more common when the heart rate is increased. Aggravation of ventricular arrhythmia is a potentially fatal complication, which is, unfortunately, relatively frequent, reported in as many as 23% of patients (105,106). The incidence is higher in patients with structural heart disease, especially when congestive heart failure has been present, but aggravation also occurs in patients with less serious heart disease. Arrhythmia aggravation may be manifest as a statistical increase in spontaneous ventricular ectopic activity or may be a more serious reaction such as incessant ventricular tachycardia (105,106). In patients with AF, encainide has resulted in an incessant wide atrial flutter with a wide-complex ventricular response, resulting from the effect of the drug on ventricular conduction. This arrhythmia may be confused with ventricular tachycardia, resulting in inappropriate emergency cardioversion.

Flecainide

Flecainide is a class 1C antiarrhythmic agent with effects similar to those of encainide (107). The drug exerts substantial depressive action on impulse conduction in all myocardial tissue. Since it markedly slows impulse conduction in the atrium and atrioventricular node, it is effective for reversion or prevention of AF and may slow conduction through the atrioventricular node, reducing the ventricular response rate (108).

Pharmacology (Table 7)

Flecainide is only available in the United States for oral use, and the usual dose is 100 to 200 mg twice per day (109,110). It is rapidly absorbed, has a bioavailability of greater than 90%, and is only 40% protein bound. Approximately 65% of the drug is metabolized by the liver to inactive metabolites (111). The remaining 35% is excreted by the kidneys as unchanged drug. The half-life of flecainide is approximately 20 hr but is significantly prolonged to more than 27 hr in the presence of congestive heart failure or liver or renal dysfunction. In these situations, the dose must be reduced to avoid toxicity. As a result of the long half-life, 4 days are generally required to achieve steady-state therapeutic levels. Therefore, the drug dose should be increased only after this period of time. The reported therapeutic plasma level is less than 1 μg/ml, and higher levels have been associated with an increased incidence of toxic side effects.

A few drug-drug interactions have been reported. Flecainide will increase serum digoxin levels, but only to a minor degree. Serum flecainide levels are increased when amiodarone or cimetidine are administered concomitantly. Use of propranolol with flecainide causes an increase in the plasma levels of both drugs.

Hemodynamics

Flecainide is a potent negative inotropic agent (112,113). The magnitude of its depressive effect is dose related, although a reduction in left ventricular function is apparent even when small doses are administered and serum level of drug is low. Flecainide produces an increase in end diastolic pressure and pulmonary capillary wedge pressure. Stroke volume, stroke work, and cardiac output are all reduced. Congestive heart failure may be precipitated by flecainide, and the incidence is higher in patients with a previous history of congestive heart failure and a markedly reduced ejection fraction, indicative of systolic dysfunction.

TABLE 7. *Flecainide*

Dose	100–200 mg b.i.d. oral
Protein binding	40%
Clearance	75% hepatic metabolism, inactive metabolites; 25% renal unchanged
Half-life	Up to 27 hr
Blood level	<1,000 μg/ml
Drug interactions	Cimetidine, digoxin
Side effects	Central nervous system, gastrointestinal, cardiac

Side Effects

Flecainide is associated with a relatively low incidence of disturbing or minor side effects (114). Minor complaints include blurred vision, dizziness, headache, nausea, constipation, fatigue, nervousness, tremor, insomnia, paresthesias, tinnitus, rash, and urinary abnormalities. Serious cardiac side effects are relatively common, especially in patients who have significant underlying structural heart disease and left ventricular dysfunction (115,116). Congestive heart failure is worsened in those with a history of it and may be precipitated in patients without previous heart failure. Conduction abnormalities are not infrequent and include sinus node dysfunction, atrioventricular nodal abnormalities, and intraventricular conduction delay and block. While these may be observed at rest, they are often exposed at higher heart rates. The most serious toxic effect is aggravation of arrhythmia, which ranges from an increased frequency of nonsustained arrhythmia to an incessant ventricular tachycardia that can be difficult or impossible to terminate. Flecainide can occasionally provoke serious ventricular arrhythmia in patients without a history of ventricular ectopy but who are receiving the drug for AF management (117). As with encainide, an incessant atrial tachycardia or atrial flutter with a wide-complex ventricular response may occur, which may cause hypotension and has been confused with ventricular tachycardia.

Propafenone

Propafenone, another member of the 1C subclass, has effects on cardiac tissue similar to those produced by encainide and flecainide (118,119). The drug causes a marked slowing of impulse conduction through ventricular and atrial tissue as well as the atrioventricular node. Like encainide and flecainide, the drug may revert or prevent AF because of its direct effect on the atrial myocardium and may also reduce the ventricular response to AF as a result of its action on the atrioventricular node (120). In addition to its direct effects, propafenone exerts beta-blocking activity, and it is estimated that the effect is approximately 1/40 as potent as that due to propranolol (121,122). Clinically, the beta-blocking activity is manifest as a blunting of peak heart rate during exercise, but it may also play a role in the electrophysiologic actions of the drug on the myocardium and the atrioventricular node. Propafenone also exerts mild calcium channel blocking activity, and the drug reportedly has 1/100 the potency of verapamil (123). The clinical significance of this property is, however, uncertain.

Pharmacology (Table 8)

Propafenone is currently available in the United States only for oral use at a recommended dose of 150 to 300 mg p.o. three times per day (124). The drug is rapidly and completely absorbed. However, bioavailability ranges from only 3% to 40% because of an extensive first-pass effect in the liver. Although hepatic metabolism is rapid and complete, it is dose dependent and therefore propafenone has nonlinear pharmacokinetics. At a higher dose, hepatic metabolic sites become saturated, the metabolic rate becomes slow, and blood levels are higher than predicted (125,126). Propafenone is 95% protein bound, and, as with encainide, its metabolism is genet-

TABLE 8. *Propafenone*

Dose	150–300 mg t.i.d. oral
Clearance	Hepatic first-pass effect, metabolites have ? activity
Half-life	6–10 hr
Blood levels	Variable
Drug interactions	Digoxin, cimetidine, warfarin
Side effects	Cardiac, central nervous system, gastrointestinal

ically determined (127). The majority of patients (93%) are rapid metabolizers, and in these patients, the propafenone levels are low, while the levels of the metabolites, primarily hydroxy-propafenone, are high (126,127). The metabolites have antiarrhythmic activity that is less than that of the parent compound, and their clinical importance has not been well studied.

Propafenone interacts with, and increases the plasma concentrations of, digoxin, warfarin, and propranolol, but these increases are not clinically important (128). Cimetidine insignificantly increases the serum levels of propafenone. When administered along with food, there is a delay in the absorption of the drug but not the total amount absorbed, and there are no important clinical consequences as a result of this interaction.

Hemodynamics

Propafenone is a negative inotrope (129). This effect is usually dose dependent but may occur even when low doses are administered. The drug causes an increase in left ventricular end diastolic pressure and pulmonary capillary wedge pressure and a reduction in stroke volume, stroke work, and cardiac output. Although there are no comparative trials, these negative inotropic effects appear to be more pronounced than those due to encainide, but less than those due to flecainide. While studies have not reported any significant changes in left ventricular ejection fraction measured at rest, congestive heart failure has been precipitated by the drug, primarily in patients with a clinical history of heart failure (101,129,130). Despite its negative inotropic effects, propafenone has been used safely in patients with a history of congestive heart failure and poor left ventricular systolic function.

Side Effects

Most of the side effects caused by propafenone are mild and do not require discontinuation of the drug (131). Since many are dose related, a reduction in dose is often all that is necessary. The majority are gastrointestinal and include nausea, vomiting, abdominal discomfort, constipation, and altered or metallic taste. Neurologic complaints include weakness, fatigue, tremor, paresthesias, and blurred vision. Other infrequent side effects include urinary retention, rash, bronchospasm, and abnormal liver function tests.

The most serious side effects are cardiovascular and are similar to those caused by the other 1C agents (132). Conduction abnormalities are not uncommon and are usually dose related. These include sinus node dysfunction, atrioventricular nodal abnormalities, and intraventricular block. They may be more common when underlying conduction abnormalities are present. Congestive heart failure may be precipitated in patients with a history of heart failure, but is rare in those with intact left ventricular systolic function (101). Aggravation of arrhythmia occurs, but the incidence is lower when compared to that reported with encainide and flecainide therapy, although the type of aggravation is similar and includes incessant ventricular tachyarrhythmia (133).

Moricizine

Moricizine, a phenothiazine derivative, is a new antiarrhythmic agent that exhibits electrophysiologic effects resembling those caused by agents of classes 1A, 1B, and 1C (134). It is therefore unclassifiable. Its major effect on atrial tissue is to slow impulse conduction, similar to the action of 1A and 1C agents (135). The drug also slows conduction through the atrioventricular node. Although data are very limited, preliminary reports suggest that it may be effective in the therapy of some atrial arrhythmias. However, its role in AF remains to be defined as data are not available.

Pharmacology (Table 9)

Moricizine is available for oral use, and the recommended dose is 200 to 400 mg three times daily (136). The drug is extensively metabolized by the liver, and there is a first-pass effect (137). Some of the metabolites may have mild antiarrhythmic activity, but this has not been thoroughly investigated. The drug is highly protein bound (>90%) and has a half-life of approximately 9 hr. Serum levels are variable and a therapeutic level has not be clearly established. Therefore, drug levels are probably of no value.

The only reported drug interactions with moricizine have been with cimetidine, which reduces the rate of moricizine metabolism, and with theophylline (138). Moricizine increases the metabolism of theophylline and lowers the expected levels.

Hemodynamics

Moricizine exerts only mild negative inotropic effects on myocardial function (139). It does not cause any significant changes on left ventricular ejection fraction, left ventricular end diastolic or systolic pressures, pulmonary artery or capillary wedge pressures, systemic arterial pressure, stroke volume, stroke work, or cardiac output. Congestive heart failure is infrequently observed and occurs only in those with a previous history of it (140).

TABLE 9. *Moricizine (ethmozine)*

Dose	200–400 mg t.i.d. oral
Protein binding	95%
Clearance	Hepatic; first-pass effect; ? metabolite activity
Half-life	3–4 hr normal, up to 13 hr in patients
Blood levels	?
Drug interactions	Cimetidine
Side effects	Gastrointestinal, central nervous system, anticholinergic, cardiac

Side Effects

Side effects caused by moricizine are generally mild and rarely is drug discontinuation necessary (141–144). Some effects are dose related and may require dose reduction. Most often reported are neurologic complaints including dizziness, headache, fatigue, sleep disturbances, perioral numbness, euphoria, tinnitus, and memory loss. Gastrointestinal complaints include nausea, anorexia, and diarrhea. Phenothiazine- or atropine-like side effects are uncommon and include dry mouth and urinary difficulties. Less commonly reported are hepatitis, rash, and thrombocytopenia. Cardiac side effects are infrequent and include atrioventricular nodal blockade, intraventricular conduction blockade, worsening of congestive heart failure, and arrhythmia aggravation.

Amiodarone

Although not approved in the United States for use in atrial arrhythmia, amiodarone is in widespread use in Europe and elsewhere for atrial arrhythmias and is often the first drug administered. Amiodarone is a very complicated drug that exerts a number of actions affecting all cardiac tissue. Its major effect is "antifibrillatory," resulting from a prolongation of action potential duration or repolarization time (145). On the surface ECG, this is associated with JT prolongation. The drug also produces mild sodium channel blocking activity and causes membrane stabilizing actions similar to those of the class 1 antiarrhythmic drugs, i.e., primarily a slowing of impulse conduction. Prolongation of the PR interval on the ECG is often observed and QRS widening may be seen.

Amiodarone is also a noncompetitive beta blocker and a calcium channel blocker. Although these effects are only mild, they may be clinically important. Last, the drug contains substantial amounts of iodine (75 mg iodine/200 mg drug), and as a result, it interacts with thyroid metabolism. Amiodarone blocks the peripheral conversion of thyroxin (T_4) to the active form of the thyroid hormone triiodothyronine (T_3) (146). It is possible that iodine, by interfering with thyroxin metabolism, is responsible for some of the drug's antiarrhythmic activity. Since amiodarone exerts substantial activity on atrial tissue as well as the atrioventricular node, the drug may be effective for prevention of AF and for controlling the ventricular response rate.

Pharmacology (Table 10)

Amiodarone has very unusual pharmacokinetic properties. When given orally, the absorption of the drug is slow, variable, and incomplete (147). As a result of its absorption characteristics and its extensive liver metabolism, its bioavailability is approximately 50% (147,148). The drug may also be given intravenously. Its major metabolite, desethylamiodarone, also possesses significant antiarrhythmic activity (149). As part of its metabolism, the drug undergoes deiodination. Although amiodarone is highly bound to serum proteins (96%), it is widely distributed throughout the body, binding avidly to all adipose tissue to which it is rapidly distributed. Indeed, the adipose stores of the drug are vast, and this tissue must be saturated before there are measurable concentrations of amiodarone in the serum and target organs,

TABLE 10. *Amiodarone*

Dose	600–1,800 mg oral loading
Clearance	Hepatic, active metabolite, deiodination
Half-life	Up to 120 days
Blood levels	1–2 µg/ml
Drug interactions	Digoxin, warfarin, antiarrhythmic drugs, beta blockers, calcium channel blockers, anesthetic agents
Side effects	Cardiac, neurologic, gastrointestinal, hematologic, dermatologic, pulmonary, thyroid, ophthalmologic

particularly the heart (150). Therefore, therapy with amiodarone requires the use of a loading dose, which may be taken as long as 1 to 3 months when administered orally. Since bioavailability is greater with intravenous administration, the loading period may be shorter. For treatment of ventricular arrhythmia, the initial oral loading dose is 600 to 1,800 mg for 1 to 2 weeks, followed by 800 to 1,200 mg for 1 to 2 weeks, and 200 to 600 mg thereafter. In general, the loading and maintenance doses necessary for prevention of atrial fibrillation are lower, and since AF is not a life-threatening arrhythmia requiring immediate control, very large doses are not usually administered for loading or for maintenance therapy. The most common loading dose for the treatment or prevention of AF is 600 mg daily administered for 2 to 3 weeks, followed by 400 mg for 2 to 4 weeks, and 200 mg daily thereafter. Not infrequently, the dose can be reduced further, sometimes to 200 mg one to three times per week.

It is estimated that 15 g of drug are necessary to saturate the adipose stores and therefore 30 g must be given orally. Although there is an intravenous preparation, amiodarone is usually only given by the intravenous route for several days, at a dose of 15 mg/kg/day (generally 1,000 mg). Thereafter, the drug is continued by oral administration. As a result of avid binding of amiodarone to adipose tissue, which is poorly perfused, the elimination of the drug from the body is very slow. The drug has an elimination half-life of 26 to 107 days, although this is variable and may be prolonged to 180 days or longer in some patients. Therapeutic blood levels have been reported as 1 to 2 µg/ml, but these vary widely and blood levels have not been predictive of efficacy or toxicity (151). It has been suggested that reverse T_3 levels may be more reliable for guiding dose, but this is not well established. Additionally, the blood levels of the active metabolite desethylamiodarone must be considered.

A number of important drug-drug interactions have been reported with amiodarone (152). These include a significant increase in serum digoxin levels and potentiation of the anticoagulant effect of warfarin. Amiodarone also elevates the levels of other antiarrhythmic drugs including quinidine, procainamide, flecainide, and phenytoin, which increases the risk of toxicity. Hypotension, bradycardia, and other conduction abnormalities may result when anesthetic agents, beta blockers, or calcium channel blockers are administered to patients receiving amiodarone.

Hemodynamics

Amiodarone produces many effects on the cardiovascular system. It is a direct-acting arterial vasodilator that reduces peripheral vascular resistance and afterload (143,153). It also dilates the coronary arteries, increasing coronary artery blood flow.

Although the drug does have direct negative inotropic actions and can depress left ventricular function, the reduction in afterload usually offsets this direct depressant myocardial action. By virtue of its direct effect, as well as a result of its beta-blocking and calcium channel-blocking actions, there is a decrease in sinus node automaticity and a reduction in heart rate. This bradycardia is not usually reversed by therapy with atropine or sympathomimetic agents.

Side Effects

A major limitation to the use of amiodarone is the frequency of the associated toxicity, which can affect many organ systems (154–156). While some side effects are dose related, others do not appear to be so, although it has been suggested that some of these side effects are related to total dose received or perhaps total duration of drug exposure. The occurrence of many of the side effects may be delayed, and their incidence increases over time. Gastrointestinal complaints include constipation, nausea, abdominal discomfort, and anorexia. Liver function test abnormalities are very common, but hepatitis is rare. Neurologic complaints include headache, weakness, myalgias, tremor, ataxia, paresthesias, nystagmus, depression, insomnia, hallucinations, and nightmares. A peripheral neuropathy may occur or symptoms of proximal muscle weakness may develop. Abnormalities of thyroid hormone levels are common and include mild elevations of T_4 or thyroid-stimulating hormone and slight decreases of T_3 levels (146). Clinically significant hypo- or hyperthyroidism is less common, each occurring in 5% to 10% of patients.

Pulmonary toxicity, which has two patterns of presentation, is the most serious side effect (157,158). Less common is an early hypersensitivity or allergic reaction, which is acute, occurring shortly after treatment is begun. This presents with diffuse pulmonary infiltrates. More commonly, pulmonary toxicity occurs later during chronic therapy, is insidious in onset, and is progressive. This form presents with bilateral and diffuse pulmonary fibrosis or, less frequently, with infiltrates. Clinically, the patient may report only mild symptoms of fatigue and malaise, slight fever, shortness of breath, or nonproductive cough. In some patients, symptoms are more severe and include respiratory difficulties or respiratory arrest. A chest x-ray is the best way to definitely establish the diagnosis, since pulmonary function tests are generally abnormal in all patients receiving amiodarone and do not predict the occurrence of pulmonary fibrosis. Unfortunately, the patient at risk cannot be accurately identified.

Skin reactions are frequent and include allergic reactions, photodermatitis, and blue-gray skin discoloration. Ophthalmologic abnormalities include asymptomatic corneal microdeposits and, possibly, macular degeneration, photophobia, and reduced visual activity.

Cardiac toxicity is not frequent and includes sinus bradycardia, atrioventricular or intraventricular conduction block, hypotension, and congestive heart failure. Aggravation of arrhythmia does occur, although the incidence is unknown because of the unusual pharmacology of the drug. Although the drug prolongs the JT interval, torsades de pointes is rarely reported and may be the result of hypokalemia or another antiarrhythmic drug used in combination, primarily quinidine. Congestive heart failure may occur, but this is uncommon.

Beta-Adrenergic Blocking Agents

The beta-blocking drugs have their principal role in AF management by providing rate control resulting from slowing the ventricular response as a result of their depressive effect on atrioventricular nodal function (159,160). They have no direct effects on the atrial myocardium, and their only action is to blunt or prevent the stimulatory effects of catecholamines and the sympathetic nervous system (161). They may be of benefit as primary agents for arrhythmia prevention when arrhythmia is precipitated or exacerbated by an increased sympathetic state; however, this is not frequently the case. The beta-blocking agents do have an important role for arrhythmia management when they are administered along with other antiarrhythmic agents as part of combination therapy (162–164). Although there are many beta-blocking agents available, the actions of each one on the electrophysiologic properties of the heart are the same and are primarily related to beta blockade. Some of these agents exert membrane stabilizing effects, similar to the class 1 antiarrhythmic drugs, but the doses necessary to achieve this action are far in excess of those used clinically (165).

Pharmacology (Table 11)

The beta blockers currently available for clinical use in the United States are acebutolol, atenolol, betaxolol, metoprolol, nadolol, pindolol, propranolol, and timolol. These drugs are primarily administered by the oral route, although there are intravenous preparations of propranolol and metoprolol. Esmolol, an ultrashort-acting beta blocker, is only available for intravenous use.

The clinically used doses of these individual agents vary and are generally established by titration to achieve the principal pharmacologic effect, i.e., beta blockade. When used for control of the ventricular response during chronic AF, the dose is based on the degree of atrioventricular nodal blockade and slowing of the ventricular rate. When the drugs are used for prevention of AF, the dose administered is usually based on slowing of the sinus node rate.

Most of the beta blockers are rapidly and completely absorbed from the gastrointestinal tract (166,167). Some of them are rapidly metabolized by the liver to inactive metabolites and have a short half-life. Other agents are not hepatically metabolized but are completely cleared by the kidney and therefore have a long half-life. The hepatically metabolized beta blockers are generally lipophilic, while those excreted unchanged by the kidney are hydrophilic (168).

These agents also possess other pharmacologic actions that differ among the various beta blockers. The first is the property of cardioselectivity (167,169). Although some of the agents are specific blockers of the beta-1 receptor, at high doses this specificity is lost (169–171). A second property is that of intrinsic sympathomimetic activity (ISA) (169,171). Drugs with this property maintain resting sympathetic tone by partial agonist activity but blunt the effects of further sympathetic stimulation and excessive circulating catecholamines. Some of the beta blockers have membrane stabilizing (i.e., quinidine-like) effects, but this is usually apparent only at doses and blood levels higher than those used clinically (172,173).

TABLE 11. *Beta blockers*

Beta blocker	Oral dose (mg)	Potency ratio (propranolol = 1)	Bioavailability (%)	Cardioselectivity	ISA	Lipid solubility	Half-life (hr)	Clearance
Acebutolol	100–300 t.i.d.	0.3	30–50	Yes	Yes	Yes	8	Liver
Atenolol	50–200 daily	1	50	Yes	No	No	3–6	Liver
Betaxolol	10–20 daily	16	89	Yes	No	No	14–22	Liver
Metoprolol	50–100 t.i.d.	0.8	50	Yes	No	Yes	3–4	Liver
Nadolol	40–160 daily	0.8	30	No	No	No	14–17	Renal
Pindolol	2.5–20 b.i.d., t.i.d.	6	50–100	No	Yes	Yes	3–4	Liver
Propranolol	10–60 t.i.d., q.i.d.	1	30	No	No	Yes	4–6	Liver
Timolol	10–20 t.i.d.	6	75	No	No	Yes	4–5	Liver

ISA, intrinsic sympathomimetic activity.

Hemodynamics

Since the beta-receptor blockers block the effects of catecholamines and the sympathetic nervous system, they generally cause a decrease in blood pressure and heart rate (174,175). Their effect on peripheral vascular resistance is variable, however, and is, in part, related to the presence of ISA and selectivity (176–178). All beta blockers are negative inotropes and can result in congestive heart failure, especially when left ventricular contractility is maintained by sympathetic tone (179). Excessive bradycardia or atrioventricular nodal conduction abnormalities can occur, more commonly when these agents are given in combination with other drugs that depress nodal function, i.e., calcium channel blockers, or in the presence of sinus or atrioventricular node disease.

Side Effects

Each of the beta blockers is associated with the same side effects, although the incidence and severity vary (180). One of the important factors in determining the occurrence and incidence of some side effects is whether the agent is lipophilic or hydrophilic. Lipophilic agents have a wide tissue distribution and cross lipid membranes easily, and high concentrations are found in many organs, especially the central nervous system. Hydrophilic agents do not cross lipid membranes or accumulate in the central nervous system.

Gastrointestinal side effects include nausea, vomiting, abdominal discomfort, and diarrhea or constipation. Neurologic complaints include fatigue, weakness, gait disturbances, insomnia, hallucinations, and changes in mental status. Urinary retention may, rarely, occur. The precipitation or exacerbation of asthma occurs primarily with the nonselective agents but may be seen with selective agents at larger doses or in particularly susceptible patients. Cardiovascular toxicity includes hypotension, congestive heart failure, and conduction abnormalities. Aggravation of arrhythmia has been reported, but the incidence is not well established and may also relate, in part, to the presence of ISA (46).

Sotalol

Sotalol is a unique antiarrhythmic drug that exerts both beta-blocking (class 2) activity as well as class 3 properties (181), i.e., increase of the action potential duration and increase in the QT (or JT) interval. In the United States, it is undergoing investigation for both ventricular and supraventricular arrhythmias and appears to have a role for therapy of AF. It may be of particular benefit for patients with Wolff-Parkinson-White syndrome. It is in use in Europe for therapy of these arrhythmias.

Sotalol is a competitive, nonselective beta blocker that has an independent and direct membrane effect resembling that of class 3 drugs. The drug is available as a racemic mixture of its stereoisomers *d* and *l*. The *l*-isomer is primarily responsible for the beta-blocking activity, while the *d*-isomer has the class 3 properties (181,182). There are a few studies in which *d*-sotalol has been used, but most of the available data are for *d;l* sotalol.

Pharmacology (Table 12)

The oral dose of the drug is 80 to 240 mg twice daily. Dose titration should be performed slowly, the dose being increased by 80 to 160 mg daily every 3 to 4 days (181,183). Careful monitoring of hemodynamic and electrophysiologic effects are important at higher doses. The intravenous formulation is administered as an infusion of 0.2 to 2.0 mg/kg over 5 to 15 min (184).

The drug is well absorbed when administered by the oral route and plasma concentrations peak 2 to 3 hr after ingestion (181,185). It is nearly 100% bioavailable and unmetabolized by the body, with renal clearance of unchanged drug accounting for its excretion. In the presence of renal impairment, the dose must be reduced (186). Sotalol has the lowest lipid solubility of the beta blockers and there are no known metabolites (187,188). The serum half-life of the drug ranges from 6 to 18 hr. There are no known drug-drug interactions.

Hemodynamics

Although sotalol possesses beta-blocking activity, its hemodynamic effects differ from those of other beta blockers. As a result of its class 3 antiarrhythmic effects, it has less of a negative inotropic effect on left ventricular function when compared to other beta blockers (189,190). This may be the result of the prolongation of phase 3, allowing for an increased influx of calcium ions and an increase in contractility, offsetting the beta-blocking activity. However, as a beta blocker, the drug does reduce heart rate. Although stroke volume and systemic vascular resistance are unaffected, there is a reduction in cardiac output due to the decreased heart rate (190).

Side Effects

Adverse effects from sotalol are most often the result of its beta-blocking activity and have been reported in 50% of patients (181,187,191). In 20%, the drug has to be discontinued. Side effects are primarily neurologic including depression, fatigue, impotency, and headache. Other central nervous system side effects are less common because the drug is not lipophilic and does not accumulate in the brain. Gastrointestinal complaints including dry mouth, nausea, vomiting, and diarrhea are observed. Retroperitoneal fibrosis has also been reported (192). Cardiac side effects include hypotension, bradycardia, and atrioventricular nodal block. Since the drug has class 3 activity, it prolongs the JT interval and may provoke torsades de pointes (193,194). Other forms of arrhythmia aggravation have been reported as well.

TABLE 12. *Sotalol*

Dose	80–240 mg b.i.d. oral
Clearance	Renal, unchanged
Half-life	6–18 hr
Blood levels	?
Drug interactions	?
Indications	Ventricular and supraventricular arrhythmia
Side effects	Central nervous system, cardiovascular

Calcium Channel Blockers

Although there are several calcium channel blockers available for clinical use, verapamil is the agent most widely used for AF (195,196). Diltiazem, administered orally and intravenously has also been reported to be effective for rate control in AF, although it is not used as often as verapamil for this indication (197). Since these agents work only on pacemaker tissue, i.e., the sinus and atrioventricular nodes, which generates a slow, calcium-mediated action potential, their major role in AF is blockade of impulse conduction in the atrioventricular node and control of the ventricular rate (198,199). They have little if any role for termination or prevention of AF except in selected cases, such as in the postoperative patient.

Pharmacology (Table 13)

Verapamil is available for intravenous and oral use. When given by the intravenous route, the dose is 5 to 20 mg administered in increments of 5 mg (200,201). Although the drug is rapidly distributed to tissue receptors and has a short serum half-life of 15 to 20 min, the depressant effect on the atrioventricular node may be of longer duration. If necessary, a constant infusion of 0.005 mg/kg/min has been used. When given by the oral route, the dose used is higher and is not related to the intravenous dose determined to be effective as a result of variability in absorption, rapid first-pass metabolism by the liver, and a wide range of blood levels achieved. The dose used should be titrated to the desired therapeutic effect, i.e., depression of atrioventricular nodal impulse transmission and a slowing of the ventricular response rate. The usual dose is 80 to 160 mg three or four times daily. There is a long-acting preparation of verapamil now available, and the usual dose is 240 to 480 mg once daily. A number of drug interactions with verapamil have been reported. Combined use with beta blockers may result in conduction abnormalities, hypotension, and congestive heart failure. Similar adverse reactions may rarely occur when verapamil is administered along with quinidine or disopyramide. Verapamil causes an increase in digoxin levels.

Diltiazem is primarily administered by the oral route, at 30 to 120 mg three or four times daily (197). A long-acting preparation allows for dosing once or twice daily. As with verapamil, the dose is usually titrated to the effect of the drug on atrioven-

TABLE 13. *Calcium channel blockers*

	Verapamil	Diltiazem
Dose		
i.v.	5–20 mg (short-acting)	30–90 mg t.i.d. (short-acting)
Oral	80–160 mg 3 or 4 times daily (short-acting)	120–240 mg daily (long-acting)
	120–480 mg daily (long-acting)	
Protein binding	90%	70%–80%
Clearance	Hepatic (95%)	Hepatic (>95%)
Half-life	4.5–12.0 hr	3.5 hr
Therapeutic blood levels	125–400 ng/ml (variable)	50–200 ng/ml (variable)
Drug interactions	Beta blockers, digoxin, disopyramide, quinidine	Beta blockers, cimetidine
Side effects	Gastrointestinal, neurologic, cardiac	Gastrointestinal, neurologic, cardiac

tricular nodal conduction and the ventricular response rate during AF. Diltiazem causes an insignificant increase in digoxin levels. Coadministration with beta blockers may cause serious conduction problems or precipitate congestive heart failure. Cimetidine causes an increase in diltiazem levels.

Hemodynamics

Since the calcium channel blockers impair impulse generation by the sinus node, they cause a sinus bradycardia (198,201). The reduction in blood pressure, commonly seen, is primarily due to a direct action of the drug on peripheral arterial resistance. These agents are also negatively inotropic, and in some patients with impaired left ventricular function, the decreased stroke volume and bradycardia may result in a significant reduction in cardiac output. Congestive heart failure may be precipitated, although often cardiac output is partially maintained and congestive heart failure prevented because of afterload reduction.

Side Effects

Side effects of the calcium channel blockers are primarily cardiovascular and include hypotension, bradycardia, atrioventricular nodal conduction abnormalities, and congestive heart failure (198,201). Constipation is common with verapamil. Headache, peripheral edema, nausea, lightheadedness, and dizziness may also occur.

Digoxin

Digoxin is the most frequently used drug for management of chronic AF and is administered primarily for control of the ventricular rate (202,203). Although it is often administered for acute termination of AF and its long-term prevention, it has no proven benefit for this indication. Although it has some direct effect on the atria and the atrioventricular node, the primary electrophysiologic actions of digoxin important for AF management are mediated by digoxin's vagotonic effects (204,205). Consequently, its major effects are on cardiac structures innervated by the vagus nerve, primarily the sinus and atrioventricular nodes (206). Digoxin, by enhancing vagal tone, slows the rate of sinus node discharge, slows impulse conduction through the atrioventricular node, and prolongs the atrioventricular nodal refractory period (193). Its major role in AF is to slow the ventricular rate.

Vagal innervation of the atrial myocardium is sparse and nonhomogeneous, affecting some, but not all, parts of the atrial myocardium (207,208). When vagal tone is increased, there is an increase in the velocity of impulse conduction through atrial tissue and a shortening of its refractory period. Since these changes occur only in the areas of atrial myocardium innervated by the vagus, an enhancement of vagal tone results in marked disparity of electrophysiologic properties of the atrial myocardium, an important precondition for the precipitation of AF (209). Digoxin may occasionally aggravate AF in susceptible patients (210).

Digoxin is a positive inotropic drug and improves left ventricular hemodynamics (211). It is a first-line drug for therapy of congestive heart failure, often the underlying abnormality responsible for precipitating AF. If the AF is a result of congestive heart failure, digoxin may produce reversion to sinus rhythm as a result of its beneficial effect on hemodynamics, left ventricular function, and left atrial pressure.

Pharmacology (Table 14)

Digoxin may be administered by the intravenous or oral route (212). Intramuscular digoxin, although occasionally used, is unreliably absorbed. When therapy is first initiated, a loading dose of digoxin may be necessary. If rapid digitalization is required, the usual loading dose is 1.5 mg administered over 24 hr. Alternatively, a dose of 0.5 to 1.0 mg can be administered for 2 to 3 days with a maintenance dose of 0.25 to 0.5 mg daily thereafter. In patients with AF, the dose is usually titrated to the effect on the ventricular response. Digoxin is cleared by the kidney in an unchanged form with a half-life of 36 hr. There are no important metabolites.

The only important role of digoxin in patients with AF is for ventricular rate control mediated by enhanced vagal tone at the atrioventricular node. However, the sympathetic nervous system also innervates the atrioventricular node and may interact with vagal activity, negating its action. Although digoxin is effective for reducing the heart rate response while the patient is at rest and catecholamine levels are low, the rate may become excessive when the sympathetic nervous system is activated, such as during exercise, and the depressive effect of the vagus negated. Therefore, many patients may require the combined use of digoxin with a beta blocker or calcium channel blocker to achieve optimal rate control during physical activity (213).

There are a number of drugs that interact with digoxin and can elevate its serum levels. These include quinidine, propafenone, flecainide, amiodarone, and verapamil.

Hemodynamics

Digoxin is a positive inotropic agent and is usually the first agent administered to patients with congestive heart failure (211). The drug increases left ventricular contractility, stroke volume, stroke work, and cardiac output. As a result, peripheral vascular resistance due to vasoconstriction, often abnormally increased in congestive heart failure, is reduced (214). Left ventricular end diastolic and left atrial pressures decrease during therapy with digoxin. Occasionally, rapidly administered intravenous digoxin may transiently increase peripheral vascular resistance and in rare cases may acutely exacerbate congestive heart failure.

TABLE 14. *Digoxin*

Dose	0.125–0.50 mg daily oral
Protein binding	20%–25%
Clearance	70% renal; unchanged
Half-life	36–48 hr
Blood levels	<2.0 ng/ml
Drug interactions	Quinidine, verapamil, amiodarone, antibiotics
Side effects	Cardiac, gastrointestinal, neurologic

Side Effects

The most frequent side effects from digoxin are those affecting the gastrointestinal system including nausea, vomiting, anorexia, and abdominal discomfort (215). Weakness, fatigue, irritability, and confusion may also be seen. Cardiac toxicity includes bradycardia, atrioventricular nodal blockade, intraventricular blockade, and atrial or ventricular arrhythmia (216).

REFERENCES

1. Vaughan Williams EM. Classification of antiarrhythmic drugs. In: Sandoe EM, Flensted-Jensen T, Olsen E, eds. *Symposium on cardiac arrhythmias.* Sodertalje, Sweden: AB Astra, 1970;449–472.
2. Hauswirth O, Singh BN. Ionic mechanisms in heart muscle in relation to the genesis and the pharmacologic control of cardiac arrhythmias. *Pharmacol Rev* 1979;39:5–63.
3. Hoffman BF, Rosen MR. Cellular mechanisms for cardiac arrhythmias. *Circ Res* 1981;49:1–15.
4. Rosen MR, Wit AL. Electropharmacology of antiarrhythmic drugs. *Am Heart J* 1983;106:829–859.
5. Gilmour RF, Heger JJ, Prystowsky EN, Zipes DP. Cellular electrophysiologic abnormalities of diseased human ventricular myocardium. *Am J Cardiol* 1983;51:137–144.
6. Mason JW, Winkle RA, Rider AK, Stenson EB, Harrison DC. The electrophysiologic effects of quinidine in the transplanted human heart. *J Clin Invest* 1977;59:481–489.
7. Moore EN, Spear JF. Effect of autonomic activity on pacemaker function and conduction. In: Wellens HJJ, Lie KI, Janse MJ, eds. *The conduction system of the heart. Structure, function and clinical implications.* The Hague: Martinus Nijhoff, 1978;100–110.
8. Josephson ME, Caracta AR, Lau SH, Gallagher JJ, Damato AN. Electrophysiological evaluation of disopyramide in man. *Am Heart J* 1973;86:771–780.
9. Josephson ME, Caracta AR, Ricciutti MA, Lau SH, Damato AN. Electrophysiologic properties of procainamide in man. *Am J Cardiol* 1974;33:596–603.
10. Josephson ME, Seides SF, Batsford WP, et al. The electrophysiological effects of intramuscular quinidine on the atrioventricular conducting system in man. *Am Heart J* 1974;87:55–64.
11. Harrison DC. Antiarrhythmic drug classification: New science and practical applications. *Am J Cardiol* 1985;56:185–190.
12. Hoffman BF, Rosen MR, Wit AL. Electrophysiology and pharmacology of cardiac arrhythmias. VII. cardiac effects of quinidine and procainamide. *Am Heart J* 1975;90:117–122.
13. McComish M, Kitson D, Robinson C, Jewitt DE. Clinical electrophysiologic effects of mexiletine. *Postgrad Med J* 1977;53(suppl 1):85–91.
14. Anderson JL, Mason JW, Winkle RA, et al. Clinical electrophysiologic effects of tocainide. *Circulation* 1978;57:685–691.
15. Hammill SC. Use of propafenone in patients with supraventricular tachycardia. *J Electrophysiol* 1987;1:561–567.
16. Anderson JL, Pritchett ELL, eds. International symposium on supraventricular arrhythmias: focus on flecainide. *Am J Cardiol* 1988;62:suppl D.
17. Naccarelli GV, Wellens HJJ, eds. A symposium: the use of encainide in supraventricular tachycardias. *Am J Cardiol* 1988;62:suppl C.
18. Wit AL, Hoffman BF, Rosen MR. Electrophysiology and pharmacology of cardiac arrhythmias. IX. Cardiac electrophysiologic effects of beta adrenergic receptor stimulation and blockade. Part A. *Am Heart J* 1975;90:521–533.
19. Wit AL, Hoffman BF, Rosen M. Electrophysiology and pharmacology of cardiac arrhythmias IX. Cardiac electrophysiologic effects of beta adrenergic receptor stimulation and blockade. Part B. *Am Heart J* 1975;90:665–675.
20. Wit AL, Hoffman BF, Rosen MR. Electrophysiology and pharmacology of cardiac arrhythmias. IX. Cardiac electrophysiologic effects of beta adrenergic receptor stimulation and blockade. Part C. *Am Heart J* 1975;90:797–805.
21. Lubbe WF, McFadyen ML, Muller CA, Worthington M, Opie LH. Protective action of amiodarone against ventricular fibrillation in the isolated perfused rat heart. *Am J Cardiol* 1979;43:533–540.
22. Zipes DP, Prystowsky EN, Heger JJ. Amiodarone: electrophysiologic actions, pharmacokinetics and clinical effects. *J Am Coll Cardiol* 1984;3:1059–1071.

23. Graboys TB, Podrid PJ, Lown B. The efficacy of amiodarone for refractory supraventricular tachyarrhythmias. *Am Heart J* 1983;106:870–876.
24. Rosen MR, Wit AL, Hoffman BF. Electrophysiology and pharmacology of cardiac arrhythmias. VI. Cardiac effects of verapamil. *Am Heart J* 1975;89:665–673.
25. Noma A, Irisawa H, Kokobun S, Kotake H, Nishimura M, Watanabe Y. Slow current systems in the AV node of the rabbit heart. *Nature* 1980;285:228–229.
26. Rosen MR, Wit AL, Hoffman BF. Electrophysiology and pharmacology of cardiac arrhythmias. IV. Cardiac antiarrhythmic and toxic effects of digitalis. *Am Heart J* 1975;89:391–399.
27. Weingart R, Kass RS, Tsien RW. Is digitalis inotropy associated with enhanced slow inward calcium current? *Nature* 1978;273:389–392.
28. Cranefield PF. Action potentials, afterpotentials and arrhythmias. *Circ Res* 1977;41:415–423.
29. Weld FM, Coromilas J, Rottman JN, Bigger JT. Mechanism of quinidine induced depression of maximum upstroke velocity in ovine cardiac Purkinje fibers. *Circ Res* 1982;50:369–376.
30. Hoffman BF. The action of quinidine and procainamide in single fiber of drug ventricle and specialized conducting system. *Ann Acad Bras Clin* 1958;29:365–368.
31. Watanabe Y, Dreifus LS. Interactions of quinidine and potassium in atrioventricular transmission. *Circ Res* 1967;20:434–446.
32. Schmid PG, Nelson LD, Mark AC, Heistad DD, Abboud FM. Inhibition of adrenergic vasoconstriction by quinidine. *J Pharmacol Exp Ther* 1974;188:124–129.
33. Swerdlow CD, Yu JO, Jacobson E, et al. Safety and efficacy of intravenous quinidine. *Am J Med* 1983;75:36–41.
34. Greenblatt DJ, Pfeifer HJ, Ochs HR, et al. Pharmacokinetics of quinidine in humans after intravenous, intramuscular and oral administration. *J Pharmacol Exp Ther* 1977;202:365–378.
35. Palmer KH, Martin B, Baggett B, Wall ME. The metabolic fate of orally administered quinidine gluconate in humans. *Biochem Pharmacol* 1969;18:1845–1860.
36. Morganroth J, Hunter H. Comparative efficacy and safety of short acting and sustained release quinidine in the treatment of patients with ventricular arrhythmia. *Am Heart J* 1985;110:1176–1181.
37. Conn HL, Luchi RJ. Some quantitative aspects of the binding of quinidine and related quinoline compounds by human serum albumin. *J Clin Invest* 1961;40:509–516.
38. Kessler KM, Lowenthal DT, Warner H, Gibson T, Briggs W, Reidenberg MM. Quinidine elimination in patients with congestive heart failure or poor renal function. *N Engl J Med* 1974;290:706–709.
39. Leahey EB, Reiffel JA, Giardina EGV, Bigger JT. The effects of quinidine and other oral antiarrhythmic drugs in serum digoxin. *Ann Intern Med* 1980;92:605–608.
40. Data JL, Wilkinson GR, Nies AS. Interaction of quinidine with anticonvulsant drugs. *N Engl J Med* 1976;294:699–702.
41. Koch-Weser J. Quinidine-induced hypoprothrombinemic hemorrhage in patients on chronic warfarin therapy. *Ann Intern Med* 1968;68:511–517.
42. Angelakos ET, Hastings EP. The influence of quinidine and procainamide on myocardial contractility in vivo. *Am J Cardiol* 1960;5:791–798.
43. Markiewicz W, Winkle R, Binitti G, Kernoff R, Harrison DC. Normal myocardial contractile state in the presence of quinidine. *Circulation* 1976;53:101–106.
44. O'Rourke RA, Horowitz LD. Effects of chronic oral quinidine on left ventricular performance. *Am Heart J* 1981;101:769–773.
45. Cohen IS, Jick H, Cohen SI. Adverse reactions to quinidine in hospitalized patients: findings based on data from the Boston Collaborative Drug Surveillance Program. *Prog Cardiovasc Dis* 1977;20:151–163.
46. Velebit V, Podrid PJ, Cohen B, Graboys TB, Lown B. Aggravation and provocation of ventricular arrhythmias by antiarrhythmic drugs. *Circulation* 1982;65:886–894.
47. Seltzer A, Wray HW. Quinidine syncope paroxysmal ventricular fibrillation occurring during treatment of chronic atrial arrhythmias. *Circulation* 1964;30:17–26.
48. Koster RW, Wellens HJJ. Quinidine induced ventricular flutter and fibrillation without digitalis therapy. *Am J Cardiol* 1976;38:519–523.
49. Roden DM, Woosley RL, Primm RK. Incidence of clinical features of the quinidine-associated long QT syndrome: Implications for patient care. *Am Heart J* 1986;111:1088–1093.
50. Bellet S, Hamden G, Somlyo A, Lara R. The reversal of cardiotoxic effects of quinidine by molar sodium lactate. An experimental study. *Am J Med Sci* 1959;237:165–176.
51. Tzivoni D, Keren A, Cohen AJ, et al. Magnesium therapy for torsades de pointes. *Am J Cardiol* 1984;53:528–530.
52. Kus T, Sasyniuk BI. Electrophysiologic actions of disopyramide phosphate on canine ventricular muscle and Purkinje fibers. *Circ Res* 1975;37:844–854.
53. Wilkinson PR, Desai J, Hollister J, Gonzalez R, Abbott JA, Scheinman MM. Electrophysiologic effects of disopyramide in patients with atrioventricular nodal dysfunction. *Circulation* 1982;66:1211–1216.

54. LaBarre A, Strauss HC, Scheinman MM, et al. Electrophysiologic effects of disopyramide phosphate on sinus node function in patients with sinus node dysfunction. *Circulation* 1979;59:226–235.
55. Birkhead JS, Vaughan Williams EM. Dual effect of disopyramide on atrial and atrioventricular conduction and refractory periods. *Br Heart J* 1977;39:657–660.
56. Siddoway LA, Barbey JT, Roden DM, Woosley RL. Pharmacologic evaluation of standard and controlled-release disopyramide. *Angiology* 1987;38:184–187.
57. Hinderling PH, Garrett ER. Pharmacokinetics of the antiarrhythmic disopyramide in healthy humans. *J Pharmacokinet Biopharm* 1976;4:199–230.
58. Haughey DB, Lima JJ. Influence of concentration dependent protein binding on serum concentrations and urinary excretion of disopyramide and its metabolite following oral administration. *Biopharm Drug Dispos* 1983;4:103–112.
59. Kapil RP, Axelson JE, Mansfield IL, et al. Disopyramide pharmacokinetics and metabolism: effect of inducers. *Br J Clin Pharmacol* 1987;24:781–791.
60. Burk M, Peters U. Disopyramide kinetics in renal impairment: determinants of interindividual variability. *Clin Pharmacol Ther* 1983;34:331–340.
61. Mathur PP. Cardiovascular effects of a newer antiarrhythmic agent, disopyramide phosphate. *Am Heart J* 1972;84:764–770.
62. DiBianco R, Gottdiener JS, Singh SN, Fletcher RD. A review of the effects of disopyramide phosphate on left ventricular function and the peripheral circulation. *Angiology* 1987;38:174–183.
63. Podrid PJ, Schoeneberger A, Lown B. Precipitation of congestive heart failure by oral disopyramide. *N Engl J Med* 1980;302:614–617.
64. Kowey PR, Friedman PL, Podrid PJ, et al. Use of radionuclide ventriculography for assessment of changes in myocardial performance induced by disopyramide phosphate. *Am Heart J* 1982;104:769–774.
65. Willis PW III. The clinical scope of disopyramide seven years after introduction. An overview. *Angiology* 1987;38:165–173.
66. Morady F, Scheinman MM, Desai J. Disopyramide. *Ann Intern Med* 1982;96:337–343.
67. Bauman JL, Gallastegui J, Strasberg B, et al. Long term therapy with disopyramide phosphate: side effects and effectiveness. *Am Heart J* 1986;111:654–660.
68. Teichman SL, Fisher JD, Matos JA, Kim SG. Disopyramide—pyridostigmine: report of a beneficial drug interaction. *J Cardiovasc Pharmacol* 1985;7:108–113.
69. Desai JM, Scheinman MM, Hirschfeld D, Gonzalez, R, Peters RW. Cardiovascular collapse associated with disopyramide therapy. *Chest* 1981;79:545–551.
70. Riccioni N, Castiglioni M, Bartolomei C. Disopyramide induced QT prolongation and ventricular tachyarrhythmias. *Am Heart J* 1983;105:870–871.
71. Tzivoni D, Keren A, Stern S, Gottleib S. Disopyramide-induced torsades de pointes. *Arch Intern Med* 1981;141:946–947.
72. Worske H, Belford J, Fastier FN, Brooks CMcC. The effect of procainamide on excitability, refractoriness and conduction in the mammalian heart. *J Pharmacol Exp Ther* 1953;107:134–140.
73. Shenasa M, Gilbert CJ, Schmidt DH, Akhtar M. Procainamide and retrograde atrioventricular nodal conduction in man. *Circulation* 1982;65:355–362.
74. Goldberg D, Reiffel JA, Davis JC, Gang E, Livelli F, Bigger JT Jr. Electrophysiologic effects of procainamide on sinus function in patients with and without sinus node disease. *Am Heart J* 1982;103:75–79.
75. Giardina EGV, Heissenbuttel RH, Bigger JT. Intermittent intravenous procainamide to treat ventricular arrhythmias: correlation of plasma concentration with effect on arrhythmia, electrocardiogram and blood pressure. *Ann Intern Med* 1973;78:183–193.
76. Greenspan AM, Horowitz LN, Spielman SR, Josephson ME. Large dose procainamide therapy for ventricular tachyarrhythmia. *Am J Cardiol* 1980;46:453–462.
77. Giardina EGV, Fenster PE, Bigger JT Jr, Mayersohn M, Perrier D, Marcus FI. Efficacy, plasma concentrations and adverse effects of a new sustained release procainamide preparation. *Am J Cardiol* 1980;46:855–862.
78. Giardina EGV, Dreyfuss J, Bigger JT, Shaw JM, Schreiber EC. Metabolism of procainamide in normal cardiac subjects. *Clin Pharmacol Ther* 1970;19:339–351.
79. Strong JM, Dutcher JS, Lee WK, Atkinson AJ. Pharmacokinetics in man of the N-acetylated metabolite of procainamide. *J Pharmacokinet Biopharm* 1975;3:223–235.
80. Woosley RL, Drayer DE, Reidenberg MM, Nies AS, Carr K, Oates JA. Effect of acetylator phenotype on the rate at which procainamide induces antinuclear antibodies and the lupus syndrome. *N Engl J Med* 1978;298:1157–1159.
81. Drayer DE, Lowenthal DT, Woosley RL, Nies AS, Schwartz A, Reidenberg MM. Cumulation of N-acetylprocainamide, an active metabolite of procainamide in patients with impaired renal function. *Clin Pharmacol Ther* 1977;22:63–69.

82. Lertora JJL, Gock D, Stec GP, Atkinson AJ Jr, Goldberg LI. Effects of N-acetylprocainamide and procainamide on myocardial contractile force, heart rate and blood pressure. *Proc Soc Exp Biol Med* 1979;161:332–336.

83. Paton WDM, Thompson JW. The ganglion blocking action of procainamide. *Br J Pharmacol* 1964;22:143–153.

84. McClendon RL, Hansen WR, Kinsman JM. Hemodynamic changes following procainamide administered intravenously. *Am J Med Sci* 1951;222:375–381.

85. Burton JR, Mathew MT, Armstrong PW. Comparative effects of lidocaine and procainamide on acutely impaired hemodynamics. *Am J Med* 1976;61:215–220.

86. Kayden HJ, Brodie BB, Steele JM. Procainamide: a review. *Circulation* 1957;15:118–126.

87. Bigger JT, Heissenbuttel RH. The use of procainamide and lidocaine in the treatment of cardiac arrhythmias. *Prog Cardiovasc Dis* 1969;11:515–534.

88. Lawson DH, Jick H. Adverse reactions to procainamide. *Br J Clin Pharmacol* 1977;4:507–511.

89. Strasberg B, Sclarovsky S, Erdberg A, et al. Procainamide-induced polymorphous ventricular tachycardia. *Am J Cardiol* 1981;47:1309–1314.

90. Kosowsky BD, Taylor J, Lown B, Ritchie RF. Long term use of procainamide following acute myocardial infarction. *Circulation* 1973;47B:1204–1210.

91. Sami M, Mason JW, Oh G, Harrison DC. Canine electrophysiology of encainide, a new antiarrhythmic drug. *Am J Cardiol* 1979;43:1149–1154.

92. Naccarelli GV, Wellens HJJ, eds. A symposium: the use of encainide in supraventricular tachycardias. *Am J Cardiol* 1988;62:suppl C.

93. Winkle RA, Peters F, Kates RE, Tucker C, Harrison DC. Clinical pharmacology and antiarrhythmic efficacy of encainide in patients with chronic ventricular arrhythmias. *Circulation* 1981;64:290–296.

94. Barbey JT, Thompson KA, Echt DS, Woosley RL, Roden DM. Antiarrhythmic activity, electrocardiographic effects and pharmacokinetics of the encainide metabolites 0-desmethyl encainide and 3-methoxy-0-desmethyl encainide in man. *Circulation* 1988;77:380–391.

95. Wang T, Roden DM, Wolfenden HT, Woosley RL, Wood AJ, Wilkinson GR. Influence of genetic polymorphism on the metabolism and disposition of encainide in man. *J Pharmacol Exp Ther* 1984;228:605–611.

96. Roden DM, Stots BR, Higgins JB, et al. Total suppression of ventricular arrhythmias by encainide. *N Engl J Med* 1980;302:877–882.

97. Quart BD, Gallo DG, Sami MH, Wood AJ. Drug interaction studies and encainide use in renal and hepatic impairment. *Am J Cardiol* 1986;58:104C–113C.

98. Bergstrand RH, Wang T, Roden DM, et al. Encainide disposition in patients with chronic cirrhosis. *Clin Pharmacol Ther* 1986;40:148–154.

99. Sami MH, Derbekyan VA, Lisbona R. Hemodynamic effects of encainide in patients with ventricular arrhythmia and poor ventricular function. *Am J Cardiol* 1983;52:507–511.

100. Gottlieb SS, Kukin ML, Yusak M, Medine N, Packer M. Adverse hemodynamic and clinical effects of encainide in severe chronic heart failure. *Ann Intern Med* 1989;110:505–509.

101. Ravid S, Podrid PJ, Lampert S, Lown B. Congestive heart failure induced by six of the newer antiarrhythmic drugs. *J Am Coll Cardiol* 1989;14:1326–1330.

102. Morganroth J, Pool PE, Miller R, Hsu PH, Lee IK, Clark DM. Dose response range of encainide for benign and potentially lethal ventricular arrhythmias. *Am J Cardiol* 1986;57:769–774.

103. Soyka LF. Safety of encainide for the treatment of ventricular arrythmias. *Am J Cardiol* 1986;58:96C–103C.

104. Tordjman T, Podrid PJ, Raeder E, Lown B. Safety and efficacy of encainide for malignant ventricular arrhythmias. *Am J Cardiol* 1986;58:87C–95C.

105. Horowitz LN. Encainide in lethal ventricular arrhythmias evaluated by electrophysiologic testing and decrease in symptoms. *Am J Cardiol* 1986;58:83C–86C.

106. Winkle RA, Mason JW, Griffin JC, Ross D. Malignant ventricular tachyarrhythmias associated with the use of encainide. *Am Heart J* 1981;102:857–864.

107. Hodess AB, Follansbee WP, Spear JF, Moore EM. Electrophysiologic effects of a new antiarrhythmic drug, flecainide, on the intact canine heart. *J Cardiovasc Pharmacol* 1979;1:427–439.

108. Anderson JL, Pritchett ELL, eds. International symposium on supraventricular arrhythmias: focus on flecainide. *Am J Cardiol* 1988;62:suppl D.

109. Anderson JL, Stewart JR, Perry BA, et al. Oral flecainide acetate for the treatment of ventricular arrhythmias. *N Engl J Med* 1981;305:473–477.

110. Hodges M, Haugland JM, Granrud G, Conard GJ, Asinger RW, Mikell FL. Suppression of ventricular ectopic depolarizations by flecainide acetate, a new antiarrhythmic agent. *Circulation* 1982;65:879–885.

111. Conard GJ, Ober RE. Metabolism of flecainide. *Am J Cardiol* 1984;53:41B–51B.

112. Josephson MA, Ikeda N, Singh BN. Effects of flecainide on ventricular function: clinical and experimental correlations. *Am J Cardiol* 1984;53:95B–100B.

113. Josephson MA, Kaul S, Hopkins J, Kvam D, Singh BN. Hemodynamic effects of intravenous flecainide relative to the level of ventricular function in patients with coronary artery disease. *Am Heart J* 1985;109:41–45.

114. Gentzkow GD, Sullivan JY. Extracardiac adverse effects of flecainide. *Am J Cardiol* 1984; 53:101B–105B.

115. Reid PR, Griffith LSC, Platia EV, Ord SE. Evaluation of flecainide acetate in management of patients at high risk of sudden cardiac death. *Am J Cardiol* 1984;53:108B–111B.

116. Flecainide Ventricular Tachycardia Study Group. Treatment of resistant ventricular tachycardia with flecainide acetate. *Am J Cardiol* 1986;57:129–130.

117. Falk RH. Flecainide induced ventricular tachycardia and fibrillation in patients treated for atrial fibrillation. *Ann Intern Med* 1989;111:107–111.

118. Kohlhardt M. Block of sodium currents by antiarrhythmic agents: analysis of the electrophysiologic effects of propafenone in heart muscle. *Am J Cardiol* 1984;54:13D–19D.

119. Connolly SJ, Kates RE, Lebsack CS, Echt DS, Mason JW, Winkle RA. Clinical efficacy and electrophysiology of oral propafenone for ventricular tachycardia. *Am J Cardiol* 1983;52:1208–1213.

120. Hammill SC. Use of propafenone in patients with supraventricular tachycardia. *J Electrophysiol* 1987;1:561–567.

121. Muller-Peltzer H, Greger G, Neugebauer G, Hollmann M. Beta-blocking and electrophysiological effects of propafenone in volunteers. *Eur J Clin Pharmacol* 1983;25:831–833.

122. McLeod AA, Stiles GL, Shand DG. Demonstration of beta adrenoceptor blockade by propafenone hydrochloride: clinical pharmacologic, radioligand binding and adenylate cyclase activation studies. *J Pharmacol Exp Ther* 1984;228:461–466.

123. Ledda F, Mantelli L, Manzini S, Amerini S, Mugelli A. Electrophysiological and antiarrhythmic properties of propafenone in isolated cardiac preparations. *J Cardiovasc Pharmacol* 1981; 3:1162–1173.

124. Smith NA, Kates RE, Harrison DC. The clinical pharmacology of propafenone. *J Electrophysiol* 1987;1:517–526.

125. Connolly SJ, Kates RE, Lebsack CS, Harrison DC, Winkle RA. Clinical pharmacology of propafenone. *Circulation* 1983;68:589–596.

126. Siddoway LA, Roden DM, Woosley RL. Clinical pharmacology of propafenone: Pharmacokinetics, metabolism and concentration-response relations. *Am J Cardiol* 1984;54:9D–12D.

127. Siddoway LA, Thompson KA, McAllister CB, et al. Polymorphism propafenone metabolism and disposition in man: clinical and pharmacokinetic consequences. *Circulation* 1987;75:785–791.

128. Stohler JL, Kowey PR, Marinchak RA, Friehling TD. Drug interactions with propafenone. *J Electrophysiol* 1987;1:568–574.

129. Baker BJ, Dinh H, Kroskey D, de Soyza NDB, Murphy ML, Franciosa JA. Effect of propafenone on left ventricular ejection fraction. *Am J Cardiol* 1984;54:20D–22D.

130. Brodsky MA, Allen BJ, Abate D, Henry WL. Propafenone therapy for ventricular tachycardia in the setting of congestive heart failure. *Am Heart J* 1985;110:794–799.

131. Ravid S, Podrid PJ, Novrit B. Safety of long term propafenone therapy for cardiac arrhythmia: experience with 774 patients. *J Electrophysiol* 1987;1:580–590.

132. Cueni L, Podrid PJ. Propafenone therapy in patients with serious ventricular arrhythmia. Noninvasive evaluation of efficacy. *J Electrophysiol* 1987;1:548–560.

133. Podrid PJ, Lampert S, Graboys TB, Blatt CM, Lown B. Aggravation of arrhythmia by antiarrhythmic drugs. Incidence and predictors. *Am J Cardiol* 1987;59:38E–44E.

134. Rosenshtraukh LV, Anyukhovsky EP, Nesterenko VV, et al. Electrophysiologic aspects of moricizine HCL. *Am J Cardiol* 1987;60:27F–34F.

135. Smetnev AS, Shugushev KK, Rosenshtraukh LV. Clinical, electrophysiologic and antiarrhythmic efficacy of moricizine HCl. *Am J Cardiol* 1987;60:40F–44F.

136. Morganroth J. Dose efficacy of moricizine on suppression of ventricular arrhythmias. *Am J Cardiol* 1990;65:26D–31D.

137. Woosley RL, Morganroth J, Fogoros RN, et al. Pharmacokinetics of moricizine HCl. *Am J Cardiol* 1987;60:35F–39F.

138. Kennedy HL, Wood AJJ, MacFarland RT. Drug interactions with ethmozine (moricizine HCl). *Am J Cardiol* 1987;60:79F–82F.

139. Pratt CM, Podrid PJ, Seals AA, et al. Effects of ethmozine (moricizine HCl) on ventricular function using echocardiographic, hemodynamic and radionuclide assessments. *Am J Cardiol* 1987;60:73F–78F.

140. Pratt C, Podrid PJ, Greatrix B, Borland MR, Mahler S. Efficacy and safety of moricizine in congestive heart failure: experience in the United States. *Am Heart J* 1989;119:1–7.

141. Singh SN, DiBianco R, Gottdiener JS, Ginsberg R, Fletcher RD. Effects of moricizine hydrochloride in reducing chronic high-frequency ventricular arrhythmia: results of a prospective, controlled trial. *Am J Cardiol* 1984;53:745–750.

142. Podrid PJ, Lyakishev A, Lown B, Mazur N. Ethmozine, a new antiarrhythmic drug for suppressing ventricular premature complexes. *Circulation* 1980;61:450–457.
143. Pratt CM, Young JB, Francis MJ, et al. Comparative efficacy of disopyramide and ethmozine in suppressing complex ventricular arrhythmias by use of a double blind placebo-controlled longitudinal crossover design. *Circulation* 1984;69:288–297.
144. Kennedy HL. Noncardiac adverse effects and organ toxicity of moricizine during short and long term studies. *Am J Cardiol* 1990;60:47D–50D.
145. Singh BN. Amiodarone: historical development and pharmacologic profile. *Am Heart J* 1983;106:788–797.
146. Singh BN, Nademanee K. Amiodarone and thyroid function: clinical implications during antiarrhythmic therapy. *Am Heart J* 1983;106:857–868.
147. Holt DW, Tucker GT, Jackson PR, Storey GCA. Amiodarone pharmacokinetics. *Am Heart J* 1983;106:840–846.
148. Andreasen F, Agerback H, Bjerregaard P, Gotzsche H. Pharmacokinetics of amiodarone after intravenous and oral administration. *Eur J Clin Pharmacol* 1981;19:293–299.
149. Adams PC, Holt DW, Storey CA, Morley AR, Callaghan J, Campbell WF. Amiodarone and its desethyl metabolite: tissue distribution and morphologic changes during long-term therapy. *Circulation* 1985;72:1064–1075.
150. Siddoway LA, McAllister CB, Wilkinson GR, Roden DM, Woosley RL. Amiodarone dosing: a proposal based on its pharmacokinetics. *Am Heart J* 1983;106:951–956.
151. Haffajee CI, Love JC, Canada AT, Lesko LJ, Adourian G, Alpert JS. Clinical pharmacokinetics and efficacy of amiodarone for refractory tachyarrhythmias. *Circulation* 1983;67:1347–1355.
152. Marcus FI. Drug interactions with amiodarone. *Am Heart J* 1983;106:924–929.
153. Kosinski EJ, Albin JB, Young E, Lewis SM, LeLand OS Jr. Hemodynamic effects of intravenous amiodarone. *J Am Coll Cardiol* 1984;4:565–570.
154. Fogoros RN, Anderson KP, Winkle RA, Swerdlow CD, Mason JW. Amiodarone: clinical efficacy and toxicity in 96 patients with recurrent drug refractory arrhythmias. *Circulation* 1983;63:88–94.
155. Raeder EA, Podrid PJ, Lown B. Side effects and complications of amiodarone therapy. *Am Heart J* 1985;109:975–983.
156. Harris L, McKenna WJ, Rowland E, Holt DW, Storey GCA, Krikler DM. Side effects of long-term amiodarone therapy. *Circulation* 1983;67:45–51.
157. Rakita L, Sobol SM, Mostow N, Vrobel T. Amiodarone pulmonary toxicity. *Am Heart J* 1983;106:906–914.
158. Adams PC, Gibson GJ, Morley AR, et al. Amiodarone pulmonary toxicity: clinical and subclinical features. *Q J Med* 1986;59:449–471.
159. Brorson L, Reele S, Dupont W, Woosley R, Shand D, Smith R. Effects of concentration and steric configuration of propranolol on AV conduction and ventricular repolarization in the dog. *J Cardiovasc Pharmacol* 1981;3:692–703.
160. Jaillon P, Weissenburger J, Heckle J, Cheymol G. Cardiac electrophysiologic effects of quinidine and propranolol isomers in anesthetized dogs: concentration-response relationships. *J Cardiovasc Pharmacol* 1981;3:431–445.
161. Szekely P, Jackson F, Wynne NA, Vohra JK, Batson GA, Dow WM. Clinical observations in the use of propranolol in disorder of cardiac rhythm. *Am J Cardiol* 1966;18:426–430.
162. Korte DW, Nash LB. The effect of the combination of quinidine and propranolol upon atrial and ventricular automaticity in dogs. *J Pharmacol Exp Ther* 1978;204:303–311.
163. Madan BR, Pendse VK. Interaction of quinidine and propranolol in experimental cardiac arrhythmias in the dog. *Arch Int Pharmacodyn Ther* 1977;225:287–293.
164. Lown B, Graboys TB. Management of patients with malignant arrhythmia. *Am J Cardiol* 1977;39:910–916.
165. Woosley RL, Kornhauser D, Smith R, et al. Suppression of chronic ventricular arrhythmias with propranolol. *Circulation* 1979;60:819–827.
166. Frishman W. Clinical pharmacology of the new beta-adrenergic blocking drugs. Part I. Pharmacodynamic and pharmacokinetic properties. *Am Heart J* 1979;97:663–670.
167. Prichard BNC, Owens CWI. Clinical pharmacology of beta-adrenoceptor blocking drugs. In: Kostis JB, De Felice EA, eds. *Beta blockers in the treatment of cardiovascular disease.* New York: Raven Press, 1984;1–56.
168. Woods PB, Robinson ML. An investigation of the comparative liposolubilities of beta-adrenoceptor blocking agents. *J Pharm Pharmacol* 1981;33:172–173.
169. Cruickshank JM. The clinical importance of cardioselectivity and lipophilicity in beta blockers. *Am Heart J* 1980;100:160–178.
170. Lertora JJL, Mark AL, Johanusen UJ, Wilson WR, Abboud FM. Selective beta-1 receptor blockade with oral practolol in man. *J Clin Invest* 1975;56:719–724.
171. Clark BJ. Pharmacologic properties of beta adrenoceptor blocking agents with special reference

to beta-1 selectivity and intrinsic sympathomimetic activity. *Br J Clin Pharmacol* 1982;13:1495–1585.

172. Singh BN. Clinical aspects of the antiarrhythmic action of beta-receptor blocking drugs. 2. Clinical pharmacology. *N Z Med J* 1973;78:529–535.
173. Woosley RL, Kornhauser D, Smith R, et al. Suppression of chronic ventricular arrhythmia with propranolol. *Circulation* 1979;60:819–827.
174. Leclerq JF, Rosengarten MD, Kurae S, Attuel P, Coumel P. Effects of intrinsic sympathetic activity of beta blockers on SA and AV nodes in man. *Eur J Cardiol* 1981;12:367–375.
175. Boudoulas H, Dervenagas S, Lewis RP, Kates RE, Dalamangas G. Time course of the blockade effect of propranolol on sinus node and atrioventricular node. *J Clin Pharmacol* 1979;19:95–99.
176. Rieckert H, Kattwinkel W, Riechelmann H, Kuss A, Sierau R. Peripheral haemodynamic effects of beta-adrenoceptor blocking drugs with ISA or relative beta 1-selectivity at rest and during physical exercise. *Br J Clin Pharmacol* 1982;13(suppl 12) 227S–228S.
177. Robinson BF, Wilson AO. Effect on forearm arteries and veins of attenuation of the cardiac response to leg exercise. *Clin Sci* 1968;35:143–152.
178. Man in't Veld AJ, Schalekamp MADH. Effects of 10 different beta-adrenoceptor antagonists on hemodynamics, plasma renin activity and plasma norepinephrine in hypertension: the key role of vascular resistance changes in relation to partial agonist activity. *J Cardiovasc Pharmacol* 1983;5:530–545.
179. Man in't Veld AJ, Schalekamp MADH. Hemodynamics of beta blockers. In: Kostes JB, De Felice EA, eds. *Beta blockers in the treatment of cardiovascular disease*. New York: Raven Press, 1984;229–251.
180. Frishman W, Silverman R, Strom J, Elkayam U, Sonnenblick E. Clinical pharmacology of the new beta-adrenergic blocking drugs. Part 4. Adverse effects. Choosing a beta-adrenoreceptor blocker. *Am Heart J* 1979;98:256–262.
181. Singh BN, Deedwania P, Nademanee K, Ward A, Sorkin EM. Sotalol: a review of its pharmacodynamic and pharmacokinetic properties, and therapeutic use. *Drugs* 1987;34:311–349.
182. Kato R, Yabe KS, Ikeda N, Kannan R, Singh BN. Electrophysiologic effects of the levo-4 isomers and dextrorotatory of sotalol in isolated cardiac muscle and their in vivo pharmacokinetics. *J Am Coll Cardiol* 1980;7:116–125.
183. Wang T, Bergstrand RH, Thompson KA, et al. Concentration-dependent pharmacologic properties of sotalol. *Am J Cardiol* 1986;57:1160–1165.
184. Touboul P, Atallah G, Kirkorian G, Lamaud M, Moleur P. Clinical electrophysiology of intravenous sotalol, a beta-blocking drug with class III antiarrhythmic properties. *Am Heart J* 1984;107:888–895.
185. Schnelle K, Klein G, Schinz A. Studies on the pharmacokinetics and pharmacodynamics of the beta-adrenergic blocking agent sotalol in normal man. *J Clin Pharmacol* 1979;19:516–522.
186. Sundquist K, Anttila M, Forsstrom J, Kasanen A. Serum levels and half-life of sotalol in chronic renal failure. *Ann Clin Res* 1975;7:442–446.
187. Singh BN, Nademanee K. Sotalol: a beta blocker with unique antiarrhythmic properties. *Am Heart J* 1987;114:121–139.
188. Cruickshank JM. The clinical importance of cardioselectivity and lipophilicity in beta blockers. *Am Heart J* 1980;100:160–178.
189. Hutton I, Lorimer AR, Hillis WS, McCall D, Reid JM, Lawrie TDV. Haemodynamics and myocardial function after sotalol. *Br Heart J* 1972;34:787–790.
190. Mahmarian JJ, Verani MS, Hohmann T, et al. The hemodynamic effects of sotalol and quinidine: analysis by use of rest and exercise gated radionuclide angiography. *Circulation* 1987;76:324–331.
191. Anderson JL, Askins JC, Gilbert EM, et al. Multicenter trial of sotalol for suppression of frequent, complex ventricular arrhythmias: a double-blind, randomized, placebo-controlled evaluation of two doses. *J Am Coll Cardiol* 1986;8:752–762.
192. Laakso M, Arvala I, Tervonen S, Sotarauta M. Retroperitoneal fibrosis associated with sotalol. *Br Med J* 1982;285:1085–1086.
193. Kuck KH, Kunze KP, Roewer N, Bleifeld W. Sotalol-induced torsades de pointes. *Am Heart J* 1984;107:179–180.
194. Gossinger HD, Siostrzonek P, Schmoliner R, Grimm G, Jager U, Mosslacher H. Sotalol-induced torsades de pointes in a patient with pre-existent normal response to programmed ventricular stimulation. *Eur Heart J* 1987;8:1351–1353.
195. Klein HO, Kaplinsky E. Digitalis and verapamil in atrial fibrillation and flutter. Is verapamil now the preferred agent? *Drugs* 1986;31:185–197.
196. Klein HO, Pauzner H, DiSegni E, David D, Kaplinsky E. The beneficial effects of verapamil in chronic atrial fibrillation. *Arch Intern Med* 1979;139:747–749.
197. Roth A, Harrison E, Mitani G, Cohen J, Rahimtoola SH, Elkayam U. Efficacy and safety of medium- and high-dose diltiazem alone and in combination with digoxin for the control of heart

rate at rest and during exercise in patients with chronic atrial fibrillation. *Circulation* 1986; 73:316–324.

198. Singh BN, Collett J, Chew CYC. New perspectives in the pharmacologic therapy of cardiac arrhythmias. *Prog Cardiovasc Dis* 1980;22:243–301.

199. Zipes DP, Fischer JC. Effects of agents which inhibit the slow channel on sinus node automaticity and atrioventricular conduction in the dog. *Circ Res* 1974;34:184–192.

200. Schamroth L. Immediate effects of intravenous verapamil on atrial fibrillation. *Cardiovasc Res* 1971;5:419–424.

201. Singh BN, Ellrodt G, Peter CT. Verapamil: a review of its pharmacological properties and therapeutic use. *Drugs* 1978;15:169–197.

202. Antman EM, Friedman PL. Use of digitalis glycosides in the management of cardiac arrhythmias. In: Smith TW, ed. *Digitalis glycosides*. Orlando: Grune and Stratton, 1985;127–138.

203. Simpson RJ, Foster JR, Woelfel AK, Gettes LS. Management of atrial fibrillation and flutter. A reappraisal of digitalis therapy. *Postgrad Med* 1986;79:241–253.

204. Gillis RA, Quest JA. The role of the nervous system in the cardiovascular effects of digitalis. *Pharmacol Rev* 1979;31:19–97.

205. Gaffney TE, Kahn JB Jr, VanMaanen EF, Acheson GH. A mechanism of the vagal effect of cardiac glycosides. *J Pharmacol Exp Ther* 1958;122:423–429.

206. Takahashi N, Zipes DP. Vagal modulation of adrenergic effects on canine sinus and atrioventricular nodes. *Am J Physiol* 1983;244:H775–H781.

207. Kassebaum DG. Electrophysiological effects of strophanthin in the heart. *J Pharmacol Exp Ther* 1963;140:329–338.

208. Zipes DP, Mihalick MJ, Robbins GT. Effects of selective vagal and stellate ganglion stimulation on atrial refractoriness. *Cardiovasc Res* 1974;8:647–655.

209. Leveque PE. Production of atrial fibrillation in dogs by thyroid administration and acetylcholine injection. *Circ Res* 1956;4:108–111.

210. Nahum LH, Hoff HE. Auricular fibrillation in hyperthyroid patients produced by acetyl-beta-methylcholine chloride, with observations on the role of the vagus and some exciting agents in the genesis of auricular fibrillation. *JAMA* 1935;105:254–257.

211. Braunwald E. Effects of digitalis on the normal and the failing heart. *J Am Coll Cardiol* 1985;5:51A–59A.

212. Antman EM, Smith TW. Pharmacokinetics of digitalis glycosides. In: Smith TW, ed. *Digitalis glycosides*. Orlando: Grune and Stratton, 1985;45–59.

213. Schwartz JB, Keefe D, Kates RE, Kirsten E, Harrison DC. Acute and chronic pharmacodynamic interaction of verapamil and digoxin in atrial fibrillation. *Circulation* 1982;65:1163–1170.

214. Mason DT, Braunwald E. Studies on digitalis. X. Effects of ouabain on forearm vascular resistance and venous tone in normal subjects and in patients in heart failure. *J Clin Invest* 1964;43:532–543.

215. Beller GA, Smith TW, Abelmann WH, Haber E, Hood WB Jr. Digitalis intoxication: a prospective clinical study with serum level correlations. *N Engl J Med* 1971;284:989–997.

216. Fisch C, Zipes DP, Noble RJ. Digitalis toxicity: mechanism and recognition. In: Yu PN, Goodwin JF, eds. *Progress in cardiology* vol 4. Philadelphia: Lea and Febiger, 1975;37–70.

*Atrial Fibrillation: Mechanisms
and Management*, edited by
R. H. Falk and P. J. Podrid.
Raven Press, Ltd., New York © 1992.

13

Pharmacologic Therapy for Reversion of Atrial Fibrillation and Maintenance of Sinus Rhythm

*Therese Fuchs and †Philip J. Podrid

*Cardiology Section, Boston City Hospital, Boston, Massachusetts 02118;
†Arrhythmia Service, University Hospital, Boston, Massachusetts 02118
and Boston University School of Medicine, Boston, Massachusetts 02118

Atrial fibrillation is a common sustained arrhythmia that frequently requires termination and/or prevention with antiarrhythmic therapy. However, arrhythmia occurrence is quite variable, it is difficult to prevent, and because of the high recurrence rate, atrial fibrillation presents a major challenge to the clinician (1,2). Although the usual indication for therapy is the treatment of symptoms, there are other reasons for therapy. Atrial fibrillation is associated with increased risk of stroke (3); it may precipitate congestive heart failure and it is associated, in some studies, with decreased survival (4,5). The prevalence of atrial fibrillation varies with the population studied but is estimated to occur in 2% to 4% of adults older than 60 years of age (4). Mechanisms vary and include atrial stretch, atrial disease, or altered autonomic tone, i.e., an increase in sympathetic or vagal inputs to the heart (7,8). This review discusses the pharmacologic management of paroxysmal and chronic atrial fibrillation.

CONVERSION OF ATRIAL FIBRILLATION TO SINUS RHYTHM

Atrial fibrillation of recent onset, which may be idiopathic or associated with a specific precipitating factor, commonly converts spontaneously to sinus rhythm or may easily convert with drug therapy. Chronic forms of atrial fibrillation, frequently due to underlying cardiac abnormalities, may convert to sinus rhythm with pharmacologic therapy but are often resistant, especially when the arrhythmia is of long duration. It has been reported that 80% to 90% of patients with chronic atrial fibrillation have sinus rhythm restored with electrocardioversion, although long-term maintenance usually requires antiarrhythmic therapy (9–12).

If feasible, an attempt should be made to restore normal sinus rhythm in most patients, especially if underlying heart disease is present or if the ventricular rate is difficult to control. However, maintenance of sinus rhythm after electric cardioversion may not be successful in patients who have been in atrial fibrillation for more than 1 to 2 years. The presence of an enlarged left atrium, often due to chronic mitral regurgitation or left heart failure, is a substrate for chronic atrial fibrillation, and restoration and maintenance of sinus rhythm are less likely. "Lone atrial fibrillation," which occurs in the absence of demonstrable heart disease, is often difficult to prevent and the maintenance of sinus rhythm may be impossible. Patients with atrial fibrillation in whom the ventricular response is slow, even without drug therapy to block the atrioventricular (AV) node, usually have associated disease of the AV- and His-Purkinje conduction system. In such patients, atrial fibrillation is probably the rhythm of choice since they may develop profound and symptomatic sinus bradycardia or prolonged periods of asystole after cardioversion. In patients who are intolerant of antiarrhythmic drugs for the maintenance of sinus rhythm, atrial fibrillation should also be accepted as the rhythm of choice (13). If the drug-resistant patient is symptomatic when in atrial fibrillation even at a slow rate or if ventricular rate control is impossible, nonpharmacologic therapy, although still investigational, is a consideration (14). However, for the vast majority of patients, pharmacologic therapy is the approach most often used initially for attempted reversion of atrial fibrillation and for the maintenance of sinus rhythm after successful cardioversion.

DIGITALIS

Digitalis is one of the oldest cardiac drugs in use and has been traditionally prescribed as the first pharmacologic intervention for the treatment of atrial fibrillation. Primarily as a result of its vagal effect, digitalis increases the refractory period of the AV node and increases the amount of concealed conduction within the node (15). As a result, it slows the rate of the ventricular response to atrial fibrillation (15,16). This is the best established use for this agent. Although the drug is sometimes given in an attempt to terminate atrial fibrillation, its use for this indication is less well established. Digitalis shortens the refractory period of the atrial myocardium and enhances conduction through this tissue, occasionally promoting the initiation and perpetuation of atrial fibrillation. The effect on atrial tissue may also increase the atrial fibrillation rate and, by augmenting the number of atrial impulses reaching the AV node, enhance concealed conduction and slow the ventricular response (16).

Although digitalis is one of the most widely used drugs for heart rate control in atrial fibrillation, there have not been large controlled trials investigating the value of this agent in terminating or preventing atrial fibrillation. Falk et al. (17), in a randomized, double-blind trial, studied 36 patients presenting with atrial fibrillation of 7 days or less duration. Patients were not on digitalis glycoside or antiarrhythmic agents and had no evidence for a reversible provoking factor such as heart failure. The patients were treated with encapsulated digoxin elixir or placebo, i.e., Lanoxicaps (0.2 mg is equivalent to 0.25 mg of oral digoxin tablets), in a dose of 0.6, 0.4, 0.2, and 0.2 mg administered at 0, 4, 8, and 14 hr, respectively. Therapy was continued until conversion to sinus rhythm occurred or the maximal dose was administered. Of 18 patients receiving digitalis, nine (50%) converted to sinus rhythm, while in nine, atrial fibrillation continued. In the group of patients receiving placebo, eight (44%) reverted to sinus rhythm, while 10 (56%) remained in atrial fibrillation. The authors concluded that digitalization was no more effective than placebo for the reversion of atrial fibrillation to sinus rhythm. In an observational study, Rawles et al. (18) evaluated the effect of digoxin on episodes of paroxysmal atrial fibrillation.

There were 139 episodes of atrial fibrillation identified from ambulatory monitor recordings in 72 patients. In 41 patients not receiving digoxin, there were 79 episodes of atrial fibrillation, and in 31 patients who were taking digoxin, there were 60 episodes (p = N.S.). More episodes lasting over 30 min (n = 13) occurred in patients taking digoxin compared to those not using this drug (n = 4; $p < 0.01$). The relative risk of having a prolonged episode of atrial fibrillation while receiving digitalis was 4.3. Importantly, there was no difference in the ventricular response rate at the onset of atrial fibrillation in those on digoxin (140 beats/min) compared to those not receiving this drug (134 beats/min; p = N.S.). The authors concluded that digoxin therapy was associated with longer paroxysms of atrial fibrillation and did not seem to reduce the frequency of the paroxysms or their ventricular rate.

In contrast, Weiner et al. (19) reported on 45 patients who had 47 episodes of acute atrial fibrillation. These patients underwent rapid intravenous digitalization. In 40 of the 47 episodes, reversion to sinus rhythm occurred within 1 to 96 hr after the initiation of digitalis therapy. In 32 patients, conversion occurred within 8 hr. The authors concluded that if reversion to sinus rhythm with digoxin does not occur by 16 to 24 hr, this drug will not be effective and additional measures to restore normal rhythm are indicated. However, this study contained no control group; some patients received additional antiarrhythmic drugs, and the relationship of restoration of sinus rhythm to digoxin use is unclear.

In conclusion, the data on conversion of recent onset atrial fibrillation to sinus rhythm with digitalis are limited but suggest that digitalis is not effective in converting acute episodes of atrial fibrillation to sinus rhythm. There are few data about the role of this drug administered chronically for preventing recurrent episodes. Most of the data are based on patients receiving digoxin after coronary artery bypass surgery for prophylaxis against atrial fibrillation and demonstrate conflicting results (20,21). These are reviewed in more detail in the chapter by Lauer and Eagle.

CLASS 1A ANTIARRHYTHMIC AGENTS

Quinidine

In the United States, quinidine is usually the first antiarrhythmic drug used for therapy of atrial fibrillation and is still the most frequently used agent (Fig. 1). There have been numerous studies reporting the efficacy of quinidine for maintaining sinus rhythm after electrocardioversion. Most of these studies involve patients with various heart diseases including valvular, hypertensive, ischemic, congenital, and idiopathic. Often, patients with thyroid disease are included. Hall and Wood (22) studied 84 patients with rheumatic heart disease. Fifty patients received quinidine after electroversion of atrial fibrillation and 34 patients were used as a control group. Quinidine did not appear to be effective for preventing recurrent arrhythmia, as approximately 45% of the patients in the two groups were still in sinus rhythm after 1 year. Radford and Evans (23) administered quinidine to 34 patients after conversion of atrial fibrillation to sinus rhythm, while 85 patients were without treatment. The follow-up was limited to only 1 month, at which time sinus rhythm was still present in 65% of the patients on quinidine and 52% of the patients not receiving therapy. In a study by Byrne-Quinn and Wing (11), in which follow-up ranged from 5 to 15 months, there was a significantly longer period of sinus rhythm in the quinidine-

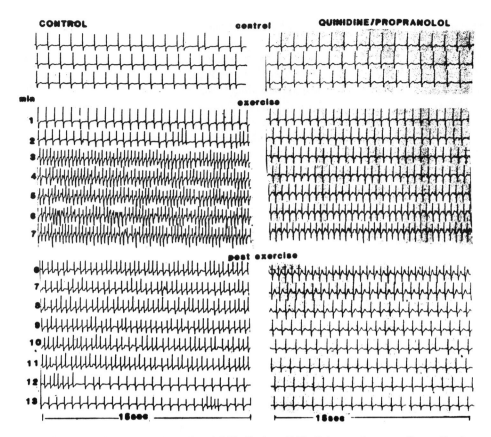

FIG. 1. Quinidine for prevention of atrial fibrillation (AF). Prior to therapy, the patient reproducibility had AF provoked by exercise. Beta blocker or quinidine used alone failed to prevent the arrhythmia. However, the combination of beta blocker and quinidine was effective.

treated group compared to the control group, and at 1 year, 60% of quinidine-treated patients were in sinus rhythm, while only 24% of the control group were still in sinus rhythm. Similar findings were reported by Sodermark et al. (24) in a study involving 176 patients. After 1 year of follow-up, 52% of the patients in the quinidine group remained in sinus rhythm compared to 30% in the placebo group ($p<0.001$). There were, however, five deaths in the quinidine group and two in the control group, although details of their deaths are not known. In a study by Hartel et al. (25) 175 patients were either randomized to therapy with quinidine after electrocardioversion or left untreated. Patients primarily had valvular disease, while a small number had either ischemic heart disease or lone atrial fibrillation. Of the 75 patients remaining on quinidine, 52 (69%) were still in sinus rhythm after 3 months, while only 30 of the 73 patients (41%) on no therapy were still in sinus rhythm.

Hillestad et al. (26) evaluated quinidine in 82 patients after electrocardioversion. As with other studies, the majority of these patients had rheumatic heart disease. Forty patients received quinidine and 42 were not treated. After 1 year, 40% of the patients on quinidine remained in sinus rhythm compared to 19% in the control group ($p<0.01$).

Boissel et al. (27) randomized 207 patients after electrocardioversion. Most patients had valvular disease or lone atrial fibrillation. The study was randomized but not blinded. After a follow-up of 3 months, 77 of the 103 patients receiving quinidine (75%) maintained sinus rhythm compared to only 58 of the 104 patients (56%) in the control group ($p<0.01$). However, in this study there were two deaths reported in the treatment group, while nine patients discontinued quinidine because of side effects (9%).

Long-acting quinidine preparations may be more effective than conventional quinidine sulfate for preventing a recurrence of atrial fibrillation (28), possibly due to the more sustained blood levels seen with the long-acting preparation. Sokolow et al. (29) observed that after a mean follow-up of 209 days, patients receiving daily maintenance doses of quinidine sulfate of 1.6 g or more had a 26% recurrence rate of atrial fibrillation compared to 45% recurrence in patients receiving less than 1.6 g of quinidine. This suggests that higher doses and blood levels of quinidine improve the efficacy of the drug and are helpful for preventing recurrences even if lower doses are ineffective.

A major concern in quinidine therapy is the potential for increased mortality. In a recent report by Coplan and co-workers (30), a meta-analysis of previous randomized, controlled trials of quinidine for prevention of atrial fibrillation was performed. In these studies, different quinidine preparations were used (bisulfate, sulfate, gluconate, and arabogalactone sulfate) and drug doses were variable. Included for analysis were six trials involving 808 patients. At 3, 6, and 12 months after cardioversion, sinus rhythm was maintained in 69%, 58%, and 50%, respectively. In the control group, the proportion of patients remaining in sinus rhythm at each interval was 45%, 35%, and 25%, respectively ($p<0.001$ at all intervals). The total mortality in the quinidine-treated patients was 2.9% compared to 0.8% in the control group, or an odds ratio of 2.98 ($p<0.05$). However, the cause of death was known in only seven of the 12 quinidine-treated patients and in only three was death sudden. It appears that quinidine is effective for preventing recurrent atrial fibrillation. It is unclear, however, if this therapy is associated with an increased mortality.

Disopyramide

Disopyramide is also a class 1A agent that is effective for reverting and preventing atrial fibrillation (Fig. 2), but because of its negative inotropic effects, its use is limited and most studies of disopyramide only include patients with intact left ventricular function. Indeed, it is possible that response to disopyramide is better in such patients.

Hartel et al. (31) compared disopyramide with placebo in a randomized, double-blind study involving 38 patients entered after successful electrocardioversion. Most patients had ischemic heart disease and were also being treated with a digitalis drug. After a 3-month follow-up, 72% of the patients receiving disopyramide remained in sinus rhythm compared to 30% of patients in the placebo group ($p<0.05$). Karlson et al. (32) studied 90 patients randomized to disopyramide or placebo after electrocardioversion. All patients also received treatment with digitalis, and unlike the previous study, most had lone atrial fibrillation and no structural heart disease. After 1 year of follow-up, sinus rhythm was maintained in 54% of the patients on disopyramide and 30% of the patients on placebo ($p<0.01$). Woo and Kong (33) randomized 31 patients following electrocardioversion to no treatment (10 patients), therapy with

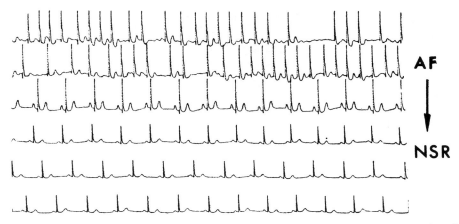

FIG. 2. Disopyramide for reversion of atrial fibrillation (AF). The patient was in AF for about 12 hr. Within 2 hr of receiving a single dose of disopyramide (300 mg), normal sinus rhythm (NSR) was restored.

disopyramide (11 patients), or to quinidine (10 patients). Atrial fibrillation recurred in eight, two, and three patients, respectively. The authors concluded that active drug treatment was effective for preventing recurrent atrial fibrillation in these patients and that quinidine and disopyramide were equally effective. In a study by Ito et al. (34) electrophysiologic studies were performed in 40 patients before and after intravenous administration of disopyramide. This study involved patients with both documented and "suspected" atrial fibrillation. After disopyramide, the induction of atrial fibrillation was completely prevented in 18 patients, whereas the ability to initiate the arrhythmia was enhanced during drug therapy in 22 patients. The authors suggested that disopyramide may alter the atrial electrophysiologic substrate in such a way as to eliminate the potential for atrial fibrillation in some patients, while in others, the drug may enhance the ability of the atrial myocardium to generate and sustain this arrhythmia. However, the definition of enhanced inducibility is questionable. Fujimura et al. (35) studied the effect of intravenous disopyramide in 54 patients with Wolff-Parkinson-White syndrome and associated atrial fibrillation. The drug was infused during an episode of sustained atrial fibrillation in 45 patients and during sinus rhythm in the remaining nine patients in whom the arrhythmia was self-terminating. Atrial fibrillation converted to sinus rhythm within 15 min after disopyramide in 37 (82%) of the 45 patients. In the remaining patients, the drug slowed the ventricular response to atrial fibrillation.

Procainamide

Procainamide is another class 1A antiarrhythmic agent. It has been used for prevention of atrial fibrillation, but long-term use is limited because of serious side effects, including a drug-induced lupus-like syndrome and, rarely, agranulocytosis. There are only a few controlled trials involving this drug. Aberg (36) evaluated 43 patients after electroversion to sinus rhythm. Twenty-three were treated with procainamide and 20 patients comprised the control group. After a 3-month follow-up, nine patients (39%) on procainamide and three patients (15%) from the control group maintained sinus rhythm. Szekely et al. (37) evaluated drug therapy for preventing atrial fibrillation after electrocardioversion in 258 patients with rheumatic heart disease. All patients were treated with digitalis, procainamide was administered to 166 patients, 73 received quinidine, while 19 were on no antiarrhythmic drug treatment. After 1 year of follow-up, 25% of the procainamide-treated patients, 23% of the quinidine-treated patients, and none of the control group patients remained in sinus rhythm. There was a significant difference in maintenance of sinus rhythm between the two treatment groups and the control group ($p < 0.05$) but no difference between quinidine and procainamide.

CLASS 1C AGENTS

Flecainide

Flecainide is a class 1C agent that has not yet been approved by the Food and Drug Administration for use in patients with supraventricular arrhythmias. There are, however, several studies in which flecainide was evaluated in patients with atrial fibrillation. Hellestrand (38) administered intravenous flecainide to patients with a variety of supraventricular arrhythmias. The dose was 2 mg/kg body weight and the rate of infusion was 10 mg/min. The drug was administered while the supraventricular arrhythmia was present. Flecainide successfully reverted atrial flutter in two of nine patients (22%) and atrial fibrillation in nine of 11 patients (82%). Suttorp et al. (39) compared intravenous flecainide to verapamil for the acute conversion of atrial fibrillation or atrial flutter to sinus rhythm. The study was a randomized, single-blind trial involving 40 patients. The intravenous dose of flecainide was 2 mg/kg administered over 10 min, and for verapamil it was 10 mg over 1 min. Treatment was considered successful if conversion occurred within 1 hr of beginning the infusion. Of 20 patients receiving flecainide, 14 of 17 (82%) with atrial fibrillation but none of three with flutter converted to sinus rhythm. All of the 20 patients treated with verapamil (17 with atrial fibrillation and three with atrial flutter) had a slower ventricular rate at 1 hr, but only one patient (6%) with atrial fibrillation converted to sinus rhythm as did one patient with atrial flutter. Fifteen of these patients initially receiving intravenous verapamil were subsequently treated with intravenous flecainide and nine reverted to sinus rhythm. Thus, overall, 23 of 32 patients with atrial fibrillation reverted with flecainide, while none of the seven with atrial flutter responded. Conversion to sinus rhythm was more likely to occur when the duration of atrial fibrillation was less than 24 hr (19 of 22 patients). When atrial fibrillation lasted longer than 24 hr, only four of 10 patients responded. The authors concluded that flecainide is effective for converting paroxysmal atrial fibrillation to sinus rhythm but is ineffective for atrial flutter.

Berns et al. (40) evaluated the efficacy of oral flecainide in 30 patients with atrial fibrillation (paroxysmal in 25 and chronic in five) and in nine patients with ectopic atrial tachycardia. During the follow-up period of 5.4 months, a complete response, defined as no recurrence of symptomatic atrial arrhythmia, was achieved in 22 patients (56%). A partial response, defined as greater than 95% reduction in the frequency of arrhythmia recurrence, was noted in three patients (8%) and there was no response in 14 (36%). The left atrial size, ejection fraction, underlying heart disease, duration of symptoms before treatment, and drug levels were not useful for predicting the clinical response. Goy et al. (41) studied the efficacy of flecainide for conversion of atrial fibrillation to sinus rhythm in 69 patients. The mean duration that arrhythmia was present prior to therapy was 49 ± 45 days. Flecainide at a dose of 2 mg/kg was initially administered intravenously over 10 min. Therefore, therapy with oral drug was continued with a dose of 200 to 300 mg/day. Conversion to sinus rhythm occurred in 49 patients (71%). The response rate was higher in patients who had atrial fibrillation of less than 10 days duration (79%) compared to patients with chronic atrial fibrillation in whom the conversion rate was 38% ($p<0.05$). Additionally, the left atrial diameter was smaller in patients who had successful conversion compared to those who did not respond (40 vs 46 mm; $p<0.05$). Anderson et al. (42) reported a multicenter, double-blind crossover study of flecainide and placebo in 64 patients with paroxysmal atrial fibrillation. Efficacy of drug was judged by relief of symptoms as well as by the use of intermittent transtelephonic monitoring. The dose of flecainide used was 200 to 400 mg/day and was based on the occurrence of side effects and patient tolerance. The patients entered into this study had failed an average of 3.8 previous drug trials. Only the data from 48 patients who met all protocol inclusions and completed the trial were analyzed. Paroxysmal atrial fibrillation was prevented in 15 patients (31%) during therapy with flecainide, while only four patients (9%) were free of arrhythmia during placebo therapy ($p=0.013$). The first attack of paroxysmal atrial fibrillation occurred after a median of 3 days on placebo compared to 14.5 days on flecainide ($p<0.001$). The time interval between attacks was also lengthened from a median of 6.2 days on placebo to 27 days on flecainide ($p<0.001$). In a comparative trial of the efficacy of flecainide or quinidine for conversion of atrial fibrillation to sinus rhythm in 60 patients, Borgeat et al. (43) administered either flecainide intravenously at a dose of 2 mg/kg followed by oral drug or quinidine administered orally up to 1.2 g/day. Atrial fibrillation was terminated in 18 of 30 patients (60%) treated with quinidine and 20 of 30 patients (67%) treated with flecainide. In patients with atrial fibrillation of less than 10 days duration, the conversion rate was 86% with flecainide and 80% with quinidine ($p=$N.S.). In patients with atrial fibrillation of more than 10 days duration, the conversion rate was 22% with flecainide and 40% with quinidine. The authors concluded that quinidine is more effective than flecainide in patients with chronic atrial fibrillation, while the drugs are equally effective for recent onset atrial fibrillation. Rasmussen et al. (44) followed 28 patients with atrial fibrillation who were treated with flecainide and 28 patients treated with disopyramide for 6 months after cardioversion. Of the patients receiving flecainide, sinus rhythm was maintained in 81% compared to a 44% response rate with disopyramide therapy. One patient on flecainide died suddenly during the study. In a review of the literature, Anderson and co-workers (45) summarized data on 577 patients with atrial fibrillation or atrial flutter. Intravenous flecainide was administered to 341 patients, and 211 (62%) had conversion to sinus rhythm. Oral therapy was administered to 225 patients of whom 137 (61%) were judged to have responded to the drug.

Flecainide has also been used in patients with atrial tachyarrhythmias associated with preexcitation syndrome. In a study by Kim et al. (46) 16 patients who had ventricular preexcitation complicated by atrial fibrillation or atrial flutter were treated with intravenous flecainide after having failed a mean of five drug trials. Intravenous flecainide prevented induction of atrial fibrillation in four of nine patients and eliminated anterograde conduction along the accessory pathway in nine of the 16 patients. In the five patients still inducible into atrial fibrillation, the shortest preexcited RR interval increased from 185 to 281 msec ($p<0.01$). Fourteen patients who had a favorable response to the intravenous drug were continued on oral flecainide. The drug was discontinued because of proarrhythmic effects in two patients and because of headaches in one patient. Eleven patients continued on the drug for a mean follow-up of 21 months. Seven patients were free of all recurrences and four patients had rare recurrences that were of briefer duration.

Encainide

The electrophysiologic properties and benefits of encainide are well established for the treatment of supraventricular tachycardias associated with AV nodal reentry and AV reentrant tachycardias using an accessory pathway (47). Little is known about its efficacy for atrial fibrillation as there are no long-term trials reported in patients with this arrhythmia and underlying structural heart disease. A relatively small but promising experience has been reported in patients with atrial fibrillation associated with Wolff-Parkinson-White syndrome. In a study of 30 patients, Naccarelli and co-workers (48) reported that oral or intravenous encainide blocked anterograde accessory pathway conduction in half of the patients and slowed the ventricular response rate by prolonging the anterograde refractory period in the other patients. Markel et al. (49) studied 16 patients with Wolff-Parkinson-White syndrome complicated by atrial fibrillation and found the efficacy of encainide for reversion and prevention of arrhythmia to be 88%. All patients had an increase in the shortest preexcited RR interval by more than 75 msec or had complete anterograde block in the accessory pathway. Similar results were found by Rinkenberger et al. (50) who reported on 36 patients with atrial fibrillation associated with Wolff-Parkinson-White syndrome. Only three patients also had structural heart disease. Nine patients had only atrial fibrillation, while 27 patients also had an AV reentrant tachycardia. The mean duration of symptomatic arrhythmia prior to encainide therapy was 195 months and an average of 2.7 drugs were previously ineffective. The dose of encainide was 175 mg/day. After a follow-up period of 30.1 ± 25 months, 24 patients (67%) continued to take encainide. Encainide was completely effective in 14 of these 24 patients and partially effective in another seven patients. Similar to the results with flecainide, encainide caused anterograde or retrograde block or decreased conduction velocity in the accessory pathway as well as prolongation of the AV nodal conduction time. In half of the patients, there was complete anterograde block in the accessory pathway. Unfortunately, there are no published data about the role of encainide for therapy of atrial fibrillation in patients without Wolff-Parkinson-White syndrome.

Propafenone

Propafenone is a recently available antiarrhythmic drug with class 1C actions as well as mild beta-blocking activity. Although most of the data about the drug are on patients with ventricular arrhythmia, there are several reports of its efficacy for atrial fibrillation. Bianconi et al. (51) studied the efficacy of intravenous propafenone at a dose of 2 mg/min in 83 patients with recent onset atrial fibrillation or atrial flutter. Conversion to sinus rhythm was achieved in 47 patients (57%), including 42 of 68 patients (62%) with atrial fibrillation and five of 15 (33%) of those with atrial flutter. Conversion occurred in 40 of 56 patients (71%) with arrhythmia of longer than 48 hr duration, but in only seven of 27 patients (26%) with arrhythmia of longer duration ($p<0.0005$). The left atrial size determined by echocardiography was larger in patients with drug failure. As with other drugs, the success rate was related to arrhythmia duration and left atrial size. In this study, propafenone was more effective for the conversion of atrial fibrillation compared to atrial flutter, an observation reported with other antiarrhythmic drugs. Propafenone did produce a low output state in three patients who were already hemodynamically compromised as a result of the atrial fibrillation. In contrast to this study, Vita et al. (52) reported on a different population of patients who had atrial fibrillation of longer duration (average 8.2 months) and a larger left atrial dimension (average 5.0 cm) and who were more resistant to therapy, as 65% had a history of previous drug failure. Intravenous propafenone was ineffective in all 24 patients and there was no conversion of atrial fibrillation to sinus rhythm during the short-term infusion. Antman et al. (53) studied the efficacy of long-term oral propafenone for preventing frequent paroxysmal episodes of symptomatic atrial fibrillation in 35 patients with drug refractory arrhythmia and for reverting chronic atrial fibrillation in 25 patients. The patients in this study had failed one to five prior drug trials (mean = 2), and the duration of arrhythmia prior to entry into the study was 30 months. The mean maximal total tolerated dose of propafenone was 795 mg/day. Propafenone was ineffective for converting chronic atrial fibrillation to sinus rhythm in all 25 patients. However, direct current (DC) cardioversion was successful in 21 of these patients (84%). All 60 patients were continued on long-term oral propafenone. After a 1-month follow-up, 54% of patients were free of recurrent atrial fibrillation, after 3 months 44% were without arrhythmia, and at 6 months 40% of patients were free of recurrent episodes of atrial fibrillation. Side effects from propafenone were reported in 22% of the patients, but the drug was discontinued in only 5% of the patients. In this study, there was no correlation between response to propafenone and duration of atrial fibrillation, left atrial size, number of previous drug trials, left ventricular ejection fraction, or nature of the underlying cardiac abnormality. In a review of the experience of propafenone for atrial arrhythmias, similar results have been reported by other investigators (54,55).

Coumel and co-workers (56) reported on 17 patients with structurally normal hearts and neurally provoked atrial fibrillation or flutter treated with propafenone. The drug was less effective than quinidine or amiodarone in the nine patients with arrhythmia that was provoked by enhanced vagal tone, while propafenone was more effective than beta-blockers or amiodarone in the eight patients with adrenergically mediated arrhythmia. In a study of patients experiencing atrial fibrillation after bypass surgery, Connolly and co-workers (57) administered intravenous propafenone (2 mg/kg over 10 min) to eight patients. This was a double-blind placebo study. One patient reverted with placebo, while three reverted to sinus rhythm with propafenone. The mean ventricular response rate was significantly reduced in the remaining patients.

CLASS 3 AGENTS

Amiodarone

Amiodarone is a class 3 agent that is approved in the United States only for use in patients with refractory ventricular arrhythmia. It is, however, also used in patients with atrial fibrillation, especially in those with arrhythmia refractory to other

TABLE 1. *Amiodarone for refractory atrial fibrillation*

Study	N	Effective (%)	Partially effective (%)[a]	Ineffective (%)
Rosenbaum	30	29(97)	1(3)	0
Ward	21	12(57)	5(24)	4(19)
Wheeler	13	7(54)	6(46)	0
Lubbe	11	4(36)	6(55)	1(9)
Rosenbaum	5	5(100)	0	0
Leak	2	0	0	2(100)
Graboys/Podrid	95	74(78)	6(6)	15(16)
Haffajee	77	54(70)	6(8)	17(22)
Peter	42	24(57)	15(38)	3(7)
Wellens[b]	17	13(76)	—	4(24)
Overall	313	222(71)	45(14)	46(15)

[a]Atrial fibrillation episodes less frequent or of shorter duration.
[b]All patients had Wolff-Parkinson-White syndrome.

drugs (Table 1), and in Europe, this agent is often the drug of choice for patients with atrial fibrillation (Fig. 3). Because of the numerous side effects of amiodarone, it is infrequently prescribed for atrial fibrillation in the United States. However, evidence suggests that some of the most serious side effects may be dose related and less commonly seen at doses prescribed for supraventricular arrhythmias. Vitolo and co-workers (58) examined the effect of amiodarone on the frequency of recurrence of atrial fibrillation after DC electrocardioversion. The authors randomized 28 patients to therapy with amiodarone and 26 patients to quinidine therapy. After a 6-month follow-up, 79% of the patients on amiodarone and 46% of the patients receiv-

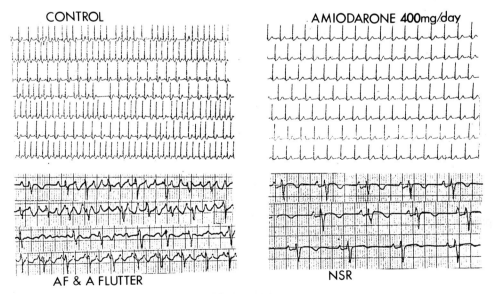

FIG. 3. Amiodarone for long-term prevention of atrial fibrillation (AF). The patient had a 4-year history of paroxysmal AF occurring several times per week. Previous antiarrhythmic therapy including quinidine, disopyramide, flecainide, and propafenone failed to prevent the arrhythmia. After 2 months of amiodarone therapy, AF was suppressed and did not recur during a 6-year follow-up. NSR, normal sinus rhythm.

ing quinidine remained in sinus rhythm ($p = 0.014$). Gold et al. (59) studied 68 patients with paroxysmal or chronic atrial fibrillation that was refractory to conventional antiarrhythmic agents. The patients were followed for 21 months. The maintenance doses of amiodarone after loading were 200 to 400 mg/day. Amiodarone therapy was effective for preventing recurrent atrial fibrillation in 54 of 68 patients (79%). Left atrial diameter, age, gender, and etiology of atrial fibrillation were not helpful in predicting success or failure of amiodarone therapy. However, as with other drugs, duration of atrial fibrillation was important. The presence of chronic atrial fibrillation for longer than 1 year was the only predictor of drug failure ($p = 0.007$), although the success rate in this group was still relatively high (57%). However, 35% of the patients had side effects that required discontinuation of the drug in 10%. Brodsky et al. (60) studied the efficacy of amiodarone for the maintenance of sinus rhythm after conversion of atrial fibrillation when a dilated left atrium was present. The study included 28 patients with a left atrial dimension greater than 45 mm. Thirteen patients (46%) had valvular heart disease, 10 (36%) dilated cardiomyopathy, and five (18%) miscellaneous disorders. Twenty-five patients (89%) had previously failed quinidine therapy. Amiodarone therapy was completely successful in 10 patients who continued in sinus rhythm after 1 year of follow-up, partially successful in 11 patients who maintained sinus rhythm for at least 6 months, but who had less frequent episodes thereafter, and the drug was ineffective in seven. Therapy was completely successful in nine of 18 patients with a left atrial dimension between 46 and 60 mm, but in only one of 10 patients with left atrial dimension greater than 60 mm. Although amiodarone was initially effective in patients with a left atrial size between 46 and 60 mm, the recurrence rate after a year was directly related to left atrial size. Similar efficacy data have been obtained by other investigators (61,62).

In one of the largest experiences, Graboys and co-workers (63) treated 95 patients with chronic or paroxysmal atrial fibrillation of long duration. These patients were resistant to an average of 3.2 previous drug trials. After a loading dose of 600 to 1,200 mg, most patients (54%) were maintained on 200 mg/day, while the remaining patients received 1,400 to 4,200 mg/week. Complete suppression of arrhythmia was achieved in 74 patients (78%). In this study, amiodarone did not revert the arrhythmia in patients with chronic atrial fibrillation but prevented recurrence after electrocardioversion. In six patients (6%), there was partial efficacy, defined as a reduction in the frequency or duration of paroxysmal episodes, while in 15 patients (16%), the drug was ineffective. These authors also summarized the reported literature up to that point. There were 82 patients with atrial fibrillation reported by several authors. Various dosing regimens were used, but overall, 57 patients (70%) were effectively controlled by the drug, 18 patients (22%) had a partial response, while the drug was ineffective in seven patients (8.5%).

Amiodarone may be particularly effective in patients with Wolff-Parkinson-White syndrome associated with atrial fibrillation (Fig. 4). Wellens et al. (64) evaluated 17 such patients with amiodarone therapy. After a 50-month follow-up (13–78 months), 13 patients (76%) were free of arrhythmia while four patients continued to have atrial fibrillation and required surgery. The dose of amiodarone effective in these 13 patients was 200 mg/day in six and 2,100 to 2,800 mg/week (average 300–400 mg/day) in seven. These authors also reported that the use of intravenous ajmaline or procainamide was a reliable method for predicting the effect of antiarrhythmic drugs, particularly amiodarone, on the anterograde effective refractory period of the accessory pathway and, hence, would predict efficacy of this agent. The loss of the delta

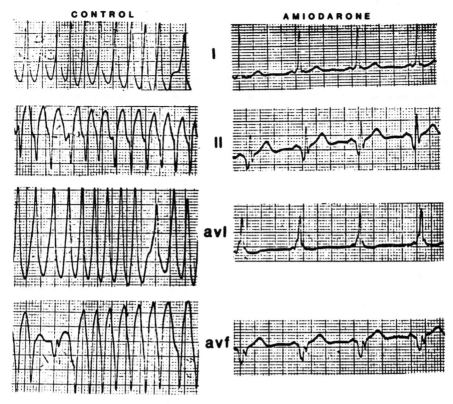

FIG. 4. Amiodarone for prevention of atrial fibrillation (AF) in a patient with Wolff-Parkinson-White syndrome. The patient presented with multiple episodes of AF and a rapid ventricular response associated with presyncope. The arrhythmia was easily induced with electrophysiologic testing. After 1 month of amiodarone therapy, AF could no longer be induced and the patient was clinically free of AF during an 8-year follow-up.

wave during infusion of these drugs, indicating complete blockade of anterograde conduction in the accessory pathway, correlated with an increase in the refractory period of greater than 100 msec, while the persistence of the delta wave was associated with no significant change. Amiodarone was more effective in patients who responded to ajmaline or procainamide.

Feld et al. (65) studied the clinical electrophysiologic effects of amiodarone in patients with atrial fibrillation associated with Wolff-Parkinson-White syndrome. The study included 10 patients with a history of spontaneous atrial fibrillation occurring with a rapid ventricular response. Seven patients underwent electrophysiologic studies before and during amiodarone therapy. After a mean follow-up of 30 months, there were no recurrences of atrial fibrillation, although one patient did have a recurrence of supraventricular tachycardia. Arrhythmia suppression was associated with a 38% prolongation of the anterograde refractory period of the accessory pathways and 34% prolongation of the atrial refractory periods. Amiodarone also slowed the ventricular rate of induced atrial fibrillation by an average of 50%.

Bepridil

Bepridil is a class 3 agent with calcium channel-blocking activity approved for treatment of angina in the United States. It has also been found to be effective for converting atrial fibrillation to sinus rhythm. A study by Perelman et al. (66) comparing bepridil with amiodarone included 14 patients with chronic atrial fibrillation present for at least 3 months who failed other conventional antiarrhythmic drug therapy. The ventricular response during atrial fibrillation was equally well controlled by bepridil and amiodarone at rest and during exercise. However, bepridil was more effective than amiodarone for converting atrial fibrillation to sinus rhythm (64% vs 40%). Bepridil was associated with the development of new ventricular arrhythmias in eight of 14 patients, including torsades de pointes in two patients. This is not unexpected since, like other agents that significantly prolong repolarization time, bepridil produces prolongation of the QT and corrected QT intervals, a finding associated with torsades. While prolongation of the QT interval occurs with other class 3 antiarrhythmic agents, particularly amiodarone, arrhythmia aggravation and torsades de pointes are rarely seen. This seems to be a problem with this class 3 agent, however. Because of its arrhythmogenic actions, bepridil is not recommended for the treatment of atrial fibrillation.

Sotalol

Sotalol is a class 3 antiarrhythmic agent currently under investigation in the United States, but clinically available in other countries. Trials evaluating the efficacy of this drug in patients with atrial fibrillation are limited. Campbell et al. (67) compared *d*-sotalol therapy to a combination of digoxin and disopyramide in a randomized study involving patients with acute atrial fibrillation occurring after open heart surgery. The authors reported that sotalol was as effective as the digoxin-disopyramide combination, but its onset of action was significantly faster in this patient population. A recent study by Sahar et al. (68) suggests a beneficial long-term effect of *d*-sotalol in a small group of patients. Jull-Moller and co-workers (69) reported a multicenter study comparing sotalol with quinidine for maintenance of sinus rhythm after electrocardioversion of atrial fibrillation. Ninety-eight patients were randomized to sotalol and 85 received quinidine. After 6 months, 52% of patients receiving sotalol and 48% receiving quinidine remained in sinus rhythm ($p = $N.S.). In the patients who relapsed to atrial fibrillation, the ventricular rate during atrial fibrillation was significantly slower in the sotalol-treated group (78 beats/min) compared to those on quinidine (109 beats/min; $p < 0.001$), and the sotalol-treated patients were less symptomatic at the time of arrhythmia recurrence. Side effects were less commonly reported by patients receiving sotalol (28% vs 50%; $p < 0.01$). One of the problems with sotalol therapy reported in studies involving patients with ventricular arrhythmia is QT prolongation and ventricular arrhythmia aggravation, particularly torsades de pointes. Thus, more clinical trials are needed to investigate the efficacy and potential toxicity of this drug in patients with atrial fibrillation.

BETA BLOCKERS

Only a small number of studies have evaluated the efficacy of beta blockers in preventing recurrence of atrial fibrillation. Szekely et al. (37) treated 23 patients with propranolol, and only three (13%) maintained sinus rhythm for 1 year as compared to a control group, in which there were no patients who maintained a normal rhythm ($p = $ N.S.). Tsolakas et al. (70) treated 18 patients after electrocardioversion for atrial fibrillation with propranolol. After 2 months, nine patients had a recurrence, one developed pulmonary edema, and four patients had to discontinue the medication because of abnormal liver enzymes. Only three patients maintained sinus rhythm and were free of side effects. Bath (71) reported that only four of 12 patients with atrial fibrillation had restoration of sinus rhythm as a result of propranolol therapy. More impressive is the low success rate reported by Gibson and Sowton (72). Of 334 patients with atrial fibrillation, only 20 reverted to sinus rhythm with beta blocker, while in 277, there was a significant reduction in ventricular response rate. It does not appear, therefore, that beta blockers are an effective therapy for reversion of atrial fibrillation or its prevention during long-term maintenance therapy. There are a few notable exceptions, including atrial fibrillation induced by an increase in sympathetic neural activity or elevated circulating catecholamines as may be seen during exercise. A few studies have suggested that they may have a beneficial role in the patient who has undergone coronary artery bypass surgery, another situation in which sympathetic activation may be important for the occurrence of atrial fibrillation. Stephenson and co-workers (73) administered low-dose propranolol several days after bypass surgery. Propranolol reduced the incidence of postoperative atrial fibrillation from 18% to 8% in controls. Limberg and co-workers (74) administered intravenous propranolol to 18 patients with atrial fibrillation after acute myocardial infarction. All patients were receiving digoxin. Sinus rhythm was restored in 14 patients, while the remaining four had significant rate slowing. Efficacy of the beta blocker may be difficult to establish since atrial fibrillation in such patients may be transient. In this regard, Jewett and Singh (75) reported that only five of 18 digitalized patients with atrial fibrillation had sinus rhythm restored by propranolol, although as expected, there was significant rate slowing. In a report by Allen and co-workers (76), beta blockers were ineffective for reverting atrial fibrillation and restoring sinus rhythm, although interestingly, these patients were not digitalized.

Although beta blockers have a limited role for reversion or prevention of atrial fibrillation when administered as monotherapy, they may be important when used in combination with the conventional class 1 antiarrhythmic drugs (Fig. 1) (77,78). Several studies have reported that beta blockers will potentiate the effects of class 1 (membrane active) agents. Class 1 antiarrhythmic drugs slow conduction, decrease membrane excitability, and reduce automaticity. In contrast, catecholamines produce opposite electrophysiologic effects, and there are growing data that catecholamines and sympathetic stimulation may reverse the beneficial effects of antiarrhythmic drugs (79,80) and that the beta blockers can prevent these catecholamine-mediated changes.

Additionally, beta blockers have an important role in controlling the ventricular rate during atrial fibrillation as a result of their effects on the AV node (Fig. 5). By interfering with sympathetic actions, they block impulse conduction through the node. This results in slowing of the ventricular response at rest, and, more importantly, during exercise.

CALCIUM BLOCKERS

Similar to the role of beta blockers, calcium channel blockers, especially verapamil, are very effective for slowing the ventricular response rate during atrial fibril-

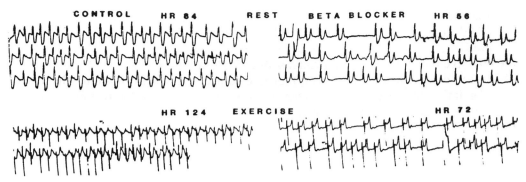

FIG. 5. Effect of beta blocker on the ventricular rate during atrial fibrillation. While receiving digoxin alone, the resting heart rate is 84 beats/min but accelerates to 124 beats/min after 2 min of exercise on a bicycle. With the addition of a beta blocker, heart rate is better controlled at rest and with exercise.

lation. When intravenous verapamil is administered, the most common response is inhibition of AV nodal conduction and slowing of the ventricular response (81). This effect is usually short-lived after the intravenous administration of drug and either a constant infusion or the use of oral drug is necessary for maintaining rate control. Also noted with verapamil is "regularization" of the ventricular rate (82) (Fig. 6). This may be particularly common at night when enhanced vagal tone working in concert with the effect of verapamil causes significant AV nodal blockade. The regularization may be due to complete AV block and an escape junctional rhythm or the result of a more uniform conduction through the AV node, causing apparent or "pseudoregularization." Regularization may be more common in patients receiving digoxin along with verapamil. It does not represent toxicity from either digoxin or

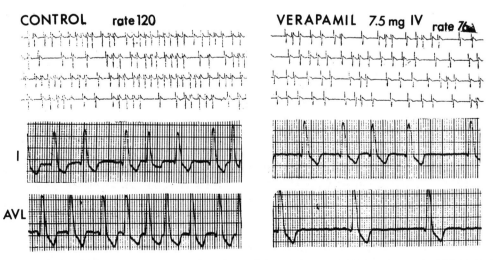

FIG. 6. Effect of verapamil on atrial fibrillation. Prior to therapy, the heart rate is 120 beats/min. After an intravenous bolus of verapamil, the heart rate slows to 76 beats/min. Evidence of "regularization" of the rhythm is seen in lead AVL.

verapamil, but rather a physiologic response to the drug and other factors that affect AV nodal conduction.

Although most of the data involve verapamil, diltiazem has also been reported to be effective for rate control of atrial fibrillation. Roth and co-workers (83) evaluated diltiazem (doses 240 and 360 mg/day) for rate control of atrial fibrillation. The lower dose of diltiazem was equivalent to digoxin alone for rate control at rest but superior with exercise, while the higher dose resulted in better rate control both at rest and with exercise. However, the frequency of side effects was significantly increased with the higher dose. Combined therapy with digoxin and low-dose diltiazem resulted in good control of heart rate at rest and with exercise. Although there are no comparative trials, diltiazem appears to be as effective as verapamil for rate control.

While the calcium channel blockers are generally useful for rate control of atrial fibrillation, one exception is the patient with Wolff-Parkinson-White syndrome. In this setting, the use of verapamil or digoxin may result in an acceleration of the ventricular rate and may provoke an episode of ventricular fibrillation (81,84). This is discussed in more detail elsewhere in this volume.

While verapamil and diltiazem are effective for rate control, their role for reverting or preventing atrial fibrillation is less well established. There are only a small number of studies that evaluate the efficacy of verapamil for converting patients with atrial fibrillation to sinus rhythm, and, therefore, data are limited. In an uncontrolled study, Tommaso et al. (85) administered intravenous verapamil to 17 patients with atrial fibrillation ($n=8$) or flutter ($n=9$), all of whom were receiving digoxin. Five patients converted to sinus rhythm (two with atrial flutter and three with atrial fibrillation). Twelve patients, seven with atrial flutter and five with atrial fibrillation, had a marked reduction of the ventricular rate after receiving intravenous verapamil, but the rhythm did not revert to sinus in these patients. The average heart rate decreased from 120 to 83 beats/min within 20 min. Three patients with atrial fibrillation of less than 1 month duration who did not convert with the intravenous preparation, converted within 24 hr of beginning oral medication. As with studies involving other antiarrhythmic drugs, the patients who converted to sinus rhythm had arrhythmia for a briefer period of time (median = 3 hr) and tended to have a smaller left atrial size (3.8 cm) compared to patients who did not convert to sinus rhythm. Haft et al. (86) studied the effectiveness of verapamil for atrial fibrillation when therapy was preceded by calcium infusion. Intravenous verapamil was used for 63 episodes of atrial fibrillation and flutter. Calcium chloride was given intravenously prior to verapamil in 41 episodes of atrial fibrillation or flutter. All the patients in this trial had a reduction in the ventricular response rate, but in no case did the arrhythmia revert to sinus rhythm. Patients treated with verapamil alone had a mean decrease in systolic pressure of 8 mmHg, while there was no change in blood pressure in the patients pretreated with calcium. The mean dose of verapamil required for rate control in these patients pretreated with calcium was lower than in the patients treated with verapamil alone. Basu and co-workers (87) reported that only one of 24 patients reverted to sinus rhythm with verapamil. However, after electrical reversion, sinus rhythm was maintained in 40% of patients receiving oral verapamil. There is no comparison group, however.

There are two studies in which oral verapamil has been compared to quinidine for maintaining sinus rhythm after electrocardioversion of atrial fibrillation. After reversion, Edhag et al. (88) randomized 29 patients to quinidine and 22 to therapy with oral verapamil. After 1 year, 46% of the patients receiving quinidine and 41% of the patients taking verapamil maintained sinus rhythm. In one patient, quinidine was discontinued because of side effects, while no side effects were reported in the group of patients on verapamil. In an open-label study, Rasmussen et al. (89) treated 41 patients with quinidine and 33 patients with verapamil. After 1 year, 24% of the patients on quinidine and 15% of the patients on verapamil remained in sinus rhythm, but this was not a statistically significant difference. Eleven patients receiving quinidine were withdrawn because of side effects and two patients died from unclear reasons. There were no withdrawals in the verapamil group. There are no studies that report the effect of diltiazem for maintenance of sinus rhythm, but it is likely that the results with this drug would be similar to those of verapamil.

Overall, there are few controlled data indicating that verapamil has any significant effect in converting atrial fibrillation to sinus rhythm, although it may improve left ventricular hemodynamics by decreasing the ventricular rate, thereby favoring spontaneous conversion.

CONCLUSION

Although DC cardioversion can restore normal sinus rhythm, at least transiently, in the majority of patients with atrial fibrillation, the recurrence rate is high when maintenance antiarrhythmic therapy is not administered. However, the long-term efficacy of antiarrhythmic drugs for preventing a recurrence of atrial fibrillation is far from ideal. It is difficult to interpret the results from different studies because the patient groups are heterogeneous and differ in regard to the nature of the underlying disease, left atrial size, and duration of atrial fibrillation before therapy is initiated. Quinidine has been reported in many studies to be effective for preventing recurrent atrial fibrillation. It is the most frequently prescribed antiarrhythmic agent for this arrhythmia, but unfortunately, quinidine frequently causes side effects and is often not well tolerated by patients. While the recent meta-analysis of several randomized, controlled trials with quinidine reported this agent to be more effective than no antiarrhythmic therapy for preventing recurrences of atrial fibrillation, it appeared to be associated with increased total mortality (2.9% in the quinidine-treated group vs 0.8% in the control group) (30). Although there are certain problems with this analysis, especially in regard to the etiology of the deaths, it does highlight the fact that, as with all antiarrhythmic drugs, quinidine should be used with caution. In patients without a clinical history of congestive heart failure, disopyramide is a good choice since it is probably as effective as quinidine but has fewer side effects.

Class 1C agents including encainide, flecainide, and propafenone are also very effective for maintaining sinus rhythm after electrocardioversion. However, these drugs have a high potential for aggravating arrhythmia in patients with serious ventricular arrhythmia who have poor left ventricular function and congestive heart failure. Although they have been safely administered to patients with atrial fibrillation, the recent report from the Cardiac Arrhythmia Suppression Trial (CAST) has raised a number of concerns about the use of these agents (90). The patients in CAST had a recent myocardial infarction complicated by VPBs, but no VT and no congestive heart failure. The mortality on encainide or flecainide was significantly higher than that observed in the placebo group. The reason for the increased incidence of sudden death was arrhythmia aggravation. While this study involved one specific group of patients, there is growing concern about the use of this class of antiarrhythmic drug in any patient with underlying heart disease, regardless of the nature of the arrhythmia disorder. These agents are therefore reserved for patients with atrial fibrillation who have a structurally normal heart, preserved left ventricular function, no congestive heart failure, and no evidence of ischemia. Amiodarone is the most effective drug for the prevention of recurrent atrial fibrillation, but because of concerns about its often serious side effects, it is generally used as a drug of last resort in the United States. When antiarrhythmic drugs fail to maintain sinus rhythm or are poorly tolerated, atrial fibrillation may be the accepted rhythm of choice. However, if the ventricular response in atrial fibrillation cannot be controlled or if the patient is symptomatic despite rate control, a nonpharmacologic approach is indicated. Because of the paucity of well-controlled trials, large, randomized clinical trials are needed to determine the efficacy, hazards, and comparative efficacy of the various antiarrhythmic drugs in patients with atrial fibrillation.

REFERENCES

1. Morris JJ, Peter RH, McIntosh HD. Electrical conversion of atrial fibrillation: immediate and long-term results and selection of patients. *Ann Intern Med* 1966;65:216–231.
2. Warris E, Kreus KE, Salokannel J. Factors influencing persistence of sinus rhythm after DC shock treatment of atrial fibrillation. *Acta Med Scand* 1971;189:161–166.
3. Wolf PA, Dawber TR, Thomas HE, Kannel WB. Epidemiologic assessment of chronic atrial fibrillation and risk of stroke: the Framingham study. *Neurology* 1978;28:973–977.
4. Kannel WB, Abbott RD, Savage DD, McNamara PM. Epidemiologic features of chronic atrial fibrillation: Framingham study. *N Engl J Med* 1982;306:1018–1022.
5. Kerr CR, Chung DC. Atrial fibrillation. Fact, controversy and future. *Clin Prog Electrophysiol Pacing* 1985;3:319–337.
6. Peterson P, Godtfredsen J. Atrial fibrillation: a review of course and prognosis. *Acta Med Scand* 1984;216:5–9.
7. Killip T, Gauet JH. Mode of onset of atrial fibrillation in man. *Am Heart J* 1965;70:172–179.
8. Bennett MA, Pentecost BL. The pattern of onset and spontaneous cessation of atrial fibrillation in man. *Circulation* 1970;41:981–88.
9. Lown B. Electrical reversion of cardiac arrhythmias. *Br Heart J* 1967;29:469–489.
10. Oram S, Davies JPH. Further experience of electrical conversion of atrial fibrillation to sinus rhythm: analysis of 100 patients. *Lancet* 1964;1:1294–1298.
11. Byrne-Quinn E, Wing AJ. Maintenance of sinus rhythm after DC reversion of atrial fibrillation. *Br Heart J* 1970;32:370–376.
12. Lown B, Perlroth MG, Kraidbey S, Abe T, Harken E. "Cardioversion" of atrial fibrillation. A report on the treatment of 65 episodes in 50 patients. *N Engl J Med* 1963;269:325–331.
13. Kowey PR, DeSilva RA, Lown B. Sustained atrial fibrillation as a rhythm of choice. *Circulation* 1979;59/60(suppl II):II-253.
14. Leitch JW, Guiraudon GM, Klein GJ, Yu R, Murdock CJ. The corridor operation for atrial fibrillation. Initial results and long-term followup. *Circulation* 1990;82(suppl III):III-472.
15. Cohen SI, Lau SH, Berkowitz WD, Damato AN. Concealed conduction during atrial fibrillation. *Am J Cardiol* 1970;25:416–419.
16. Meijler FF. An "account" of digitalis and atrial fibrillation. *J Am Coll Cardiol* 1985;5:60A–68A.
17. Falk RH, Knowlton AA, Bernard SA, Gotlieb NE, Battinelli NJ. Digoxin for converting recent-onset atrial fibrillation to sinus rhythm. A randomized, double-blinded trial. *Ann Intern Med* 1987;106:503–506.
18. Rawles JM, Metcalfe MJ, Jennings K. Time of occurrence, duration, and ventricular rate of paroxysmal atrial fibrillation: the effect of digoxin. *Br Heart J* 1990;63:225–227.
19. Weiner P, Bassan MM, Jarchovsky J, Iusim S, Plavnick L. Clinical course of acute atrial fibrillation treated with rapid digitalization. *Am Heart J* 1983;105:223–227.
20. Johnson LW, Dickstein RA, Freuhan CT. Prophylactic digitalization for coronary artery bypass surgery. *Circulation* 1976;53:819–822.
21. Tyras DH, Stothert JC, Kaiser GC. Supraventricular tachyarrhythmias after myocardial revascularization: a randomized trial of prophylactic digitalization. *J Thorac Cardiovasc Surg* 1979;77:310–314.
22. Hall JI, Wood DR. Factors affecting cardioversion of atrial arrhythmias with special reference to quinidine. *Br Heart J* 1968;30:84–90.

23. Radford MD, Evans DW. Long-term results of DC reversion of atrial fibrillation. *Br Heart J* 1968;30:81–83.
24. Sodermark T, Yansson B, Olson A, et al. Effect of quinidine on maintaining sinus rhythm after conversion of atrial fibrillation or flutter. A multicenter study from Stockholm. *Br Heart J* 1975;37:486–492.
25. Hartel G, Louhija A, Konttinern A, Halomen PI. Value of quinidine in maintenance of sinus rhythm after electric conversion of atrial fibrillation. *Br Heart J* 1970;32:57–60.
26. Hillestad L, Bjerkelund C, Dale J, Maltau J, Storstein O. Quinidine in maintenance of sinus rhythm after electroversion of chronic atrial fibrillation. A controlled clinical study. *Br Heart J* 1971;33:518–521.
27. Boissel JP, Wolf E, Gillet J, et al. Controlled trial of a long-acting quinidine for maintenance of sinus rhythm after conversion of sustained atrial fibrillation. *Eur Heart J* 1981;2:49–55.
28. Normand JP, Legendre M, Kahn JC, Bourdarias JP, Mathivat A. Comparative efficacy of short-acting and long-term quinidine for maintenance of sinus rhythm after electrical conversion of atrial fibrillation. *Br Heart J* 1976;38:381–387.
29. Sokolow M, Ball RE. Factors influencing conversion of chronic atrial fibrillation with special reference to serum quinidine concentration. *Circulation* 1956;14:568–583.
30. Coplan SE, Antman EM, Berlin JA, Hewitt P, Chalmers TC. Efficacy and safety of quinidine therapy for maintenance of sinus rhythm after cardioversion. A meta analysis of randomized control trials. *Circulation* 1990;82:1106–1116.
31. Hartel G, Louhija A, Konttinen A. Disopyramide in the prevention of recurrence of atrial fibrillation after electroversion. *Clin Pharmacol Ther* 1974;15:551–555.
32. Karlson BW, Torstensson I, Abjorn C, Yansson GO, Peterson LE. Disopyramide in the maintenance of sinus rhythm after electroversion of atrial fibrillation—a placebo controlled one year followup study. *Eur Heart J* 1988;9:284–290.
33. Woo KS, Kong SM. Disopyramide and quinidine in maintenance of sinus rhythm after electroversion—a controlled study. *Hong Kong Cardiol Soc* 1979;6:137.
34. Ito M, Omodera S, Hashimoto J, et al. Effect of disopyramide on initiation of atrial fibrillation and relation to effective refractory period. *Am J Cardiol* 1989;63:561–566.
35. Fujimura O, Klein GJ, Sharma AD, Yee R, Szabo T. Acute effect of disopyramide on atrial fibrillation in the Wolff-Parkinson-White syndrome. *J Am Coll Cardiol* 1989;13:113–117.
36. Aberg H. Prokainamid som profylax mot formaksflimmer, En kontrollerad studie. *Nord Med* 1969;82:1011.
37. Szekely P, Sideris DA, Batson GA. Maintenance of sinus rhythm after atrial fibrillation. *Br Heart J* 1970;32:741–746.
38. Hellestrand KJ. Intravenous flecainide acetate for supraventricular tachycardias. *Am J Cardiol* 1988;62:16D–22D.
39. Suttorp MJ, Kingma JH, Lie AHL, Mast EG. Intravenous flecainide versus verapamil for acute conversion of paroxysmal atrial fibrillation or flutter to sinus rhythm. *Am J Cardiol* 1989;63:693–696.
40. Berns E, Rinkenberger RL, Yeang MK, Dougherty AH, Yenkins M, Naccarelli GV. Efficacy and safety of flecainide acetate for atrial tachycardia or fibrillation. *Am J Cardiol* 1987;59:1337–1341.
41. Goy JJ, Kaufmann V, Kappenberger L, Sigwart V. Restoration of sinus rhythm with flecainide in patients with atrial fibrillation. *Am J Cardiol* 1988;62:38D–40D.
42. Anderson JL, Gilbert EM, Alpert BL, et al. Prevention of symptomatic recurrences of paroxysmal atrial fibrillation in patients initially tolerating antiarrhythmic therapy. A multicenter double-blind, crossover study of flecainide and placebo with transtelephonic monitoring. Flecainide Supraventricular Tachycardia Study Group. *Circulation* 1989;80:1557–1570.
43. Borgeat A, Goy JJ, Maendly R, Kaufman V, Grbic M, Sigwart W. Flecainide versus quinidine for conversion of atrial fibrillation to sinus rhythm. *Am J Cardiol* 1986;58:496–498.
44. Rasmussen K, Anderson A, Abrahamsen AM, Overskeid K, Bathen J. Flecainide versus disopyramide in maintaining sinus rhythm following conversion of chronic atrial fibrillation. *Eur Heart J* 1989;9(suppl 1):52 (abstract).
45. Anderson JL, Jolivette DM, Fredell PA. Summary of efficacy and safety of flecainide for supraventricular arrhythmias. *Am J Cardiol* 1988;62:62D–66D.
46. Kim SS, Smith P, Ruffy R. Treatment of atrial tachyarrhythmia and preexcitation syndrome with flecainide acetate. *Am J Cardiol* 1988;62:29D–34D.
47. Kunze KP, Kuck KH, Schluter M, Kuch B, Bleifeld W. Electrophysiologic and clinical effects of intravenous and oral encainide in accessory atrioventricular pathway. *Am J Cardiol* 1984;54:323–329.
48. Naccarelli GV, Rinkenberger RL, Dougherty AH, Giebel RA. Use of encainide in treating atrial fibrillation in the Wolff-Parkinson-White syndrome. *Circulation* 1984;70(suppl II):II-445 (abstract).
49. Markel ML, Prystowsky EN, Heger JJ, Miles WM, Fineberg N, Zipes DP. Encainide for treat-

ment of supraventricular tachycardia associated with the Wolff-Parkinson-White syndrome. *Am J Cardiol* 1986;58:41C–48C.

50. Rinkenberger RL, Naccarelli GV, Miles WH, et al. Encainide for atrial fibrillation associated with Wolff-Parkinson-White syndrome. *Am J Cardiol* 1988;62:26L–30L.
51. Bianconi L, Boccadame R, Pappabardo A, Gentili C, Pistolese M. Effectiveness of intravenous propafenone for cardioversion of atrial fibrillation and flutter of recent onset. *Am J Cardiol* 1989;64:335–338.
52. Vita J, Friedman PC, Cautillon C, Antman EM. Efficacy of intravenous propafenone for acute management of atrial fibrillation. *Am J Cardiol* 1989;63:1275–1278.
53. Antman EM, Beamer AD, Cautillon C, McGowan N, Goldman L, Friedman PL. Long-term oral propafenone therapy for suppression of refractory symptomatic atrial fibrillation and atrial flutter. *J Am Coll Cardiol* 1988;12:1005–1011.
54. Hammil SC. Use of propafenone in patients with supraventricular tachycardia. *J Electrophysiol* 1987;1:561–567.
55. Kerr CR, Mason MA, Chung DC. Propafenone: an effective drug for prevention of recurrent atrial fibrillation. *Circulation* 1985;72(suppl III):III-1 (abstract).
56. Coumel P, Leclerq JF, Assayag P. European experience with the antiarrhythmic efficacy of propafenone for supraventricular and ventricular arrhythmias. *Am J Cardiol* 1984;60D–64D.
57. Connolly JJ, Mulji AJ, Rogers DA. The effect of intravenous propafenone on rapid atrial fibrillation. *Circulation* 1985;72(suppl III):III-253 (abstract).
58. Vitolo E, Tronci M, Larovere MT, Rumolo R, Morabito A. Amiodarone versus quinidine in the prophylaxis of atrial fibrillation. *Acta Cardiol* 1981;36:431–444.
59. Gold RL, Haffajee CL, Charos G, Solan K, Baker S, Alpert JS. Amiodarone for refractory atrial fibrillation. *Am J Cardiol* 1986;57:124–127.
60. Brodsky MA, Allen BJ, Walker CJ III, Casey TP, Lucket CT, Henry WL. Amiodarone for maintenance of sinus rhythm after conversion of atrial fibrillation in the setting of a dilated left atrium. *Am J Cardiol* 1987;60:572–575.
61. Blevins RD, Kerin NZ, Benaderet D, et al. Amiodarone in the management of refractory atrial fibrillation. *Arch Intern Med* 1987;147:1401–1404.
62. Horowitz LN, Spielman SR, Greenspan AM, et al. Use of amiodarone in the treatment of persistent and paroxysmal atrial fibrillation resistant to quinidine therapy. *J Am Coll Cardiol* 1985;6:1402–1407.
63. Graboys TB, Podrid PJ, Lown B. Efficacy of amiodarone for refractory supraventricular tachyarrhythmias. *Am Heart J* 1983;106:870–876.
64. Wellens HJJ, Brugada P, Abdollah H. Effect of amiodarone in paroxysmal supraventricular tachycardia with or without Wolff-Parkinson-White syndrome. *Am Heart J* 1983;106:876–880.
65. Feld GK, Nademance K, Stevenson W, Weiss J, Kliznen T, Singh BN. Clinical and electrophysiologic effects of amiodarone in patients with atrial fibrillation complicating the Wolff-Parkinson-White syndrome. *Am Heart J* 1988;115:102–107.
66. Perelman MS, McKenna WJ, Rowland E, Krikler DM. A comparison of bepridil with amiodarone in the treatment of established atrial fibrillation. *Br Heart J* 1987;58:339–344.
67. Campbell TJ, Gavaghan TP, Morgan JJ. Intravenous sotalol for the treatment of atrial fibrillation and flutter after cardiopulmonary bypass comparison with disopyramide and digoxin in a randomized trial. *Br Heart J* 1985;54:86–90.
68. Sahar DI, Raffel JA, Bigger JT Jr, Squatrito A, Kidwell GA. Efficacy, safety and tolerance of d-sotalol in patients with refractory supraventricular tachyarrhythmias. *Am Heart J* 1989;117:562–568.
69. Jull-Moller S, Edvardsson N, Rehnqvist-Ahlberg N. Sotalol versus quinidine for the maintenance of sinus rhythm after direct current conversion of atrial fibrillation. *Circulation* 1990;82:1932–1939.
70. Tsolakas TC, Davies JPH, Oram S. Propranolol in attempted maintenance of sinus rhythm after electrical defibrillation. *Lancet* 1964;2:1064.
71. Bath JCJL. Treatment of cardiac arrhythmias in unanesthetized patients. Role of adrenergic beta receptor blockade. *Am J Cardiol* 1966;18:415–425.
72. Gibson D, Sowton E. The use of beta adrenergic receptor blocking drugs in dysrhythmias. *Prog Cardiovasc Dis* 1964;12:16–39.
73. Stephenson LW, MacVaugn H, Tomasello DN, Josephson ME. Propranolol for prevention of postoperative cardiac arrhythmias: a randomized study. *Ann Thorac Surg* 1980;29:113–116.
74. Limberg L, Castellanos A, Arcebal A. The use of propranolol in arrhythmias complicating acute myocardial infarction. *Am Heart J* 1970;80:479–487.
75. Jewett DE, Singh BN. Role of beta adrenergic blockade in myocardial infarction. *Prog Cardiovasc Dis* 1974;16:421–438.
76. Allen JD, Pantridge JF, Shanks DG. The effects of practotol on the dysrhythmias complicating acute ischemic heart disease. *Am J Med* 1975;58:199–208.

77. Podrid PJ, Vendetti F, Levine P, Klein M. Role of drug combinations for the treatment of arrhythmias. *Pract Cardiol* 1988;14:35–54.
78. Fors WJ, Vanderark CR, Reynolds LW. Evaluation of propranolol and quinidine in the treatment of quinidine resistant arrhythmias. *Am J Cardiol* 1971;27:190–194.
79. Brugada P, Facchine M, Wellens HJJ. Effects of isoproterenol and amiodarone and the role of exercise in initiation of circus movement tachycardia in the accessory atrioventricular pathway. *Am J Cardiol* 1986;57:146–149.
80. Niazi I, Naccarelli G, Dougherty A, Rinkenberger R, Tchou P, Akhtar M. Treatment of atrioventricular nodal reentrant tachycardia with encainide: reversal of drug effect with isoproterenol. *Am J Coll Cardiol* 1989;13:904–910.
81. Singh BN, Nademanee K, Baky J. Calcium antagonists: clinical uses in treating arrhythmias. *Drugs* 1983;25:125–153.
82. Schamroth LD, Krikler DM, Garrett C. Immediate effects of intravenous verapamil in cardiac arrhythmias. *Br Heart J* 1972;1:660–664.
83. Roth A, Harrison E, Mitani G, Cohen J, Rahimtoola SH, Elkayam U. Efficacy and safety of medium and high dose diltiazem alone and in combination with digoxin for control of heart rate at rest and during exercise in patients with chronic atrial fibrillation. *Circulation* 1986;73:316–324.
84. Sellers TD, Bashore TM, Gallagher JJ. Digitalis in the pre-excitation syndrome: analysis during atrial fibrillation. *Circulation* 1977;56:260–266.
85. Tommaso C, McDonough T, Parker M, Talano JV. Atrial fibrillation and flutter. Immediate control and conversion with intravenously administered verapamil. *Arch Intern Med* 1983;143:877–881.
86. Haft JI, Habbab MA. Treatment of atrial arrhythmias. Effectiveness of verapamil when preceded by calcium infusion. *Arch Intern Med* 1986;146:1085–1089.
87. Basu B, Cherian G, Abraham KA. Oral verapamil as maintenance therapy after cardioversion for atrial fibrillation. *Inn J Chest Dis Allud Sci* 1977;19:170–176.
88. Edhag O, Erhardt LR, Lundman T, Sodermark T, Sjogren A. Verapamil and quinidine in maintaining sinus rhythm after electroconversion of atrial fibrillation. *Opascula Med* 1982;27:22.
89. Rasmussen K, Wang H, Fausa D. Comparative efficacy of quinidine and verapamil in the maintenance of sinus rhythm after DC conversion of atrial fibrillation. A controlled clinical trial. *Acta Med Scand* 1981(suppl 645):23–28.
90. Cardiac Arrhythmia Suppression Trial (CAST) Investigators. Preliminary report: effect of encainide and flecainide on mortality in a randomized trial of arrhythmia suppression after myocardial infarction. *N Engl J Med* 1989;321:406–412.

Atrial Fibrillation: Mechanisms and Management, edited by
R. H. Falk and P. J. Podrid.
Raven Press, Ltd., New York © 1992.

14

Control of the Ventricular Rate in Atrial Fibrillation

Rodney H. Falk

*Division of Cardiology, Boston City Hospital, Boston, Massachusetts 02118
and Boston University School of Medicine, Boston, Massachusetts 02118*

Since William Withering's observations more than two centuries ago on the salutary effects of the leaf of the purple foxglove (digitalis purpurea) (1), digoxin has been the mainstay for slowing the ventricular rate in patients with atrial fibrillation. In the early part of the 20th century Mackenzie (2) noted that atropine reversed the effects of digitalis in atrial fibrillation and suggested that the effects of the glycoside were mediated by the vagus nerve. Further support for this concept was garnered by Blumgart (3) in 1924, who noted that the control of the resting heart rate by digoxin could be overcome by exercise (Fig. 1). The concept that a controlled resting ventricular rate in atrial fibrillation is no guarantee of control during daily activities or vigorous exertion is now well accepted (4), but the assessment of adequacy of rate control and the determination of who and how to treat are less well established. This chapter will review the assessment of adequate ventricular rate control in atrial fibrillation, starting with a brief overview of basic aspects, and concentrating on the clinical management.

DETERMINANTS OF VENTRICULAR RATE IN ATRIAL FIBRILLATION

The atrioventricular (AV) node is generally considered to be the primary structure determining the heart rate response to atrial fibrillation. The classical theory of AV nodal conduction in atrial fibrillation suggests that the node acts as a "filter" protecting the ventricles from extremely rapid rates. For the purpose of this chapter, this theory will be accepted, since most published studies base their conclusions on this concept. However, it should be pointed out that Meijler and Fisch (5) have recently presented elegant arguments against the classical concept of AV nodal conduction and suggested that the AV node does not conduct but rather acts as an electrotonically modulated autonomous pacemaker. These arguments and alternative theories are described in detail in the contribution by Meijler and Wittkampf elsewhere in this volume.

The ventricular response to atrial fibrillation is dependent on several factors including the refractory period of the AV node, the amount of concealed conduction within the node, and the relative degree of sympathetic and vagal tone and/or en-

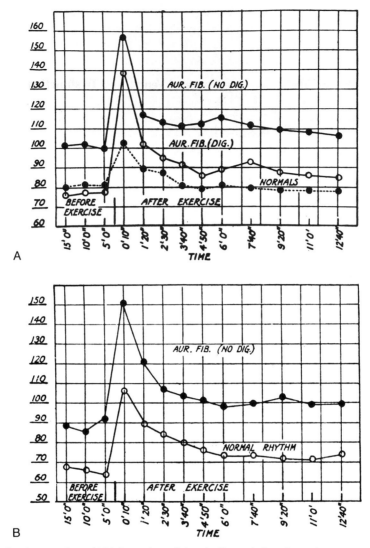

FIG. 1. Early observations (1924) on the minimal effect of digoxin on heart rate control during exercise (repeatedly stepping on a chair). **A:** Comparison of six normal subjects in sinus rhythm with nine patients with atrial fibrillation (AUR. FIB.) receiving digitalis (DIG.) or on no therapy (NO DIG.). Digoxin controls resting rate, but peak heart rate exceeds that of subjects in sinus rhythm by 40 beats per minute. **B:** Heart rate with exercise in five undigitalized patients before (AUR. FIB., NO DIG.) and after (normal rhythm) conversion to sinus rhythm to show that it is the arrhythmia and not the underlying heart disease that produces the disproportionate tachycardia. (From ref. 3.)

dogenous catecholamines. In addition to the loss of atrial contribution to ventricular filling that occurs with atrial fibrillation, an uncontrolled ventricular response results in a decreased diastolic filling time and an increased myocardial oxygen demand either or both of which may have serious clinical consequences. Decreased diastolic filling time may cause significant elevation of left atrial pressure, particularly in subjects with restriction to ventricular filling such as those with mitral stenosis or hypertrophic cardiomyopathy (6), and in patients with coronary artery disease the combination of a shortened diastole and increased oxygen demand may precipitate myocardial ischemia (Fig. 2).

Atrial Fibrillation as a Cause of Ventricular Dysfunction

Although incessant atrial tachycardia is the most commonly reported cause of tachycardia-induced left ventricular dysfunction, occasional cases of atrial fibrillation with poorly controlled ventricular rate have been described in which reversion to sinus rhythm is associated with improvement in ejection fraction. Peters and Kiezle (7) reported the case of a 56-year-old man with a 10-year history of chronic atrial fibrillation and congestive heart failure. The resting ventricular response was 150 beats per minute rising to 200 beats per minute with exercise. He was electrically converted to sinus rhythm and maintained on amiodarone therapy, and over a 6-month period the ejection fraction rose from 18% to 54% with resolution of all symptoms.

Subtle improvement in ventricular function may also occur after cardioversion of atrial fibrillation in patients with relatively well-controlled heart rates, whose ejection fraction during atrial fibrillation was only minimally impaired. Left ventricular fractional shortening increased significantly immediately after cardioversion ($23 \pm 8\%$–$29 \pm 8\%$) and increased further by 7 days (8). A similar improvement over a period of 1 week was noted by other investigators (9). However, these findings may be more related to restoration of atrial systole than to improved rate control, as heart rates prior to conversion were less than 100 beats per minute.

Strong support for the concept that ventricular rate control alone may improve ventricular function in poorly controlled atrial fibrillation comes from data on catheter ablation of the AV junction. As discussed in the chapter by Rosenqvist and Scheinman, evaluation of serial ventricular function for a large group of patients undergoing ablation apparently showed no effects (10). However, four of five patients with an ejection fraction less than 35% who underwent ablation for poorly controlled atrial fibrillation had a rise in the mean ejection fraction from 25% to 45% after a median follow-up of 28 months, suggesting that clinical improvement may occur in the more severely affected patients.

What Is the Expected Resting Heart Rate in Uncomplicated Atrial Fibrillation?

Patients with untreated atrial fibrillation may present with a wide range of ventricular responses to the arrhythmia, although the usual mean ventricular rate in the resting untreated patient is between 100 and 160 beats per minute. Ventricular rates slower than 90 beats per minute suggest intrinsic AV nodal disease (although high vagal tone may occasionally be responsible), whereas more rapid rates may indicate a high catecholamine state such as thyrotoxicosis, fever, dehydration, acute blood loss, or congestive heart failure.

Most studies of atrial fibrillation include patients with acute conditions that may elevate the ventricular response, and thus data on "pure" ventricular rates in atrial fibrillation are rare. After excluding patients with medical conditions likely to accelerate the ventricular response, we found a mean ventricular rate of 120 beats per minute (range 95–170) in 36 patients with atrial fibrillation of less than 7 days dura-

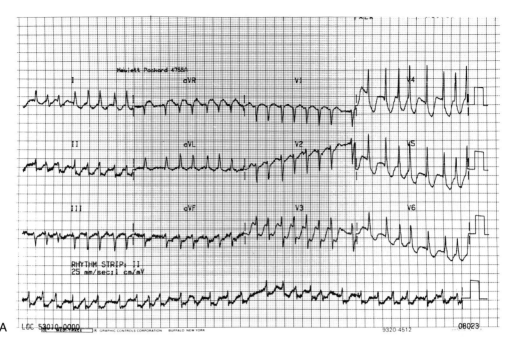

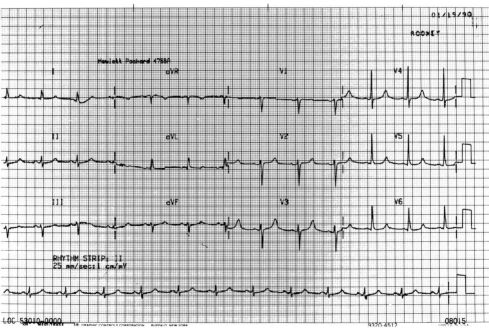

FIG. 2. Effects of atrial fibrillation with uncontrolled ventricular response in a middle-aged woman with nonexertional angina. **A:** Presentation to emergency room with atrial fibrillation and angina. There is extensive ST segment depression due to myocardial ischemia. **B:** After spontaneous conversion to sinus rhythm, the chest pain resolved and the ST segments rapidly returned to baseline.

tion (11). In a controlled trial of the effect of digoxin on ventricular rate, Beasley et al. (12) reported a mean heart rate of 108 beats per minute (range 82–170) in 12 men with nonvalvular heart disease who were receiving placebo therapy. Similar ventricular responses to induced atrial fibrillation have been found at electrophysiology study of patients with normal AV nodal conduction (13).

The above studies in noninduced atrial fibrillation describe the ventricular rate in patients presenting with atrial fibrillation but are unable to examine the heart rate at the onset of the arrhythmia. In a study of Holter monitor recordings from patients with paroxysmal atrial fibrillation, Rawles et al. (14) noted a mean ventricular response of 134 ± 22 beats per minute in subjects receiving no digoxin. Kawakubo and co-workers (15) reported similar findings from 14 apparently healthy subjects with paroxysmal atrial fibrillation receiving no therapy. The mean ventricular rate at the onset of 18 episodes of arrhythmia lasting 5 min or more was 124 ± 20 beats per minute. Two distinct trends were seen in relation to arrhythmia course. In seven paroxysms, with a mean rate at onset of 107 ± 18 beats per minute, the heart rate remained stable throughout the arrhythmia, which terminated within 2 hr in all cases (mean rate at termination 106 ± 19 beats per minute). The heart rate in the remaining 11 paroxysms gradually fell from onset (133 ± 14 beats per minute) to termination (86 ± 9 beats per minute) and in all but one episode, the atrial fibrillation lasted more than 2 hr. The authors concluded that the onset of arrhythmia may produce or be produced by an increased sympathetic tone, which is commonly subject to modulating influences in longer paroxysms.

The atrial rate of the fibrillating atrium is in the region of 400 to 600 beats per minute and thus the relatively slow ventricular response in untreated patients suggests that the AV node is an efficient filter. In atrial flutter, the atrial rate is 280 to 320 beats per minute and the ventricular response is commonly half this rate, i.e., 140 to 160 beats per minute. The observation that the mean ventricular response in patients with atrial fibrillation is less than 150 beats per minute despite a higher atrial rate than flutter suggests a role for concealed conduction in the AV node—a hypothesis supported by the observation that the ventricular rate often decreases when atrial flutter converts to fibrillation (16). In an attempt to study the relative contribution of concealed conduction and AV nodal refractoriness on the ventricular response to atrial fibrillation, Toivonen and co-workers (13) measured standard electrophysiologic parameters in 52 patients undergoing electrophysiologic testing during sinus rhythm. Concealed AV nodal conduction was assessed by two separate atrial extrastimulus techniques (17,18), following which atrial fibrillation was induced by rapid atrial pacing. The effective and functional refractory periods of the AV node and the shortest atrial pacing cycle length correlated most strongly with the mean ventricular rate during induced fibrillation, whereas indices of concealed conduction did not improve the prediction of heart rate. The same relationship held after isoproterenol or propranolol infusion. Fujiki et al. (19) reported similar findings with regard to factors influencing the mean ventricular rate. In addition, a strong correlation was noted between the coefficient of variation of the ventricular response and the concealment index, suggesting that concealed conduction is responsible, in large part, for the irregularity of the ventricular rate.

Neither of these authors measured atrial rates during induced atrial fibrillation. Allessie et al. (20) have demonstrated that, as atrial fibrillation terminates, it is associated with a decrease in the number of wavelets within the atrium. This is manifest in the intra-atrial electrogram as a coarsening of the fibrillatory waves (21) and is associated on the surface ECG with an increase in ventricular response (22). We have noted that, prior to conversion of atrial fibrillation to sinus rhythm, there is frequently an acceleration in ventricular rate (23) (Fig. 3). This is unlikely to be caused by changes in the AV nodal refractory period and is best explained by organization of atrial activity, resulting in a fall in the number of impulses reaching the AV with a consequent decrease in the degree of concealed conduction. In a parallel observation Meijler (24) has shown that the decrease in ventricular response to atrial fibrillation following digoxin therapy cannot be fully explained by increases in the refractory period of the AV node, although he dismisses the theory of concealed conduction as an explanation for the decreased rate.

The suggestion that AV nodal refractory period correlates more strongly with the ventricular response during atrial fibrillation than do measures of concealed conduction is not necessarily at odds with our observation of preconversion rate acceleration. The studies quoted above do not quantify atrial rate, and extrapolation of indices of concealment derived during sinus rhythm to events during atrial fibrillation may not be fully valid. It is also possible that, for a group, indices of AV nodal refractoriness may correlate well with ventricular response, whereas changes in degree of concealment may predominate at an individual level and account for a proportion of the observed swings in heart rate seen throughout the day.

Although the effect on heart rate of sudden changes in autonomic tone is well known during atrial fibrillation, little has been written about the effects of circadian variation. Using a sophisticated statistical analysis of 24-hr Holter monitors from 63 patients with atrial fibrillation, Raeder (25) showed that the heart rate manifests a circadian variation with a peak at about 11:30 A.M. and a nadir at 2:40 A.M. This

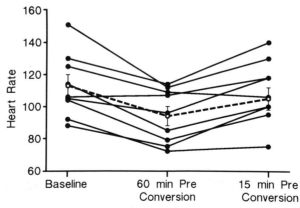

FIG. 3. Ventricular response to atrial fibrillation in nine patients spontaneously converting to sinus rhythm after receiving a loading dose of digoxin. All patients were in atrial fibrillation ≥ 5 hr. There is a slowing of the ventricular rate from baseline (predigoxin) to 1 hr prior to conversion ($p < 0.005$) due to the effect of the drug. The mean ventricular rate then significantly accelerates again ($p < 0.005$) 15 min prior to conversion to a heart rate that is not statistically significantly different from baseline (109 ± 6 vs 113 ± 7). This is attributed to the organization of atrial activity resulting in a decreased degree of anterograde concealed conduction. *Solid lines* are individual patients; *broken line* is mean for the group. (From ref. 23, with permission.)

response is similar to the circadian variation in sinus rhythm and indicates the effect of autonomic tone on the AV node during atrial fibrillation.

Ventricular Response to Exercise in Atrial Fibrillation

Patients with atrial fibrillation generally have a more rapid ventricular rate during exercise than do age-matched subjects in sinus rhythm as discussed in detail in the chapter by Atwood. Early in exercise the ventricular rate increases as a result of withdrawal of vagal tone, and as the level of exertion increases there is an increase in neurally released and endogenous catecholamines. Since AV nodal conduction during atrial fibrillation is sensitive to the level of vagal and sympathetic tone, these changes result in a steep heart rate increase (Figs. 1 and 4). As indicated below, control of resting ventricular rate by digoxin is little or no guarantee of adequate control with exertion since the predominant effect of digoxin is neurally mediated.

Optimal Heart Rate in Atrial Fibrillation

Pharmacologic therapy in chronic atrial fibrillation is often prescribed to maintain a resting heart rate in the range of 60 to 90 beats per minute, similar to the range found in most patients with sinus rhythm. Persistent resting tachycardia is inappropriate because of the potential for elevation of left atrial filling pressures, increased myocardial oxygen demand, and decreased left ventricular filling. In sinus rhythm, the atrial systolic contribution to ventricular filling contributes from under 10% to over 40% of ventricular filling, depending on the state of the mitral valve and the filling properties of the left ventricle (26,27). Thus, loss of atrial systole in atrial fibrillation might be expected to decrease stroke volume, necessitating an increase in heart rate to maintain resting cardiac output.

To examine the optimal resting heart rate required to produce maximal stroke volume in atrial fibrillation, Rawles (28) performed Doppler examinations of aortic

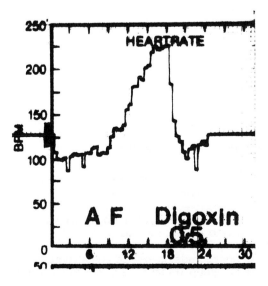

FIG. 4. Heart rate response to treadmill exercise (modified Bruce protocol) in a 28-year-old woman with chronic atrial fibrillation and a mitral valve replacement who was experiencing exertional palpitations and fatigue. Her resting heart rate while lying down was 70 beats per minute when receiving digoxin 0.5 mg daily. With exercise the heart rate remained relatively well controlled until 9 min of exercise (approximately equivalent to 7 MET or climbing stairs) and then accelerates abruptly to 225 beats per minute. At cessation of exercise there is an abrupt fall in heart rate. The addition of propranolol blunted the heart rate rise and abolished her symptoms (not shown).

valve flow velocity integrals in a group of 60 patients with atrial fibrillation of various etiologies. The flow velocity integral, a measurement proportional to stroke volume, was correlated with the preceding two R-R intervals to determine the effect of heart rate on stroke volume. The calculated maximal stroke volume in individual patients occurred at widely differing R-R intervals (equivalent to heart rates of 60 to 200 beats per minute) with a mean for the group of 122 beats per minute. Importantly, the mean resting ventricular rate in 27% of patients exceeded that predicted for the production of maximal cardiac output, and all of this group had a ventricular rate greater than 90 beats per minute. Although some patients with heart rates greater than 90 beats per minute did not exceed the predicted heart rate for maximal cardiac output, all seven patients in whom the ventricular rate was grater than 140 beats per minute were in excess of their calculated optimal rate. These data indicate that, while maximal resting cardiac output in atrial fibrillation may occur over a wide range in individual patients with atrial fibrillation, a heart rate less than 90 beats per minute is unlikely to be excessive, whereas one greater than 140 beats per minute is generally too high. It should be stressed that the author of this study did not intend to suggest that patients with atrial fibrillation necessarily benefit from a resting tachycardia, since other considerations such as myocardial oxygen demand and left atrial pressure may be adversely affected by higher heart rates.

Controversy exists regarding the importance of heart rate control for improving exercise duration in atrial fibrillation. Atwood et al. (29) have examined the response of heart rate to exercise in patients with lone atrial fibrillation compared to that in patients with atrial fibrillation and intrinsic heart disease. A higher peak heart rate and maximal O_2 uptake during exercise were reached in the lone fibrillator group than in the group with intrinsic heart disease. When lone fibrillators were compared to equivalent age-matched controls, there was no difference in gas exchange variables or functional capacity, suggesting that the "excessive" heart rate rise was not deleterious. However, no comparison was made between those with organic heart disease who had atrial fibrillation and a comparable group in sinus rhythm.

In summary, it is probably not possible to generalize about an optimal resting or exercise heart rate in atrial fibrillation since interpatient variability is great, partly as a result of the presence and type of underlying disease. Nevertheless, it is clinically appropriate to aim for a resting heart rate under 90 beats per minute and to carefully assess and treat patients for objective evidence of symptoms related to exertional tachycardia.

DRUG THERAPY FOR RATE CONTROL IN ATRIAL FIBRILLATION
(TABLE 1)

In discussing therapy for the control of ventricular rate in atrial fibrillation it is helpful to consider three aspects in patients with sustained arrhythmia and a fourth in subjects with paroxysmal atrial fibrillation. These are (a) acute control of the ventricular response in an untreated patient presenting with the arrhythmia, (b) chronic maintenance of adequate ventricular response during rest and normal low-level daily activities, and (c) prevention of disproportionate exertional tachycardia. In the patient with intermittent arrhythmia, consideration should be given to prevention of excessive tachycardia during a paroxysm.

TABLE 1. *Effective agents for slowing ventricular rate in atrial fibrillation (in absence of preexcitation)*

Drug	Acute dose	Maintenance dose	Comments
Digoxin	1.0–1.5 mg i.v. or oral over 24 hr in increments of 0.25–0.5 mg	0.125–0.5 mg daily	Loading takes several hours to slow the rate and can be avoided if no urgency. Minimally effective during exercise, fever, and other high catecholamine states. Caution in elderly patients or those with renal impairment.
Propranolol[a]	1–5 mg i.v. (1 mg every 2 min)	10–120 mg three times daily	Extreme caution in patients with congestive heart failure. May be adequate chronically in twice-daily dose.
Esmolol	0.5 mg i.v./kg/min	0.05–0.2 mg/kg/min i.v.	Very short half-life. Only available intravenously. Hypotension common.
Xamoterol[b]	No information	200 mg twice daily	Beta-1 stimulant at low levels of activity. Competitive beta antagonist at higher stimulation. Increases mortality in severe congestive heart failure.
Verapamil	5–20 mg in 5-mg increments i.v. i.v. boluses of 5–10 mg every 30 min or 0.005 mg/kg/ min infusion	40–120 mg three times daily or 120–360 mg of the slow-release form once daily	May be synergistic with digoxin but also increases digoxin levels. Peripheral edema may mimic congestive heart failure.
Diltiazem[c]	0.25–0.35 mg/kg i.v. followed by 5–15 mg infusion i.v. per hour	60–90 mg three or four times daily (or single dose of 120–240 mg slow release)	Synergistic with digoxin; no significant effects on digoxin levels. May cause ankle edema

[a]Propranolol is given as representative example of beta-blockers. Doses of other oral beta-blockers for maintenance include metoprolol 25 to 100 mg twice daily, atenolol 50 to 100 mg daily, nadolol 40 to 320 mg daily.
[b]Not available in the United States.
[c]Intravenous diltiazem not currently available in the United States.

The key to successful management of patients with atrial fibrillation lies in the individualization of these goals on a patient-by-patient basis. Clearly, a patient presenting with minor palpitations and atrial fibrillation with a rapid ventricular response does not require the same urgency for heart rate control as does one with mitral stenosis who has pulmonary edema precipitated by the arrhythmia. Similarly one would give little consideration to vigorously assessing daily variations in heart rate in a symptomatic, sedentary, elderly patient with atrial fibrillation, but might aim for careful assessment in a young patient who regularly exercises or performs a physically demanding job.

In clinical practice it is not uncommon to find a significant proportion of patients with atrial fibrillation who experience exertional palpitations despite adequate resting heart rates or, more subtly, who may manifest symptoms of easy fatigability, exertional dyspnea, or limitation of exercise. In such patients rate control may be the key to marked symptomatic improvement. Digoxin, calcium channel blockers, and beta-blocking agents have been extensively evaluated for heart rate control at rest and during exercise in subjects with atrial fibrillation. Despite the clear-cut efficacy of the last two groups of drugs in blunting exertional tachycardia, few studies show any benefit of drug therapy for the improvement of exercise tolerance. Never-

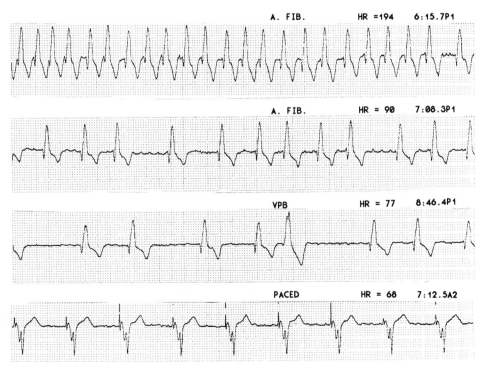

FIG. 5. Representative Holter monitoring rhythm strips from a middle-aged male who had a tricuspid valve prosthesis and an epicardial pacemaker system because of atrial fibrillation with prolonged symptomatic ventricular pauses. He was receiving digoxin 0.25 mg daily. **A:** While taking out the garbage at work, the mean ventricular rate is over 190 beats per minute. **B:** Driving home, mean rate 80 to 100 beats per minute. **C:** Relaxing at home. **D:** Prior to arising in morning; the pacemaker is capturing at 68 beats/minute.

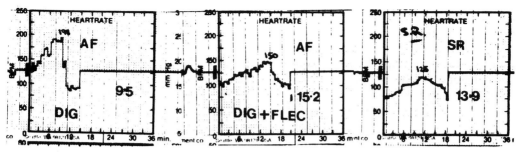

FIG. 6. Effect of heart rate control on a 50-year-old woman with atrial fibrillation and congestive heart failure secondary to an atrial septal defect. **Left panel:** During exercise on digoxin alone (0.25 mg) there is a rapid, excessive heart rate rise. Exercise was stopped at a heart rate of 198 beats per minute after 9.5 min due to dyspnea and fatigue. **Middle panel:** The addition of flecainide 100 mg twice daily for 2 weeks as part of a research study (ref. 88) results in a blunting of the peak heart rate response to 150 beats per minute and an improvement in exercise tolerance to 15.2 min. **Right panel:** Following electrical cardioversion to sinus rhythm the peak heart rate is reduced further compared to flecainide-treated atrial fibrillation with little effect on exercise duration (13.9 min). Such a dramatic response following heart rate control is unusual but may occasionally be seen in individual patients.

theless maximal exercise tolerance may be a poor predictor of clinical improvement, since few patients perform vigorous physical exertion during daily activities. In addition individual patients may benefit considerably from careful heart rate control even though benefit for large groups cannot be demonstrated.

An example of the daily wide swings in heart rate in a patient with a resting controlled ventricular response is shown in Fig. 5, and the effect of heart rate control on exercise tolerance in a symptomatic individual is demonstrated in Fig. 6.

In the remainder of this chapter the three main classes of drugs commonly used for heart rate control in atrial fibrillation are discussed, and data on alternative, less commonly used, agents are considered. The discussion is limited to heart rate control in patients without preexcitation since therapy of atrial fibrillation in the preexcitation syndromes is discussed in detail elsewhere in the book. As most trials of beta-blockers and calcium channel blockers show similar results, only representative studies will be presented.

DIGOXIN

Acute Control of Heart Rate

Although the onset of the inotropic action of intravenous digoxin may be apparent as early as 15 to 30 min after administration (30), its effect on the heart rate in atrial fibrillation may take considerably longer to be apparent. Many patients presenting with an acute episode of atrial fibrillation have evidence of associated congestive failure. In these patients concomitant treatment with digoxin and diuretics may rapidly lower filling pressures and improve systolic function, resulting in secondary control of heart rate. However, in a series of patients with recent-onset atrial fibrillation carefully selected to exclude subjects with heart failure or other conditions likely to aggravate the ventricular rate (11), we found the heart rate in actively digitalized patients (given as 0.6 mg encapsulated digoxin elixir at 0 hr, 0.4 mg at 4 hr, 0.2 mg at 8 hr, and 0.2 mg at 14 hr) took an average of 5.5 hr to fall below a control group given placebo. Although intravenous digoxin might have acted a little more quickly, the encapsulated elixir preparation used is fully and rapidly absorbed (31), and blood levels at 4 hr were well within the therapeutic range.

Despite the relatively slow effect of digoxin for control of ventricular rate, it remains an important drug for patients in whom rate control is not urgent and/or in those in whom systolic dysfunction coexists with their arrhythmia. In the latter group, control of heart failure may also help to slow heart rates. Failure to control the ventricular rate with adequate doses of digoxin (1.0–1.2 mg i.v. or 1.25–1.5 mg orally over 24 hr) usually indicates an intrinsic or drug-induced hyperadrenergic state (e.g., fever, thyrotoxicosis, theophylline), and additional doses may lead to toxicity without clinical efficacy (32).

Evidence exists that hypomagnesemia may result in relative digoxin resistance in subjects with atrial fibrillation. De Carli et al. (33) found that 20% of 45 consecutive patients with symptomatic atrial fibrillation had a serum magnesium level less than 1.5 mEq/liter. Control of ventricular rate in these subjects required twice the amount of intravenous digoxin as the normomagnesemic subjects. Support for the role of magnesium in slowing AV nodal conduction comes from DiCarlo et al. (34) who found that 6 g of magnesium sulfate administered intravenously over 6 min followed by a continuous infusion of 1 g over 1 hr resulted in significant increases in AV nodal conduction time and refractory periods. Fananapazir et al. (35) demonstrated that the effects of magnesium (74 mg/kg) on AV nodal conduction were more marked at higher atrial pacing rates, compatible with a use-dependent effect.

Chronic Control of Ventricular Rate During Daily Activity

Digoxin remains an important and effective drug for resting heart rate control in atrial fibrillation. As detailed in the chapter by Pollak and Falk, it is important to recognize that nocturnal pauses of up to 3 sec are both common and of no consequence in digitalized subjects with atrial fibrillation (36). Most sedentary and elderly patients requiring digoxin for initial rate control can be maintained on the drug as monotherapy.

Exertional Heart Rate

It has long been recognized that digoxin has little effect on controlling peak heart rate during vigorous exertion (3,37–39), and in some patients the ventricular response may be poorly controlled even at low levels of exercise. In a study to determine the optimal digoxin dose for resting and exercise heart rate control in patients with atrial fibrillation, Redfors (39) administered daily doses of digoxin (0.125, 0.25, 0.5, 0.75, and 1.0 mg/day) increasing every 2 weeks until toxicity occurred or the maximal dose was reached. Patients underwent symptom-limited bicycle ergometry at low (150 kpm/min) medium (300 kpm/min) and high (450 kpm/min) workloads. Seven of the 14 patients studied tolerated 0.75 mg or more of digoxin per day. Resting heart rate decreased by a mean of 21% at rest as the dose was increased to the optimal (best tolerated) dose, whereas the maximal exertional ventricular rate was only reduced by 6%. At low and medium workloads with optimal digoxin levels, the corresponding reductions were 19% and 16%, respectively.

Similar findings were reported by Beasley and co-workers (12), who studied 12 patients with chronic nonvalvular atrial fibrillation. Subjects underwent treadmill exercise testing while receiving either placebo or an individualized dose of digoxin tailored to produce a low (0.8 ± 0.2 mEq/liter) or higher (1.8 ± 0.7 mEq/liter) serum digoxin level. At low levels of exercise, equivalent to walking at 3 mph on the flat, the mean heart rates when receiving placebo, and low and high doses of digoxin, respectively, were 171, 161, and 140 beats per minute, and the corresponding heart rates for a moderate level of exercise were 191, 182, and 164. Despite high doses of digoxin the mean exercise heart rate was still considerably higher at low and medium workloads than it was in control subjects in sinus rhythm (140 vs 105 and 164 vs 118 beats per minute, respectively). Thus, while digoxin does have some effect on exertional heart rate control, its effect is limited, and it should not be assumed that an adequately controlled resting ventricular response is indicative of good control during daily activities.

Rate Control During Paroxysmal Atrial Fibrillation

Patients who have had one or more episodes of paroxysmal atrial fibrillation with a rapid ventricular response are often maintained on digoxin in the belief that the ventricular rate will be slowed in the event of a recurrence. Since digoxin therapy in sustained atrial fibrillation chronically controls the ventricular rate, it seems logical that chronic therapy should prevent excessive tachycardia in paroxysmal arrhythmia. However, the onset of a paroxysm of atrial fibrillation may be provoked by or may provoke a surge in sympathetic nervous system activity that, similar to the situation during exercise, counters the effects of digoxin.

Data supporting the lack of efficacy of chronic digoxin therapy for preventing tachycardia during paroxysmal fibrillation come both from Holter monitor studies and, indirectly, from studies of other agents for preventing paroxysmal arrhythmia. In their study of Holter monitor recordings, Rawles et al. (14) found no difference in ventricular rates at the onset of a paroxysm of atrial fibrillation in patients taking or not taking digoxin (140 ± 25 vs 134 ± 22 beats per minute). Patients with higher serum levels of digoxin showed no difference in rate from those with lower levels or those receiving no drug. Anderson et al. (40) in a trial of the efficacy of flecainide for paroxysmal atrial fibrillation found no difference in heart rate at relapse between placebo patients who were receiving digoxin and those who were not.

Similarly in a group of patients receiving quinidine for maintenance of sinus rhythm (41), the mean ventricular rate at the time of relapse to sinus rhythm was 109 beats per minute whether patients were receiving digoxin or not.

Summary

In summary, digoxin is an effective agent for ventricular rate control in the resting subject without any concomitant factors likely to increase sympathetic nervous activities. It is usually sufficient therapy for elderly or less active patients but may not prevent disproportionate tachycardia in more active subjects, who may therefore need additional or alternative drug therapy. It is probably not of value for preventing tachycardia at the onset of paroxysmal atrial fibrillation and its use as a sole agent for this indication, although widespread, has no basis. Despite these caveats about the use of digoxin, the majority of patients with chronic atrial fibrillation are elderly and may be successfully treated with digoxin alone.

BETA-BLOCKING AGENTS

Acute Control

A large number of beta-blocking agents are available in the United States, although only three (esmolol, metoprolol, and propranolol) are available as intravenous preparations. Both the intravenous and oral beta-blocking agents are highly effective for controlling a rapid ventricular response to atrial fibrillation. Generally, however, beta-blocking agents tend not to be used as first-line agents for acute rate control since unsuspected heart failure may be severely exacerbated by their negative inotropic effects and and/or by blockade of endogenous catecholamine stimulation. An exception is the patient with thyrotoxicosis-associated atrial fibrillation and a rapid ventricular response in whom beta-blockade is the treatment of choice (42). In such cases oral therapy, e.g., propranolol 40–120 mg t.i.d., is generally satisfactory until the thyroid disease is controlled.

Esmolol, an intravenous beta-blocker with a half-life of 9 min in normal subjects (43) is a useful drug for the short-term control of ventricular rate in atrial fibrillation (44). Therapy is initiated with a bolus of 0.5 mg/kg given over 1 min, followed by an infusion of 0.05 to 0.3 mg/kg/min titrated to heart rate. The disadvantage of esmolol is the necessity to give it by continuous infusion, but the advantage is that side effects dissipate very rapidly after infusion discontinuation (45). Esmolol has been shown to be as effective as verapamil for the control of ventricular response in recent onset atrial fibrillation (46), with a mean reduction in heart rate from 139 to 100 beats per minute during esmolol infusion of 8 to 16 mg/min.

Resting Heart Rate Control

Most studies of beta-blockade in atrial fibrillation have concentrated on the effects of this class of drugs on exercise. However, resting and daily heart rates are often recorded and consistently show a reduction, which is generally most marked during waking hours (47).

Rate Control During Exercise

Beta-blocking agents are highly effective in slowing the ventricular response to exercise both in patients with sinus rhythm and in those with atrial fibrillation. Several studies, using a variety of beta-blockers, demonstrated a heart rate reduction at all levels of exercise, but failure to show improvement in exercise tolerance is almost universal. Indeed some studies (47,48) show a decreased exercise tolerance despite a "normalization" in the excessive heart rate rise. DiBianco et al. (47) evaluated the effect of nadolol (mean dose 87 ± 43 mg/day) on resting and exercise heart rates in patients with atrial fibrillation who were also receiving digoxin therapy. Daily mean heart rates decreased from 92 to 73 beats per minute and heart rates at submaximal exercise fell from a mean of 153 to 111 beats per minute. However, the total exercise time fell from 466 sec to 380 sec—a decrease of almost 20%. A similar result was noted by Atwood et al. (48), who investigated the effect of the beta-1 selective adrenergic blocker celiprolol. The heart rate response to exercise was markedly blunted, with a mean peak heart rate during therapy of 118 beats per minute—a 53 beats per minute reduction. Using gas exchange analysis, oxygen uptake at maximal exertion was found to be significantly reduced by the beta-blocker, and this corresponded to a significant reduction in treadmill time.

One problem with these studies is that the dose of beta-blocker may have been too great for optimal heart rate control during exercise, resulting in an excessive slowing and consequent decrease in cardiac output at each level of exercise. Although specifically avoiding conclusions regarding the optimal exertional heart rate in atrial fibrillation, the data by Rawles (28), discussed previously, regarding resting heart rates imply that a certain degree of exertional tachycardia might be beneficial in atrial fibrillation. Alternatively, beta-blockade may have impaired exercise capacity by means of a negative inotropic effect. The negative inotropic effects of propranolol have been demonstrated even in normal subjects (49), and it is likely that, in subjects with atrial fibrillation in whom myocardial disease often exists, the effect might be more marked.

Control of Heart Rate During Paroxysmal Atrial Fibrillation

Beta-blocking agents are generally ineffective in preventing paroxysmal atrial fibrillation. Coumel, in this volume, suggests that sympathetic triggering of atrial fibrillation is less common than vagal triggers, whereas Rawles et al. (14) suggested that sympathetic triggers predominate in paroxysmal atrial fibrillation. In either case, the onset of atrial fibrillation may be associated with a surge in sympathetic activity secondary to the sudden tachycardia, due to the fall in stroke volume and/or to anxiety generated by the palpitations. In such cases beta-blockers might be expected to be beneficial. Margolis et al. (50) reported on 14 patients with paroxysmal atrial fibrillation or flutter treated with a combination of antiarrhythmic drugs taken only at the onset of arrhythmia. Propranolol was frequently used in combination with other agents, and for the group the intermittent use of combination antiarrhythmics was documented to successfully reduce hospital admissions and decrease symptom severity.

Although few published data exist, we frequently combine a low dosage of beta-blocker with an antiarrhythmic agent in patients in whom paroxysmal atrial fibrillation is only partially controlled. The combination is effective in controlling ventricular rate during a paroxysm and is particularly useful when atrial antiarrhythmic agents, such as quinidine or disopyramide, are used, which have minimal or no effect on AV nodal conduction. If such a combination is contemplated, care must be taken to assess the risks of combining two agents with negative inotropic properties, such as propranolol and disopyramide.

CALCIUM CHANNEL BLOCKERS

The calcium channel-blocking drugs verapamil and diltiazem both increase the refractory period and probably the conduction time of the AV node (51). At the time of writing, only verapamil is clinically available in an intravenous form in the United States, although intravenous diltiazem is undergoing clinical studies (52). Both agents are available in regular or slow-release oral preparations.

The calcium channel-blocking agents have some advantage over beta-blockade for the control of ventricular rate in atrial fibrillation because they have vasodilator properties that partially offset any negative inotropic effects. In addition, because they act directly on the heart to slow ventricular rate rather than blocking the effects of circulating catecholamines, there may be some advantage to choosing one of these agents for heart rate control in a patient in whom myocardial contractility is impaired and is partly dependent on sympathetic drive.

Studies in animals indicate that the slowing of AV nodal conduction by diltiazem and verapamil is frequency dependent, i.e., the effect is more pronounced at higher stimulation rates (53,54). This observation may indicate why calcium channel blockers have salutary effects during atrial fibrillation, despite relatively small changes in AV nodal properties during sinus rhythm.

Acute Control of Ventricular Rate

Intravenous verapamil is highly effective for slowing the ventricular rate in atrial fibrillation (55). A maximal response is seen within 2 to 3 min after administration of the drug, which may be given in 5-mg increments up to a total of 20 mg. The effect of verapamil is independent of the level of sympathetic tone, but it is relatively short lived. A verapamil infusion of 0.005 mg/kg/min has been found to be effective for maintaining rate control, although the use of the drug in this manner is not widespread.

Intravenous diltiazem is also highly effective for the rapid control of ventricular rate in atrial fibrillation. In a double-blind study of 113 patients with atrial fibrillation or flutter and a ventricular rate greater than or equal to 120 beats per minute, 75% of patients responded to 0.25 mg/kg diltiazem (given over 2 min) with at least a 20% reduction in heart rate or a reduction in ventricular rate to less than 100 beats per minute (52). An additional 18% responded to a higher dose (0.35 mg/kg) administered 15 min after the initial dose. The median time from the onset of drug use to rate control was 4.3 min, and side effects were mild and uncommon, most often related to hypotension. Maintenance of ventricular rate control with intravenous diltiazem has been successfully obtained with a bolus dose of 20 mg (followed, if necessary, by a second bolus of 25 mg after 15 min) then an infusion of 10 to 15 mg/hr *(unpublished observations)*.

Daily Heart Rate (Fig. 7)

As with beta-blocking agents, most trials of calcium channel blockers concentrate on the effect of the drugs on maximal exercise heart rate, although resting rates and heart rate during daily activity are generally reported to be slightly reduced. Several trials have estimated the effects of either verapamil or diltiazem compared to digoxin

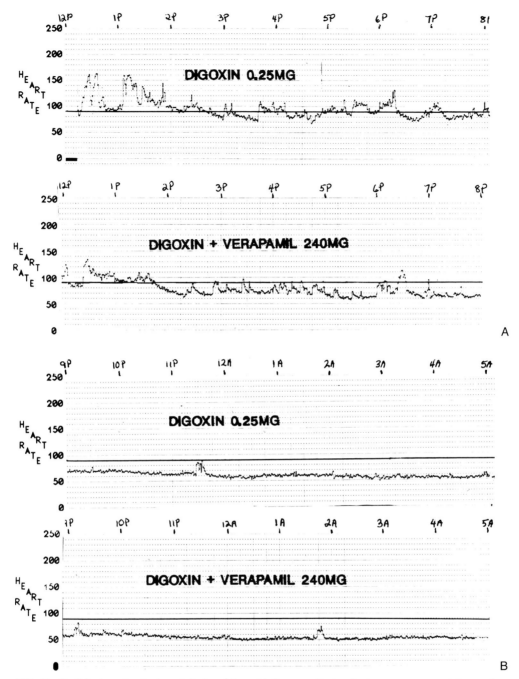

FIG. 7. A: 8-hr heart rate trend derived from Holter monitoring between noon and 8 P.M. in a patient with chronic atrial fibrillation receiving 0.25 mg digoxin. The peak heart rate exceeds 160 beats per minute, and considerable tachycardia occurs between noon and 2 P.M. The heart rate exceeds 90 beats per minute (*solid line*) for most of the 8-hr period. After addition of 240 mg slow-release verapamil to the digoxin, the symptomatic episodes of tachycardia are abolished and there is a fall in overall heart rate to less than 90 beats per minute (peak 140 beats per minute). **B:** Heart rates at night, during same 24-hr period. The heart rate swings are absent and mean heart rate on digoxin alone is approximately 60 beats per minute, falling slightly to about 55 beats per minute after addition of verapamil.

alone, but few have directly compared the two calcium channel blockers. An exception is the study of Lundstrom and Ryden (56), who examined the effects of verapamil, diltiazem, and placebo in 19 patients with chronic atrial fibrillation (17 of whom were also receiving digoxin). Diltiazem (90 mg three times a day) and verapamil (80 mg three times a day) both reduced resting heart rates to a similar degree (mean of 100 beats per minute on digoxin reduced to 75 beats per minute with addition of either calcium channel blocker). Similarly the mean hourly heart rates derived from Holter monitoring were also reduced throughout the 24-hr period, with maintenance of the normal diurnal variation.

Verapamil may elevate serum digoxin levels and precipitate toxicity, which may be manifest only days to weeks after the drug combination is started (57). While the elevation in digoxin levels may partly explain a synergistic effect of the drugs on the resting heart rate, synergism is also seen with diltiazem, an agent with minimal effects on digoxin levels (58). In a controlled trial of medium- (240 mg/day) and high-dose diltiazem (360 mg/day) alone or in combination with digoxin, Roth et al. (58) found that medium-dose diltiazem was equivalent to digoxin for control of resting heart rate (88 ± 19 vs 86 ± 12 beats per minute, respectively). At the higher dose, diltiazem had a greater effectiveness on resting heart rate (79 ± 17 beats per minute), but 75% of subjects experienced one or more side effects. The combination of digoxin and medium-dose diltiazem was as effective as the higher dose combination and better than any monotherapy. A similar effect of combination therapy was found by Steinberg et al. (59), who also noted symptomatic improvement in 11 of 16 patients treated with diltiazem.

Effects on Exercise Duration and Tolerance

Heart rate at all levels of exercise is significantly blunted by both verapamil and diltiazem compared to digoxin alone. In the study of Roth et al. (58), cited earlier, the synergistic effects of diltiazem and digoxin were seen on exertion as well as at rest, with mean peak hearts for those on digoxin alone, 240 mg diltiazem alone, and combination therapy of 170 ± 20, 154 ± 23, and 132 ± 32 beats per minute, respectively.

In contrast to the consistently negative or adverse results of beta-blocking agents on exercise duration in atrial fibrillation, several studies utilizing calcium channel blockers have shown a modest improvement in exercise tolerance and/or maximal oxygen uptake (56,58,60,61). While others have failed to show improvement (62), no studies have reported a decreased tolerance, as sometimes seen with beta-blockade.

Effects on Heart Rate During Paroxysmal Atrial Fibrillation

Few data exist regarding the efficacy of chronic therapy with calcium channel blockers alone or in combination with digoxin for controlling heart rate during paroxysmal atrial fibrillation. Generally calcium channel blockers are ineffective for preventing paroxysmal atrial fibrillation and, in some cases, may increase the duration of the arrhythmia (63). In one study of flecainide for preventing paroxysmal atrial fibrillation, verapamil was prescribed to reduce the ventricular response in the event that the arrhythmia recurred (64). While this combination was well tolerated, no details were given regarding efficacy. Certainly there is a theoretical basis for using a calcium channel blocker in a patient with troublesome tachycardia due to paroxysmal atrial fibrillation, although if chronic therapy is required and beta-blockers are tolerated, the latter group of drugs might be preferable in view of their anti-sympathetic effects.

SUMMARY AND GUIDELINES FOR THERAPY WITH DIGOXIN, BETA-BLOCKERS, AND CALCIUM CHANNEL BLOCKERS TO CONTROL HEART RATE IN ATRIAL FIBRILLATION

From the preceding review, several general guidelines can be derived. At this stage it must be reemphasized that this discussion is limited to patients without overt preexcitation syndrome—a group in whom the use of digoxin or calcium channel blockers, and, rarely, beta-blockers for atrial fibrillation may have life-threatening adverse effects.

Digoxin therapy remains the mainstay of monotherapy for chronic atrial fibrillation in most asymptomatic patients. The dose necessary to achieve an adequate resting heart rate is often more than the standard 0.25 mg daily dose, particularly in young patients with normal renal function. Digoxin levels are of little value in assessing adequate dose (65) but may be helpful if low or when toxicity is clinically suspected. Generally Holter monitoring and/or exercise testing to determine adequacy of rate control are unnecessary in the asymptomatic, relatively sedentary older patients with a resting rate under 90 beats per minute. In younger, active patients with chronic atrial fibrillation, particularly those with reduced exercise tolerance, Holter monitoring is of great value to determine the range of heart rate throughout the day. Often symptoms attributed to underlying heart disease (particularly mitral valve disease) are found to be related to disproportionate tachycardia at low levels of exertion and the addition of another agent may dramatically improve well-being.

Treadmill exercise testing is most useful for assessing the efficacy of treatment in patients in whom Holter monitoring has revealed excessive periods of disproportionate tachycardia during daily activity. We (66) have demonstrated the reproducibility of exercise testing for assessing heart rate control in atrial fibrillation, and although a minor learning effect may blunt heart rate on successive tests (67), treadmill exercise is still a valuable tool. Although we favor a modified Bruce protocol, other protocols are equally effective, providing the level of exertion is not too severe too early in the test.

Trials of beta-blockers do not seem to indicate a significant effect of therapy on exercise duration, but the doses used were rarely individually titrated and may have been too high, resulting in excessive heart rate slowing in many patients. In addition, maximal exercise tolerance is a poor indicator of drug efficacy, since most patients do not routinely perform such vigorous exertion and require therapy only for symptoms such as palpitations. An example of the discrepant benefit of beta-blockade on well-being and exercise tolerance is indicated in an early study (68) in which 50% of patients experienced symptomatic relief when timolol was added to digoxin, despite the failure to prolong exercise duration. Presumably this was due to the blunting of heart rate at lower levels of exertion.

Thus, beta-blockers do have a role in selected patients with poorly controlled atrial fibrillation and may be the first-line agent to add to digoxin if the rate is poorly controlled. This is particularly so in anxious patients with symptomatic palpitations, in whom only a small dose (as low as 10 mg twice daily of propranolol) may be required.

The choice of a calcium channel blocker over a beta-blocker depends on a number of factors, but calcium channel blockers may have fewer side effects. Subjects with bronchospasm, diabetes, or peripheral vascular disease should, if possible, avoid beta-blockers, and in such patients the addition of a calcium channel-blocking agent is the treatment of choice if digoxin alone fails. Although there are no published data on the efficacy of the slow-release preparations of verapamil or diltiazem for rate control in chronic atrial fibrillation, personal experience suggests that a good response may be anticipated with either of these agents (Fig. 7). If verapamil is chosen over diltiazem, the patient should be carefully monitored for evidence of digoxin toxicity and serum digoxin levels should be measured before and approximately 7 to 10 days after the institution of therapy with appropriate dose adjustments as required.

An issue related to the optimal dose of either beta-blockers or calcium channel blockers is the dosing intervals used for shorter acting agents such as propranolol, diltiazem, and verapamil. Usually these drugs have been prescribed three times daily, frequently in conjunction with digoxin (47,57,69). However, nocturnal heart rates during atrial fibrillation are generally low and frequently associated with ventricular pauses (25,36). Thus, there appears to be little value in prescribing an evening dose of medication specifically for the purpose of rate control. When using short-acting agents for this purpose, it is appropriate to prescribe only a morning and midday dose and to confirm the efficacy of this regime with Holter monitoring.

OTHER AGENTS EFFECTIVE FOR HEART RATE CONTROL IN ATRIAL FIBRILLATION

A number of other cardioactive agents have effects on the AV node that indicate a possible beneficial effect for rate control in atrial fibrillation. These include xamoterol, amiodarone, sotalol, and the type IC agents, particularly propafenone. Because of the risk of serious side effects with some of these agents, they have not generally been systematically studied for this indication. However, data derived from studies related to attempted maintenance of sinus rhythm give useful information (Table 2).

Xamoterol

Xamoterol (Corwin) is a unique agent with selective beta-1 adrenoceptor partial agonist properties that has been used in Europe in patients with mild to moderate congestive heart failure (70). At low levels of sympathetic activity the drug acts as a beta-1 stimulant and produces positive chronotropic effects (71). However, at the higher levels of activity occurring with exercise, xamoterol acts as a competitive antagonist and heart rate is blunted (72). These actions make xamoterol an attractive agent for exertional heart rate control in atrial fibrillation in patients in whom excessive resting bradycardia may be problematic.

Molajo et al. (73) performed a double-blind crossover trial of xamoterol (200 mg twice daily or placebo) in 10 patients with chronic atrial fibrillation who were receiving digoxin and found that the drug blunted both peak daily heart rates (documented by Holter monitoring) and peak treadmill exercise heart rates. Resting heart rate, when receiving xamoterol in combination with digoxin, was slightly but significantly

TABLE 2. *Effective atrial antiarrhythmics that may control heart rate during reversion of sinus rhythm to atrial fibrillation[a]*

Drug	Acute dose	Maintenance dose	Comments
Sotalol	—	80–160 mg twice daily	Combined beta-blocker and type 3 activities. May cause torsades de pointes.
Amiodarone	5–7 mg/kg up to 1,500 mg over 24 hr (but not recommended for this use)	100–300 mg daily as single dose	Multiple, long-term side effects, most commonly seen at higher doses.
Propafenone	2 mg/kg i.v. (not recommended for this use)	150–300 mg three times daily	1C agent with weak beta-blocking properties.
Flecainide	—	100–200 mg twice daily	Avoid in patients with prior myocardial infarction. Negative inotrope.
Encainide	—	Usual dose 25–50 mg three times daily	Minimal data on efficacy for rate control, except in Wolff-Parkinson-White syndrome. Avoid in patients with prior myocardial infarction.

[a]Not recommended for heart rate control alone owing to potential for toxicity.

higher than when receiving digoxin alone. Five subjects were in New York Heart Association Class 2 and two in Class 3, and all 7 showed improvement in exercise tolerance. In contrast, none of the three with Class 1 symptoms improved. Similar effects on heart rate at rest and exercise were found by Ang and co-workers (74) in a 12-patient comparison of xamoterol, digoxin, or placebo as sole therapy. However, the majority of their patients had Class 1 symptoms, and no statistical difference was found between the three groups in terms of exercise duration. It is unlikely that this agent will be released in the United States since a large-scale, multicenter trial of xamoterol in heart failure was associated with increased mortality despite symptomatic improvement (75).

Sotalol

Sotalol is a beta-blocking drug with class 3 antiarrhythmic properties. It has not been systematically studied for heart rate control in atrial fibrillation, although it is effective in maintaining atrial fibrillation after cardioversion to sinus rhythm (76). Jull-Moller et al. (41) reported on the efficacy of sotalol (80–160 mg twice daily) or quinidine (600 mg slow release, twice daily) for the maintenance of sinus rhythm after conversion from atrial fibrillation in 183 patients. Thirty-two of 95 patients able to tolerate sotalol reverted to atrial fibrillation during follow-up with a mean ventricular rate of 78 beats per minute. This was significantly less than the heart rate in the 17 of 79 patients receiving quinidine who relapsed (mean 109 beats per minute). Subjects relapsing while on sotalol had fewer symptoms than those on quinidine at the time of arrhythmia recurrence, presumably related to the lower heart rate.

It is likely that the predominant effect of sotalol on ventricular rate in atrial fibrillation is due to its beta-blocking properties, and thus it has no obvious advantages in chronic atrial fibrillation over standard beta-blocking agents that do not have significant antiarrhythmic properties. Furthermore, sotalol's propensity to cause torsades de pointes makes it a less desirable choice for rate control alone. However, when a drug is needed for attempted maintenance of sinus rhythm in a patient with frequent paroxysms of atrial fibrillation associated with a rapid, symptomatic, ventricular response, sotalol may be of value. An additional setting in which the combined beta-blocking and antiarrhythmic properties of the agent may play a role is the case in which rapid heart rate control is required prior to attempting to convert recent-onset atrial fibrillation (77).

Amiodarone

The use of amiodarone in the United States is generally limited to patients with life-threatening ventricular arrhythmias. However, as discussed elsewhere in this volume, the drug is highly effective in low doses for maintaining sinus rhythm after conversion of atrial fibrillation. Since the drug prolongs refractoriness in all cardiac tissue (78), it might be expected to slow the ventricular response to atrial fibrillation. In a small group of patients with chronic atrial fibrillation (79), the mean resting ventricular rate fell from 139 beats per minute on no therapy to 100 beats per minute after 1 month of amiodarone therapy (800 mg/day for 1 week followed by 400 mg daily). Heart rate at peak exercise fell from 190 to 160 beats per minute. A similar fall in resting heart rate during chronic amiodarone therapy has been noted by other authors and may be associated with symptomatic improvement (80,81).

In a comparative trial of amiodarone and digoxin in patients with acute atrial fibrillation complicating suspected acute myocardial infarction, Cowan et al. (82) found that intravenous amiodarone effectively terminated atrial fibrillation in the majority of cases. Intravenous amiodarone was administered as 7 mg/kg over 30 min followed by an infusion over 23 hr for a total dose of 1,500 mg. In subjects remaining in atrial fibrillation who received amiodarone, the ventricular rate was more rapidly controlled than in patients receiving digoxin (at a dose of 0.5 mg i.v. over 30 min repeated 30 min later), with a decrease in mean ventricular rate of approximately 30 beats per minute at 1 hr in the amiodarone group compared to six beats per minute in patients receiving digoxin. By 6 hr the two treatments had comparable rate reductions.

In summary, amiodarone is not only a potent atrial antiarrhythmic agent but is also effective for the acute and chronic control of ventricular rate in atrial fibrillation. While the long-term side effects of the drug severely curtail its use for ventricular rate control, it may occasionally be effective when other agents fail or cannot be used and when AV nodal ablation therapy is not an option.

Type IC Agents

The type IC agents propafenone and flecainide are effective for the termination and prevention of atrial fibrillation (83–85), and encainide, although not systematically studied, is likely to have similar effects. These agents have a relatively slight electrophysiologic effect on the AV node during sinus rhythm but manifest a prominent use-dependent effect and may slow ventricular response during atrial fibrillation (86). Conversion of fibrillation to flutter during treatment with type IC drugs has been associated with relatively slow atrial rate and 1:1 AV nodal conduction may occur, resulting in hemodynamic deterioration (87).

Anderson et al. (40) reported a multicenter trial of flecainide or placebo prescribed for prevention of paroxysmal atrial fibrillation. Thirty patients experienced recurrent arrhythmia while receiving the study drug (flecainide 200–400 mg daily [mean 295 mg] or placebo). During a recurrence of atrial fibrillation the rate on placebo was 123 ± 4 beats per minute and on flecainide it was 118 ± 4 beats per minute—a small but statistically significant difference. For patients receiving concomitant digoxin therapy, the mean ventricular rates were 120 ± 6 beats per minute on placebo and 112 ± 4 on flecainide compared to 128 ± 6 on placebo and 124 ± 5 on flecainide in the nondigoxin group. The authors noted a trend toward better control with a combination of digoxin and flecainide, but this did not reach statistical significance.

In a study of the effects of flecainide on ventricular rate in patients with chronic atrial fibrillation (88), we found that flecainide 100 mg twice daily produced poorer heart rate control at rest when compared to standard doses of digoxin. The combination of flecainide 100 mg twice daily with digoxin resulted in an unchanged resting heart rate but caused a blunted response to all stages of exercise, with a 17 beats per minute reduction at peak exercise. Increasing the dose to 150 mg twice daily in combination with digoxin produced further rate control. No effect was seen on exercise tolerance, although some individuals reported improved well-being. A major problem with this therapy was the development of rapid, regular, wide-complex tachycardia in two of 12 patients, which occurred immediately following exercise and required defibrillation in one case (89). Thus, flecainide, although demonstrating a beneficial effect on heart rate control in atrial fibrillation when combined with digoxin, cannot generally be recommended for the control of chronic arrhythmia.

Encainide

Encainide has electrophysiologic properties similar to those of flecainide, and its effect on ventricular rate in atrial fibrillation would be anticipated to be similar. Other than a report of good efficacy in Wolff-Parkinson-White syndrome (90), no published systematic studies exist to show encainide's effect on ventricular rate in atrial fibrillation. However, in our experience, it is effective in slowing ventricular rate, and patients relapsing from sinus rhythm to atrial fibrillation during encainide therapy tend to have relatively well-controlled heart rates.

Propafenone

Propafenone is a type IC agent with mild beta-blocking properties. The beta-blocking effects may make propafenone a better choice of agent for prevention of paroxysmal atrial fibrillation in order to prevent excessive tachycardia during recurrences. Bianconi et al. (86) evaluated propafenone in 68 patients with atrial fibrillation of recent onset, 42 (82%) of whom converted to sinus rhythm 4 to 95 min (mean 29 ± 24 min) after 2 mg/kg propafenone was infused intravenously. The ventricular rate fell before conversion in most patients. In the nonconvertors heart rate fell significantly from 138 ± 31 to 109 ± 24 beats per minute. A similar beneficial effect in heart rate during paroxysmal atrial fibrillation has been reported by Kerr et al. (83) during oral therapy with propafenone.

In summary, the type IC agents may slow the ventricular response to atrial fibrillation, but for flecainide and probably encainide this effect is minor even when combined with digoxin. Because of its mild beta-blocking properties, the rate-slowing effects of propafenone may be somewhat more apparent. However, the IC agents are associated with serious proarrhythmic effects (91) and have no role in the chronic control of ventricular rate in atrial fibrillation. When used for prevention of paroxysmal atrial fibrillation, their rate-slowing effects may reduce symptoms at time of recurrence, but rate control should not be an argument to use the drugs in this situation as the potential for rate acceleration also exists (87).

CONCLUSION

Although the majority of patients with chronic atrial fibrillation are elderly and can have heart rate control managed with digoxin alone (or no therapy), younger subjects frequently have wide swings in daily heart rates, which may produce a variety of troublesome symptoms. The physician faced with a patient with symptomatic chronic atrial fibrillation should evaluate heart rates with 24-hr Holter monitoring during normal daily activities and if excessive tachycardia is found, consider the addition of a beta-blocking agent, verapamil or diltiazem, to digoxin. Treadmill exercise testing may be a helpful way to assess response to therapy as well as to determine any effect (positive or negative) that therapy has on exercise duration.

In the patient with paroxysmal atrial fibrillation the ideal goal is elimination of all paroxysms. Unfortunately this is not always possible and thus a two-pronged approach can be taken: reduction in frequency of palpitations and reduction in heart rate when a paroxysm of atrial fibrillation occurs. While the newer agents may be effective for both of these goals, their side-effect profile warrants caution and their use should probably be limited to patients failing standard therapy with type IA drugs. If tolerated, quinidine plus a beta-blocking agent remains a useful regime for reducing the frequency of paroxysmal atrial fibrillation and decreasing the heart rate should a paroxysm occur. The use of diltiazem or verapamil offers an alternative to a beta-blocker. While digoxin as monotherapy is a poor agent for ventricular rate control, except at rest (4), it may be of value in combination with other agents (58).

As with many things in medicine, the routine treatment of a common problem may be an acceptable standard most of the time. However, atrial fibrillation, although a common problem, occasionally poses a more difficult challenge, such as the appropriate control of heart rate. Careful evaluation of the patient and his symptoms combined with knowledge of the therapeutic options and their risks can markedly improve the quality of life in symptomatic subjects.

REFERENCES

1. Withering W. *An account of the foxglove and some of its medical uses*. London: Paternoster-Row, 1785.
2. Mackenzie J. *Disease of the heart*, 3rd ed. London: Oxford Medical, 1914;211–236.
3. Blumgart H. The reaction to exercise of the heart affected by auricular fibrillation. *Heart* 1924;11:49.
4. Falk RH, Leavitt JI. Digoxin for atrial fibrillation: a drug whose time has gone? *Ann Intern Med* 1991;114:573–575.
5. Meijler FL, Fisch C. Does the atrioventricular node conduct? *Br Heart J* 1989;61:309–315.
6. Robinson K, Frenneaux MP, Stockins B, Karatasakis G, Poloniecki JD, McKenna WJ. Atrial

fibrillation in hypertrophic cardiomyopathy: a longitudinal study. *J Am Coll Cardiol* 1990;15:1279–1285.

7. Peters KG, Kienzle MG. Severe cardiomyopathy due to chronic rapid atrial fibrillation: complete recovery after reversion to sinus rhythm. *Am J Med* 1988;85:242–244.

8. Shite J, Yokota Y, Takeuchi Y, et al. Echocardiographic evaluation of serial amelioration of left ventricular function after defibrillation of chronic atrial fibrillation. *Circulation* 1990;82(suppl 3):III-129.

9. Miwa H, Arakawa M, Kagawa K, Noda T, Kawade T. Long-term follow-up of left atrial and ventricular function after conversion of chronic atrial fibrillation sinus rhythm. *Circulation* 1990;82(suppl 3):III-749.

10. Abbott JA, Schiller NB, Ilvento JB, et al. Catheter ablation of atrioventricular conduction may improve left ventricular function and cause minimal aortic valve damage. *PACE* 1987;10:411.

11. Falk RH, Knowlton AA, Bernard S, Gotlieb NE, Battinelli NJ. Digoxin for converting recent onset-atrial fibrillation—a randomized, double-blind trial. *Ann Intern Med* 1987;106:503–506.

12. Beasley R, Smith DA, McHaffie DJ. Exercise heart rates at different serum digoxin concentrations in patients with atrial fibrillation. *Br Med J (Clin Res)* 1985;290:9–11.

13. Toivonen L, Kadish A, Kou W, Morady F. Determinants of the ventricular rate during atrial fibrillation. *J Am Coll Cardiol* 1990;16:1194–1200.

14. Rawles JM, Metcalfe MJ, Jennings K. Time of occurrence, duration and ventricular rate of paroxysmal atrial fibrillation: the effect of digoxin. *Br Heart J* 1990;63:225–227.

15. Kawakubo K, Murayama M, Itai T, et al. Heart rate at onset and termination of paroxysmal atrial fibrillation in apparently healthy subjects. *Jpn Heart J* 1986;27:645–651.

16. Langendorf R, Pick A, Katz L. Ventricular response in atrial fibrillation: role of concealed conduction in the AV node. *Circulation* 1965;32:69–75.

17. Wu D, Denes P, Dhingra RC, Wyndham CR, Rosen KM. Quantification of human atrioventricular nodal concealed conduction utilizing S1, S2, S3 stimulation. *Circulation* 1976;39:659–665.

18. Steinman RT, Lehmann MH. Beat-to-beat changes in atrioventricular nodal excitability and its modulation by concealed conduction during functional 2:1 block in man. *Circulation* 1987;76:759–767.

19. Fujiki A, Tani M, Mizumaki K, Yoshida S, Sasayama S. Quantification of human concealed atrioventricular nodal conduction: relation to ventricular response during atrial fibrillation. *Am Heart J* 1990;120:598–603.

20. Allessie MA, Rensma PL, Brugada J, Smeets JLRM, Penn O, Kirchrof CJHJ. Pathophysiology of atrial fibrillation. In: Zipes DP, Jalife J, eds. *Cardiac electrophysiology: from cell to bedside.* Philadelphia: WB Saunders, 1990;548–549.

21. David D, Long RM, Neumann A, Borow KM, Akselrod S, Mor-Avi V. Parasympathetically modulated antiarrhythmic action of lidocaine in atrial fibrillation. *Am Heart J* 1990;119:1061–1068.

22. Bennett MA, Pentecost BL. The pattern of onset and spontaneous cessation of atrial fibrillation in man. *Circulation* 1970;41:981–988.

23. Knowlton AA, Falk RH. Paradoxical increase in heart rate before conversion to sinus rhythm in patients with recent-onset atrial fibrillation. *Ann J Cardiol* 1990;65:930–932.

24. Meijler FL. An "account" of digitalis and atrial fibrillation. *J Am Coll Cardiol* 1985;5(suppl A):60A–68A.

25. Raeder EA. Circadian fluctuations in ventricular response to atrial fibrillation. *Am J Cardiol* 1990;66:1013–1016.

26. Graettinger JS, Carleton RA, Muenster JJ. Circulatory consequences of changes in cardiac rhythm produced in patients by transthoracic direct-current shock. *J Clin Invest* 1964;43:2290–2302.

27. Killip T, Baer RA. Hemodynamic effects after reversion from atrial fibrillation to sinus rhythm by precordial shock. *J Clin Invest* 1966;45:658–671.

28. Rawles JM. What is meant by a "controlled" ventricular rate in atrial fibrillation? *Br Heart J* 1990;63:157–161.

29. Atwood JE, Myers J, Sullivan M, et al. Maximal exercise testing and gas exchange in patients with chronic atrial fibrillation. *J Am Coll Cardiol* 1988;11:508–513.

30. Smith TW. Digitalis glycosides. *N Engl J Med* 1973;288:719–722.

31. Mallis GI, Schmidt GH, Lindenbaum J. Superior bioavailability of digoxin solution in capsules. *Clin Pharmacol Ther* 1976;18:761–768.

32. Goldman S, Probst P, Selzer A, Cohn K. Inefficacy of therapeutic serum levels of digoxin in controlling the ventricular rate in atrial fibrillation. *Am J Cardiol* 1975;35:651–655.

33. DeCarli C, Sprouse G, LaRosa JC. Serum magnesium levels in symptomatic atrial fibrillation and their relation to rhythm control by intravenous digoxin. *Am J Cardiol* 1986;57:956–959.

34. DiCarlo LA, Morady F, deBuitlier, Krol RB, Schurig L, Annesley TM. Effect of magnesium sulfate on cardiac conduction and refractoriness in human. *J Am Coll Cardiol* 1986;7:1356–1362.

35. Fananapazir L, Cannon RO, Winkler JB, Cropp A, Elin RJ. Frequency-dependent effects of magnesium on atrioventricular nodal conduction in man. *Circulation* 1989;80(suppl II):II-653.

36. Pitcher DW, Papouchado M, James MA, Rees JR. Twenty-four hour ambulatory electrocardiography in patients with chronic atrial fibrillation. *Br Med J* 1986;292:594.
37. Modell W, Gold H, Rothendler HH. Use of digitalis to prevent exaggerated acceleration of the heart. *JAMA* 1941;116:2241.
38. Knox JAC. The heart rate with exercise patients with auricular fibrillation. *Br Heart J* 1949; 11:119.
39. Redfors A. Digoxin dosage and ventricular rate at rest and exercise in patients with atrial fibrillation. *Acta Med Scand* 1971;190:321–333.
40. Anderson JL, Gilbert EM, Alpert BL, et al. Prevention of symptomatic recurrences of paroxysmal atrial fibrillation in patients initially tolerating antiarrhythmic therapy. A multicenter, double-blinded, crossover study of flecainide and placebo with transtelephonic monitoring. *Circulation* 1989;80:1557–1570.
41. Jull-Moller S, Edvardsson N, Rehnqvist-Alzberg N. Sotalol versus quinidine for the maintenance of sinus rhythm after direct-current cardioversion of atrial fibrillation. *Circulation* 1990;82:1932–1939.
42. Wilkinson R, Burr WA. A comparison of propranolol and nadolol pharmacokinetics and clinical effects in thyrotoxicosis. *Am Heart J* 1984;108:1160–1167.
43. Sum CY, Yacobi A, Kartzinal R, et al. Kinetics of esmolol an ultrashort-acting beta-blocker, and of its major metabolite. *Clin Pharmacol Ther* 1983;47:427–444.
44. Anderson S, Blansky L, Byrd R, et al. Comparison of the efficacy and safety of esmolol, a short-acting beta-blocker, with placebo in the treatment of supraventricular tachyarrhythmias. *Am Heart J* 1986;111:46–48.
45. Abrams J, Allen J, Allin D, et al. Efficacy and safety of esmolol versus propranolol in the treatment of supraventricular tachyarrhythmias. A multicenter double-blind clinical trial. *Am Heart J* 1985;110:913–922.
46. Platia EV, Michelson EL, Porterfield JK, Das G. Esmolol versus verapamil in the acute treatment of atrial fibrillation or atrial flutter. *Am J Cardiol* 1989;63:925–929.
47. DiBianco R, Morganroth J, Freitag RJ, et al. Effects of nadolol on the spontaneous and exercise-provoked heart rate in patients with chronic atrial fibrillation receiving stable doses of digoxin. *Am Heart J* 1984;108:1121–1127.
48. Atwood JE, Sullivan M, Forbes S, et al. Effect of beta-adrenergic blockade on exercise performance in patients with chronic atrial fibrillation. *J Am Coll Cardiol* 1987;10:314–320.
49. Clifton GD, Harrison MR, DeMaria AN. Influence of beta-adrenergic blockade upon hemodynamic response to exercise assessed by Doppler echocardiography. *Am Heart J* 1990;120:579–585.
50. Margolis B, DeSilva RA, Lown B. Episodic drug treatment in the management of paroxysmal arrhythmias. *Am J Cardiol* 1980;45:621–626.
51. Rowland E, McKenna WJ, Gullzer H, Krikler DM. The comparative effects of diltiazem and verapamil on atrioventricular conduction and atrioventricular reentry tachycardia. *Circulation* 1983;52:163–168.
52. Salerno DM, Dias VC, Kleiger RE, et al. Efficacy and safety of intravenous diltiazem for treatment of atrial fibrillation and atrial flutter. The diltiazem-atrial fibrillation/flutter study group. *Am J Cardiol* 1989;63:1046–1051.
53. Talajic M, Nattel S. Frequency-dependent effects of calcium antagonists on atrioventricular conduction and refractoriness: demonstration and characterization in anesthetized dogs. *Circulation* 1986;74:1156–1167.
54. Talajic M, Nayebpour M, Jing W, Nattel S. Frequency-dependent effects of diltiazem on the atrioventricular node during experimental atrial fibrillation. *Circulation* 1989;80:380–389.
55. Waxman HL, Myerburg RJ, Appel R, et al. Verapamil for control of ventricular rate in paroxysmal supraventricular tachycardia and atrial fibrillation or flutter: a double-blind randomized crossover study. *Ann Intern Med* 1981;94:1–61.
56. Lundstrom T, Ryden L. Ventricular rate control and exercise performance in chronic atrial fibrillation: effects of diltiazem and verapamil. *J Am Coll Cardiol* 1990;16:86–90.
57. Panidis LP, Morganroth J, Baessler C. Effectiveness and safety of oral verapamil to control exercise-induced tachycardia in patients with atrial fibrillation receiving digitalis. *Am J Cardiol* 1983;52:1197–1201.
58. Roth A, Harrison E, Mitani G, Cohen J, Rahimtoola SH, Elyakam U. Efficacy of medium and high-dose diltiazem alone and in combination with digoxin for control of heart rate at rest and during exercise in patients with chronic atrial fibrillation. *Circulation* 1986;73:316–324.
59. Steinberg JS, Katz RJ, Bren GB, Buff LA, Varghese PF. Efficacy of oral diltiazem to control ventricular response in chronic atrial fibrillation at rest and during exercise. *J Am Coll Cardiol* 1987;9:405–411.
60. Lang R, Klein H, Segni E, et al. Verapamil improves exercise capacity in chronic atrial fibrillation: double-blind crossover study. *Am Heart J* 1983;105:820–824.
61. Lang R, Klein HO, Weiss E, et al. Superiority of oral verapamil therapy to digoxin in treatment of chronic atrial fibrillation. *Chest* 1983;83:491–499.

62. Atwood JE, Myers JN, Sullivan MJ, Forbes SM, Pewes WF, Froelicher VF. Diltiazem and exercise performance in patients with chronic atrial fibrillation. *Chest* 1988;93:20–25.

63. Shenasha M, Kus T, Fromer M, LeBlanc RA, Dubuc M, Nadean R. Effect of intravenous and oral calcium antagonists (diltiazem and verapamil) on sustenance of atrial fibrillation. *Am J Cardiol* 1988;62:403–407.

64. Van Gelder IC, Crijns HJGM, Van Gilst WH, Van Wijk LN, Hamer HPM, Lie KI. Efficacy and safety of flecainide acetate in the maintenance of sinus rhythm after electrical cardioversion of chronic atrial fibrillation or atrial flutter. *Am J Cardiol* 1989;64:1317–1321.

65. Chamberlain DA, White RJ, Howard MR, Smith TW. Plasma digoxin concentrations in patients with atrial fibrillation. *Br Med J* 1970;3:429–432.

66. Falk RH, Knowlton AA, Battinelli NJ, Huntington M. Reproducibility of the heart rate response to exercise in patients with atrial fibrillation. *J Am Coll Cardiol* 1988;(suppl A):247A.

67. Kraemer MD, Sullivan M, Atwood JE, Forbes S, Myers J, Froelicher V. Reproducibility of treadmill exercise data in patients with atrial fibrillation. *Cardiology* 1989;76:234–242.

68. David D, DiSegni E, Klein HV, Kaplinsky E. Inefficacy of digitalis in the control of heart rate in patients with chronic atrial fibrillation: beneficial effect of an added beta adrenergic blocking agent. *Am J Cardiol* 1979;44:1378–1382.

69. Brown RW, Goble AJ. Effect of propranolol on exercise tolerance in patients with atrial fibrillation. *Br Med J* 1969;2:279–280.

70. Anonymous. Xamoterol: revised indications. *Lancet* 1990;335:1394–1395.

71. Hashimoto T, Shiina A, Toyo-Oka T, Hosoda S, Kondo K. The cardiovascular effects of xamoterol, a beta-1 adrenoceptor partial agonist, in healthy volunteers at rest. *Br J Clin Pharmacol* 1986;21:259–265.

72. Harry JD, Marlow HF, Wardelworth AG, Young J. The action of ICI 118,587 (a beta 1 partial agonist) on the heart rate response to exercise in man. *Br J Clin Pharmacol* 1981;12:266P–267P.

73. Molajo AO, Coupe MO, Bennett DH. Effect of Corwin (ICI 118587) on resting and exercise heart rate and exercise tolerance in digitalized patients with chronic atrial fibrillation. *Br Heart J* 1984;52:392–395.

74. Ang EL, Chan WL, Cleland JGF, et al. Placebo controlled trial of xamoterol versus digoxin in chronic atrial fibrillation. *Br Heart J* 1990;64:256–260.

75. The Xamoterol in Severe Heart Failure Study Group. Xamoterol in severe heart failure. *Lancet* 1990;336:1–6.

76. Antman EM, Beamer AD, Cantillon C, McGowan N, Friedman PL. Therapy of refractory symptomatic atrial fibrillation and atrial flutter: a staged care approach with new antiarrhythmic drugs. *J Am Coll Cardiol* 1990;15:698–707.

77. Campbell T, Gavaghan TP, Morgan JJ. Intravenous sotalol for the treatment of atrial fibrillation and flutter after cardiopulmonary bypass: comparison with disopyramide and digoxin in a randomized trial. *Br Heart J* 1985;54:86–90.

78. Shenasa M, Denker S, Mahmud R, et al. Effect of amiodarone on conduction and refractoriness of the His-Purkinje system in the human heart. *J Am Coll Cardiol* 1984;4:105–110.

79. Perelman MS, McKenna WJ, Rowland E, Krikler DM. A comparison of bepridil with amiodarone in the treatment of established atrial fibrillation. *Br Heart J* 1987;58:339–344.

80. Blevins RD, Kerin NZ, Benaderet D, et al. Amiodarone in the management of refractory atrial fibrillation. *Arch Intern Med* 1987;147:1401–1404.

81. Horowitz LN, Spielman SR, Greenspan AM, et al. Use of amiodarone in the treatment of persistent and paroxysmal atrial fibrillation resistant to quinidine therapy. *J Am Coll Cardiol* 1985;6:1402–1407.

82. Cowan JC, Gardiner P, Reid DS, Newell DJ, Campbell RWF. A comparison of amiodarone and digoxin in the treatment of atrial fibrillation complicating suspected acute myocardial infarction. *J Cardiovasc Pharmacol* 1986;8:252–256.

83. Kerr CR, Klein GH, Axelson JF, Cooper JC. Propafenone for prevention of recurrent atrial fibrillation. *Am J Cardiol* 188;61:914–916.

84. Chouty F, Coumel P. Oral flecainide for prophylaxis of paroxysmal atrial fibrillation. *Am J Cardiol* 1988;62(suppl D):35D–37D.

85. Suttorp MJ, Kingma JH, Lie AHL, Mast EG. Intravenous flecainide versus verapamil for acute conversion of paroxysmal atrial fibrillation or flutter to sinus rhythm. *Am J Cardiol* 1989;63:693–698.

86. Bianconi L, Boccadamo R, Pappalardo A, Gentili C, Pistolese M. Effectiveness of intravenous propafenone for conversion of atrial fibrillation and flutter of recent onset. *Am J Cardiol* 1989;64:335–338.

87. Marcus FI. The hazards of using type IC antiarrhythmic agent for the treatment of paroxysmal atrial fibrillation. *Am J Cardiol* 1990;66:366–367.

88. Timm CT, Knowlton AA, Battinelli NJ, Falk RH. Flecainide for heart rate control in atrial fibrillation. *J Am Coll Cardiol* 1989;13:164A.

89. Falk RH. Flecainide-induced ventricular tachycardia and fibrillation in patients treated for atrial fibrillation. *Ann Intern Med* 1989;111:107–111.

90. Reinkenberger RL, Naccarelli GV, Miles WM, et al. Encainide for atrial fibrillation associated with Wolff-Parkinson-White syndrome. *Am J Cardiol* 1988;62:26L–30L.
91. The Cardiac Arrhythmia Suppression Trial (CAST) Investigators. Increased mortality due to encainide or flecainide in a randomized trial of arrhythmia suppression after myocardial infarction. *N Engl J Med* 1989;321:406–412.

Atrial Fibrillation: Mechanisms and Management, edited by
R. H. Falk and P. J. Podrid.
Raven Press, Ltd., New York © 1992.

15

Proarrhythmic Responses to Atrial Antiarrhythmic Therapy

Rodney H. Falk

*Division of Cardiology, Boston City Hospital, Boston, Massachusetts 02118
and Boston University School of Medicine, Boston, Massachusetts 02118*

The concept of arrhythmia aggravation by antiarrhythmic agents, commonly termed "proarrhythmia," has received much attention over the past decade in patients being treated for ventricular arrhythmia. Since the study by Velebit et al. (1) in 1982, which documented 6% to 16% worsening of arrhythmia in patients undergoing acute drug testing for the treatment of ventricular arrhythmia, several investigations have examined the phenomenon of proarrhythmia and have defined subgroups of patients at high and low risk, as well as associated factors and specific antiarrhythmic agents more likely to cause arrhythmia aggravation (2–5).

Two relatively distinct types of ventricular proarrhythmia exist, either the worsening of a preexisting arrhythmia or the occurrence of an arrhythmia not previously experienced. The most serious new arrhythmias are monomorphic and polymorphic ventricular tachycardia (VT), either of which may degenerate into ventricular fibrillation (VF). Until recently the profile of patients treated for ventricular arrhythmia who developed drug-induced monomorphic VT or VF was considered to consist predominantly of those with prior significant ventricular arrhythmia particularly in the presence of a reduced ejection fraction (2–5). Patients treated for asymptomatic "benign" ventricular arrhythmias were generally considered to tolerate antiarrhythmic therapy well, although they are the group for whom potential clinical benefit is least apparent.

The results of the Cardiac Arrhythmia Suppression Trial (CAST) study raised doubts about these observations (6). Until the premature termination of the flecainide and encainide arms of this study in 1989, proarrhythmia was thought to be a phenomenon occurring early after initiation of drug therapy or after a change in dosage. The CAST study demonstrated that, for the class IC agents encainide and flecainide, the risk of sudden death was not clustered at the onset of therapy but appeared ongoing throughout the follow-up period. In addition, the excess of deaths occurred in a group of patients who had premature ventricular contractions but had never previously experienced malignant ventricular arrhythmias. As a result of this study there has been a major reconsideration of the approach to patients with ventricular arrhythmias, particularly those with nonsustained VT or isolated, frequent premature ventricular contractions (7–10).

Many authorities consider patients with supraventricular arrhythmias to be at extremely low risk of arrhythmia aggravation by antiarrhythmic agents. However, a distinction should be made between patients treated for reentrant atrioventricular (AV) nodal or AV tachycardia and atrial flutter or fibrillation. In the former group, structural abnormality of the heart (other than the electrophysiologic abnormality) is uncommon, whereas patients with atrial fibrillation/flutter not infrequently have underlying heart disease and, consequently, may be at greater risk of adverse cardiac effects of antiarrhythmic agents. Indeed, the earliest reports of quinidine-induced VT were in patients treated for atrial fibrillation (11–13).

In addition to the potential for provocation of ventricular arrhythmia, a number of other adverse effects on cardiac rhythm may occur in patients treated for atrial fibrillation (Table 1). Conversion of atrial fibrillation to atrial flutter with a relatively slow atrial rate may decrease or abolish anterograde concealed conduction within the AV node resulting in an increase in ventricular response associated with hemodynamic compromise. In patients treated for paroxysmal atrial fibrillation, antiarrhythmic agents may suppress the sinus node following a run of tachycardia resulting in prolonged post-tachycardia sinus arrest. Rarely, AV block may be provoked by antiarrhythmic agents. Finally, evidence exists that occasional cases of paroxysmal atrial fibrillation may be converted into sustained arrhythmia by digoxin or calcium channel-blocking agents. For the purpose of this chapter all of the above events are considered as arrhythmia aggravation in patients with atrial fibrillation.

TORSADES DE POINTES

The provocation of polymorphic or monomorphic VT by antiarrhythmic drugs is the most serious complication of pharmacologic treatment of atrial fibrillation. Un-

---

TABLE 1. *Types of proarrhythmia produced by drugs used for atrial fibrillation*

Ventricular arrhythmias
  Torsades de pointes
  Monomorphic ventricular tachycardia
Atrial arrhythmias
  Conversion of atrial fibrillation to atrial flutter
  Increased frequency/duration of paroxysmal atrial fibrillation
  Conversion of paroxysmal to sustained atrial fibrillation
  Incessant atrial tachycardia (rare)
Conduction disturbances
  Acceleration of ventricular rate due to
  1. Enhanced AV nodal conduction
  2. Slowing of atrial rate
  3. Conversion of atrial fibrillation to atrial flutter
  4. Preferential conduction down accessory pathway
  Development of AV block manifest as
  1. Atrial fibrillation with symptomatic bradycardia
  2. AV block after reversion to sinus rhythm
  Aggravation of sinus node disease
  1. Prolonged offset pause after cardioversion or after termination of paroxysmal atrial fibrillation
  2. Sinus bradycardia/arrest after reversions to sinus rhythm

like monomorphic VT, polymorphic VT associated with QT prolongation (known as torsades de pointes) commonly occurs in patients with a normal or near-normal ventricle (14) (Fig. 1). Most commonly seen with type IA antiarrhythmics (quinidine, procainamide, and disopyramide) torsades may be provoked by other agents such as amiodarone and sotalol (which also markedly prolong the QT interval), but it is rarely caused by the IB or IC agents, whose effects on the T wave are minimal.

The prevalence of and risk factors for development of proarrhythmia in patients treated for atrial fibrillation have not been as well studied as in patients receiving therapy for ventricular arrhythmia. Although many patients with atrial fibrillation have abnormal ventricles, a considerable number have normal or near-normal ventricular function. It is therefore perhaps not surprising that a high proportion of cases of ventricular arrhythmia provoked by atrial antiarrhythmic agents are due to torsades de pointes. However, while torsades is proportionately a more common side effect than monomorphic VT in this group of patients, there is no evidence to suggest that the absolute risk of torsades is greater in patients receiving antiarrhythmic therapy for atrial fibrillation than in patients receiving similar therapy for ventricular arrhythmia.

Quinidine

In an early, nonrandomized British study of quinidine prophylaxis following electrical cardioversion for atrial fibrillation, Radford and Evans (15) noted two deaths and one new episode of sustained VT among 34 patients receiving quinidine compared to no deaths in a group of 85 patients receiving no prophylactic therapy. As a

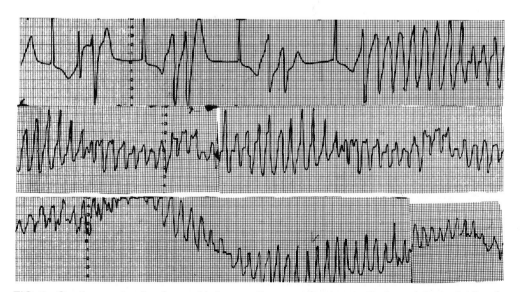

FIG. 1. Continuous tracing from a Holter monitor recording in a patient receiving quinidine for the maintenance of sinus rhythm after cardioversion for atrial fibrillation. A prolonged episode of torsades de pointes is seen, which occurred during sleep when the sinus rate was low. This terminated spontaneously (not shown).

result of these events, the trial was prematurely terminated and quinidine prophylaxis rapidly fell into disfavor in the United Kingdom (16). Campbell (17) in 1980
pooled the data from 11 studies (both randomized and nonrandomized) and noted
six deaths among 693 quinidine-treated patients, compared to a "very low" mortality
in the untreated group, suggesting that quinidine was the cause of deaths in these
subjects.

A recent, meta-analysis of six randomized, controlled trials of quinidine prophylaxis published between 1970 and 1984 totaling 808 patients has led to renewed concerns about the safety of quinidine in atrial fibrillation. Coplen and colleagues (18)
found an unadjusted total mortality rate of 2.9% in quinidine-treated patients (12 of
413) compared to 0.8% (3 of 387) in the control groups—a threefold increase. It is
important to note that these figures represent all modes of death and that the precise
cause of death was documented in only seven of the 12 quinidine-treated patients.
Three of these seven deaths were sudden, two were due to stroke, one to suicide,
and one to myocardial infarction. Of the remaining five deaths, two patients had
cancer, one pneumonia, and one hepatic failure as contributing causes, and one died
of undocumented causes. Assuming that the sudden deaths were due to ventricular
arrhythmia, the overall prevalence of malignant arrhythmia in the quinidine group
(including two nonfatal cardiac arrests) was 1.2% (1.5% if the unclassified death was
arrhythmic) compared to 0% (or 0.25%) in the control group.

Quinidine-induced torsades has a number of predisposing factors (14). Roden et
al. (19) reviewed their experience with quinidine therapy and described 20 patients
with torsades de pointes. They noted that half of these patients received the drug for
atrial arrhythmias, and, while most developed torsades within 48 hr of starting quinidine, four subjects had been receiving the therapy for more than 1 year. Based on
their overall experience, they estimated a minimal annual risk for the development
of torsades de pointes of 1.5%. Several risk factors for the development of this arrhythmia were noted, specifically low serum potassium levels and excessive bradycardia. Two-thirds of patients had a serum potassium level less than 4.0 mEq/liter,
and hypomagnesemia was present in one-third of the cases in which this electrolyte
was measured. Of note, a clear-cut complicating feature was present in each of the
four patients who developed torsades after more than 1 year of therapy: hypokalemia
in three and AV block in the fourth. Six of the eight patients receiving quinidine for
atrial fibrillation developed torsades only after conversion of AF to sinus rhythm,
and the rhythm prior to torsades was unknown in two.

The finding that restoration of sinus rhythm after an episode of atrial fibrillation
may have been a factor in precipitating torsades is not surprising. Bradycardia as a
precipitating factor of this arrhythmia is well recognized, and its propensity for producing torsades has been attributed, among other causes, to the provocation of early
afterdepolarizations (20). These abnormal cellular oscillatory phenomena are believed to be due to an imbalance between the inward sodium current and the repo-
larizing potassium current and, when present, are more prominent at slower stimulation rates. Bradycardia, low extracellular potassium, and quinidine (particularly at
low concentrations) may all affect potassium flux more than sodium flux, resulting
in early afterdepolarizations. Indeed, it has been suggested that a low serum quinidine may be more likely to result in torsades than higher levels, since higher serum
levels depress sodium current and restore the sodium-potassium balance, potentially
reducing the likelihood of the development of early afterdepolarizations (21).

Procainamide

Torsades in patients treated for atrial fibrillation has been noted with procainamide and, as with quinidine, hypokalemia is considered to be a major precipitating factor (22–24). Although quinidine-associated torsades is not related to drug levels and may occur at subtherapeutic doses, it has been suggested that procainamide-induced torsades may be more common in patients with elevated levels of N-acetylprocainamide, the first metabolite of procainamide (23,24). No study has attempted to systematically assess the incidence of procainamide-induced torsades.

Sotalol

Sotalol, a class III agent with beta-blocking properties also causes torsades (25,26). Unlike the QT prolongation seen with quinidine, which may be prominent at low serum levels, that due to sotalol is primarily concentration dependent (27) and sotalol overdose is commonly complicated by torsades (26). As with the type IA agents, sotalol-induced torsades is aggravated by hypokalemia, and the combination of sotalol with a diuretic in a single tablet has been implicated as a serious risk factor for this arrhythmia in patients receiving therapy for hypertension (25).

High sotalol levels may be a precipitating factor for torsades, an observation noted by several authors. In a comparative study of slow-release quinidine sulfate 600 mg twice daily for the maintenance of sinus rhythm following electrical cardioversion, Jull-Moller et al. (28) noted one episode of drug-induced VF in 85 patients receiving quinidine and one episode of torsades among 97 patients receiving sotalol (this occurred in a patient receiving 80 mg twice daily). Both episodes occurred during sinus rhythm and within 24 hr of commencing therapy. In contrast to the above study, four episodes of torsades and four sudden deaths were seen among a similar number of patients receiving higher doses of sotalol for the maintenance of sinus rhythm after an episode of atrial fibrillation. Three of the deaths and three episodes of torsades occurred in patients receiving 640 mg daily of sotalol and one death and one case of torsades occurred in patients receiving 480 mg daily (R. Saini, *personal communication*). Almost all events occurred after reversion to sinus rhythm (Fig. 2). As a result of these findings, it is recommended that the maximal dose of sotalol for maintenance of sinus rhythm should not exceed 480 mg daily.

Other Agents

Many of the antiarrhythmic agents less commonly used in the United States for maintenance of sinus rhythm in patients with prior atrial fibrillation have occasionally been implicated in the genesis of torsades. These include amiodarone (29,30), which had also been used successfully to terminate torsades (14). The arrhythmia is said to be very uncommon with the IC agents, which have minimal effects on the QT interval (31).

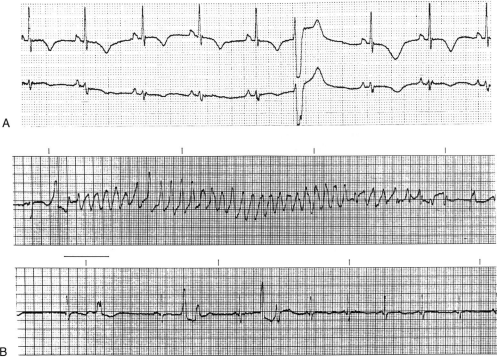

FIG. 2. A: Simultaneous leads from a Holter recording 24 hr after DC conversion from atrial fibrillation in a patient receiving sotalol 640 mg daily. Note the excessive QT prolongation in the sinus beat following a PVC, suggesting a pathologic abnormality of repolarization. **B:** Transtelephonic ECG from the same patient 2 days later during a dizzy spell. The basic rhythm is sinus. A 9-sec run of torsades de pointes occurs. (Top and bottom strips are same lead recorded within seconds of one another.) Neither symptoms nor arrhythmia occurred while the patient was in atrial fibrillation, during 9 days of sotalol therapy.

MONOMORPHIC VENTRICULAR TACHYCARDIA/VENTRICULAR FIBRILLATION

In patients treated with antiarrhythmic agents for nonsustained ventricular arrhythmias, the development of sustained VT or VF temporally related to drug therapy is not uncommon and is considered a proarrhythmic response. Patients with atrial fibrillation associated with ventricular dysfunction may have concomitant ventricular arrhythmia, and provocation of sustained ventricular arrhythmia during therapy for atrial fibrillation is most probably a function of the underlying ventricular

FIG. 3. A: Twelve-lead ECG at peak exercise in a patient with atrial fibrillation in the absence of underlying heart disease receiving digoxin 0.25 mg and flecainide 100 mg twice daily. The ventricular response is close to 200 beats per minute, with a shortest R-R interval (*arrow*) of 240 msec (paper speed 25 mm/sec). **B:** Immediately postexercise (18.5 min on a modified Bruce protocol) ventricular flutter (VF) occurs (note paper speed of 50 mm/sec). **C:** Twelve-lead ECG of ventricular flutter/fibrillation immediately before defibrillation. (From ref. 35, with permission.)

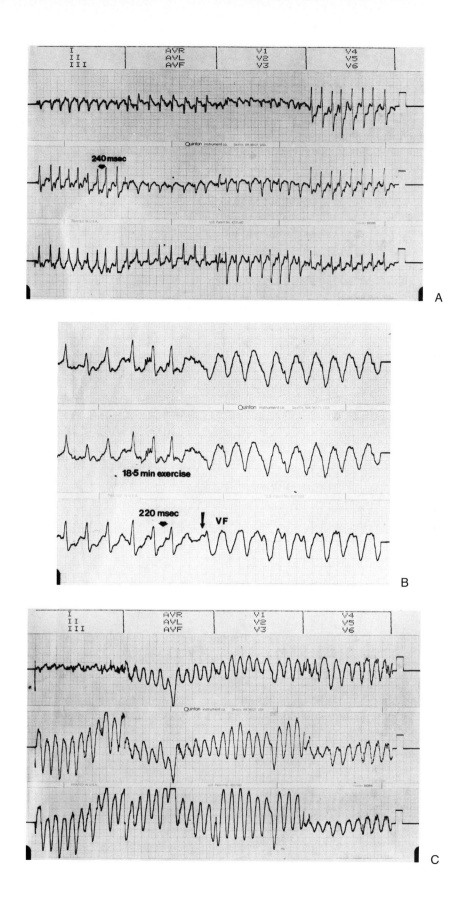

disease. Other than polymorphic VT, reports of significant drug-induced ventricular arrhythmias in patients treated for atrial fibrillation are rare, presumably because of the relatively low prevalence of significant ventricular dysfunction in many series. The type IC agents, which have been implicated in causing an increased risk of sudden death when used after myocardial infarction, have generally had a good safety profile for treatment of atrial fibrillation (32–34). However, a small series of cases suggested that, in the setting of chronic atrial fibrillation, the use of flecainide may cause life-threatening ventricular arrhythmias during vigorous exertion in patients without significant ventricular dysfunction (35) (Fig. 3). It is hypothesized that the very rapid and irregular ventricular rate, combined with the use-dependent properties of these drugs and the high levels of circulating catecholamines, may result in enough inhomogeneity of conduction in a minimally diseased ventricle to produce a substrate suitable for sustained ventricular arrhythmia (36,37).

ABERRANT VENTRICULAR CONDUCTION

Rate-related bundle branch block is a well-recognized phenomenon in supraventricular tachycardia and in patients with conduction system disease (38). Although bundle branch block may be precipitated by a variety of classes of antiarrhythmic agents in susceptible patients, the IC agents are especially prone to this phenomenon, particularly at high heart rates (Fig. 4). Rate-related widening of the QRS with IC agents may occur in the absence of prior conduction system disease as it is related to the use-dependent characteristics of these drugs. The QRS complexes may appear bizarrely widened and can have a surface ECG characteristic of VT (Fig. 5) (37,39).

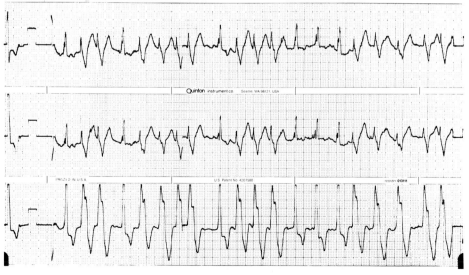

FIG. 4. Simultaneous leads 2, AVF and V5 during exercise in a patient with chronic atrial fibrillation receiving digoxin 0.25 mg daily and flecainide 100 mg twice daily. The majority of beats are conducted aberrantly with a left bundle branch block configuration. On digoxin alone, no aberration occurred even at a higher ventricular rate than illustrated.

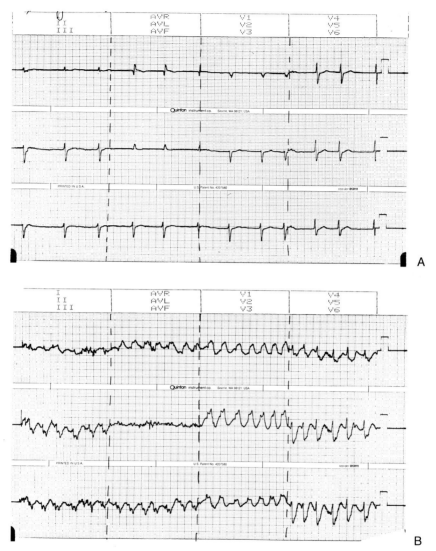

FIG. 5. A: Resting 12-lead ECG in a patient with chronic atrial fibrillation receiving digoxin 0.25 mg daily and flecainide 100 mg twice daily. **B:** Same patient at peak exercise. The rapid ventricular response is conducted with a very wide bizarre QRS morphology, resulting from the use-dependent properties of flecainide.

In patients with atrial fibrillation treated with IC agents, QRS widening frequently increases modestly at faster heart rates but may also show intermittent profound aberration precipitated by long-short cycles. In a small series of patients, Crijns et al. (39) noted that runs of aberrantly conducted ventricular complexes during atrial fibrillation were always irregular, giving a clue to their supraventricular origin.

As described below, the conversion of atrial fibrillation to atrial flutter during treatment with flecainide or encainide has been associated with 1:1 AV nodal transmission with aberrant ventricular conduction.

DRUG-INDUCED ACCELERATION OF VENTRICULAR RESPONSE TO ATRIAL FIBRILLATION

Acceleration of the ventricular response to atrial fibrillation or flutter may result in hemodynamic deterioration. Heart rate acceleration may occur as a result of the conversion of atrial fibrillation to flutter, the vagolytic effect on the AV node of certain agents, sympathetic nervous system activation, or drug-induced preferential conduction down an accessory pathway.

Quinidine

Quinidine-induced ventricular rate acceleration in patients with atrial flutter has been recognized for many years and is due to a critical combination of slowing of the flutter rate and a vagolytic-mediated increase in AV conduction. The recognition of this potentially hazardous effect led, almost half a century ago, to the recommendation to use digitalis glycosides concomitantly with quinidine in order to increase AV nodal block (40,41). However, the use of digoxin prior to quinidine therapy is not a guarantee against 1:1 AV nodal conduction, which, although rare, may be associated with severe hemodynamic impairment (42) (Fig. 6).

Organization of atrial fibrillation into atrial flutter may occur during pharmacologic therapy of atrial fibrillation and may be associated with a significant heart rate increase. The exact prevalence of this complication during therapy of atrial fibrillation with currently used doses of quinidine (e.g., 800–1,200 mg of quinidine sulfate daily) is not known, but prior to the advent of electrical cardioversion, when a dose of 3,200 mg daily was routinely used in attempts to convert atrial fibrillation to sinus rhythm (43), the development of atrial flutter was common. In a series of 115 patients with atrial fibrillation treated with this dose of quinidine, in conjunction with digitalis (44), sinus rhythm was restored in 72 patients, 27 of whom developed atrial flutter prior to restoration of sinus rhythm. An additional 39 patients converted from atrial fibrillation to flutter without subsequent restoration of sinus rhythm. The mean atrial rate during flutter was 188, and three patients developed 1:1 conduction (2.6% of all patients treated and 4.5% of those with flutter).

Controversy exists regarding the necessity of concomitant digoxin use when quinidine is used for the maintenance of sinus rhythm. Grande et al. (45) have suggested that the combination of digoxin and quinidine may slightly reduce the efficacy of the latter drug, whereas other investigators have found no adverse effect (28). In the comparative study of quinidine sulfate and sotalol for the maintenance of sinus rhythm described above (28), eight patients receiving sotalol reverted to atrial fibrillation and the mean ventricular response was slower than that prior to cardioversion when they were receiving either no therapy or digoxin alone. However, quinidine-treated subjects reverting to atrial fibrillation had a statistically higher ventricular rate than at baseline, and the presence or absence of concomitant digoxin therapy did not affect the mean ventricular rate. No details of digoxin dose or serum levels were given, and therefore inadequate dosage of digoxin as a cause of the increased rate cannot be excluded.

Conversion of atrial fibrillation to flutter in patients treated with the lower doses of quinidine currently in use appears relatively infrequent and 1:1 conduction is very rarely seen. At most, any increase in ventricular response to atrial fibrillation pro-

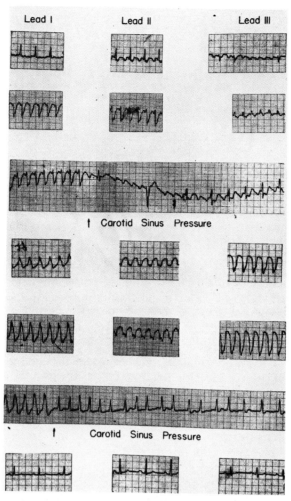

FIG. 6. Drug-induced 1:1 AV conduction in a patient receiving quinidine. **A:** ECG on admission showing atrial flutter with variable block. **B:** After 0.3 mg digitoxin and 100 mg quinidine sulfate, a rapid wide-complex tachycardia develops, associated with hemodynamic collapse. **C:** Carotid sinus massage revealing atrial flutter with transient high degree of block, reverting to 2:1 block at exactly half the rate of the wide-complex tachycardia. The flutter rate has slowed, compared to admission, as a result of the quinidine. **D:** Recurrence of wide-complex tachycardia despite adequate digitalization occurring 12 hr later after a total of 3,400 mg quinidine. This terminates with carotid pressure. **E:** Further episode at 7 days. **F:** Conversion of flutter with 1:1 conduction to atrial fibrillation with a slower ventricular response. **G:** Reversion to sinus rhythm on no antiarrhythmic therapy (day 45). (From ref. 42, with permission.)

voked by quinidine is modest and rarely of clinical significance. Nevertheless, it is frequent practice to prescribe digoxin concomitantly with quinidine prior to attempted cardioversion and to continue it as maintenance therapy after reversion to sinus rhythm. In a patient who has demonstrated poor rate control during atrial fibrillation while receiving digoxin or who has a tendency to develop atrial flutter alternating with fibrillation, serious consideration should be given to combining quinidine with a small dose of a beta-blocking agent rather than with digoxin, as the latter agent may be ineffective under conditions of heightened sympathetic tone.

Other IA Agents

Both disopyramide (46) and procainamide (47) have been associated with an accelerated ventricular response during atrial flutter and presumably may cause a paradoxical heart rate increase should atrial fibrillation convert to flutter with a relatively slow rate during therapy. The negative inotropic effect of disopyramide (48) in conjunction with a rapid ventricular response may be particularly harmful.

Lidocaine

Lidocaine therapy is generally considered of value only for ventricular arrhythmias. A mild and inconsistent increase in AV conduction has been demonstrated (49), but the effects of lidocaine on the atrium are not well recognized. In an animal model of atrial fibrillation, in which atrial fibrillation was induced by mechanical stimulation of the atrium in alpha-chloralose-anesthetized dogs, lidocaine was uniformly effective in terminating the arrhythmia (50). Alpha-chloralose is a powerful parasympathetomimetic agent, and its use in animals is associated with sinus bradycardia and AV block. Atrial fibrillation induced under these conditions was associated with a rapid intra-atrial electrogram and a slow ventricular response. The use of lidocaine decreased the atrial rate during atrial fibrillation and was associated with a marked increase in ventricular response due, presumably, to decreased anterograde concealed AV nodal conduction. This observation suggests that, at least under conditions of enhanced vagal tone, lidocaine decreases the rate or number of fibrillatory waves in the atrium.

Isolated case reports in humans have documented an increase in ventricular response during lidocaine therapy given for ventricular arrhythmias to patients who also have atrial flutter (51,52). In a systematic study of this phenomenon, Danahy and Aronow (53) reported on 18 patients with atrial flutter and 35 patients with atrial fibrillation who received 100 mg of intravenous lidocaine. A prompt decrease in atrial rate, peaking at 1 to 2 min and resolving by 20 min, occurred in all patients with atrial flutter. Three patients with flutter (17%) increased their ventricular response by more than 20 beats per minute (maximal increase 47 beats per minute) due to an increased degree of AV nodal conduction. In the patients with atrial fibrillation given lidocaine, the mean ventricular rate for the group increased by only six beats per minute. However, three patients (8.6%) developed a heart rate increase of more than 20 beats per minute with a maximal increase of 40 to 50 beats per minute. Of note, the concomitant use of quinidine in 15 patients with atrial fibrillation appeared to be associated with a lidocaine-induced increase in ventricular response. In view of these observations, it appears prudent to be cautious about lidocaine use for treating ventricular arrhythmias in patients with atrial fibrillation, particularly if quinidine therapy has been started.

Since aberrant ventricular conduction may mimic VT and since a rapid ventricular response to atrial fibrillation may itself predispose to ventricular arrhythmias, lidocaine may not necessarily be appropriate therapy for suspected VT occurring in association with atrial fibrillation. Heart rate control by digoxin or beta-blocking or calcium-channel-blocking agents (or electrical cardioversion if the hemodynamic status is precarious) may be the preferred choice for suspected ventricular arrhythmias in this setting.

Encainide, Flecainide, and Propafenone

The type IC agents encainide, flecainide, and propafenone present a rather unique problem when used for the treatment of atrial fibrillation. Clinical trials have demonstrated efficacy of these agents for terminating recent-onset atrial fibrillation or maintaining sinus rhythm following cardioversion (32–34,54,55), and they are generally well tolerated. The IC drugs manifest the phenomenon of use-dependence in which their effect on blockade of the fast-channel sodium current is increasingly prominent with increasing rates of stimulation (37). This phenomenon, although not unique to type IC agents, is most prominent with this class of drug and may result in a marked QRS widening at rapid ventricular rates, making electrocardiographic differentiation between supraventricular and ventricular tachycardia extremely difficult (39).

As with other antiarrhythmic drugs, flecainide, encainide, and propafenone may organize and slow the rate of atrial fibrillation and convert it to atrial flutter with a slow enough atrial rate for 1:1 conduction to occur. When this happens, the rapid ventricular response is often aberrantly conducted with bizarre wide complexes similar to those that may occur with atrial fibrillation and a rapid ventricular response (Fig. 5).

Murdock et al. (56) noted the occurrence of atrial flutter in 14 of 82 patients treated with propafenone for atrial fibrillation. Eight of the 14 patients had never before had documented flutter. Three patients (one receiving concomitant quinidine therapy) developed 1:1 AV conduction with ventricular rates of 200 to 275 beats per minute and QRS widths of up to 160 msec. An additional two patients developed a wide-complex ventricular response during atrial flutter with 2:1 AV block. A similar phenomenon has been observed during therapy with flecainide and encainide (57,58) and has been described in 3.5% of patients receiving the investigational IC agent recainam (58).

The overall incidence of the transformation of atrial fibrillation to flutter appears to be in the range of 3.5% to 5%, and it may result in significant hemodynamic compromise in the setting of 1:1 AV nodal conduction. Consequently, it has been suggested that it is wise to use concomitant beta-blocking agents, digoxin, or calcium blockers when using IC agents for the treatment of atrial fibrillation, particularly if atrial flutter has previously occurred (39,56). The safety of verapamil combined with flecainide has been shown in a small, selected series of patients (34), but caution is warranted in subjects with reduced ventricular function in view of the potential for additive negative inotropic effects. Digoxin in combination with flecainide has a modest effect in controlling the ventricular rate during exercise in patients with atrial fibrillation (59), but there is no firm evidence that its use will be adequate to prevent 1:1 conduction should atrial flutter occur. As with verapamil, beta-blocking agents are potentially negatively inotropic when used in conjunction with IC agents (60), but we believe this combination to be safe in the presence of normal ventricular function. In selected patients, beta-blockers have been shown to be effective in preventing the ventricular proarrhythmic effects of flecainide and to be well tolerated despite a reduced ejection fraction (61).

AGGRAVATION OF ATRIAL ARRHYTHMIA

The recognition of arrhythmia aggravation by antiarrhythmic agents is confounded by many variables, including the spontaneous variability of "stable" arrhythmia (62), changes in myocardial substrate, and shifts in electrolyte balance. In patients treated pharmacologically for nonsustained ventricular arrhythmia, the development of sustained VT or VF is highly suggestive of a proarrhythmic response (3,5). Other probable manifestations include an increase in the frequency of arrhythmia, increased ease of inducibility of ventricular arrhythmia during electrophysiology testing, and the degeneration of a previously relatively slow VT into a poorly tolerated tachycardia of shorter cycle length (62).

Clearly, in patients with chronic atrial fibrillation, true aggravation of atrial arrhythmia is not a consideration, and isolated atrial premature beats so rarely need therapy that no data exist on the likelihood of converting them to a sustained atrial tachycardia, flutter, or fibrillation. Even the examples of conversion of fibrillation to flutter with increased ventricular response, described above, are not true examples of proarrhythmia but rather reflect an incomplete manifestation of the desired properties of the drug, i.e., organization of atrial activity.

Paroxysmal atrial fibrillation offers a possibility to examine the incidence of aggravation of arrhythmia in terms of increased frequency and duration of episodes, although the sporadic nature of this arrhythmia defies attempts to formalize criteria for an exact definition of atrial proarrhythmia (63,64). Elsewhere in this volume, Coumel describes his experience with a variety of antiarrhythmic agents in neurally mediated atrial fibrillation and notes a potential for increased paroxysms of arrhythmia with the use of propafenone, digoxin, and beta-blocking agents when vagotonia is the precipitating event.

Digoxin

Digoxin is often used in paroxysmal atrial fibrillation in an attempt to reduce the frequency of paroxysms or to slow the ventricular response should an episode of atrial fibrillation occur. However, the role of digoxin in paroxysmal atrial fibrillation when heart failure is absent is controversial. Although proposed as having an atrial antiarrhythmic effect by some authors (65), we have found no benefit from digoxin over placebo in terminating atrial fibrillation of less than 1 week duration unassociated with heart failure (66). Indeed patients receiving digoxin who converted to sinus rhythm had a tendency to remain in atrial fibrillation prior to conversion longer than those who converted after receiving placebo. A similar observation was made by Rawles and co-workers (67), who examined Holter monitor tracings in 72 patients with one or more paroxysms of atrial fibrillation. Although the mean number of paroxysms and the ventricular rate did not differ between the digoxin and nondigoxin groups, significantly more episodes of arrhythmia lasting for 30 min or longer occurred in the patients receiving digoxin. The investigators calculated a relative risk of 4.3 (confidence intervals 1.6–11.9) for having a prolonged episode of atrial fibrillation associated with digoxin use.

Occasionally the tendency of digoxin to prolong episodes of atrial fibrillation in certain patients may transform paroxysmal to sustained atrial fibrillation, and this has been used therapeutically to reduce symptoms associated with the paroxysmal onset of the arrhythmia (68). In a patient with troublesome, drug-resistant atrial fibrillation receiving maintenance digoxin, it is our practice to stop digoxin and reassess the arrhythmia, with occasionally gratifying results.

Verapamil and Diltiazem

Calcium channel blockers have also been incriminated in prolonging, and occasionally precipitating, atrial fibrillation, although the exact mechanism remains unclear. We have described the development of atrial fibrillation in a normal subject following a 10-mg injection of verapamil (69), and in animals verapamil has been demonstrated to increase the inducibility and persistence of induced atrial fibrillation (70).

Shenasa et al. (71) studied 35 patients at electrophysiology study, 17 of whom had never had documented paroxysmal atrial fibrillation. Atrial fibrillation induction was attempted by single, double, and triple atrial extrastimuli at two drive cycle lengths, followed if necessary by rapid atrial pacing. The arrhythmia was induced at baseline in 17 of 18 patients with prior atrial fibrillation and lasted for a mean of 31 ± 12 min. Following intravenous verapamil or diltiazem, atrial fibrillation in this group persisted for 112 ± 49 min. In patients given oral verapamil, the induced arrhythmia lasted 69 ± 35 min. Both of these values (after intravenous or oral drug) were highly significant compared to baseline ($p < 0.001$). A similar phenomenon of prolonged episodes of atrial fibrillation was noted in patients who had never experienced spontaneous arrhythmia, although the ease of induction and duration of sustained arrhythmia were less than in those with spontaneous paroxysmal fibrillation.

Calcium channel blockers have little demonstrable effect on the intact human atrium (72,73), and it has been suggested that changes in sympathetic tone due to acute vasodilation may be the cause of provocation of atrial fibrillation. However, the finding that the oral forms of diltiazem and verapamil cause persistence of induced atrial fibrillation suggests that the mechanism cannot be fully explained on the basis of autonomic changes. Aizawa et al. (74) have suggested that the mechanism of increased inducibility of the arrhythmia after verapamil may be related to augmented fragmentation of atrial activity resulting from premature atrial extrastimuli, and this may be partly responsible for persistent arrhythmia.

ADVERSE EFFECTS OF DRUGS IN ATRIAL FIBRILLATION ASSOCIATED WITH WOLFF-PARKINSON-WHITE SYNDROME

The management of atrial fibrillation in Wolff-Parkinson-White (WPW) syndrome is dealt with in detail by Wellens elsewhere in this volume and will be considered here only briefly. In patients with a short refractory period of the accessory pathway, the ventricular response to atrial fibrillation may be exceedingly rapid and spontaneous VF may occasionally ensue (75). Agents such as calcium channel blockers, which are highly effective in slowing the ventricular rate to atrial fibrillation in patients without preexcitation, have minimal effects on the accessory pathway and their use may seriously aggravate a patient's condition by producing an acceleration in ventricular response, resulting in marked hemodynamic deterioration (Fig. 7).

Several reports have documented the adverse effects of verapamil in preexcited atrial fibrillation (75–77). McGovern et al. (77) reported on five patients referred for

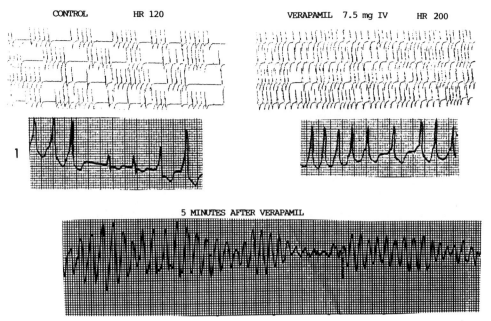

FIG. 7. Adverse effects of verapamil in Wolff-Parkinson-White syndrome. The *upper left panels* show atrial fibrillation conducted with intermittent preexcitation. After 7.5 mg of intravenous verapamil (*right*) the ventricular response markedly increases and all beats are preexcited. Five minutes later, ventricular fibrillation occurs (*lower trace*).

evaluation because of atrial fibrillation associated with WPW who had developed VF or profound hypotension following 5 to 10 mg of intravenous verapamil. Review of tracings available before and after verapamil administration revealed the sudden development of VF in three patients and a marked increase in ventricular response in two. Subsequent electrophysiologic testing in a drug-free state indicated that the shortest R-R interval in induced atrial fibrillation was 160 to 220 msec. Garratt et al. (78) reviewed 18 cases of WPW presenting to an emergency room with preexcited atrial fibrillation, 10 of whom were treated with intravenous verapamil. Six of the 10 patients became hypotensive after intravenous verapamil, of whom four needed urgent direct-current cardioversion.

The exact mechanism of clinical deterioration following intravenous verapamil in WPW syndrome with atrial fibrillation is unclear but is probably multifactorial. Acceleration of the ventricular response may occur as a result of increased AV nodal blockade, which secondarily causes decreased retrograde concealed conduction in the accessory pathway. Alternatively, the rate increase may be secondary to increased sympathetic tone provoked by drug-induced vasodilation. The negative inotropic effect of verapamil may also contribute to hemodynamic deterioration in patients who are barely compensating for the extremely rapid rate and a decrease in an already reduced stroke volume, resulting from ventricular dyssynergy in preexcited beats, may play a role. Whatever the reason, it is clear that verapamil has no role in the management of atrial fibrillation in WPW patients. Unfortunately, the study by Garratt et al. (78) indicates that the diagnosis of preexcited atrial fibrillation is often not considered in patients presenting to an emergency room, and verapamil still continues to be given in error, with serious consequences.

Digoxin

Digoxin, a traditional agent for rate control in atrial fibrillation, has minimal effects on an accessory pathway and acceleration of ventricular response and/or VF is not uncommon (75,79). Consequently digoxin should be studiously avoided for this arrhythmia.

Beta-Blockers

Although beta-blocking agents also have no significant effects on accessory pathway conduction (80) and are thus not indicated in atrial fibrillation associated with WPW, reports of significant adverse effects are rare. Nevertheless, ventricular response acceleration has been reported and may be considerable (81).

Lidocaine

Lidocaine presents an interesting therapeutic problem in patients with preexcited atrial fibrillation, since this arrhythmia is often misdiagnosed as VT, for which lidocaine may be highly effective. Although early reports suggested that lidocaine was effective in slowing conduction through an accessory pathway (80) and in controlling the ventricular response to preexcited atrial fibrillation (82), subsequent studies have found no consistent effects on accessory pathway conduction (83). Indeed Akhtar et al. (83) noted a decrease in the R-R interval following lidocaine during induced atrial fibrillation in five of eight patients with WPW, two of whom had significant hemodynamic deterioration. The exact incidence of serious hemodynamic effects of lidocaine given for WPW in clinical practice is not known, but the absence of published reports suggests that it is rare, and this agent is still considered of value by some authorities.

Amiodarone

An unusual case of ventricular rate acceleration has been reported following intravenous amiodarone therapy for preexcited atrial fibrillation in a patient with a previous inferior wall infarction (84). Amiodarone has been widely and successfully used for WPW patients and such an occurrence appears distinctly unusual.

DIGOXIN CARDIOTOXICITY

Digoxin is still the mainstay for heart rate control in atrial fibrillation. However, digoxin toxicity has been considered to be one of the most common drug reactions seen by practitioners (85,86). Arrhythmias are a well-known manifestation of digoxin toxicity and include paroxysmal atrial tachycardia with block, ventricular bigeminy, VT and VF, and various degrees of AV block.

In a prospective study of digitalis intoxication in admissions to a single hospital undertaken in 1969, 135 patients were determined to be receiving some form of digoxin, representing 15% of all admissions (87). Forty-seven (35%) patients were in atrial fibrillation. The diagnosis of digoxin toxicity was based primarily on ECG rhythm abnormalities and was correlated with serum digoxin levels. Twenty-three percent of patients were considered to be definitely and 6% possibly digoxin toxic, and the predominant toxic arrhythmia was an AV junction escape rhythm. Of note, digoxin toxicity was considered more common (50%) in patients with atrial fibrillation than those with sinus rhythm (13%). Although this paper may have overestimated the prevalence of digoxin toxicity, it is likely that there has been a true reduction in prevalence over the past 20 years. In a retrospective study of digoxin toxicity at a large urban hospital conducted for the period 1980–1988, Mahdyoon et al. (88) concluded that definite criteria for toxicity occurred in only 20% of patients with suspected toxicity. In a 1-year period (1987), 563 patients taking digoxin were admitted to the hospital and only four (0.8%) met criteria for definite digoxin toxicity. The authors attribute this dramatic fall from the 23% estimate of Beller et al. (87) in 1970 to the widespread availability of serum digoxin assays and awareness of the effects of such agents as quinidine, verapamil, and amiodarone on serum digoxin levels.

Despite the marked reduction in the prevalence of digoxin toxicity, it remains a challenging problem in patients with atrial fibrillation in whom the emergence of junctional rhythm, manifest as regularization of cardiac rhythm, may represent the first manifestation of digoxin overdose (85). Progression to junctional rhythm with Wenckebach block leads to a regularly irregular rhythm, which, to the untrained eye, may be mistaken for the irregularly irregular ventricular response of atrial fibrillation. As in sinus rhythm, ventricular bigeminy and VT may occur, progressing, rarely, to a classical biventricular tachycardia (Fig. 8). Recognition of digoxin toxicity is particularly important in patients undergoing cardioversion, since the electric shock may expose serious ventricular arrhythmias (Fig. 9).

The diagnosis of digoxin toxicity may be particularly difficult in patients with atrial fibrillation receiving verapamil or diltiazem, as these agents may cause regularization of the ventricular response even in absence of digoxin (90) and verapamil may elevate serum digoxin levels (91). Although serum digoxin levels correlate poorly with digoxin toxicity, particularly in atrial fibrillation, a high digoxin level in conjunction with a suspicious rhythm is suggestive of toxicity and should mandate a

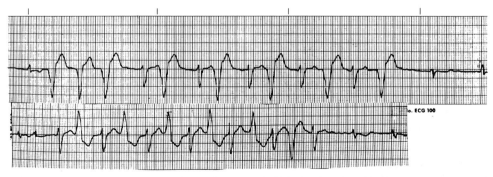

FIG. 8. Noncontinuous, nonsimultaneous tracing. Biventricular tachycardia in a patient with chronic atrial fibrillation and digoxin toxicity. The normal QRS morphology can be seen at the beginning and end of each strip.

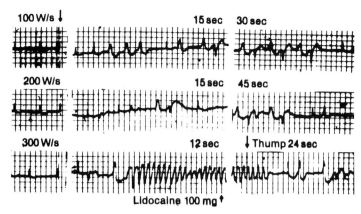

FIG. 9. Attempted cardioversion of atrial fibrillation in a patient with unrecognized digoxin toxicity. After 100-Wsec, short runs of ventricular tachycardia occur, followed at 30 sec by biventricular tachycardia. Similar rhythms occur after 200 Wsec, and after a 200-Wsec shock, polymorphic ventricular tachycardia occurs, terminated with lidocaine and chest thump. (Courtesy of Dr. M. Klein.)

trial of dose reduction. Careful attention to serum levels of potassium, and probably of magnesium, with maintenance well within the normal range is mandatory to reduce the risk of digoxin-induced arrhythmia.

DRUG-INDUCED BRADYCARDIA

Since atrial fibrillation is generally associated with a rapid ventricular response, the aim of therapy is often to normalize the ventricular rate. Not infrequently digoxin, beta-blockers, or calcium channel-blocking agents may be required because of symptomatic exertional tachycardia in a patient whose resting ventricular response is normal. Occasionally, this may result in excessive rate slowing at rest requiring permanent pacing in order to safely administer a drug.

Atrial fibrillation is commonly a concomitant manifestation of sinus node disease, and under these circumstances paroxysmal atrial fibrillation may be followed by symptomatic periods of sinus arrest (Fig. 10). While pharmacologic control of tachycardia may prevent the post-tachycardia pauses (92), incomplete tachycardia control may result in worsening of bradycardia because of further drug-induced sinus node depression. Virtually all antiarrhythmic agents including digoxin, beta-blockers, and calcium channel blockers have been implicated in the aggravation of sick sinus syndrome (93–99), and the aggravation or precipitation of post-tachycardia pauses should be considered in the differential diagnosis of patients treated for paroxysmal atrial fibrillation who develop dizziness or syncope, particularly if excessive pauses have previously been noted. Finally, since atrial fibrillation may be one manifestation of widespread disease of the conduction system, heart block may occasionally be precipitated by atrial antiarrhythmic agents within or, less commonly, below the AV node.

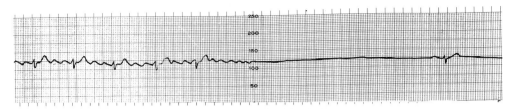

FIG. 10. Termination of an episode of atrial fibrillation in a patient on no therapy with dizziness due to tachycardia-bradycardia syndrome. Attempted pharmacologic suppression of the atrial fibrillation may aggravate the offset pauses if the paroxysms are not totally controlled.

CONCLUSION

As in the case of patients with ventricular arrhythmias, pharmacologic treatment of atrial fibrillation may be associated with serious cardiac toxicity. While the incidence of cardiotoxicity of most drugs used for the therapy of atrial fibrillation is not known, the risk is probably less than that of the same treatment prescribed for ventricular arrhythmia, as the underlying heart disease is often less severe. Nevertheless, the practitioner should be attuned to the potentially serious effects of these agents, which may occasionally manifest themselves after therapy has been well tolerated for weeks or months. It should also be borne in mind that the course and prognosis of atrial fibrillation are more benign than that of sustained ventricular arrhythmias and therefore that any decision to treat should include careful consideration of the relatively small but serious risks of certain agents, which may be weighed against the potential long-term benefits in an individual patient.

REFERENCES

1. Velebit V, Podrid P, Lown B, Cohen BH, Graboys TB. Aggravation and provocation of ventricular arrhythmias by antiarrhythmic drugs. *Circulation* 1982;65:886–894.
2. Morganroth J, Anderson JL, Gentzkow GD. Classification by type of ventricular arrhythmia predicts frequency of adverse cardiac events from flecainide. *J Am Coll Cardiol* 1986;8:607–615.
3. Horowitz LN, Zipes DP, Bigger JT, et al. Proarrhythmia: arrhythmogenesis or aggravation of arrhythmia: a status report, 1987. *Am J Cardiol* 1987;59:54E–56E.
4. Minardo JD, Heger JJ, Miles WM, Zipes DP, Prystowsky EN. Clinical characteristics of patients with ventricular fibrillation during antiarrhythmic drug therapy. *N Engl J Med* 1988;319:257–262.
5. Stanton MS, Prystowsky EN, Fineberg NS, Miles WM, Zipes DP, Heger JJ. Arrhythmogenic effects of antiarrhythmic drug: a study of 506 patients treated for ventricular tachycardia or fibrillation. *J Am Coll Cardiol* 1989;14:209–215.
6. The Cardiac Arrhythmia Suppression Trial (CAST) Investigators. Increased mortality due to encainide or flecainide in a randomized trial of arrhythmia suppression after myocardial infarction. *N Engl J Med* 1989;321:406–412.
7. Ruskin JN. The Cardiac Arrhythmia Suppression Trial (CAST). *N Engl J Med* 1989;321:386–387.
8. Wellens HJJ, Brugada P. Treatment of cardiac arrhythmias: when, how and where? *J Am Coll Cardiol* 1989;14:1417–1428.
9. Bigger JT Jr. Implications of the Cardiac Arrhythmia Suppression Trial for antiarrhythmic drug treatment. *Am J Cardiol* 1990;65:3D–10D.
10. Pratt CM, Brater CD, Harrell FE, et al. Clinical and regulatory implications of the Cardiac Arrhythmia Suppression Trial. *Am J Cardiol* 1990;65:103–105.
11. Kerr WG, Bender WL. Paroxysmal ventricular fibrillation with cardiac recovery in a case of auricular fibrillation and complete heart block while under quinidine sulfate therapy. *Heart* 1922;9:269–278.

12. Binder MJ, Rosene L. Paroxysmal ventricular tachycardia and fibrillation due to quinidine. *Am J Med* 1952;12:491–497.
13. Selzer A, Wray W. Quinidine syncope. Paroxysmal ventricular fibrillation occurring during treatment of chronic atrial arrhythmias. *Circulation* 1964;30:17–26.
14. Nguyen PT, Scheimman MM, Seger J. Polymorphous ventricular tachycardia: clinical characterization, therapy and the QT interval. *Circulation* 1986;74:340–349.
15. Radford MD, Evans DW. Long-term results of DC reversion of atrial fibrillation. *Br Heart J* 1968;30:91–96.
16. Oram S. The dysrhythmias. In: Oram S, ed. *Clinical heart disease,* 2nd ed. London: Heineman Medical Books, 1981;585–657.
17. Campbell R. Drug prophylaxis of atrial fibrillation. In: Kulbertus HE, Olsson SB, Schlepper M, eds. *Atrial fibrillation.* Molndal, Sweden: AB Hassle, 1982;274–284.
18. Coplen SE, Antman FM, Berlin JA, Hewitt P, Chalmers TC. Efficacy and safety of quinidine therapy for maintenance of sinus rhythm after cardioversion. *Circulation* 1990;82:1106–1116.
19. Roden DM, Woosley RL, Primm RK. Incidence and clinical features of the quinidine-associated long QT syndrome: implications for patient care. *Am Heart J* 1986;111:1088–1093.
20. Roden DM, Hoffman BF. Action potential prolongation and induction of abnormal automaticity by low quinidine concentrations in canine Purkinje fibers. Relation to potassium and cycle length. *Circ Res* 1985;56:857–867.
21. Jackman WM, Friday KJ, Anderson JL, et al. The long QT syndromes: a critical review, new clinical observations and a unifying hypothesis. *Prog Cardiovasc Dis* 1988;31:115–172.
22. Strasberg B, Sclaarovsky S, Erdberg A, et al. Procainamide-induced polymorphic ventricular tachycardia. *Am J Cardiol* 1981;47:1309–1314.
23. Stratmann HG, Walter KE, Kennedy HL. Torsades de pointes associated with elevated N-acetylprocainamide levels. *Am Heart J* 1985;109:375–376.
24. Herre JM, Thompson JA. Polymorphic ventricular tachycardia and ventricular fibrillation due to N-acetyl procainamide. *Am J Cardiol* 1985;55:227–228.
25. McKibbin JK, Pocock W, Barlow JM, Scottmillar RN, Obel IWP. Sotalol, hypokalemia, syncope and torsades de pointes. *Br Heart J* 1984;51:157–162.
26. Neuvonen PJ, Elonen E, Vuorenmaa T, et al. Prolonged Q-T interval and severe tachyarrhythmias; common features of sotalol intoxication. *Eur J Clin Pharmacol* 1981;20:85–89.
27. Wang T, Bergstrand RH, Thompson KA, et al. Concentration dependent pharmacologic properties of sotalol. *Am J Cardiol* 1986;57:1160–1165.
28. Jull-Moller S, Edvardsson N, Rehngvist-Alzlberg N. Sotalol versus quinidine for the maintenance of sinus rhythm after direct current conversion of atrial fibrillation. *Circulation* 1990;82:1932–1939.
29. Keren A, Tzivoni D, Gottlieb S, et al. Atypical ventricular tachycardia (torsades de pointes) induced by amiodarone. *Chest* 1982;81:384–386.
30. Brown MA, Smith WM, Lubbe WF, Norris RM. Amiodarone-induced torsades de pointes. *Eur Heart J* 1986;7:234.
31. Woosley RL, Wood AJJ, Roden DM. Drug therapy: encainide. *New Engl J Med* 1988;318:1107–1115.
32. Chouty F, Coumel P. Oral flecainide for prophylaxis of paroxysmal atrial fibrillation. *Am J Cardiol* 1988;62:35D–37D.
33. Anderson JL, Gilbert EM, Alpert BL, et al. Prevention of symptomatic recurrences of paroxysmal atrial fibrillation in patients initially tolerating antiarrhythmic therapy. A multicenter, double-blind, crossover study of flecainide and placebo with transtelephonic monitoring. *Circulation* 1989;80:1557–1570.
34. Van Gelder IC, Crijns HJGM, Van Gilst WH, Van Wijk LN, Hamer HPM, Lie KI. Efficacy and safety of flecainide acetate in the maintenance of sinus rhythm after electrical cardioversion of chronic atrial fibrillation or atrial flutter. *Am J Cardiol* 1989;64:1317–1321.
35. Falk RH. Flecainide-induced ventricular tachycardia and fibrillation in patients treated for atrial fibrillation. *Ann Intern Med* 1989;111:107–111.
36. Anastasiou-Nana MI, Anderson J, Stewart JR, et al. Occurrence of exercise-induced and spontaneous wide-complex tachycardia during therapy with flecainide for complex ventricular arrhythmias: a probable proarrhythmic effect. *Am Heart J* 1087;113:1071–1077.
37. Ranger S, Talajic M, Lemerey R, Roy D, Nattel S. Amplification of flecainide-induced ventricular conduction slowing by exercise. *Circulation* 1989;79:1000–1008.
38. Fisch C. Aberration: seventy five years after Sir Thomas Lewis. *Br Heart J* 1983;50:297–302.
39. Crijns HJ, van Gelder IC, Lie KI. Supraventricular tachycardia mimicking ventricular tachycardia during flecainide treatment. *Am J Cardiol* 1988;62:1303–1306.
40. Tandowsky RM, Oyster JM, Silverglade A. The combined use of Lanatoside C and quinidine sulphate in the abolition of auricular flutter. *Am Heart J* 1946;32:617–633.
41. Herrmann GR, Hejtmancik M. Atrial flutter. *Am Heart J* 1951;41:182–191.

42. London F, Howell M. Atrial flutter: 1 to 1 conduction during treatment with quinidine and digitalis. *Am Heart J* 1954;48:152–156.
43. Cheng TO, Sutton GC, Swisher WP, Sutton DC. Effect of quinidine on the ventricular complex of the electrocardiogram with special reference to the duration of the Q-JT interval. *Am Heart J* 1956;51:417–444.
44. Cheng TO. Atrial flutter during quinidine therapy of atrial fibrillation. *Am Heart J* 1956;52:273–289.
45. Grande P, Sonne B, Pedersen A. A controlled study of digoxin and quinidine in patients DC reverted from atrial fibrillation to sinus rhythm (abstract). *Circulation* 1986;74:II-101.
46. Robertson CE, Miller HC. Extreme tachycardia complication the use of disopyramide in atrial flutter. *Br Heart J* 1980;44:602–603.
47. McGeehin FC III, Michelson EL. Procainamide. In: Messerli FZ, ed. *Cardiovascular drug therapy*. Philadelphia: WB Saunders, 1990;1202–1211.
48. Podrid PJ, Schoenberger A, Lown B. Precipitation of congestive heart failure by oral disopyramide. *N Engl J Med* 1980;302:614–617.
49. Rosen KM, Lau SH, Weiss MB. The effect of lidocaine on atrioventricular and intraventricular conduction in man. *Am J Cardiol* 1970;25:1–6.
50. David D, Long RM, Neumann A, Borow KM, Akselrod S, Mor-Avi V. Parasympathetically modulated antiarrhythmic action of lidocaine in atrial fibrillation. *Am Heart J* 1990;119:1061–1068.
51. Adamson AR, Spracklen FHN. Atrial flutter with block—contraindication to the use of lignocaine. *Br Med J* 1968;2:223–224.
52. Marriott HJL, Bieza CF. Alarming ventricular acceleration after lidocaine administration. *Chest* 1972;61:682–683.
53. Danahy DT, Aronow WS. Lidocaine-induced cardiac rate changes in atrial fibrillation and atrial flutter. *Am Heart J* 1978;95:474–482.
54. Bianconi L, Boccadomo R, Pappalarido A, Gentili C, Pistolese M. Effectiveness of intravenous propafenone for conversion of atrial fibrillation and flutter of recent onset. *Am J Cardiol* 1989;64:335–338.
55. Porterfield JG, Porterfield LM. Therapeutic efficacy and safety of oral propafenone for atrial fibrillation. *Am J Cardiol* 1989;63:114–116.
56. Murdock CJ, Kyles AE, Yeung-Lai-Wah JA, Qi A, Vorderbrugge S, Kerr CR. Atrial flutter in patients treated for atrial fibrillation with propafenone. *Am J Cardiol* 1990;66:755–757.
57. Feld GK, Chen PS, Nicod P, Fleck P, Meyer D. Possible atrial proarrhythmic effects of Class IC antiarrhythmic agents. *Am J Cardiol* 1990;66:378–383.
58. Marcus FI. The hazards of using type IC antiarrhythmic drugs for the treatment of paroxysmal atrial fibrillation. *Am J Cardiol* 1990;66:366–367.
59. Timm CT, Knowlton AA, Battinelli NJ, Falk RH. Flecainide for heart rate control in atrial fibrillation (abstr). *J Am Coll Cardiol* 1989;13:164A.
60. Lewis GP, Holtzman JL. Interaction of flecainide with digoxin and propranolol. *Am J Cardiol* 1984;53:89B–94B.
61. Myerburg RJ, Kessler KM, Cox MM, et al. Reversal of proarrhythmic effects of flecainide acetate and encainide hydrochloride by propranolol. *Circulation* 1989;80:1571–1579.
62. Rae AP. Proarrhythmic responses during electrophysiology testing. *Cardiol Clinics* 1986;4:487–496.
63. Greer GS, Wilkinson WE, McCarthy EA, Pritchett ELC. Random and nonrandom behavior of symptomatic paroxysmal atrial fibrillation. *Am J Cardiol* 1989;64:339–342.
64. Pritchett ELC, Lee KL. Designing clinical trials for paroxysmal atrial tachycardia and other paroxysmal arrhythmia. *J Clin Epidemiol* 1988;41:851–858.
65. Weiner P, Bassan MM, Jarchovsky J, Iusin S, Plavnick L. Clinical course of acute atrial fibrillation treated with rapid digitalization. *Am Heart J* 1983;105:223–227.
66. Falk RH, Knowlton AA, Bernard SA, Gotlieb NE, Battinelli NJ. Digoxin for converting recent-onset atrial fibrillation to sinus rhythm. A randomized double-blinded trial. *Ann Intern Med* 1987;106:503–506.
67. Rawles JM, Metcalfe MJ, Jennings K. Time of occurrence, duration and ventricular rate of paroxysmal atrial fibrillation on the effect of digoxin. *Br Heart J* 1990;63:225–227.
68. Kowey PR, DeSilva RA, Lown B. Sustained atrial fibrillation as a rhythm of choice. *Circulation* 1979;60(suppl 2):II-253.
69. Falk RH, Knowlton AA, Manaker S. Verapamil-induced atrial fibrillation (letter). *N Engl J Med* 1988;318:640–641.
70. Kasanuki H, Ohnishi S. Verapamil increasing inducibility and persistence of atrial fibrillation (abstract). *Circulation* 1986;74:II-105.
71. Shenasa M, Kus T, Fromer M, LeBlanc RA, DuBuc M, Nadean R. Effect of intravenous and oral calcium antagonists (diltiazem and verapamil) on sustenance of atrial fibrillation. *Am J Cardiol* 1988;62:403–407.
72. Shenasa M, Denkes S, Mahmud R, Lehmann M, Murthy US, Akhtar M. Effect of verapamil on

retrograde atrioventricular nodal conduction in the human heart. *J Am Coll Cardiol* 1983;3:545–550.

73. Singh BN, Ellrodt G, Peter CT. Verapamil: a review of its pharmacologic properties and therapeutic uses. *Drugs* 1978;15:169–197.
74. Aizawa Y, Miyajima S, Niwana S, Tamura M, Shibata A. Augmented fragmentation of atrial activity upon premature electrical stimuli by verapamil. *Angiology* 1989;40:94–100.
75. Klein GJ, Bashore TM, Sellers TD, Pritchett ELC, Smith WM, Gallagher JJ. Ventricular fibrillation in the Wolff-Parkinson-White syndrome. *N Engl J Med* 1979;301:1080–1085.
76. Gulamhusein S, Ko P, Klein GJ. Ventricular fibrillation following verapamil in the Wolff-Parkinson-White syndrome. *Am Heart J* 1983;106:145–147.
77. McGovern B, Garan H, Ruskin JN. Precipitation of cardiac arrest by verapamil in patients with Wolff-Parkinson-White syndrome. *Ann Intern Med* 1986;104:791–794.
78. Garratt C, Antonio A, Ward D, Cannon AJ. Misuse of verapamil in pre-excited atrial fibrillation. *Lancet* 1989;1:367–369.
79. Sellers TD, Bashore TM, Gallagher JJ. Digitalis in the pre-excitation syndrome. *Circulation* 1977;56:260–267.
80. Rosen KM, Barwolf C, Ehsani A, Rahimtoola S. Effects of lidocaine and propranolol on the normal and anomalous pathways in patients with pre-excitation. *Am J Cardiol* 1972;30:801–809.
81. Morady F, DiCarlo L, Berman JM. Effect of propranolol on ventricular rate during atrial fibrillation in the Wolff-Parkinson-White syndrome. *PACE* 1987;10:492–496.
82. Barrett PA, Laks MM, Mandel WJ, Yamaguchi I. The electrophysiologic effects of intravenous lidocaine in the Wolff-Parkinson-White syndrome. *Am Heart J* 1980;100:23–33.
83. Akhtar M, Gilbert CJ, Shenasha M. Effect of lidocaine on atrioventricular response via the accessory pathways in patients with Wolff-Parkinson-White syndrome. *Circulation* 1981;63:435–441.
84. Sheinman BD, Evans T. Acceleration of ventricular rate by amiodarone in atrial fibrillation associated with the Wolff-Parkinson-White syndrome. *Br Med J* 1982;285:999–1000.
85. Smith TW, Antman EM, Friedman PL, Blatt CM, Marsh JG. Digitalis glycosides: mechanisms and manifestations of toxicity. *Prog Cardiovasc Dis* 1984;28:413–458.
86. Fisch C, Knoebel SB. Digitalis cardiotoxicity. *J Am Coll Cardiol* 1985;5:91A–98A.
87. Beller GA, Smith TW, Abelmann WH, Haber E, Hood WB. Digitalis intoxication: a prospective clinical study with serum level correlations. *N Engl J Med* 1971;284:989–997.
88. Mahdyoon H, Battilana G, Rosman H, Goldstein S, Gheorghiade M. The evolving pattern of digoxin intoxication: observations at a large urban hospital from 1980 to 1988. *Am Heart J* 1990;94:1189–1200.
89. Kastor JA, Yurchak P. Recognition of digitalis intoxication in the presence of atrial fibrillation. *Ann Intern Med* 1967;67:1045–1054.
90. Khalsa A, Olsson SB. Verapamil-induced ventricular regularity in atrial fibrillation. *Acta Med Scand* 1979;205:509–515.
91. Piepho RW, Culbertson VL, Rhodes RS. Drug interactions with the calcium-entry blockers. *Circulation* 1987;75(suppl 5):V-181–V-194.
92. Brown AK, Primhak RA, Newton P. Use of amiodarone in bradycardia-tachycardia syndrome. *Br Heart J* 1978;40:1149–1152.
93. Talley JD, Wathen MS, Hurst JW. Hyperthyroid-induced atrial flutter-fibrillation with profound sinoatrial nodal pauses due to small doses of digoxin, verapamil and propranolol. *Clin Cardiol* 1989;12:45–47.
94. Grayzel J, Angeles J. Sino-atrial block in man provoked by quinidine. *J Electrocardiol* 1972;5:289–294.
95. Margolis JR, Strauss HC, Miller HC, et al. Digitalis and the sick sinus syndrome. Clinical and electrophysiologic documentation of a severe toxic effect on sinus node function. *Circulation* 1975;52:162–169.
96. Strauss HC, Gilbert M, Svenson RH, et al. Electrophysiologic effects of propranolol on sinus node function in patients with sinus node dysfunction. *Circulation* 1976;54:452–459.
97. LaBarre A, Strauss HC, Scheinman MM, et al. Electrophysiologic effects of disopyramide phosphate on sinus node function in patients with sinus node dysfunction. *Circulation* 1979;59:226–235.
98. Touboul P, Atallah G, Gressard A, et al. Effects of amiodarone on sinus node in man. *Br Heart J* 1979;42:573–578.
99. Vik-Mo H, Ohm OJ, Lund-Johansen P. Electrophysiologic effects of flecainide acetate in patients with sinus nodal dysfunction. *Am J Cardiol* 1982;50:1090–1094.
100. Roden DM, Hoffman BF. Action potential prolongation and induction of abnormal automaticity by low quinidine concentration in canine Purkinje fibers. Relationship to potassium and cycle length. *Circ Res* 1985;56:857–867.

Atrial Fibrillation: Mechanisms and Management, edited by
R. H. Falk and P. J. Podrid.
Raven Press, Ltd., New York © 1992.

16

Anticoagulant Therapy for Atrial Fibrillation

Palle Petersen

*Department of Neurology, University Hospital, Rigshospitalet,
DK-2100 Copenhagen, Denmark*

Atrial fibrillation (AF) is found in 0.4% of the adult population (1,2). Prevalence increases with age to a high of 2% to 4% in those over 60 years old (1–3).

The prognosis for AF is a subject of growing interest due to the increase of elderly persons in the population, increased mortality among patients with AF versus patients with sinus rhythm, and the risk of thromboembolic complications (2,4,5). The primary aim of this chapter is to discuss the current knowledge of treatment with anticoagulants or aspirin to prevent thromboembolic complications in patients with AF, with attention to the risk of stroke and systemic embolism in chronic versus paroxysmal AF and rheumatic versus nonrheumatic AF.

THROMBOEMBOLIC COMPLICATIONS IN ATRIAL FIBRILLATION

It is important to differentiate between chronic and paroxysmal AF as increasing evidence suggests that paroxysmal AF is associated with a significantly lower risk of thromboembolic events than is chronic AF. The true distribution of chronic versus paroxysmal AF is difficult to establish because of the different methods used and the difficulties in verifying the paroxysms of AF, especially in outpatients (6). Among 1,212 hospitalized patients with AF, paroxysmal AF occurred in 35% (4). Two other hospital-based series found that 40% of 234 patients (7) and 33% of 414 patients (8) with AF had the paroxysmal form. In contrast, a study of life insurance records from 3,099 younger patients with AF found that 90% had the paroxysmal form (9), a distribution similar to that found in studies of airmen (10). The differing prevalences of chronic and paroxysmal AF in the above studies are obviously related to the type of population studied.

Chronic Atrial Fibrillation

The risk of stroke in patients with nonrheumatic chronic AF is increased more than fivefold over that in controls with sinus rhythm, as shown in the Framingham study (11), corresponding to a 4% to 5% annual incidence of stroke. The risk was increased 17-fold when the etiology of AF was rheumatic heart disease. This is in accordance with results from other studies of chronic AF (12–14). Thus, Szekely (12) retrospectively investigated 754 patients with rheumatic heart disease, of whom 219 patients had AF. In this study the incidence of thromboembolic events was increased sevenfold in AF as compared to patients in sinus rhythm. Fleming and Bailey (13) retrospectively investigated 500 patients with mitral valve disease, among whom 57% had AF. A total of 125 patients suffered a systemic embolus during the 9.5-year study period. Of the 125 embolic events, 101 occurred during AF, i.e., 35% of the patients with AF had a thromboembolic event during the follow-up period compared to 11% of patients in sinus rhythm. A Japanese epidemiologic study (14) found the incidence of stroke among patients with AF to be 5.0%, corresponding to a 5.6-fold increased risk as compared to the population in sinus rhythm, and a recent study of patients with nonrheumatic chronic AF (median age 74 years) found the annual incidence of thromboembolic complications to be 5.5% without protective treatments (15). The British Whitehall and Regional Heart Studies found the total annual stroke incidences to be lower, 1.5% and 0.4%, respectively (16). However, the relative risks were 6.9 and 2.3, respectively, in the two studies, close to the 5.6 found in both the Framingham study (11) and the study by Tanaka et al. (14). The two British studies investigated a total of 111 men with chronic nonrheumatic AF aged 40 to 69 years at entry, corresponding to an approximate mean age of 55 years. In the British Whitehall Study, patients were enrolled between 1967 and 1969 and 21% of the patients with AF had evidence of rheumatic heart disease, i.e., they were excluded from the study. In the British Regional Heart Study patients were enrolled in 1979 to 1980 and 11% of the patients with AF had rheumatic heart disease. Thus, the incidence of rheumatic heart disease has declined during the past decades (7,16–18), but the magnitude of the problem of stroke in AF is considerable because so many elderly patients have AF (5,6,8). Thus, approximately 15% to 20% of all ischemic strokes are attributed to AF, that is, cardiogenic embolism is assumed to be the cause (19,20). However, the proportion of cardiogenic embolism among stroke patients with AF can only be roughly estimated, as it at present is impossible to distinguish precisely between a thrombotic and a thromboembolic stroke, i.e., the differentiation is based on clinical evaluation. This can explain why the estimated proportions of cardioembolic strokes in patients with AF vary to a great extent, being as high as 75% in some studies and as low as 19% in others (20). In patients with AF, however, it is reasonable to believe that a subsequent stroke can be due to cardiogenic embolism, although it sometimes could be due to a thrombotic event.

That chronic AF in fact is associated with increased intracardiovascular clotting has been shown recently by Kumagai et al. (21), who investigated plasma D-dimer levels in 73 patients with chronic AF and in 21 patients without. They found that the plasma D-dimer level was significantly higher in AF than in sinus rhythm, despite that, in both groups, there were no significant differences in plasma D-dimer levels between patients with and without organic heart disease. These findings indicate that AF itself may be more important than factors predisposing to AF in the development of intracardiovascular clotting, although the clinical implications of the investigation need to be more clarified in future studies.

Paroxysmal Atrial Fibrillation

Since Parkinson and Campbell (22) published their clinical data on 200 patients with paroxysmal AF in 1930, there has been no further evidence that paroxysmal

AF is a risk factor for stroke compared to chronic AF or sinus rhythm (8). In that study paroxysmal AF was classified on clinical evaluation as (a) typical recurrent paroxysmal AF (more than half of the cases), (b) a few paroxysms of AF preceding the onset of chronic AF, and (c) single or very occasional paroxysms. However, the verification of paroxysmal AF may be difficult, and long-term ambulatory monitoring is essential in proper documentation of paroxysmal AF (6). The definition of paroxysmal AF in recent studies includes at least one episode of AF with a documented conversion to sinus rhythm (6–8,23), but it is important to emphasize that the number of paroxysms is most likely to be underestimated (6), particularly in retrospective studies (23).

In a retrospective study of 94 patients with paroxysmal AF (7), six cerebrovascular complications were noted, but no exact data were available about incidence rate. As follow-up was several years, it is likely that the annual frequency of stroke was low. It was not stated whether the events occurred before or after transition to chronic AF, which occurred in 19 of 75 patients with an observation period of more than 1 year. Treseder et al. (8) retrospectively investigated 414 elderly inpatients, 276 with chronic AF and 138 with paroxysmal AF, with a mean age in both groups of approximately 80 years. The prevalence of AF was reported to be about 10%, reflecting the advanced age of the patients. These authors found a significantly lower risk of stroke in the group with paroxysmal AF. A retrospective study of 426 patients found the incidence of embolic complications during paroxysmal AF to be 2%, but after transition to chronic AF the incidence rose to 5% (23). The rate of transition to chronic AF was 33%, with a median time to transition of 34 months. Important factors in the incidence of embolic complications were determined using Cox's regression model; Table 1 shows that only occurrence of chronic AF was a significant risk factor for an embolic complication. Surprisingly, the number of paroxysms of AF was of no significance in the risk of embolization. As mentioned, the number of paroxysms of AF is probably underestimated in a retrospective study, but this does not change the fact that few embolic complications occurred during paroxysmal AF. That paroxysmal AF is associated with a lower risk of embolization than chronic AF is supported by a recent study by Wiener (24), who found that chronic AF was the only clinical factor that separated AF patients with thromboemboli from those without. A total of 115 patients with nonrheumatic AF were evaluated, 17 of whom had emboli in the past or at admission. Age, sex, systemic hypertension heart failure, and left atrial size were all without statistical importance.

The above studies found the risk of embolic complications in patients with paroxysmal AF to be lower than that in patients with chronic AF. This does not seem to be explained by difference in age or underlying etiologies (7,8), the only important

TABLE 1. *Factors of importance for embolic complications in 426 patients with initial paroxysmal atrial fibrillation (AF)*

	p Values	
	Forward selection	Backward selection
Sex	0.42	0.25
Age	0.33	0.28
Etiology	0.24	0.24
Occurrence of chronic AF	<0.00005	<0.00005

Ref. 23.

factor being transition to chronic AF (23). It is therefore possible that more intensive treatment of patients with paroxysmal AF with antiarrhythmic agents may postpone the development of chronic AF and thereby reduce their risk of stroke, but future studies are needed to show whether this is true (23).

No studies of stroke prevention in patients with paroxysmal AF are available, and considering their relatively low incidence of embolic complications, such a study will require many patients to show any effect of treatments.

Cerebral Blood Flow in Atrial Fibrillation

Lavy et al. (25) found cerebral blood flow to be less in patients with AF than in controls in sinus rhythm. They investigated 31 patients with chronic AF without symptoms of heart failure and free from neurologic diseases. In 27 of 31 patients regional cerebral blood flow was found to be lower than for age-matched normal control subjects. Another study found that decreased cerebral blood flow during chronic AF normalized after electrical cardioversion to sinus rhythm (26). Nine patients with AF of less than 3 months duration had their cerebral blood flow measured the day before and after and again 30 days after electrical cardioversion therapy to sinus rhythm. None of the patients had congestive heart failure or systemic hypertension. After correction for changes in end-tidal pCO_2, the median cerebral blood flow had increased significantly from 35.8 to 40.3 ml/100g/min on day 1 and to 46.7 on day 30. Thus, reduced cerebral blood flow could contribute to the development of stroke in persons with AF, but studies of more patients are needed before it will be possible to outline the clinical implications of these findings.

The concentration of atrial natriuretic peptide is elevated during AF and normalizes after sinus rhythm is obtained (27). Atrial natriuretic peptide increases hematocrit (28,29) as do paroxysms of AF (30). Chabrier et al. (31) found atrial natriuretic peptide receptors in the microvessels of the brain, and although the importance of this finding is unknown, there might be a relation between elevated atrial natriuretic peptide concentration, decreased cerebral blood flow, and the occurrence of cerebrovascular complications in patients with AF (26). However, future studies will have to show whether this is true.

SILENT CEREBRAL INFARCTION IN ATRIAL FIBRILLATION

A preliminary report by Norrving and Nilsson (32) detected a high frequency of silent cerebral infarction in patients with AF and cerebral embolism. Of 85 patients examined with brain computed tomography (CT) scan, 12 (14%) had clinically silent infarction. This subject was investigated in a controlled study, in which 30 elderly outpatients with chronic AF of greater than 1 year duration and 30 age- and sex-matched controls in sinus rhythm and with no history of cerebrovascular disease were examined with CT (33). Fourteen AF patients had abnormal CT scans, with areas of low density sharply demarcated from surrounding tissue compared with such CT scans in eight patients in sinus rhythm. This difference in prevalence of abnormal CT scans was not significant, but the number of abnormal areas was significantly higher in the AF (39 lesions) than in the control (16 lesions) group (Fig. 1). There was no correlation between the presence of low-density lesions and age, independent of rhythm disturbance. Most of the AF patients had atherosclerotic and/

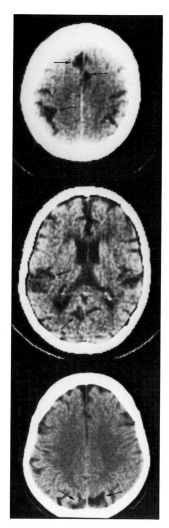

FIG. 1. Cerebral low-density areas (*arrows*) in three patients with atrial fibrillation. None of these patients had had a symptomatic neurologic event.

or hypertensive heart disease, whereas the controls considered themselves healthy. However, there was no significant difference in mean arterial blood pressure between the groups, and the controls probably had some degree of clinically silent atherosclerosis. These findings are supported by a recent preliminary study (34) and a study by Kempster et al. (35), who retrospectively investigated 54 patients with chronic AF presenting with symptoms of cerebral ischemia. A significantly higher prevalence of silent cerebral infarction was found in patients with chronic AF than in the 168 controls in sinus rhythm, although hypertension and diabetes were more common in the control group. As all subjects presented with cerebral ischemia, the degree of atherosclerosis in the two groups was probably the same. This does not exclude hypertension and generalized atherosclerosis as coexisting factors important in the occurrence of low-density areas on CT scans in patients with chronic AF. However, if these factors are of significance, it underscores the magnitude of this problem as most AF patients have systemic hypertension and/or atherosclerotic heart disease. More studies, however, are needed in patients with lone AF, i.e., those without hypertension and known atherosclerosis, and in patients with sinus rhythm, hypertension, and atherosclerosis.

Few data are available from patients with paroxysmal AF. One study compared the prevalence of cerebral low-density areas on CT scans in 30 outpatients with paroxysmal AF and 30 age- and sex-matched controls in sinus rhythm without cerebrovascular disease and found no significant difference (36). The number of subjects was relatively small, and, accordingly, it cannot be ruled out that the true risk of cerebral low-density areas on CT scans would be increased by a factor of two or three, assuming a 10% risk in the controls (36). The occurrence of cerebral abnormalities in these controls was lower than that from the study of Petersen et al. (33), but these controls were nearly 10 years younger than the others. A preliminary study by Sasaki et al. (37) found a lower prevalence of silent cerebral infarction among patients with paroxysmal AF than in those with chronic AF, thus supporting the impression that the former is associated with a lower risk of cerebral damage than the latter. That AF is associated with increased risk of cerebral low-density areas is confirmed in a recent study by Feinberg et al. (38), who also suggested the risk of such areas to be higher (34%) in chronic AF than in paroxysmal AF (22%). In this study 141 asymptomatic patients with AF were investigated with a CT scan. Thirty-six patients (26%) had one or more hypodense areas consistent with previous cerebral infarction (38).

Although the cerebral low-density areas on the CT scans were asymptomatic by definition, they might be important regarding cognition in elderly people (20,39). However, even if several studies find an increased prevalence of cerebral low-density areas on CT scans of AF patients, this new field of research needs more studies, with particular focus on the risk of developing clinically overt cerebrovascular disease (38).

PREVENTION OF EMBOLISM IN ATRIAL FIBRILLATION

Stroke prevention in patients with AF has been discussed for several decades (40–44), but preventive strategies and management have remained empiric and controversial (20). Several studies have strongly suggested a beneficial effect of oral anticoagulation in patients with rheumatic AF (12,13), but due to methodologic problems, the clinical interpretation of these studies has been difficult to outline. Thus, Szekely (12) investigated 30 patients with established AF and no history of embolism. Anticoagulation treatment was started immediately or very shortly after the onset of AF and continued for a total period of 46 patient-years. In this group no thromboembolic events were noted. In a more or less comparable group of 98 patients with AF, but without treatment with anticoagulants, 29 patients had 34 embolic episodes during a total period of 499 patient-years. In the study by Fleming and Bailey (13) 217 patients with mitral valve disease were treated with anticoagulants, and only five thromboembolic events occurred. The reported incidence of events was 0.8% during anticoagulation treatment. Overall, 120 thromboembolic events were noted in 283 patients without such treatment, i.e., the incidence of events in this group can be calculated to be about 4% to 5% per year. No separate data for patients with AF treated with anticoagulants were reported, but more than half of the 500 patients had AF and the majority of thromboembolic events occurred in patients with AF. Some authors have recommended oral anticoagulation for all patients with AF (41). Other authors have suggested anticoagulation for subgroups, including patients with recurrent stroke, rheumatic AF, thyrotoxic AF, patients with large atria, and even patients with lone AF (43,45–47).

In a retrospective study of 134 patients with nonrheumatic AF, emboli occurred in 5.9% per year among patients who were without anticoagulation, compared to only 0.7% per year among those treated with anticoagulants (48). Recently, our group published prospective data from 1,007 outpatients with nonrheumatic chronic AF (median age 74.2, range 38–91 years) (15). The patients were randomized to treatment with warfarin ($n = 335$), 75 mg aspirin per day ($n = 336$), or placebo ($n = 336$) to evaluate the effect of treatment on the occurrence of thromboembolic complications. Anticoagulation therapy was conducted openly using Normotest (NycoMed AS, Oslo, Norway) with a therapeutic range of 4.2 to 2.8 (international normalized ratio [INR]) (49); the aspirin and placebo arms were double blind. The patients were followed by the same investigator at scheduled intervals for 2 years. The primary end point was a thromboembolic complication, that is, transient cerebral ischemia, stroke, embolism to the viscera or to the extremities. A total of 20 thromboembolic complications was noted in the aspirin group, not significantly different from the 21 events in the placebo group. Five cerebrovascular complications were recorded in the warfarin group. The difference in frequency of events in the three groups was statistically significant, even when adjusted for interim analysis. Moreover, only two of the five strokes occurred during adequate anticoagulation. Two patients had strokes after temporary cessation of anticoagulant treatment due to surgical intervention or evaluation of hematuria, and one patient had a stroke on the day of randomization, that is, before anticoagulant treatment was begun. Thus, a total of 46 patients had thromboembolic events (median age 73.7, range 38–85 years). The occurrence of thromboembolism increased with the duration of AF, with no evidence of a specific vulnerable period. The yearly incidence of events was 2.0% among patients receiving warfarin (95% confidence limits 0.6%–4.8%) and 5.5% among those receiving either aspirin or placebo (95% confidence limits 2.9%–9.4%). The number of thromboembolic events occurring after cessation of treatments were six, one, and four in the three groups, respectively ($p > 0.10$). Intention-to-treat analysis of all thromboembolic complications (including those in patients receiving treatment and in those who withdrew) gave probability values of 0.056 (chi-square test) and 0.046 (likelihood ratio test) in favor of warfarin (Table 2). Vascular mortality was

TABLE 2. *Thromboembolic complications in the Copenhagen AFASAK study*

	Anticoagulation		Aspirin		Placebo	
	On ($n = 335$)	Off	On ($n = 336$)	Off	On ($n = 336$)	Off
Transient ischemic attack	0	1	2	0	3	0
Minor stroke	0	1	1	0	2	1
Nondisabling stroke	0	2	7	0	3	1
Disabling stroke	4	1	4	1	7	1
Fatal stroke	1	0	3	0	4	0
Visceral	0	1	2	0	2	1
Extremities	0	0	1	0	0	0
Total	11		21		25	

Ref. 15.

significantly lower during anticoagulation than during treatment with aspirin or placebo; however, intention-to-treat analysis of all deaths, including the patients who withdrew, showed no difference in either vascular or total mortality.

Preliminary data from a randomized, placebo-controlled study of 1,244 patients with nonrheumatic AF were recently published (50). The trial aimed to evaluate the effects of warfarin and aspirin as prophylaxis against ischemic stroke and systemic embolism. Patients eligible to receive warfarin were allocated to warfarin (open treatment), aspirin 325 mg per day, or placebo (double-blind treatment). Those who were not eligible for treatment with warfarin received either aspirin or placebo (double-blind fashion). The study showed a beneficial effect of both active treatments and the placebo arm was therefore terminated. The trial is continuing in order to address the relative benefits of aspirin and warfarin. However, the authors were unable to show a benefit of aspirin in patients over 75 years of age. Like the Danish trial (15), the North American study reported no age correlation regarding the effect of warfarin on stroke occurrence. The studies also agreed in that no effect of warfarin on mortality could be obtained (intention-to-treat methods). The two studies differed in several aspects (Table 3). However, at present it seems impossible to point out one reason of particular importance when considering the different results of treatment with aspirin. Although it is likely that the different doses of aspirin can explain some of this difference between the studies, other possibilities exist. In particular, the age differences between the studies might be of importance as the American study found no effect of aspirin in patients above 75 years, and almost half of the patients in the Danish study were above this age (Table 3). However, both studies found a beneficial effect of warfarin, and until further results are available the exact effect of aspirin remains unclear.

The Boston Area Anticoagulation Trial for Atrial Fibrillation (The BAATAF Study) was published in November 1990 (51). This study was an unblinded, randomized, placebo-controlled trial of low-dose warfarin (INR 2.7–1.5) for stroke prevention in nonrheumatic AF. The incidence of stroke among 212 patients treated with

TABLE 3. *Differences between three prospective studies of antithrombotic prophylaxis in atrial fibrillation*

	AFASAK (15)	SPAF (50)	BAATAF (51)
Age (years)	74	67	68
Type of AF	Chronic	Chronic/paroxysmal	Chronic/paroxysmal
Aspirin dose (mg/day)	75	325	—[a]
Intracerebral hemorrhage	Primary end point	Side effect	Side effect
Aspirin effective	No	Yes, in patients ≤75 years of age[b]	—[a]
Warfarin therapeutic interval (INR)	4.2–2.8	3.5–2.0	2.7–1.5
Multicenter study	No	Yes	Yes
Warfarin effect on mortality	No	No	Yes

[a]Patients in control arm allowed to take aspirin, see text for details.
[b]No effect of aspirin in patients >75 years of age.
AF, atrial fibrillation; INR, international normalized ratio.

warfarin was significantly lower as compared to that noted among 208 patients without anticoagulation (0.4% vs 3.0%, respectively), i.e., the risk reduction on warfarin was reported to be 86%. In contrast to the AFASAK (15) and the Stroke Prevention in Atrial Fibrillation (SPAF) (50) studies, the BAATAF study (51) found a significantly lower mortality among the warfarin-treated patients. The controls in that study were allowed to take aspirin. Aspirin use, both frequency and dose, was recorded at follow-up. Forty-six percent of all patient-years in the control group were contributed by patients taking aspirin regularly. Eight of 13 strokes in the control group occurred among patients taking aspirin (seven taking at least 325 mg per day), for an incidence rate of stroke of 3.99% per year. Only two of these strokes were mild, and four occurred among patients younger than 75 years of age. Although the assessment of aspirin was nonrandomized, the results are more consistent with a lack of aspirin effect, even at a dose of 325 mg per day (51).

In all three studies mentioned above, the rate of thromboembolic events rose with duration of AF, with no evidence of a particularly vulnerable period. They all showed that warfarin can reduce significantly the incidence of thromboembolic complications in AF. The risks of major bleeding complications were low as compared to benefits of warfarin. The Danish study (15) reported one fatal intracerebral hemorrhage (calculated as a primary end point) in the warfarin group and one patient had a nonfatal bleeding episode requiring blood transfusion. In the aspirin group one nonfatal bleeding complication requiring blood transfusion was noted. There were no bleeding complications in the placebo group. The SPAF study (50) also reported a low incidence of major bleeding complications during anticoagulation treatment. Thus, the yearly incidences of hemorrhagic events requiring hospital admission, blood transfusion, or surgery occurred at rates of 1.7%, 0.9%, and 1.2% among patients treated with warfarin, aspirin, and placebo, respectively. The BAATAF study (51) reported one fatal hemorrhage in each group. The frequency of bleeding events leading to hospitalization or transfusion was essentially the same in both groups. Thus, the three trials all suggested that with careful, centralized monitoring warfarin treatment can be very safe.

The intended degree of anticoagulation was less in the American studies than in the AFASAK study (Table 3). However, the actual level of anticoagulation in the Danish study was lower than initially intended (15), suggesting that warfarin is effective even when administered less intensively. This finding is of importance with regard to the risk of bleeding complications, which is related to the degree of anticoagulation (52).

Another randomized study supports the beneficial effect of warfarin in preventing arterial thromboembolic complications (53). This study was not concerned with patients with AF, but investigated a total of 1,214 patients with acute myocardial infarction. They were allocated to receive warfarin or placebo (double-blind method) in order to investigate the effect on myocardial reinfarction, mortality, and cerebrovascular complications. The study showed a beneficial effect of warfarin on all three end points, i.e., a significant risk reduction of 55% in the occurrence of cerebrovascular events (intention-to-treat model). Like the AFASAK study (15), the Norwegian study (53) included all types of cerebrovascular events, i.e., intracerebral hematomas as well as ischemic stroke.

Anticoagulation therapy is associated with a risk of bleeding complications and demands good compliance. It is therefore important to search for risk factors for stroke to identify patients at high risk who may benefit most from treatment with anticoagulants. However, there is disagreement about which risk factors are of importance in the development of thromboembolic complications in AF, and at present it is difficult to demonstrate which patients with AF might benefit most from treatment with anticoagulants (54). However, it seems as if patients with paroxysmal AF have a low risk of stroke, and this seems also to be the case for younger patients with idiopathic AF (55). Some studies have suggested that thyrotoxicosis is a significant risk factor for thromboembolic complications in AF; however, they had been criticized for not being sufficiently controlled and for not taking the follow-up period into account (56). Recently, 610 patients with untreated thyrotoxicosis, 91 of whom had AF, were studied in a retrospective fashion (56). In this study there was no significant difference in the occurrence of cerebrovascular complications between patients with AF and those in sinus rhythm (Table 4). The incidence of cerebrovascular events in thyrotoxic AF of approximately 6% was comparable to that from other studies of patients with AF including other etiologies (56). The incidence of cerebrovascular events among patients in sinus rhythm was 1.7%. That a significant difference in the occurrence of events between AF patients and those in sinus rhythm was not found can be explained by the relatively small number of AF patients. However, the study could not confirm thyrotoxicosis as an etiology of AF as a greater risk factor for embolization than other etiologies of AF.

In a reevaluation of the Copenhagen AFASAK study (54) previous myocardial infarction was the only significant risk factor for a thromboembolic complication. The yearly incidence of thromboembolic events for patients without previous myocardial infarction was 5.4% and 14% for patients with previous myocardial infarction. Age, sex, heart failure, chest pain, systemic hypertension, diabetes systolic and diastolic blood pressures, smoking, relative heart volume, and left atrial size were all without statistical importance. Aronow et al. (57) studied 110 patients with AF with and without stroke and also found previous myocardial infarction to be a significant risk factor as well as systemic hypertension, left atrial enlargement, and left ventricular hypertrophy. Age and sex were without importance for the outcome. Flegel et al. (16) found raised systolic or diastolic blood pressure to be important, while age and ischemic heart disease were without significance regarding the stroke risk in AF. However, it is unclear whether patients with ischemic heart disease included those with a history of chest pain or only patients with previous myocardial infarction. Another study found age over 75 years and raised systolic blood pressure to be significant factors for a first stroke (58). The recent BAATAF study (51) found no association between stroke and left atrial size, hypertension, and a variety of other clinical and echocardiographic features. On the other hand, age, mitral annular calcification, and, less so, coronary artery disease were significant risk factors for stroke. As pointed out (51,54), the conflicting results obtained in many studies prob-

TABLE 4. *Significance of risk factors for cerebrovascular events during first year after diagnosis of thyrotoxicosis*

Risk factor	Probability
Age	<0.005
Sex	0.09
Atrial fibrillation	0.17

Significance assessed using logistic regression methods.
Ref. 56.

ably reflect the small samples, and I agree with Walker (59) regarding the merit of combining data from ongoing studies of stroke prophylaxis in AF to obtain a sufficient number of patients to investigate the importance of the many variables. However, even though many topics regarding risk factors and stroke prevention in AF still need to be investigated, I find it reasonable, from the results of the above prospective studies, to consider patients with chronic AF for treatment with warfarin if no contraindications are present.

In summary, the data from four prospective, randomized studies strongly suggest that warfarin is effective in reducing the risk of thromboembolic events not only in patients with AF but also in patients with acute myocardial infarction. Further studies of the effects of aspirin are needed, as well as studies using even lower doses of warfarin.

ACKNOWLEDGMENT

Supported by a research fellowship from the Danish Heart Foundation and the University of Copenhagen.

REFERENCES

1. Ostrander LD Jr, Brandt RL, Kjelsberg MO, Epstein FH. Electrocardiographic findings among the adult population of a total natural community, Tecumseh, Michigan. *Circulation* 1965;31:888–898.
2. Kulbertus HE, Leval-Rutten FD, Bartsch P, Petit J. Atrial fibrillation in elderly ambulatory patients. In: Kulbertus HE, Olsson SB, Schlepper M, eds. *Atrial fibrillation, Kiruna, Sweden.* Mölndal: AB Hässle, 1982;148–157.
3. Örndahl G, Thulesius O, Hood B. Incidence of persistent atrial fibrillation and conduction defects in coronary heart disease. *Am Heart J* 1972;84:120–131.
4. Godtfredsen J. *Atrial fibrillation. Etiology, course and prognosis. A follow-up study of 1,212 cases.* Copenhagen: Munksgaard, 1975.
5. Petersen P, Godtfredsen J. Atrial fibrillation—a review of course and prognosis. *Acta Med Scand* 1984;216:5–9.
6. Martin A, Benbow LJ, Butrous GS, Leach C, Camm AJ. Five-year follow-up of 101 elderly subjects by means of longterm ambulatory cardiac monitoring. *Eur Heart J* 1984;5:592–596.
7. Takahashi N, Seki A, Imataka K, Fujii J. Clinical features of paroxysmal atrial fibrillation: an observation of 94 patients. *Jpn Heart J* 1981;22:143–149.
8. Treseder AS, Sastry BSD, Thomas TPL, Yates MA, Pathy MSJ. Atrial fibrillation and stroke in elderly hospitalized patients. *Age Ageing* 1986;15:89–92.
9. Gajewski J, Singer RB. Mortality in an insured population with atrial fibrillation. *JAMA* 1981;245:1540–1544.
10. Bennett D. Atrial fibrillation. *Eur Heart J* 1984;5(suppl A):89–93.
11. Wolf PA, Dawber TR, Thomas HE, Kannel WB. Epidemiologic assessment of chronic atrial fibrillation and risk of stroke: the Framingham study. *Neurology* 1978;28:973–977.
12. Szekely P. Systemic embolism and anticoagulant prophylaxis in rheumatic heart disease. *Br Med J* 1964;1:1209–1212.
13. Fleming HA, Bailey SM. Mitral valve disease, systemic embolism and anticoagulants. *Postgrad Med J* 1971;47:599–604.
14. Tanaka H, Hayashi M, Date C, et al. Epidemiologic studies of stroke in Shibata, a Japanese provincial city: preliminary report on risk factors for cerebral infarction. *Stroke* 1985;16:773–780.
15. Petersen P, Boysen G, Godtfredsen J, Andersen ED, Andersen B. Placebo-controlled, randomised trial of warfarin and aspirin for prevention of thromboembolic complications in chronic atrial fibrillation. The Copenhagen AFASAK Study. *Lancet* 1989;1:175–179.
16. Flegel KM, Shipley MJ, Rose G. Risk of stroke in nonrheumatic atrial fibrillation. *Lancet* 1987;1:526–529.
17. Petersen P, Godtfredsen J. Risk factors for stroke in chronic atrial fibrillation. *Eur Heart J* 1988;9:291–294.
18. Morris DC, Hurst JW. Atrial fibrillation. *Curr Probl Cardiol* 1980;5:1–51.

19. Godtfredsen J, Petersen P. Thromboembolic complications in atrial fibrillation. In: Refsum H, Sulg IA, Rasmussen K, eds. *Heart brain and brain heart*. Heidelberg: Springer-Verlag, 1989;225–229.
20. Halperin JL, Hart RG. Atrial fibrillation and stroke: new ideas, persisting dilemmas. *Stroke* 1988;19:937–941.
21. Kumagai K, Fukunami M, Ohmori M, Kitabatake A, Kamada T, Hoki N. Increased intracardio-vascular clotting in patients with chronic atrial fibrillation. *J Am Cardiol* 1990;16:377–380.
22. Parkinson J, Campbell M. Paroxysmal auricular fibrillation. A record of two hundred patients. *Q J Med* 1930;24:67–100.
23. Petersen P, Godtfredsen J. Embolic complications in paroxysmal atrial fibrillation. *Stroke* 1986;17:622–626.
24. Wiener I. Clinical and echocardiographic correlates of systemic embolization in nonrheumatic atrial fibrillation. *Am J Cardiol* 1987;59:177.
25. Lavy S, Stern S, Melamed E, Cooper G, Keren A, Levy P. Efect of chronic atrial fibrillation on regional cerebral blood flow. *Stroke* 1980;11:35–38.
26. Petersen P, Kastrup J, Videbæk R, Boysen G. Cerebral blood flow before and after cardioversion of atrial fibrillation. *J Cereb Blood Flow Metab* 1989;9:422–425.
27. Roy D, Paillard F, Cassidy D, et al. Atrial natriuretic factor during atrial fibrillation and supra-ventricular tachycardia. *J Am Coll Cardiol* 1987;9:509–514.
28. de Bold AJ, Borenstein HB, Veress AT, Sonnenberg H. A rapid and potent natriuretic response to intravenous injection of atrial myocardial extract in rats. *Life Sci* 1981;28:89–94.
29. Flückiger JP, Waeber B, Matsueda G, Delaloye B, Nussberger J, Brunner HR. Effect of atriopep-tin III on hematocrit and volemia of nephrectomized rats. *Am J Physiol* 1986;251:H880–H883.
30. Imataka K, Nakaoka H, Kitahara Y, Fujii J, Ishibashi M, Yamaji T. Blood hematocrit changes during paroxysmal atrial fibrillation. *Am J Cardiol* 1987;59:172–173.
31. Chabrier PE, Roubert P, Braquet P. Specific binding of atrial natriuretic factor in brain microves-sels. *Proc Natl Acad Sci USA* 1987;84:2078–2081.
32. Norrving B, Nilsson B. Cerebral embolism of cardiac origin: the limited possibilities of secondary prevention (abstract). *Acta Neurol Scand* 1986;73:520.
33. Petersen P, Madsen EB, Brun B, Pedersen F, Gyldensted C, Boysen G. Silent cerebral infarction in chronic atrial fibrillation. *Stroke* 1987;18:1098–1100.
34. Feinberg WM, Seeger JF, Carmody RF, Hart RG, Anderson DC, Miller VT. Asymptomatic ce-rebral infarction in patients with atrial fibrillation (abstract). *Circulation* 1988;78(suppl II):600.
35. Kempster PA, Gerraty RP, Gates PC. Asymptomatic cerebral infarction in patients with chronic atrial fibrillation. *Stroke* 1988;19:955–957.
36. Petersen P, Pedersen F, Johnsen A, et al. Cerebral computed tomography in paroxysmal atrial fibrillation. *Acta Neurol Scand* 1989;79:482–486.
37. Sasaki W, Yanagisawa S, Maki K, Onodera A, Awaji T, Kanazawa T. High incidence of silent small cerebral infarction in the patients with atrial fibrillation (abstract). *Circulation* 1987;76(suppl IV):104.
38. Feinberg WM, Seeger JF, Carmody RF, Anderson DC, Hart RG, Pearce LA. Epidemiologic fea-tures of asymptomatic cerebral infarction in patients with nonvalvular atrial fibrillation. *Arch Intern Med* 1990;150:2340–2344.
39. Ratcliffe PJ, Wilcock GK. Cerebrovascular disease in dementia: the importance of atrial fibrilla-tion. *Postgrad Med J* 1985;61:201–204.
40. Selzer A. Atrial fibrillation revisited (editorial). *N Engl J Med* 1982;306:1044–1045.
41. Fisher CM. Reducing risks of cerebral embolism. *Geriatrics* 1979;34:59–66.
42. Forfar JC, Toft AD. Thyrotoxic atrial fibrillation: an underdiagnosed condition? *Br Med J* 1982;285:909–910.
43. Dunn M, Alexander J, de Silva R, Hildner F. Antithrombotic therapy in atrial fibrillation. *Chest* 1986;89(suppl 2):68S–81S.
44. Bucknall CA, Morris GK, Mitchell JRA. Physicians' attitudes to four common problems: hyper-tension, atrial fibrillation, transient ischaemic attacks, and angina pectoris. *Br Med J* 1986;293:739–742.
45. Moss AJ. Atrial fibrillation and cerebral embolism (editorial). *Arch Neurol* 1984;41:707.
46. Is lone atrial fibrillation really benign (editorial)? *Lancet* 1986;1:305–306.
47. Cerebral Embolism Study Group. Immediate anticoagulation of embolic stroke: a randomized trial. *Stroke* 1983;14:668–676.
48. Roy D, Marchand E, Gagné P, Chabot M, Cartier R. Usefulness in anticoagulant therapy in the prevention of embolic complications of atrial fibrillation. *Am Heart J* 1986;112:1039–1043.
49. Poller L. Therapeutic ranges in anticoagulant administration. *Br Med J* 1985;290:1683–1686.
50. Stroke Prevention in Atrial Fibrillation Study Group Investigators. Preliminary report of the stroke prevention in atrial fibrillation study. *N Engl J Med* 1990;322:863–868.
51. The Boston Area Anticoagulation Trial for Atrial Fibrillation Investigators. The effect of low-

dose warfarin on the risk of stroke in patients with non-rheumatic atrial fibrillation. *N Engl J Med* 1990;323:1505–1511.

52. Saour JN, Sieck JO, Mamo LAR, Gallus AS. Trial of different intensities of anticoagulation in patients with prosthetic heart valves. *N Engl J Med* 1990;322:428–432.

53. Smith P, Arnesen H, Holme I. The effect of warfarin on mortality and reinfarction after myocardial infarction. *N Engl J Med* 1990;323:147–152.

54. Petersen P, Kastrup J, Helweg-Larsen S, Boysen G, Godtfredsen J. Risk factors for thromboembolic complications in chronic atrial fibrillation. The Copenhagen AFASAK Study. *Arch Intern Med* 1990;150:819–821.

55. Petersen P. Thromboembolic complications in atrial fibrillation. *Stroke* 1990;21:4–13.

56. Petersen P, Hansen JM. Stroke in thyrotoxicosis with atrial fibrillation. *Stroke* 1988;19:15–18.

57. Aronow WS, Gustein H, Hsieh FY. Risk factors for thromboembolic stroke in elderly patients with chronic atrial fibrillation. *Am J Cardiol* 1989;63:366–367.

58. Flegel KM, Hanley J. Risk factors for stroke and other embolic events in patients with nonrheumatic atrial fibrillation. *Stroke* 1989;20:1000–1004.

59. Walker MD. Atrial fibrillation and antithrombotic prophylaxis: a prospective metaanalysis. *Lancet* 1989;1:325–326.

Atrial Fibrillation: Mechanisms and Management, edited by
R. H. Falk and P. J. Podrid.
Raven Press, Ltd., New York © 1992.

17

Clinical Electrophysiology of the Normal and Diseased Human Atria

Ross J. Simpson, Jr.

Cardiology Section, University of North Carolina at Chapel Hill, Chapel Hill, North Carolina 27599

Atrial fibrillation, atrial flutter, and ectopic atrial tachycardia are forms of primary atrial arrhythmia that may cause congestive heart failure and stroke and may increase the risk of death (1–5). However, until recently, there has been little electrophysiologic information on what predisposes the human atrium to these arrhythmias. The difficulty in measuring atrial excitability and conduction in patients predisposed to primary atrial tachycardias has contributed to our lack of understanding of the electrophysiologic mechanism for this important class of arrhythmias.

Historically, atrial fibrillation was studied as a model for ventricular fibrillation, and many of the principles of reentry, the wavefront theory, and the importance of increased chamber size and mass in determining the potential for fibrillation were originally described in the human atrium (6–10). Electrophysiologic studies by microelectrode techniques of human atrial tissue have also contributed to our understanding of mechanisms for fibrillation. Observed abnormalities of the diseased human atria include elevation of the resting membrane potential, depression of the maximal amplitude, and decreased upstroke velocity of the action potential. These abnormalities appear related to a patient's past history of atrial tachyarrhythmia and the presence of a dilated atrium (11–15). These types of abnormalities should be detectable by clinical electrophysiologic study.

In order to determine if abnormalities of atrial excitability and conduction could explain the probability of a patient's developing atrial fibrillation, we measured strength-interval curves and strength-duration curves from the high right atrium, and conduction times within the atrium in a variety of patients undergoing clinical electrophysiologic study. We chose to measure these electrophysiologic properties because of their ease of standardization, their wide applicability to other electrophysiology laboratories, and their previous safe use in the human ventricle. We hypothesized that these techniques would be ideal for defining the clinical electrophysiology of the normal atrium and identifying electrophysiologic abnormalities of patients with the diverse pathologic abnormalities often found in patients at risk for atrial fibrillation (16,17).

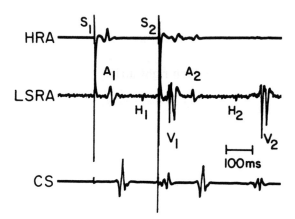

FIG. 1. Intracardiac recording from the high right atrium (HRA), low septal right atrium (LSRA), and distal coronary sinus (CS) in a patient with abnormal P-wave morphology suggestive of atrial disease. S_1 represents the last beat in the atrial pacing train and S_2 the premature beat. Latency is measured from the stimulus artifact (S_1 or S_2) to the HRA deflection (A_1 or A_2). Intraatrial conduction time is measured from the local electrogram of HRA catheter to that of the LSRA catheter, and interatrial conduction time is measured from the electrograms of the HRA to the left atrial (CS) deflection. In this patient the introduction of S_2 is associated with an increased latency, intraatrial and interatrial conduction time. (From ref. 16, with permission.)

ELECTROPHYSIOLOGIC TECHNIQUES

Our laboratory uses standard electrophysiologic pacing catheters. Following a routine electrophysiologic study for clinical indications and following research consent procedures, patients have multiple pole catheters positioned in the high lateral right atrium at the junction of the superior vena cava and the right atrium. Exact positioning of the right atrial catheter is adjusted until a stable late diastolic threshold of less than 1 mA at a pulse duration of 2 msec is obtained. An additional multiple pole catheter is positioned across the His bundle in the low septal right atrium such that an atrial electrogram, a His electrogram, and a ventricular electrogram are recorded. Whenever possible, a catheter is positioned to record the left atrium via the coronary sinus or, if the coronary sinus cannot be entered, another left atrial recording site.

Atrial strength-interval curves are measured by pacing the high right atrium for eight to 10 beats of S_1S_2 drive pacing at a rate faster than sinus rhythm. Pacing is performed at twice the late diastolic threshold for a 2-msec stimulus, and an S_2 premature stimulus is introduced late in the cardiac cycle. Threshold of the S_2 stimulus is measured by selectively decreasing the current strength of the stimulus until capture is lost. The S_1S_2 coupling interval is then decreased and the process repeated until a 10-mA current fails to induce a propagated response. The current strength of the stimulus for each impulse is measured by a calibrated voltage-to-current converter and the voltage displayed simultaneously with the standard electrograms.

Electrograms are recorded at paper speeds of 100 to 200 mm per second, and atrial conduction times are measured from the high right atrial catheter to the low septal right atrial catheter and from the high right atrial catheter to the left atrial catheter for each induced atrial beat. Conduction times include *latency,* measured from the stimulus artifact to the local electrogram on the high right atrial catheter, *intraatrial conduction time*, measured from the local electrogram of the high right atrial catheter to the low septal right atrial catheter, and *interatrial conduction time*, measured from the local electrogram of the high right atrial catheter to the left atrial catheter (Fig. 1).

PATIENTS STUDIED

We have studied approximately 60 patients in whom the added time of the procedure did not appear to pose a significant risk. Most had atrioventricular (AV) block, paroxysmal atrial fibrillation or flutter, AV nodal reentrant tachycardia, or unexplained syncope. All were in sinus rhythm. Most were men (61%), and almost half (48%) had a history of primary atrial arrhythmia, and 40% had clinically diagnosed organic heart disease.

Because of the high prevalence of atrial abnormalities in our subjects, we developed rigorous criteria for a normal atrium. A *normal atrium* was defined by the absence of a history of primary atrial tachyarrhythmia, absence of EKG conduction abnormalities suggesting sick sinus syndrome, absence of a P wave in excess of 120 msec, absence of cardiomegaly, and absence of congestive heart failure. Patients with apparently normal atria but who had a history of paroxysmal atrial fibrillation were classified as having lone atrial fibrillation (18). Patients were classified as having sick sinus syndrome if there was evidence of persistent sinus bradycardia, sinus exit block, or sinus pauses (19).

CLINICAL ELECTROPHYSIOLOGY OF THE ATRIA

We could not detect major differences in atrial excitability of the right atrium of patients with primary atrial arrhythmia or patients with sick sinus syndrome compared to normals. Characteristically, the high right atrial threshold was stable in late diastole but increased rapidly at a critical S_1S_2 coupling interval. This critical value was defined as the *total refractory period* (Fig. 2), the shortest S_1S_2 interval prior to

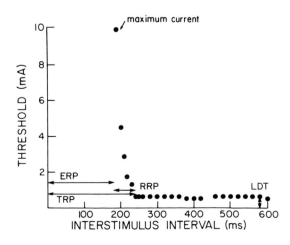

FIG. 2. Representative strength-interval curve showing threshold of shortest S_1 and S_2 to induce a propagated response (maximum current), total refractory period (TRP), effective refractory period (ERP), relative refractory period (RRP), and late diastolic threshold (LDT). (From ref. 17, with permission.)

a 25% increase in threshold current. Other refractory periods measured included the *effective refractory period,* defined as the longest S_1S_2 interval in which a stimulus of 10 mA failed to initiate a response, and the *relative refractory period,* defined as the difference between the effective refractory period and the total refractory period (Fig. 2).

We found that high currents are required to accurately measure the atrial functional and the effective refractory periods. Compared to currents of twice diastolic threshold, currents of 10 mA decrease the effective refractory period by an average of 30 msec and the functional refractory period (defined as the shortest measured A_1A_2 interval) by an average of 15 msec. In general, a minimal current strength of four times the late diastolic threshold is necessary to accurately measure the effective refractory period.

The average duration of the relative refractory period was approximately 60 msec and ranged from 20 to 130 msec. The relative refractory period did not correlate with the type or severity of atrial arrhythmia and did not separate patients with apparently normal atria from patients with primary atrial arrhythmia. Similarly, late diastolic threshold averaged 0.9 msec and did not differ among groups of patients. Moreover, the functional, total, relative, and effective refractory periods did not vary by patient group, except that the effective refractory period was shorter in patients with lone atrial fibrillation than in patients with normal atria.

The relationship between threshold current and pulse duration was measured for pulse durations from 0.1 to 10 msec. In late atrial diastole, as the pulse duration decreased below 2.0 msec, the threshold current gradually increased until at a pulse duration of 0.1 msec the threshold averaged approximately 6.6 mA. *Rheobasic current,* which is an estimate of the current threshold at wide pulse durations, was operationally estimated as the stable threshold current achieved at a wide pulse duration of 10.0 msec. The minimal pulse duration that achieves rheobasic current was defined as the shortest pulse duration at which the threshold current was within 0.2 mA of the rheobasic current.

Rheobasic current was uncommonly achieved with a pulse duration of 2 msec, and only 20% of our patients achieved rheobasic current at this pulse duration. In the remainder of patients, current threshold decreased as the pulse duration increased, with approximately 50% of patients achieving rheobasic current at a pulse duration of 4 msec.

The strength-duration curve was remeasured at a short S_1S_2 coupling interval when the threshold had increased in early diastole (Fig. 3). As expected, the strength-duration curve shifted upward with thresholds of narrow pulse duration stimuli increasing more than thresholds at longer pulse durations. However, the strength-duration relationship, whether measured in early or late diastole, did not differ across patient groups and did not separate patients who had a history of arrhythmia from those without such a history. We could not define any obvious characteristic of the strength-duration curves that correlated with clinical characteristics of our patients.

In contrast to the atrial excitability measurements, conduction time measurements appeared to be clinically useful. Conduction times were stable in late atrial diastole. However, as the atrial relative refractory period was entered, conduction times increased. Latency increased during early atrial diastole in all patients. A significant but less dramatic increase in the intraatrial and interatrial conduction times occurred in most patients, but such major atrial conduction time changes rarely occurred in patients with normal atria.

Conduction times in late diastole did not differ by clinical history of the patient

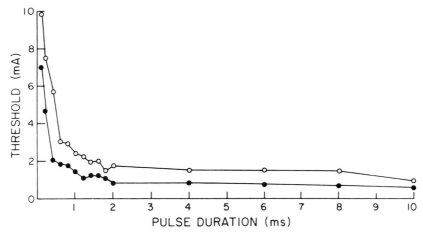

FIG. 3. Strength-duration curve measured during late diastole (*closed circles*) and during relative refractory period (*open circles*). See text for details. (From ref. 17, with permission.)

and averaged 40 msec for latency, 30 msec for the right atrial intraatrial conduction time, and 68 msec for the right to left atrial interatrial conduction time. When premature atrial beats were induced during the relative refractory period, latency increased by an average maximum of 43 msec, intraatrial conduction time increased by an average maximum of 26 msec, and interatrial conduction time by an average maximum of 35 msec. Compared to normals, patients with sick sinus syndrome, those with lone atrial fibrillation, and those with any type of previous history of primary atrial tachyarrhythmia had significantly greater increases in these latter conduction times (Fig. 4). In normal atria, the maximal increase (mean ± SD) in intraatrial and interatrial conduction times was 10 ± 2 and 11 ± 4 msec, respectively. In contrast, patients with lone atrial fibrillation increased conduction times by 29 ± 8 and 35 ± 6 msec, respectively. Patients with sick sinus syndrome had similar changes in maximal conduction times compared to patients with lone atrial fibrillation. These differences between patients with normal atria and those with lone atrial fibrillation (or sick sinus syndrome) are the more noteworthy since these patients all had virtually identical conduction times in late diastole.

We attempted to augment the increase in the maximal intraatrial conduction time by delivering a second (A_3) beat, by decreasing the drive cycle length, and by administering lidocaine or procainamide. An A_3 premature beat following an early cycle A_2 beat shortened the effective refractory period of A_2 by approximately 55 msec. However, it caused no further increase in latency or in the maximal increase in atrial conduction time of the A_3 beat compared to the A_2 beat. Furthermore, a 100-msec decrease in the S_1S_1 drive cycle length decreased the effective refractory period as expected but did not further increase the maximal change in latency or the maximal increase in intraatrial conduction time. Similarly, lidocaine had no effect on effective refractory period latency or the increase in intraatrial conduction time of early cycle premature atrial beats. Procainamide was administered in two patients and increased the effective refractory period by 40 msec without further increasing the intraatrial conduction time of early cycle premature atrial beats. The maximal increase in conduction time observed for early cycle A_2 beats thus appeared to be a

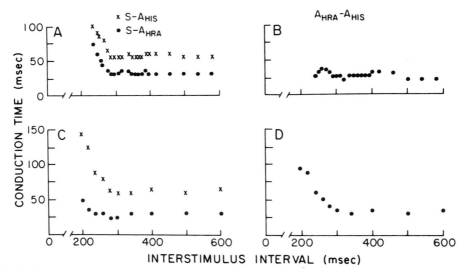

FIG. 4. Representative conduction-interval curves in a patient with normal P-wave morphology (**A** and **B**) and from the patient shown in Fig. 1 (**C** and **D**). A is a graph of the latency conduction time from stimulus to local high right atrial electrogram (S-A$_{HRA}$) and of the stimulus to the local LSRA electrogram (S-A$_{HIS}$). B shows intraatrial conduction time (A$_{HRA}$-A$_{HIS}$) determined by subtracting S-A$_{HRA}$ from S-A$_{HIS}$. As can be seen, there is little increase in intraatrial conduction time as the interstimulus interval decreases. In C and D a marked increase in intraatrial conduction time is seen, due mainly to the increase in S-A$_{HIS}$ provoked by S$_2$. (From ref. 16, with permission.)

true maximal atrial conduction time, and further increases in conduction time were not readily achieved.

These increases in conduction time of the A$_2$ beat were often associated with repetitive atrial beats (Fig. 5) and approximately 43% of our patients had induction of single, nonsustained, or sustained primary atrial tachyarrhythmia. These repetitive responses were not induced in patients with normal atria but occurred predominantly in patients with a history of sick sinus syndrome or lone atrial fibrillation. However, increases in atrial conduction time of early cycle beats were not limited to patients with a history of atrial tachyarrhythmia but occurred in many patients who had sick sinus syndrome with no previous history of atrial arrhythmia. Moreover, there was no obvious relationship between the magnitude of the change in conduction time and the frequency or type of previous episodes of atrial arrhythmia. That is, patients with more frequent episodes of atrial fibrillation were not more likely to have greater increases in atrial conduction time compared to patients who had had only one episode of atrial fibrillation. Moreover, patients who had a history of nonsustained ectopic atrial tachycardia had similar increases in intraatrial conduction time compared to patients who had a history of atrial fibrillation.

In a correlation analysis, the strongest correlate of primary atrial tachyarrhythmia was the maximal increase in interatrial or intraatrial conduction times (17). The ability to induce a primary atrial arrhythmia by a single, very early cycle atrial premature beat was also highly correlated with the maximal increase in the interatrial or intraatrial conduction time. The patient's age, functional class, left atrial size, P-wave duration, and an excessively short effective refractory period or a long latency

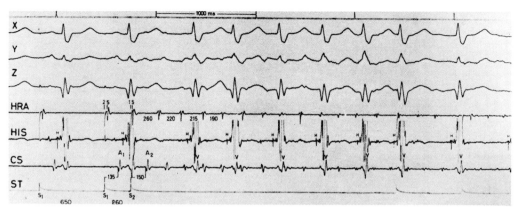

FIG. 5. Precipitation of atrial fibrillation by a single atrial extrastimulus (S_2) in a patient with a history of paroxysmal atrial fibrillation. S_2 produces a prolongation of interatrial conduction time (S_2 cannot be visualized from the His bundle catheter owing to the superimposition of the ventricular spike). Multiple, irregular atrial responses of <300 msec, best seen in the high right atrial (HRA) and coronary sinus (CS) catheter, follow S_2 and represent atrial fibrillation, which persisted until DC cardioversion, 20 min later. (From ref. 24, with permission.)

period were also correlated with the ability of an early cycle premature atrial beat to induce repetitive beats.

COMMENT

This project allowed us to develop reference tables for high right atrial threshold, high right atrial refractory periods, and conduction times in the intact human atrium and to estimate the effect of two relatively common diseases, sick sinus syndrome and lone atrial fibrillation, on atrial conduction and excitability. It led us to a tenable hypothesis to explain the mechanism of the commonly observed phenomenon whereby an early cycle atrial beat often is the initiating event in the induction of atrial fibrillation (20,21). We found a significant correlation between a patient's past history of primary atrial tachyarrhythmia and the maximal increase in atrial conduction time of early cycle premature beats. Moreover, this increase in atrial conduction time of premature beats during the relative refractory period correlated with induction of repetitive atrial beats during electrophysiologic study. However, this abnormality lacked specificity and patients with sick sinus syndrome who did not have a history of primary atrial arrhythmia had similar increases in conduction time compared to similar patients who had a history of atrial arrhythmias.

Other investigators have found results similar to ours. Cosio et al. (22) and subsequently Buxton et al. (23) described similar changes in atrial conduction time of early cycle premature atrial beats. These changes in atrial conduction time could be related to the coupling of the premature beat and whether the underlying rhythm was paced or sinus (22). Cosio et al. also related the propensity to induce slowed conduction to repetitive atrial firing and to a patient's past history of atrial fibrillation (22,24). Buxton et al. suggested that these results were nonspecific and occurred in most subjects, even normals, when the S_1S_2 drive cycle length was decreased (23).

This apparent difference in results may be partially due to differences in patients studied and the stringent criteria used for defining a normal atrium.

Other investigators have described the "fractionation" of the local atrial electrogram as closely coupled atrial premature beats are induced in the atria of patients with a history of atrial fibrillation (25) (Fig. 6). Similar fragmented electrograms were seen by us and appeared associated with the increase in conduction time observed between recording electrodes when premature beats were induced during the atrial relative refractory period. It seems reasonable to believe that the increase in atrial conduction time and fragmentation of local electrograms are due to the same electrophysiologic process that both fractionates signals recorded at a pair of recording electrodes and delays or reroutes the path of conduction between pairs of recording electrodes.

Recently, prolonged and fragmented atrial electrograms have been measured in sinus rhythm in patients with paroxysmal atrial fibrillation and sinus node disease (Fig. 7). Tanigawa et al. (26) measured atrial electrograms from 12 right atrial sites in each of 92 patients. An abnormal atrial electrogram was defined as having a duration of 100 msec or more or the presence of eight or more fragmented deflections (Fig. 8). Such abnormal electrograms were found more commonly in atrial maps of patients with a history of paroxysmal atrial fibrillation and sick sinus syndrome compared to patients with sick sinus syndrome alone (26). Although these findings need to be confirmed, they suggest that diseased atrial muscle segments can be identified and that such areas are more extreme in patients with a more extensive tachyarrhythmia history. Support for this observation comes from Fukunami et al. (27), who found prolonged, low-amplitude signals following the P wave in patients with a history of paroxysmal atrial fibrillation undergoing P wave-triggered, signal-averaged electrocardiography (Fig. 9). Other investigators have often described how repetitive atrial firing can be induced by a closely coupled early premature beat, occasionally in patients who do not have a history of atrial tachyarrhythmia (28). Our experience

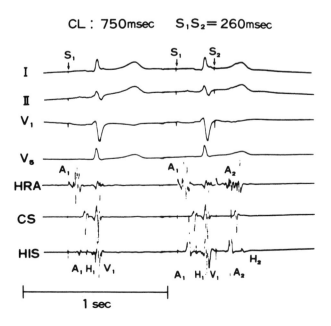

FIG. 6. Representative surface leads I, II, V_1, and V_5 and intracardiac recording in a 43-year-old woman with sick sinus syndrome and paroxysmal atrial fibrillation. Following atrial stimulation (S_1) at a basic cycle length of 750 msec, a premature stimulus (S_2) is introduced at a coupling interval of 260 msec. Prolonged, fragmented atrial activity exceeding 100 msec in duration (A_2) is seen in the high right atrium (HRA). Such a prolonged duration of fragmentation was not seen in any of 16 control subjects free of sick sinus syndrome or spontaneous atrial fibrillation. (From ref. 25, with permission.)

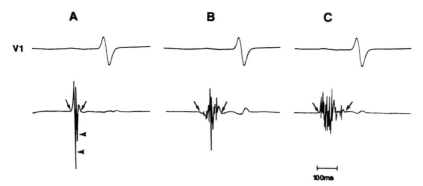

FIG. 7. Local atrial electrograms recorded during sinus rhythm from three separate sites in the right atrium of a patient with paroxysmal atrial fibrillation and sick sinus syndrome. The *diagonal arrows* mark the onset and offset of local atrial activity. **A:** Electrogram is normal with a duration of 50 msec and two fragmented deflections (defined as discrete, downward deflections, *horizontal arrows*). **B:** Electrogram is prolonged to 110 msec and nine fragmented deflections are present. Electrogram in **C** is even more abnormal with a duration of 130 msec and 13 fragmented deflections. (From ref. 26, with permission.)

is that induction of single, repetitive, or sustained atrial tachyarrhythmia is common. It occurs in patients who have any type of atrial abnormality including a prolonged P-wave duration, left atrial enlargement, congestive heart failure, or sick sinus syndrome. This phenomenon appears to be nonspecific and is both common in patients with lone atrial fibrillation but rare in the truly normal atria. It does not appear to be an artifact of stimulating current or pacing protocol, since a prolonged P-wave

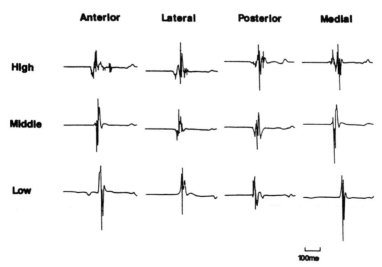

FIG. 8. Complete 12 site intraatrial map recorded from the right atrium during sinus rhythm in a patient with sick sinus syndrome and paroxysmal atrial fibrillation. The site of each recording is labeled. All four electrograms in the high right atrium exceed 100-msec duration and show many fragmented deflections. Recordings from the mid and low atrium are normal in number and duration. The abnormal high right atrial recordings demonstrate the importance of recording from multiple catheter sites to detect prolonged or fractionated electrograms. (From ref. 26, with permission.)

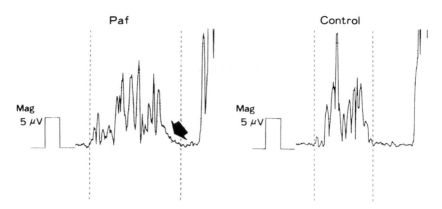

FIG. 9. P-wave triggered signal averaged electrocardiograms in a patient with paroxysmal atrial fibrillation (paf) (**left**) and a subject without this arrhythmia (control) (**right**). The *arrow-head* indicates the low-amplitude "atrial late potential" in the terminal portion of the filtered P wave. Note that the duration of the filtered P wave in the patient with paroxysmal atrial fibril-lation is considerably longer than that in the control (*dotted lines*). (From ref. 27, with permis-sion.)

duration (29,30) increased atrial size (31), and sick sinus syndrome all predispose to clinical episodes of atrial fibrillation.

Our observations are also consistent with the medical literature. Stimulus strength and duration appear to be important in estimating refractory periods. Importantly, stimulating currents of greater than twice the late diastolic threshold are required to achieve stable estimates of effective, functional, and relative refractory periods. This finding is similar to, but more pronounced than, results from the human ventricle (32). The observation implies that atrial effective refractory periods cannot be esti-mated by means of the extrastimulus technique if the stimulating current is artifi-cially limited to currents of twice the late diastolic threshold. Moreover, the atrial relative refractory period may be longer than the ventricular relative refractory pe-riod. However, due to differences in our technique compared to the studies done by Greenspan et al. (32), further studies are needed to directly compare the differences in the relative refractory period of the atrium and ventricle to clarify if such differ-ences are present.

We were surprised that there was not an association between atrial excitability and either a patient's history of atrial tachyarrhythmia or the ability of an early cycle premature beat to induce tachyarrhythmia. We expected a prolonged relative refrac-tory period or a short effective refractory period to predispose to reentrant arrhyth-mia. Some investigators have reported that a high right atrial effective refractory period is shorter in patients with a past history of atrial fibrillation or flutter; how-ever, others report conflicting results (33–35). Our observations suggest that a short-ened effective refractory period may be seen in some patients with a history of atrial fibrillation but that this property is not a sufficient cause of atrial fibrillation or re-petitive atrial firing for most patients.

Dispersion of atrial refractory periods may be measured by determining functional and effective refractory periods at three different atrial sites and measuring the dif-ference between the longest and shortest periods (35). It was not an electrophysio-logic property we measured. Dispersion of atrial refractory periods may be present in patients with sick sinus syndrome (36). However, whether such dispersion of refractory periods is present in most patients prone to atrial fibrillation is unclear, and some authors do not find abnormally dispersed refractory periods in patients with a history of atrial fibrillation (34,36).

These observations suggest that most patients with sick sinus syndrome or a history of primary atrial tachyarrhythmia have abnormal increases in atrial conduction time when early cycle premature atrial beats are induced during the atrial relative refractory period. We think that this change in conduction allows early cycle atrial beats to induce atrial fibrillation in these patients. Patients who appear prone to such induction of atrial fibrillation include patients with sick sinus syndrome and lone atrial fibrillation and may include other patients with atrial enlargement or a prolonged P-wave duration on the electrocardiogram (16). Unfortunately, detailed measurements of high right atrial refractory periods or thresholds do not appear to aid in identifying patients susceptible to primary atrial tachyarrhythmias. However, these measurements of atrial excitability may be important in estimating such commonly used measures as the atrial refractory period.

ACKNOWLEDGMENTS

The studies described in this chapter were supported in part by the National Institute of Health Awards HL26484 and HL23624, and by Program Project Grant HL2730. The research methods and results are described in detail by the author in articles in the *American Heart Journal* and the *Journal of the American College of Cardiology,* as shown in the bibliography.

REFERENCES

1. Simpson RJ Jr, Foster JR, Gettes LS. The electrophysiological substrate of atrial fibrillation. *PACE* 1983;6:1166–1170.
2. Benditt DG, Benson DW Jr, Dunnigan A, Gornick CC, Anderson RW. Atrial flutter, atrial fibrillation, and other primary atrial tachycardias. *Med Clin North Am* 1984;68:895–929.
3. Kannel WB, Abbott RD, Savage DD, McNamara PM. Epidemiologic features of chronic atrial fibrillation—the Framingham study. *N Engl J Med* 1982;30:1018–33.
4. Brand FN, Abbott RD, Kannel WB, Wolf PA. Characteristics and prognosis of lone atrial fibrillation—30 year follow-up in the Framingham study. *JAMA* 1985;254:3449–3453.
5. Feld GK. Atrial fibrillation—is there a safe and highly effective pharmacological treatment. *Circulation* 1990;82:2248–2250.
6. Garrey WE. The nature of fibrillary contraction of the heart—its relation to tissue mass and form. *Am J Physiol* 1914;33:397–414.
7. Lewis T. *Mechanism and graphic registration of the heart beat.* London: Shaw & Sons, 1925;83.
8. Han J, Millet D, Chizzonitti B, et al. Temporal dispersion of recovery of excitability in atrium and ventricle as a function of heart rate. *Am Heart J* 1966;71:481–487.
9. Moe GK, Rheinboldt WC, Abildskov JA. A computer model of atrial fibrillation. *Am Heart J* 1964;67:200–220.
10. Moe GK, Abildskov JA. Experimental and laboratory reports—atrial fibrillation as a self-sustaining arrhythmia independent of focal discharge. *Am Heart J* 1959;58:59–70.
11. Hordof AJ, Edie R, Malm JR, Hoffman BF, Rosen MR. Electrophysiologic properties and response to pharmacologic agents of fibers from diseased human atria. *Circulation* 1976;54:774–779.
12. Mary-Rabine L, Albert A, Pham TD, et al. The relationship of human atrial cellular electrophysiology to clinical function and ultrastructure. *Circ Res* 1983;52:188–199.
13. Gelband H, Bush HL, Rosen MR, Myerburg RJ, Hoffman BF. Electrophysiologic properties of isolated preparations of human atrial myocardium. *Circ Res* 1972;33:293–300.
14. Hordof AJ, Spotnitz A, Mary-Rabine L, Edie RN, Rosen MR. The cellular electrophysiologic effects of digitalis on human atrial fibers. *Circulation* 1978;57:223–229.

15. Van Dam RT, Durrer D. Excitability and electrical activity of human myocardial strips from the left atrial appendage in cases of rheumatic mitral stenosis. *Circ Res* 1961;9:509–514.

16. Simpson RJ Jr, Foster JR, Gettes LS. Atrial excitability and conduction in patients with interatrial conduction defects. *Am J Cardiol* 1982;50:1331–1337.

17. Simpson RJ Jr, Amara I, Foster JR, Woelfel A, Gettes LS. Thresholds, refractory periods, and conduction times of the normal and diseased human atrium. *Am Heart J* 1988;116:1080–1090.

18. Evans W, Swann P. Lone auricular fibrillation. *Br Heart J* 1954;16:189–194.

19. Ferrer MI. The sick sinus syndrome in atrial disease. *JAMA* 1968;206:645–646.

20. Bennett MA, Pentecost BL. The pattern of onset and spontaneous cessation of atrial fibrillation in man. *Circulation* 1970;41:981–988.

21. Killip T, Gault JH. Mode of onset of atrial fibrillation in man. *Am Heart J* 1965;70:172–179.

22. Cosio FG, Palacios J, Vidal JM. Cocina EG, Gomez-Sanchez MA, Tamargo L. Electrophysiologic studies in atrial fibrillation. *Am J Cardiol* 1983;51:122–130.

23. Buxton AE, Waxman HL, Marchlinski FE, Josephson ME. Atrial conduction: effects of extra-stimuli with and without atrial dysrhythmias. *Am J Cardiol* 1984;54:755–761.

24. Cosio FG, Llovet A, Vidal JM. Mechanism and clinical significance of atrial repetitive responses in man. *PACE* 1983;6:53–59.

25. Ohe T, Matsuhisa M, Kamakura S, et al. Relation between the widening of the fragmented atrial activity zone and atrial fibrillation. *Am J Cardiol* 1983;52:1219–1222.

26. Tanigawa M, Fukatani M, Konoe A, Isomoto S, Kadena M, Hashiba K. Prolonged and fraction-ated right atrial electrograms during sinus rhythm in patients with paroxysmal atrial fibrillation and sick sinus node syndrome. *J Am Coll Cardiol* 1991;17:403–408.

27. Fukunami M, Yamada T, Ohmori M, et al. Detection of patients at risk for paroxysmal atrial fibrillation during sinus rhythm by P wave triggered signal-averaged electrocardiogram. *Circulation* 1991;83:162–169.

28. Engel TR, Luck JC, Leddy CL, Gonzales AC. Diagnostic implications of atrial vulnerability. *PACE* 1979;2:208–214.

29. Buxton AE, Josephson ME. The role of P-wave duration as a predictor of postoperative atrial arrhythmias. *Chest* 1981;80:68–73.

30. Kawano S, Hiraoka M, Sawanobori T. Electrocardiographic features of P-waves from patients with transient atrial fibrillation. *Jpn Heart J* 1988;29:57–67.

31. Henry WL, Morganroth J, Pearlman AS, et al. Relation between echocardiographically deter-mined left atrial size and atrial fibrillation. *Circulation* 1976;53:273–278.

32. Greenspan AM, Camardo JS, Horowitz LN, Spielman SR, Josephson ME. Human ventricular refractoriness: effects of increasing current. *Am J Cardiol* 1981;47:244–250.

33. Michelucci A, Padeletti L, Fradella GA. Atrial refractoriness and spontaneous or induced atrial fibrillation. *Acta Cardiol* 1982;37:333–344.

34. Bauernfeind RA, Wyndham CR, Swiryn SP, et al. Paroxysmal atrial fibrillation in the Wolff-Par-kinson-White syndrome. *Am J Cardiol* 1981;47:562–569.

35. Sharma AD, Klein GJ, Guiraudon GM, Milstein S. Atrial fibrillation in patients with Wolff-Par-kinson-White syndrome: incidence after surgical ablation of the accessory pathway. *Circulation* 1985;72:161–169.

36. Luck JC, Engel TR. Dispersion of atrial refractoriness in patients with sinus node dysfunction. *Circulation* 1979;60:404–412.

Atrial Fibrillation: Mechanisms and Management, edited by
R. H. Falk and P. J. Podrid.
Raven Press, Ltd., New York © 1992.

18

Atrial Fibrillation in Wolff-Parkinson-White Syndrome

H. J. J. Wellens, J. L. R. M. Smeets, L. M. Rodriguez,
and A. P. M. Gorgels

*Department of Cardiology, Academic Hospital Maastricht, University of Limburg,
6202 AZ Maastricht, The Netherlands*

In other chapters of this book the causes, consequences, and management of atrial fibrillation have been discussed mainly in patients in whom conduction to the ventricles occurs via the normal atrioventricular (AV) node-His pathway. However, the presence of an accessory AV pathway can significantly influence both the risks and therapy of atrial fibrillation and may also play a role in the development of the arrhythmia itself. In this chapter we therefore discuss in detail the occurrence and management of atrial fibrillation in patients with preexcitation.

CLASSIFICATION OF PREEXCITATION

As shown in Fig. 1 several connections are possible either directly between the atrium and ventricle or between parts of the specific conduction system and atrium or ventricle. With the exception of fasciculoventricular fibers, all these connections bypass the AV node, either partially or completely. A true AV accessory pathway (Wolff-Parkinson-White [WPW] syndrome) is by far the most common of these connections. If such an AV accessory pathway is present, the ventricular rate during atrial fibrillation is not determined by the properties of the AV node-His pathway alone, but also, and sometimes exclusively, by the electrophysiological properties of the extra connection.

INCIDENCE OF ATRIAL FIBRILLATION IN PATIENTS WITH AN ACCESSORY ATRIOVENTRICULAR PATHWAY

The true incidence of atrial fibrillation in patients with an accessory AV pathway is not known. In patients having such a pathway and referred to an arrhythmia clinic because of symptomatic arrhythmia, the prevalence of atrial fibrillation has been found to vary from 10% to 35% (1–5). In a more recent series from our institution 20 of 220 patients undergoing surgical dissection of their accessory pathway had previously had clinical documentation of atrial fibrillation. This lesser prevalence of

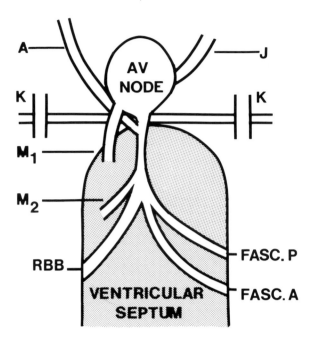

FIG. 1. Scheme of the normal atrioventricular (AV) conduction system and possible accessory connection(s) partially or totally bypassing the normal AV connections. A, atriofascicular bypass tract; J, atrionodal bypass tract; K, accessory AV pathway; M_1, nodoventricular pathway; M_2, fasciculoventricular pathway, Fasc. P, posterior fascicle of the left bundle branch; Fasc. A, anterior fascicle of the left bundle branch; RBB, right bundle branch.

atrial fibrillation probably reflects earlier referral of the WPW patient to an arrhythmia center.

The incidence of atrial fibrillation is age related. The older the patient, the higher the number of patients suffering from atrial fibrillation. In a consecutive series of 280 of our WPW patients, 35 of 212 (17%) patients had their first episode of atrial fibrillation before as compared to 20 of 68 (29%) patients after the age of 30 years.

RISK OF ATRIAL FIBRILLATION

As pointed out by several authors (6–18), sudden death may be the first arrhythmic manifestation in patients with WPW syndrome. In a recent European multicenter study (19) six of 23 patients with WPW syndrome resuscitated from ventricular fibrillation had sudden death as their first arrhythmic complaint. It seems reasonable to assume that atrial fibrillation precedes ventricular fibrillation in most of these patients.

In the human heart the ventricles are protected by the refractory period of the AV node against a very rapid ventricular rate during atrial fibrillation. In patients with an accessory AV pathway atrial fibrillation can be an extremely dangerous arrhythmia if the accessory connection has a short anterograde refractory period (Fig. 2). As shown in Fig. 3 atrial fibrillation with a very fast ventricular rate may degenerate into ventricular fibrillation. As indicated in Table 1 many factors determine the ventricular rate during atrial fibrillation (20). The table also suggests that measurements of these factors by invasive and noninvasive methods may be of help in predicting the ventricular rate during atrial fibrillation in a particular patient and therefore the possible risks if atrial fibrillation supervenes. This will be discussed later.

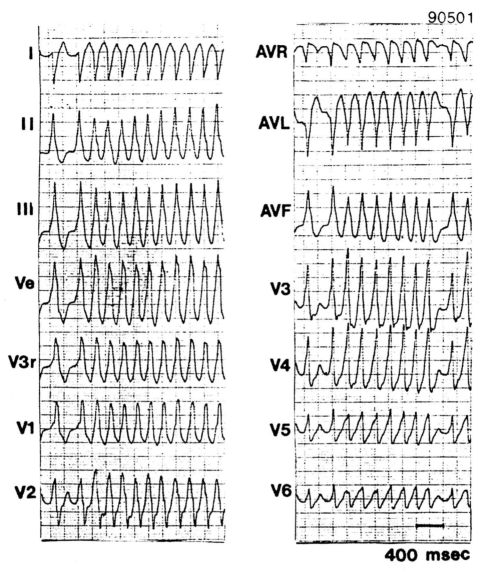

90501

400 msec

FIG. 2. Atrial fibrillation in a patient with a left free-wall accessory pathway. Note the very rapid and irregular rhythm with a wide QRS complex. These three features are typical for atrial fibrillation in the presence of an accessory pathway with a short anterograde refractory period.

MECHANISMS OF ATRIAL FIBRILLATION IN PATIENTS WITH AN ACCESSORY ATRIOVENTRICULAR PATHWAY

In an earlier publication (21), we described that in the clinical electrophysiology laboratory several mechanisms of initiation of atrial fibrillation can be observed in the WPW patient. These include a single atrial premature beat or an early ventricular premature beat that is retrogradely conducted to the atrium, as well as straight ventricular pacing (Fig. 4) or degeneration of a circus movement tachycardia (both orthodromic [Fig. 5] and antidromic [19,22,23]).

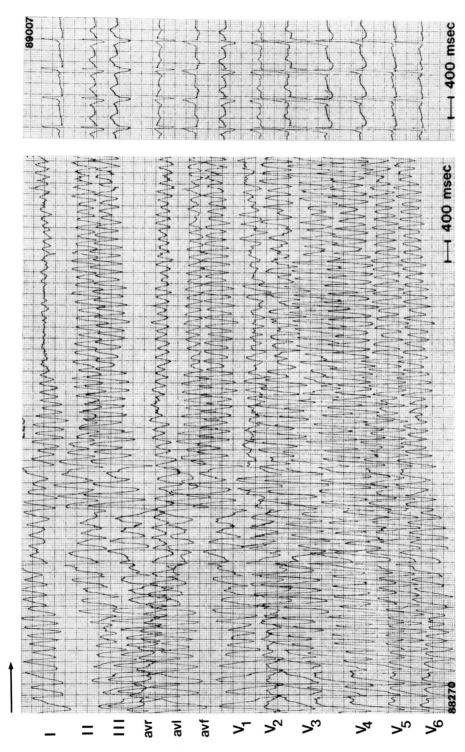

FIG. 3. Deterioration of atrial fibrillation into ventricular fibrillation in a patient with Wolff-Parkinson-White syndrome. *Right:* ECG during sinus rhythm.

TABLE 1. *Factors determining the ventricular rate during atrial fibrillation in Wolff-Parkinson-White syndrome*

Accessory pathway
1. Refractory period (influenced by heart rate and autonomic nervous system).
2. Conductive properties (related to width, length, and type of tissue of accessory pathway)
3. Concealed conduction → in atrioventricular direction
                          → in ventriculoatrial direction
4. Reentry?
AV nodal pathway
1. Refractory period (influenced by heart rate and autonomic nervous system)
2. Conductive properties
3. Concealed conduction
4. Reentry
Ventricle
1. Refractory period

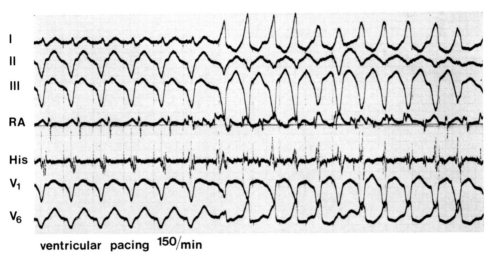

ventricular pacing 150/min

FIG. 4. Initiation of atrial fibrillation during regular ventricular pacing at a rate of 150 beats per minute. Note in the right atrial (RA) recording a change from 1 to 1 retrograde conduction into atrial fibrillation.

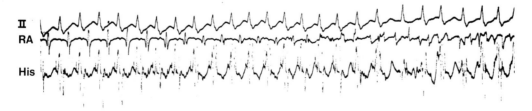

600 msec

FIG. 5. Example of orthodromic circus movement tachycardia deteriorating into atrial fibrillation. This change can best be observed in the right atrial (RA) recording.

Some authors have shown that vulnerability for induction of atrial fibrillation is greater in patients with WPW syndrome suffering from atrial fibrillation than in those without spontaneous atrial fibrillation (24). Recent observations by Fujimura et al. (25) suggest that intra-atrial conduction abnormalities are present in patients with WPW and atrial fibrillation as evidenced by a longer PA interval in patients with inducible sustained atrial fibrillation.

Several groups have indicated that the presence of anterograde conduction over an accessory pathway is a factor facilitating the occurrence of atrial fibrillation (25–28). In our own series the incidence of spontaneous atrial fibrillation was 55 of 280 patients (20%) with AV conduction over the accessory pathway in contrast to two of 98 patients (2%) having only retrograde conduction over an accessory pathway (a so-called concealed accessory pathway). Sharma et al. (26) showed a marked reduction in the incidence of atrial fibrillation after successful surgical ablation of the accessory pathway. They (26) and other investigators (27,28) demonstrated that not only does the presence of anterograde conduction over the accessory pathway play a role in the genesis of atrial fibrillation, but the duration of the anterograde refractory period of the accessory pathway is also important, as patients with both spontaneous and electrically inducible atrial fibrillation had a shorter anterograde refractory period of their accessory pathway. The presence of more than one accessory pathway is also a factor associated with atrial fibrillation. As shown by Atié et al. (29), patients with multiple accessory pathways have a higher incidence of atrial fibrillation as compared to those having only one extra connection between atrium and ventricle. An intriguing question, which has to be answered, is the possible role of anisotropy between atrial fibers and the fibers at the atrial end of the accessory pathway. Theoretically, this might affect vulnerability to atrial fibrillation.

HOW TO DETERMINE RISK IN THE WOLFF-PARKINSON-WHITE PATIENT WHEN ATRIAL FIBRILLATION OCCURS

As has been discussed, the ventricular rate during atrial fibrillation is an important determinant of hemodynamic compromise and death in the WPW patient. A short anterograde refractory period of the accessory pathway is therefore a marker of a rapid ventricular rate during atrial fibrillation. In the past we showed that there is a good correlation between the shortest R-R interval during atrial fibrillation and the anterograde refractory period of the accessory pathway (20). Thus, measuring that refractory period using the single atrial test stimulus method during atrial pacing allows an estimation of the ventricular rate during atrial fibrillation (20). It is important to realize, however, that sympathetic stimulation induced by anxiety or a fall in blood pressure following the onset of a spontaneous episode of atrial fibrillation will lead to further abbreviation of the anterograde refractory period of the accessory pathway and an increase in ventricular rate (31). Consequently, determination of the anterograde refractory period of the accessory pathway by the single stimulus method tends to underestimate the ventricular rate during atrial fibrillation.

Information about the anterograde refractory period of the accessory pathway can also be obtained noninvasively. We have observed that failure to achieve complete anterograde block in this pathway following the intravenous administration of 50 mg of ajmaline is highly suggestive of an anterograde effective refractory period of the accessory pathway of less than 270 msec (32). This also holds true for procainamide given intravenously in a dosage of 10 mg/kg body weight over a 5-min period (33).

Therefore, in patients with WPW syndrome, a positive ajmaline or procainamide test (induction of anterograde block over the accessory pathway as demonstrated in Fig. 6) indicates that the patient has a relatively long duration of the pathway's refractory period and therefore will not have a very fast ventricular rate if atrial fibrillation occurs. Using a modified ajmaline test, Chimienti et al. (34) showed that the amount of ajmaline required to block conduction over the accessory pathway correlates with the duration of its anterograde refractory period. Because both ajmaline and procainamide also prolong the refractory period of the His-Purkinje system, such testing should be performed in an area where the possible complication of complete AV block can be appropriately managed.

There are two other noninvasive tests that indicate a long duration of the refractory period of the accessory pathway in the anterograde direction. First, the finding of intermittent preexcitation (35) on the 12-lead ECG or a long-term ECG recording. Second, as shown by Levy et al. (36), disappearance of preexcitation during exer-

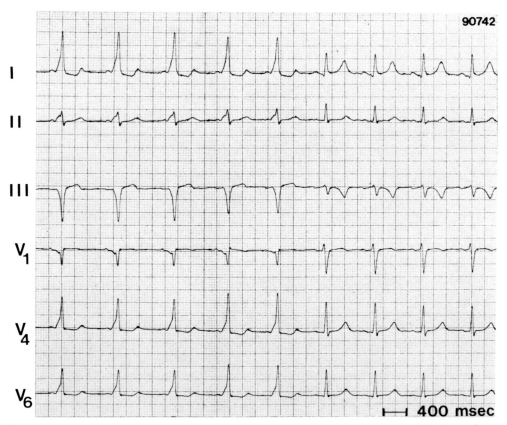

FIG. 6. Example of the creation of complete block in the accessory atrioventricular pathway by the intravenous injection of procainamide (10 mg/kg bodyweight over 5 min). Note disappearance of preexcitation in the middle of the figure.

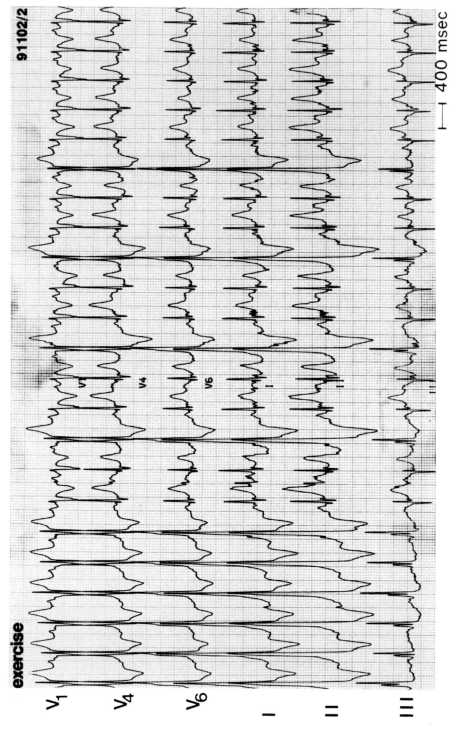

FIG. 7. Disappearance of preexcitation during exercise. As shown on reaching a critical heart rate of 140 beats per minute, block occurs in the accessory pathway. After a short period in which every third sinus beat is still conducted over the accessory pathway exclusive conduction over the atrioventricular node supervenes because of complete block in the accessory pathway.

cise, an example of which is shown in Fig. 7, indicates a long anterograde refractory period of the accessory pathway. One should be careful, however, in interpreting the results of exercise testing since sympathetic stimulation during exercise will speed up AV nodal conduction and might thereby diminish the area of the ventricles preexcited over the accessory pathway. Several ECG leads should be recorded simultaneously and special attention should be given to the ECG after exercise where, in case of exercise-induced block in the accessory pathway, a sudden marked change in the ECG takes place when preexcitation resumes.

While patients at low risk can be identified relatively easily, the asymptomatic patient in whom the results of noninvasive testing suggest a short anterograde refractory period of the accessory pathway presents a more difficult problem. The European multicenter study reported by Torner (19) showed that in an appreciable number of patients with WPW syndrome resuscitated from ventricular fibrillation, this arrhythmia was the first symptomatic arrhythmia they ever experienced.

Other studies, such as the one by Sharma et al. (37), suggest that *asymptomatic* patients with a short anterograde refractory period of their accessory pathway who are not treated with antiarrhythmic drugs have a good prognosis.

TREATMENT DURING ATRIAL FIBRILLATION

If the arrhythmia is hemodynamically poorly tolerated because of a rapid ventricular rate, direct current shock is indicated. When hemodynamically tolerated, drugs that lengthen the anterograde refractory period and have an antifibrillatory action can be injected intravenously. Our preference is for procainamide (10 mg/kg body weight over a 5-min period). Other drugs that can be given include ajmaline (1 mg/kg body weight over 3 min) and disopyramide. At the present time, insufficient information is available about the effectiveness and risks of the intravenous administration of class Ic drugs (propafenone, flecainide, encainide) for the treatment of atrial fibrillation with a rapid ventricular response in patients with WPW syndrome. It is important to stress that digitalis and verapamil should not be given during atrial fibrillation. Digitalis may shorten the anterograde refractory period of the accessory pathway (38) thereby increasing the ventricular rate during atrial fibrillation and facilitating deterioration into ventricular fibrillation. Verapamil, because of its negative inotropic effect, may also speed up the ventricular rate during atrial fibrillation.

PREVENTION OF NEW EPISODES OF ATRIAL FIBRILLATION

Following termination of atrial fibrillation one should first of all exclude other possible causes for atrial fibrillation than WPW syndrome itself by performing the appropriate tests. If additional causes are present, they should, of course, be corrected. If no other causes can be identified, our present policy in the treatment of the patient who has suffered from an episode of atrial fibrillation is to study the anterograde refractory period of the accessory pathway and to induce atrial fibrillation in the catheterization laboratory to obtain an impression of the ventricular rate during that arrhythmia. The effect of sympathetic stimulation (by giving isoproterenol) on the anterograde refractory period of the accessory pathway and the ventricular rate during electrically induced atrial fibrillation is also evaluated during the same stimulation study.

In view of the low risk and high success rate of radiofrequency current catheter ablation (39,40), this approach is suggested to the patient if a short anterograde refractory period (270 msec and less) is present or if atrial fibrillation is induced (without or during isoproterenol infusion) showing a shortest R-R interval of 250 msec or less. In patients in whom radiofrequency current catheter ablation is unsuccessful, surgical interruption of the accessory pathway or pathways is advised. In patients refusing radiofrequency current catheter ablation or surgery or in less symptomatic patients who have a relatively long anterograde refractory period of the accessory pathway, antiarrhythmic drug treatment is prescribed.

The antiarrhythmic drug should have an antifibrillatory effect and should prolong the anterograde refractory period of the accessory pathway. Class Ia (quinidine, procainamide, and disopyramide), class Ic (encainide, propafenone, and flecainide), and class III drugs (amiodarone and sotalol) all fulfill these requirements.

In our experience amiodarone has been most effective in preventing recurrent episodes of atrial fibrillation (41). It has the advantage of a single daily dose. The low dose required (usually 200 mg) is accompanied by a low incidence of side effects.

WHAT TO DO WITH THE ASYMPTOMATIC PATIENT

Considerable interest exists in the appropriate management of the asymptomatic patient discovered to have a WPW pattern on a routine electrocardiogram (42–45). In general, our policy is to withhold antiarrhythmic drug therapy in patients who show the WPW ECG without a history of arrhythmia but who have a short anterograde refractory period of the accessory pathway on noninvasive and invasive testing. We agree with Sharma et al. (37) and Klein et al. (46) that these patients have a good prognosis. However, in selected asymptomatic patients with a short anterograde refractory period of the accessory pathway, we have interrupted conduction over that structure by surgical or radiofrequency current ablation for professional reasons, for example, to be licensed to fly a commercial airliner or to be insured as a professional football player.

REFERENCES

1. Campbell RWF, Smith RA, Gallagher JJ, Pritchett ELC, Wallace AG. Atrial fibrillation in the preexcitation syndrome. *Am J Cardiol* 1977;40:514–520.
2. Bauernfeind RA, Wyndham CR, Swiryn SP, et al. Paroxysmal atrial fibrillation in the Wolff-Parkinson-White syndrome. *Am J Cardiol* 1981;47:562–569.
3. Sharma AD, Klein GJ, Guiraudon GM, Milstein S. Atrial fibrillation in patients with Wolff-Parkinson-White syndrome: incidence after surgical ablation of the accessory pathway. *Circulation* 1985;72:161–169.
4. Robinson K, Rowland E, Krikler DM. Wolff-Parkinson-White syndrome: atrial fibrillation as the presenting arrhythmia. *Br Heart J* 1988;59:578–580.
5. Wellens HJJ, Smeets JLRM, Gorgels APM, Farré J. The Wolff-Parkinson-White syndrome. In: Mandel WJ, ed. *Cardiac arrhythmias.* Philadelphia: Lippincott (*in press*).
6. Dreifus LS, Haiat R, Watanabe Y. Ventricular fibrillation: a possible mechanism of sudden death in patients with Wolff-Parkinson-White syndrome. *Circulation* 1971;43:520–527.
7. Laham J. *Actualités electrocardiographiques 1969: le syndrome de Wolff-Parkinson-White.* Paris: Libraire Maloine SA, 1969.
8. Kaplan MA, Cohen KL. Ventricular fibrillation in the Wolff-Parkinson-White syndrome. *Am J Cardiol* 1969;24:259–264.
9. Okel BB. The Wolff-Parkinson-White syndrome: report of a case with fatal arrhythmia and au-

topsy findings of myocarditis, interatrial lipomatous hypertrophy and prominent right moderator band. *Am Heart J* 1968;75:673–678.

10. Castillo-Fenoy A, Goupil A, Offenstadt G, et al. Syndrome de Wolff-Parkinson-White et mort subite. *Ann Med Intern* 1973;124:871–875.

11. Lem CH, Toh CCS, Chia BL. Ventricular fibrillation in type B Wolff-Parkinson-White syndrome. *Aust NZ J Med* 1974;4:515.

12. Dreifus LS, Wellens HJJ, Watanabe Y, et al. Sinus bradycardia and atrial fibrillation associated with the Wolff-Parkinson-White syndrome. *Am J Cardiol* 1976;38:149–156.

13. Klein GJ, Bashore TM, Sellers TD, et al. Ventricular fibrillation in the Wolff-Parkinson-White syndrome. *N Engl J Med* 1979;301:1080–1085.

14. Martin-Noel P, Denis B, Grundwald D, et al. Deux cas mortels de syndrome de Wolff-Parkinson-White. *Arch Mal Coeur* 1970;63:1647–1654.

15. Ahlinder S, Granath A, Holmer S, et al. The Wolff-Parkinson-White syndrome with paroxysmal atrial fibrillation changing into ventricular fibrillation, successfully treated with external heart massage. *Nord Med* 1963;70:1336–1343.

16. Fox TT, Weaver J, March HW. On the mechanism of arrhythmias in aberrant atrioventricular conduction (Wolff-Parkinson-White). *Am Heart J* 1952;43:507–514.

17. Touche M, Touche S, Jouvet M, et al. Eléments de prognostic dans le syndrome de Wolff-Parkinson-White. *Presse Med* 1968;76:567–570.

18. Wellens HJJ, Bär FW, Farré J, et al. Sudden death in the Wolff-Parkinson-White syndrome. In: Kulbertus KE, Wellens HJJ, eds. *Sudden death,* The Hague: Martinus Nijhoff, 1980;392–399.

19. Torner PM. Ventricular fibrillation in the Wolff-Parkinson-White syndrome. *Eur Heart J* 1991;12:144–152.

20. Wellens HJJ, Durrer D. Wolff-Parkinson-White syndrome and atrial fibrillation: relation between refractory period of the accessory pathway and ventricular rate during atrial fibrillation. *Am J Cardiol* 1974;40:514–520.

21. Wellens HJJ. The electrophysiologic properties of the accessory pathway in the Wolff-Parkinson-White syndrome. In: Wellens HJJ, Lie KI, Janse MJ, eds. *The conduction system of the heart.* Philadelphia: Lea and Febiger, 1976;567–584.

22. Pritzker MR, Kriett JM, Benditt DG. Onset of AF during antidromic tachycardia: association with sudden cardiac arrest and ventricular fibrillation in a patient with Wolff-Parkinson-White syndrome. *Am J Cardiol* 1982;50:353–359.

23. Bardy GH, Packer DL, German LD, Gallagher JJ. Preexcited reciprocating tachycardia in patients with Wolff-Parkinson-White syndrome: incidence and mechanisms. *Circulation* 1984;70:377–391.

24. Fiorenzo G, Carla G, Riccardo R, et al. Relation between spontaneous atrial fibrillation and atrial vulnerability in patients with Wolff-Parkinson-White pattern. *PACE* 1990;13:1249–1253.

25. Fujimura O, Klein GJ, Yee R, Sharma AD. Mode of onset of atrial fibrillation in the Wolff-Parkinson-White syndrome: how important is the accessory pathway? *J Am Coll Cardiol* 1990;15:1082–1086.

26. Sharma AD, Klein GJ, Guiraudon GM, Milstein S. Atrial fibrillation in patients with Wolff-Parkinson-White syndrome: incidence after surgical ablation of the accessory pathway. *Circulation* 1985;72:161–169.

27. Waspe LE, Brodman R, Kim SG, Fisher JD. Susceptibility to atrial fibrillation and ventricular tachyarrhythmia in the Wolff-Parkinson-White syndrome: role of the accessory pathway. *Am Heart J* 1986;112:1141–1152.

28. Della Bella P, Brugada P, Talajic M, et al. Atrial fibrillation in patients with an accessory pathway: importance of the conduction properties of the accessory pathway. *J Am Coll Cardiol* 1991;17:1352–1356.

29. Atié J, Brugada P, Smeets JLRM, et al. Clinical and electrophysiological characteristics of patients with antidromic circus movement tachycardia in the Wolff-Parkinson-White syndrome. *Am J Cardiol* 1990;66:1082–1091.

30. Wellens HJJ, Brugada P. Value of programmed stimulation of the heart in patients with the Wolff-Parkinson-White syndrome. In: Josephson ME, Wellens HJJ, eds. *Tachycardias.* Philadelphia: Lea and Febiger, 1984;199–222.

31. Wellens HJJ, Brugada P, Roy D, et al. Effect of isoproterenol on the anterograde refractory period of the accessory pathway in patients with the Wolff-Parkinson-White syndrome. *Am J Cardiol* 1982;50:180–184.

32. Wellens HJJ, Bär FW, Gorgels AP, et al. Use of ajmaline in identifying patients with the Wolff-Parkinson-White syndrome and a short refractory period of their accessory pathway. *Am J Cardiol* 1980;45:130–133.

33. Wellens HJJ, Braat SH, Brugada P, et al. Use of procainamide in patients with the Wolff-Parkinson-White syndrome to disclose a short refractory period of the accessory pathway. *Am J Cardiol* 1982;50:921–925.

34. Chimienti M, Moizi M, Klersy C, et al. A modified ajmaline test for prediction of the effective refractory period of the accessory pathway in the Wolff-Parkinson-White syndrome. *Am J Cardiol* 1987;59:164–165.
35. Wellens HJJ. The Wolff-Parkinson-White syndrome. Part I. *Mod Concepts Cardiovasc Dis* 1983;52:52–56.
36. Levy S, Broustet JP, Clemency J. Syndrome de Wolff-Parkinson-White. Correlations entre l'exploition electrophysiologique et l'effet de l'épreuve d'effort sur l'aspect electrocardiographique de pre-excitation. *Arch Mal Coeur* 1979;72:634–643.
37. Sharma AD, Yee R, Guiraudon G, et al. Sensitivity and specificity of invasive and noninvasive testing for risk of sudden death in Wolff-Parkinson-White syndrome. *J Am Coll Cardiol* 1987;10:373–381.
38. Wellens HJJ, Durrer D. Effect of digitalis on atrioventricular conduction and circus movement tachycardias in patients with the Wolff-Parkinson-White syndrome. *Circulation* 1973;47:1229–1233.
39. Jackman W, Wang X, Friday KJ, et al. Catheter ablation of accessory atrioventricular pathways (Wolff-Parkinson-White syndrome) by radiofrequency current. *N Engl J Med* 1991;324:1605–1611.
40. Calkins H, Sousa J, El-Atassi R, et al. Diagnosis and cure of the Wolff-Parkinson-White syndrome or paroxysmal supraventricular tachycardia during a single electrophysiologic test. *N Engl J Med* 1991;324:1612–1618.
41. Wellens HJJ, Brugada P, Abdollah H. Effect of amiodarone in paroxysmal supraventricular tachycardia with or without Wolff-Parkinson-White syndrome. *Am Heart J* 1983;106:876–880.
42. Klein GJ, Prystowsky EN, Yee R, Sharma AD, Laupacis A. Asymptomatic Wolff-Parkinson-White—should we intervene? *Circulation* 1989;80:1902–1905.
43. Leitch JW, Klein GJ, Yee R, Murdock C. Prognostic value of electrophysiologic testing in asymptomatic patients with Wolff-Parkinson-White pattern. *Circulation* 1990;82:1718–1724.
44. Fisch C. Clinical electrophysiologic studies and the Wolff-Parkinson-White pattern. *Circulation* 1990;82:1872–1873.
45. Beckman KJ, Gallastegui JL, Bauman JL, Hariman RJ. The predictive value of electrophysiologic studies in untreated patients with Wolff-Parkinson-White syndrome. *J Am Coll Cardiol* 1990;15:640–647.
46. Klein GJ, Yee R, Sharma AD. Longitudinal electrophysiologic assessment of asymptomatic patients with the Wolff-Parkinson-White electrocardiographic pattern. *N Engl J Med* 1989;320:1229–1233.

*Atrial Fibrillation: Mechanisms
and Management*, edited by
R. H. Falk and P. J. Podrid.
Raven Press, Ltd., New York © 1992.

19

The Use of Pacemakers in Atrial Fibrillation

Arthur Pollak and Rodney H. Falk

*Division of Cardiology, Boston City Hospital, Boston, Massachusetts 02118; Boston
University School of Medicine, Boston, Massachusetts 02118*

Atrial fibrillation (AF) is commonly associated with significant organic heart disease, may be a manifestation of generalized disease of the conduction system, or may require treatment with drugs that impair AV nodal conduction. Under these circumstances the ventricular response may be slow, requiring cardiac pacing. In this chapter we will review the strategies for permanent and temporary pacing in patients with AF, discuss the preferred mode of pacing in different situations, address some of the functional aspects of pacemakers used in AF, and express some newer concepts regarding the use of pacemakers for ventricular rhythm stabilization.

SLOW VENTRICULAR RATE IN ATRIAL FIBRILLATION

The ventricular response to AF is dependent on several factors including the structural integrity of the atrioventricular (AV) node, the degree of concealed AV nodal conduction, the state of autonomic tone, and the use of cardioactive medications. Ventricular rates may vary widely in an individual patient with AF, reaching slow or fast extremes depending on the net momentary effect of these factors on the AV node (Fig. 1). The heart rate variations may be much greater than those seen in sinus rhythm, and thus the range of heart rates described in normal subjects cannot be extrapolated to patients with AF.

It is important to recognize the "normal" extent and distribution of slow ventricular rates and prolonged ventricular pauses in AF, since both AF and symptoms of syncope or dizziness are common in older patients, but their coexistence does not necessarily imply that the symptoms are related to the arrhythmia. The literature in this regard is sparse, and most studies are retrospective and frequently contain subjects in whom Holter monitor recordings were obtained as part of the evaluation of diverse symptomatology.

Two uncontrolled studies concluded that pacing in patients with AF and dizziness or syncope who also had ventricular pauses during Holter monitoring was successful in abolishing symptoms in most subjects. Ector et al. (1) reviewed 24-hr Holter recordings of 2,350 consecutive patients and found 53 patients (2.3%) to have pauses of 3 sec or more. Of these patients, 42% had persistent AF. The majority of patients with pauses of 3 sec or more in this study had cerebral symptoms, and the authors concluded that such pauses therefore represent a definite indication for permanent

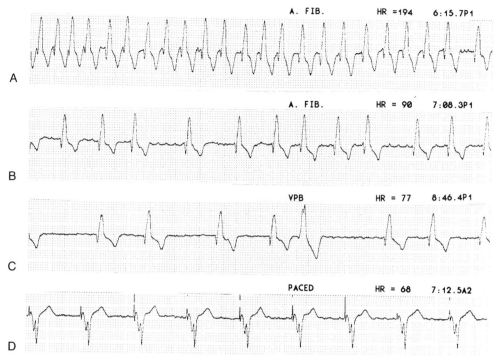

FIG. 1. Representative Holter monitor tracings from a patient with a tricuspid valve replacement and atrial fibrillation who received an epicardial pacing system for symptomatic ventricular pauses. The tracings demonstrate the wide range of heart rates during normal daily activities. **A:** While sweeping the floor. **B:** 1 hr later, driving home. **C:** Relaxing and talking to wife. **D:** Prior to waking, ventricular pacing at a rate of 68 beats per minute. Heart rates as noted above each strip.

pacing. Rebello and co-workers (2) reported on the results of permanent pacemaker insertion in 35 patients with syncope or dizziness who also had chronic AF and pauses of 2 sec or more on Holter monitoring. Despite a lack of correlation between ventricular pauses and symptoms, they found symptom resolution or improvement after pacing in all subjects and concluded that permanent pacemaker placement will help to improve or resolve cerebral symptoms in subjects with persistent AF and pauses in excess of 2 sec.

The two studies described above lacked a control group and addressed neither the expected natural history of symptoms nor the anticipated range of ventricular rates in an unselected patient population with chronic AF. This issue has been examined, and the findings cast serious doubt on the recommendations to insert a permanent pacemaker for pauses that are not correlated with symptoms in AF. Pitcher et al. (3) reviewed the Holter recordings of 66 asymptomatic patients with AF in whom the resting ventricular response was considered to be adequately controlled. The majority of subjects were receiving digoxin. Eight received beta blockers and one received verapamil. A wide rhythm distribution was found throughout 24 hr with a difference between fastest and slowest rates in individual patients ranging from 35 to 141 beats per minute (mean 86). Two-thirds of patients had pauses longer than 2 sec and 20% had pauses of 3 sec or more in duration. No significant relation between serum digoxin levels and resting heart rate, fastest heart rate, slowest heart rate, or duration of pauses was noticed. The authors concluded that daytime pauses of up to 2.8 sec and nocturnal pauses of up to 4.0 sec or longer can be regarded as being within the expected rate distribution of AF, and such findings on Holter monitoring do not require a pacemaker in an asymptomatic patient.

In a larger group of patients with AF, Saxon et al. (4) compared Holter monitor recordings from 105 patients with cerebral symptoms (dizziness or syncope) to recordings from 306 asymptomatic patients. Ventricular pauses greater than 2 sec occurred in 68% of the asymptomatic group compared to 76% of the symptomatic patients (difference not significant). In addition there was no difference in the mean duration of the longest pause in symptomatic versus asymptomatic patients (mean 2.5 vs 2.4 sec). Clinical data were available in 50 of the 105 patients with cerebral symptoms. Pauses correlated with symptoms in only three (6%) of these subjects. A permanent pacemaker was inserted in 15 patients, of whom 11 (73%) had resolution of symptoms. In the unpaced group, 31 of 35 (89%) had symptom resolution. No significant difference in survival occurred between paced and unpaced groups of patients with prolonged ventricular pauses, regardless of the presence of symptoms. A similar observation has been made by other authors in mixed groups of patients with ventricular pauses due either to sinus node disease or AF with a slow heart rate (5,6).

In summary, patients with cerebral symptoms and AF will frequently be found to have prolonged (≥ 2 sec) pauses on 24-hr monitoring. However, such pauses are equally common in asymptomatic patients, and correlation between symptoms and pauses is poor. Resolution of symptoms is common even in untreated patients and ventricular pacing has not been shown to affect survival. Consequently we would recommend that pacing generally be reserved for patients in whom a clear relationship can be established between specific complaints and bradycardia documented by monitoring.

SPECIFIC INDICATIONS FOR PACING IN ATRIAL FIBRILLATION

Drug-Induced Pauses

Patients with a slow ventricular response to AF at rest but poor rate control on exercise may need therapy that potentially further suppresses AV conduction to the point of symptomatic bradycardia. In addition, treatment of the associated myocardial condition may adversely affect heart rate. Digoxin in congestive failure, beta blockers and calcium channel blockers in hypertrophic cardiomyopathy, uncontrolled hypertension or angina pectoris, and amiodarone for certain ventricular arrhythmias are examples of clinical concerns when associated with slow AF. In such cases the necessity of the drug must be weighed against the need for a pacemaker, which would be indicated if such therapy cannot be withheld.

Tachycardia-Bradycardia Syndrome

An important and fairly clear-cut indication for permanent pacing in AF is the tachycardia-bradycardia syndrome. Episodes of paroxysmal AF, frequently with a rapid ventricular response, are followed by a period of sinus arrest after arrhythmia

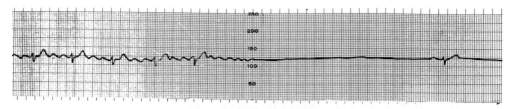

FIG. 2. Rhythm strip tortuitously recorded in a patient with recurrent syncope. Atrial fibrillation is present, which terminates with a prolonged period of sinus arrest.

termination (Fig. 2). Antiarrhythmic therapy may fail to fully control the paroxysms and may aggravate post-tachycardia pauses. Under these circumstances permanent pacing facilitates treatment and abolishes pause-related symptoms.

Pacing After Catheter Ablation

Chronically uncontrolled ventricular rates during AF may lead to symptomatic heart failure and/or severe ventricular dysfunction with a clinical picture resembling that of dilated cardiomyopathy (7–9). As described elsewhere in this volume by Rosenqvist and Scheinman, catheter ablation of the AV node provides effective rate control of drug-resistant AF (8,10). Since the AV node is deliberately damaged by ablative therapy, resulting in immediate or delayed AV block, a permanent pacemaker is generally indicated after the procedure (10).

Deliberate Provocation of Atrial Fibrillation

An unusual indication for pacemaker therapy was reported by Moreira et al. (11) in a patient with ectopic atrial tachycardia and a ventricular response up to 214 beats per minute. Secondary heart failure developed as a consequence of this long-standing supraventricular tachyarrhythmia. A specially designed implanted atrial pacemaker continuously pacing at a rate of 375 beats per minute for a 10-month period induced chronic, self-sustaining AF, permitting effective rate control with digoxin and improvement in congestive failure to the point of symptom resolution. This unusual indication for permanent pacing may be considered as an alternative for a small, well-selected group of patients in whom AV junction ablation and other antitachycardia measures are either unavailable or not feasible.

TEMPORARY PACING IN ATRIAL FIBRILLATION

Temporary use of ventricular pacing is warranted in the context of acute situations complicated by AF with AV block and hemodynamic instability. Deliberate or accidental overdose of drugs used for chronic treatment of AF (digoxin, beta blockers, calcium channel blockers), may cause profound bradycardia. An unusual situation is the development of AF during acute inferior wall myocardial infarction associated with AV nodal involvement. Under these circumstances the rapid atrial rate may provoke high-degree AV block, which was not apparent during sinus rhythm (Fig. 3).

Cardioversion of AF in the setting of suspected sinus node dysfunction, with or without accompanying AV block, may occasionally result in long asystolic periods or profound bradycardia causing clinical deterioration and lasting as long as 36 hr (12,13). It has therefore been suggested that where sick sinus syndrome has been documented or where advanced AV nodal disease is likely to be present (as indicated by a slow ventricular response), elective cardioversion should be attempted only with temporary pacemaker back-up, and perhaps only in patients who would be good candidates for permanent pacing should that need arise (13). A temporary transvenous wire can be inserted prior to cardioversion. Alternatively external noninvasive pacing may be used (14). Self-adhesive pacing electrodes are attached to a patient

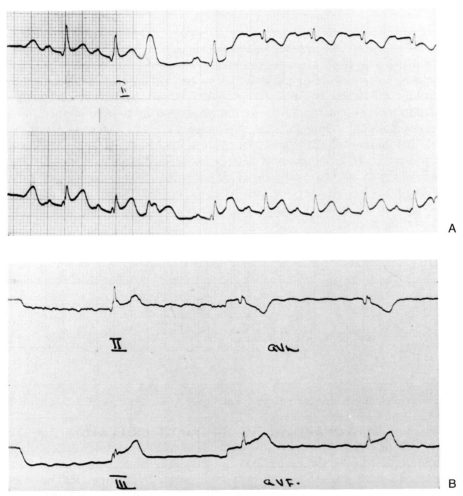

FIG. 3. Recordings from a patient with acute inferior wall myocardial infarction. **A:** (Leads II, avL, III, and aVF). Sinus rhythm with first-degree AV block is present. **B:** The onset of atrial fibrillation/atrial flutter is associated with high-degree AV block due, presumably, to concealed AV nodal conduction.

undergoing electrical cardioversion in whom the procedure is anticipated to be complicated by long periods of asystole or bradycardia, and the device can be tested immediately prior to cardioversion to establish pacing threshold (15).

PREFERRED MODE OF PACING IN ATRIAL FIBRILLATION

Dual-Chamber Pacing

In the early experience of transvenous pacing, ventricular stimulation was the only available mode. With the advent of dual-chamber stimulation, paroxysmal AF was considered a contraindication as it was believed that progression to chronic AF—a condition in which atrial stimulation is of no value—was common. Subsequently it has become apparent that AV sequential pacing may be superior to VVI pacing in a significant number of patients with known paroxysmal AF and may prevent the development of AF in chronically paced subjects.

Feuer et al. (16) studied the effect of cardiac pacing mode (DDD or DDI vs VVI) on the long-term development of chronic AF in 220 patients who were in sinus rhythm at the time of pacemaker placement. In a mean follow-up of 4 years, significantly more patients developed AF in the VVI-paced group compared to the DDD/DDI group (18% vs 8%, respectively; $p<0.05$). About one-third of patients had paroxysmal supraventricular arrhythmia known at the time of implantation. In this group, chronic AF developed in 48% of patients with VVI pacemakers compared to only 11% of patients paced in the DDD/DDI mode ($p<0.01$). In a similar study by Rosenqvist et al. (17), 168 patients with sinus node disease were treated by either VVI or AAI pacing. The incidence of development of permanent AF was much higher in the VVI compared to the AAI group (47% and 6.7%, respectively; $p<0.0005$). The incidence of AF developing among patients with reported paroxysmal atrial tachyarrhythmia before implantation was almost eight times higher in the VVI group compared to the AAI group (69% vs 9%; $p<0.001$). Atrially paced patients had a lower incidence of heart failure (37% vs 15%, VVI vs AAI groups; $p<0.005$), regardless of the development of AF, and a better survival rate compared to the ventricularly paced group ($p<0.05$).

The mechanism for the development of AF in ventricularly paced patients is probably multifactorial and includes retrograde stimulation of the atrium, increased atrial pressure due to loss of AV synchrony, and increased risk of heart failure due to loss of atrial contribution to ventricular filling. In addition, in certain patients with neurally triggered paroxysmal AF, the onset of the arrhythmia is preceded by a slowing of the sinus rate. Under these circumstances, atrial pacing at a slightly higher rate than that occurring before arrhythmia onset may reduce the frequency of, or abolish entirely, episodes of arrhythmia.

In summary, dual-chamber pacing in the DDI or DDD mode is the preferred pacing mode in patients with paroxysmal AF who need to be paced because of other disorders (16–21). Even if the paroxysms are frequent, constantly pacing the atrium and/or the addition of an atrial antiarrhythmic agent may control the AF. Not only may survival be improved by dual chamber pacing, but the incidence of heart failure is reduced, as is the development of chronic AF with its associated risks of thromboembolism.

Rate Responsive Pacing

In the presence of AF, atrial capture by an external stimulus will not occur and tracking of atrial rhythm is neither effective nor of value. Thus, persistent AF obviously precludes the use of a dual-chamber pacing system (22), narrowing the choice to a ventricular demand pacemaker with either a fixed-rate setting (VVI) or rate-modulating capabilities (VVIR).

The importance of chronotropic competence for provision of adequate cardiac output during exercise is well established (22,23,24). Data indicate that atrial synchrony, while undoubtedly of importance, may be of greater value at the lower end of the normal heart rate range (between 50–90 beats per minute). At higher ventricular rates (120–180 beats per minute) cardiac output is more critically dependent on rate and less so on AV synchrony (25). It has been demonstrated that, in the presence of complete anterograde and retrograde block, functional capacity and cardiac output during exercise are similar in patients paced to equivalent heart rates with or without AV synchrony (i.e., VDD or VVIR pacing) (23,25). VVIR pacing, while comparable to fixed-rate VVI pacing during resting conditions, was found to increase exercise tolerance by achieving a higher maximal cardiac output, thus being superior to VVI pacing during exercise (26,27). Consequently, rate responsive pacing is the preferred pacing mode in patients with AF with a slow resting heart rate and a blunted ventricular response to exercise. Fixed-rate VVI pacemakers may still be satisfactory, providing reasonable rate response is preserved during exercise and pacing is mainly needed for resting bradycardia. A practical suggestion would be to exercise AF patients and assess chronotropic competence prior to pacemaker implantation. A VVI pacemaker will usually be adequate also for the older, sedentary patient with a low activity level in daily routine.

Pacemaker Problems Resulting from Atrial Fibrillation

Patients with dual-chamber pacing systems and paroxysmal atrial arrhythmias may have pacemaker problems specifically related to the arrhythmia. During an episode of arrhythmia, irregular and unpredictable sensing of the endogenous atrial signals can occur, with triggering of the ventricular output at or near the upper rate of the pacemaker program (22,28). As a result patients may continue to be symptomatic because of periods of rapid and irregular paced ventricular rhythms during paroxysmal atrial arrhythmia (Fig. 4). Management requires careful programming of the pacemaker with a relatively long atrial refractory period (PVARP) and a low upper rate limit. An alternative measure is to change from DDD to DDI mode, thereby disabling atrial triggering of ventricular stimulation and eliminating the risk. This mode has been used successfully in patients with predominant sinus node disease (21). Nevertheless, if reprogramming and pharmacologic measures still do not control AF paroxysms, the VVIR mode is the final choice as in chronic AF patients.

ELECTRICAL CARDIOVERSION IN PATIENTS WITH PACEMAKERS

Many patients with AF require electrical cardioversion and may need it repeatedly. Patients with an implanted pacemaker who require cardioversion may be ex-

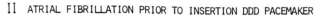

II ATRIAL FIBRILLATION PRIOR TO INSERTION DDD PACEMAKER

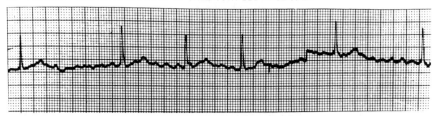

M.L. ATRIAL FIBRILLATION AFTER INSERTION DDD PACEMAKER

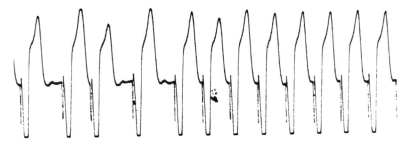

FIG. 4. Tracking of atrial fibrillation by a dual-chamber pacemaker (DDD mode) in a patient with paroxysmal atrial fibrillation. (From ref. 29, with permission.)

posed to potential adverse influences of high-energy direct currents (DC) on their pacing system. While the situation is relatively uncommon, it can prove to be a major problem when encountered; physicians should be aware of the possible consequences of this interaction and be prepared to manage them.

Damage caused by DC shock may occur to the pulse generator itself and/or the electrode-myocardial interface. Today's advanced devices incorporate protective measures designed to shield the internal circuits from excessive external currents. Once a large current surge is applied onto the system, the majority of this energy will be diverted away from the internal circuitry, thus enabling it to continue its proper performance. However, these safety features are not foolproof and malfunction or ineffectiveness may result in anywhere from an unintentional change in programmed parameters to permanent damage of the pacemaker necessitating its prompt replacement. In addition, safety features designed to protect the circuitry shunt external currents into the electrodes and potentially increase the risk of problems at the electrode-myocardial interface.

Experiments have been performed in animals with implanted unipolar pacemakers in which DC shocks were delivered with paddles placed in the anterior-anterior position on the chest wall, with one paddle directly on the skin overlying the pulse generator (30). An acute rise in pacing threshold was noted, which lasted up to several days. Pathologic examination demonstrated areas of inflammation, necrosis, and fibrosis in the myocardium adjacent to the electrode insertion point. These observations were noted both when one single high-energy (320 J) or multiple low-energy dose shocks were applied. Only when using single low-energy shock were the rise in threshold and the histologic damage minimized. The results suggest that endomyocardial damage, potentially capable of causing exit block, may result from electrical defibrillation/cardioversion procedures and that this damage is additive, related to the total amount of energy delivered.

A few cases of damage to implanted pacemakers during DC shock have been described in humans. These comprise temporary loss of capture and/or sensing in either the atrial or ventricular channel, reprogramming of the pacemaker to a faster rate or to the default fixed-rate back-up VVI mode, and permanent destruction of pulse generator components. Levine et al. (31) reported on seven patients and later summarized a total of 15 episodes with enough documentation to permit characterization of the problem in each case (30). Problems occurred mostly in unipolar systems (13 of 15) with permanent damage to the pulse generator occurring in four instances. In all cases an anterior-anterior paddle placement was utilized with one paddle at the upper right sternal border and the other over the cardiac apex. Thirteen patients had the pulse generator implanted in the right pectoral fossa, while only two had them in the left pectoral area. In a few of the patients who lost capture immediately after DC shock, subsequent measurements of thresholds were obtained and indicated that the rise in pacing thresholds may last anywhere from a few minutes to a few months or even become chronically elevated.

Directly transmitted electrical current through the electrode to the myocardium can be significantly reduced by placing the paddles as far as possible from the pulse generator and by using insulated generators as bipolar systems. However, current can be induced in a pacing lead by means of capacitive coupling (i.e., induction of current in an insulated conductor by an extrinsic energy field). The magnitude of such currents is proportional to the degree of parallel alignment of the lead to the direction of the dipole of energy flow and also proportional to the magnitude of the energy delivered at defibrillation. Such currents are independent of the polarity of the pacing system. When the electrode plane and paddle position are critically oriented, the generated currents within the system may be strong enough to either damage the pulse generator or to cause endocardial burns, thus facilitating exit block. Of note, electrocautery has been reported to induce ventricular fibrillation and to cause an increased incidence of exit block in paced patients undergoing open heart surgery. The presumed mechanism for these events is capacitive electrical current induction in the lead system produced by the cauterization.

Understanding the possible mechanisms of pacemaker malfunction following cardioversion enables the creation of a few general guidelines.

1. Paddles should be placed as far from the pulse generator as possible, preferably in the anterior-posterior position. This will minimize both the DC capable of shunting through the system and the current elicited within the wires by means of capacitive coupling.
2. The energy should be titrated, starting at the minimal anticipated effective output for cardioversion. (However, if this assessment is incorrect, multiple shocks will be required, and the cumulative influence may be equal to or greater than a single high-energy cardioversion shock.)
3. In patients who are likely to be subject to future cardioversion attempts, such as those with a history of recurrent AF, it would be preferable to use bipolar pacing systems implanted in the left pectoral area.
4. A good practice is to maximize output levels (voltage and pulse duration) as well as sensitivity in all programmable pacemakers prior to attempted elective cardio-

version. This reduces the risk of a noncapture and nonsensing period, should the threshold acutely rise.

5. In the patient who is known to be pacemaker dependent in whom cardioversion is contemplated, the physician should be ready to pace temporarily through another access site or with external stimulation, should asystole occur.

6. Whether or not problems are encountered immediately postcardioversion, a careful follow-up to assess sensing, capture, programming capability, and battery drainage should be performed periodically over the next 2 to 3 months. Once thresholds are stabilized, the pacemaker can be reprogrammed according to the new data.

THE EFFECT OF DRUGS ON PACEMAKER FUNCTION

A variety of physiologic conditions (e.g., eating, exercise, sleeping), metabolic abnormalities (e.g., hypoxemia, hyperkalemia, hyperglycemia, acid-base imbalance, hypothyroidism), and pharmacologic agents (e.g., corticosteroids) are known to influence pacing and sensing thresholds, although clinical consequences of most of these (except for extreme hyperkalemia) are negligible.

Patients with AF and permanent pacemakers are frequently receiving cardioactive drugs, some of which may potentially affect pacing thresholds. Digoxin, the most commonly prescribed agent, has no effect on pacemaker function (31). Since sympathetic stimuli and sympathomimetic drugs are known to decrease pacing thresholds (31–33), it has been postulated that beta blockers, by counteracting sympathetic influence, will increase pacing threshold. However, studies to investigate this assumption have shown variable results. Some investigators found that intravenous propranolol given to patients with transvenous pacemakers was associated with a mean rise in threshold of 40% (34), while others observed beta blockade to abolish isoproteronol-induced pacemaker threshold lowering. Administration of propranolol increased stimulation thresholds in patients after physical activity, but no effect was noted when thresholds were measured in the resting state (35). In contrast, other studies have found that neither propranolol nor sotalol had any effect on pacing threshold with either oral or intravenous administration (36). These results are inconsistent and imply that threshold changes with propranolol, if present, are minor and are of no clinical significance. Similar studies using calcium channel blockers have failed to show a significant effect on pacing thresholds (33), either in patients with transvenous pacemakers or in subjects undergoing noninvasive external pacing (37).

Amiodarone may affect defibrillation threshold and prolong the latency of evoked response to pacing after intravenous administration but does not seem to increase acute or chronic stimulation thresholds or to affect pacemaker function (33).

Class IA antiarrhythmic drugs have demonstrated variable effects on pacing in animal models and in humans. Toxicity with procainamide and disopyramide resulted in marked threshold increase with failure to capture (38,39), but no significant effects were noted at usual therapeutic dosages of quinidine, procainamide, and disopyramide in humans (32,33,35).

At present, class IC agents are the cause of greatest concern. Flecainide has been shown to raise acute and chronic pacing thresholds, both with intravenous and oral administration, with an increase of up to 200% during continuous oral therapy. The change was dose related and thresholds returned to baseline after flecainide was discontinued (40). A similar effect, although of lesser magnitude has been reported with encainide with an average increase in pacing thresholds of 75% at the higher dose range (41). These observations imply that the use of class IC drugs may considerably reduce the pacing safety margin, especially in patients whose thresholds are higher than average before institution of such therapy.

Pacemaker-sensing capabilities have not been significantly influenced by therapeutic levels of cardioactive drugs (32). Sotalol and propafenone decreased sensing thresholds by 15% in one study (42), but these changes are potentially meaningful only in individuals with borderline sensing parameters. Clinical problems regarding sensing function have not been recognized with any of the drugs discussed above.

New rate-responsive pacemakers incorporate sensors for metabolic needs. The most widely used sensor is an activity-motion sensing device that is not influenced by cardiac drugs. Other sensors depend on intracardiac measurements to function, such as QT interval, stroke volume/preejection interval, and paced depolarization integral. These parameters could potentially be affected by drug influence on ventricular function and/or depolarization-repolarization sequence. Future experience will reveal the practical problems generated by therapy on rate-modulated sensing and ways of overcoming them in the clinical setting.

It may be concluded that, although many cardiac medications may have minor effects on pacing or sensing thresholds, these changes are usually small and do not exceed the modern pacemaker safety margins and programability. Consequently, therapy with most cardioactive drugs should not be withheld when needed in a patient with a normally functioning pacemaker. A relative exception is use of IC antiarrhythmic agents, which may have a more substantial influence and, if possible, are best avoided in pacemaker-dependent patients. If no alternative exists, the pacemaker should be programmed with a wide safety margin, and these patients must be carefully followed to confirm that any further rise in pacing threshold does not exceed the pacemaker's output capabilities. Systems with output self-regulation, which automatically increase the pacemaker output when a rise in pacing threshold is detected, might prove most beneficial in this subset of patients.

REGULARIZATION OF VENTRICULAR RATE IN ATRIAL FIBRILLATION

Wittkampf and co-workers (43) have observed that right ventricular pacing in patients with AF eliminates spontaneous RR intervals shorter than the pacing cycles. Constant pacing at a rate slightly faster than the mean ventricular response to AF abolished more than 95% of spontaneous ventricular activity, thereby regulating heart rate to the actual pacing rate. Based on these observations, the investigators developed an automatic pacing algorithm that was able to regularize the otherwise random and highly irregular spontaneous rhythm of AF patients (44). Theoretical insights about the complex role of the AV junction in AF emerged from these studies. Application of these observations to clinical practice still needs to be evaluated, but they indicate that it may be possible to control a rapid ventricular response to AF by pacing the ventricle at a somewhat slower rate. Another method of ventricular rate slowing in AF was reported by Lau et al. (45), who achieved a slowing of pulse rate and a reduction of pulse-to-pulse interval variability by regularly introducing a ventricular paced stimulus after every sensed beat. A rapid improvement in cardiac hemodynamics in patients with mitral stenosis and AF, as measured by cardiac output, pulmonary arterial pressure, pulmonary wedge pressure, and transmitral gradient, was observed. The authors suggested this method to be useful in patients in whom rapid AF develops after cardiac operations and in whom temporary epicardial electrodes are still present, thus achieving immediate slowing of pulse while waiting for any concomitant antiarrhythmic agent to act. Continuous use of this method, termed intercalated pacing, to regulate heart rate in AF patients is probably not feasible, both because of the high pacing rate needed, which significantly shortens battery life, and the necessity to pace someone permanently within or near the vulnerable period of ventricular repolarization.

SUMMARY

From this review it can be concluded that pacing is indicated in patients with AF when clinical symptoms are readily attributable to slow ventricular response and prolonged ventricular pauses. When choosing a pacemaker for implantation, one should consider the importance of a reasonable chronotropic response to exercise and provide a rate responsive system (VVIR) for those patients who show chronotropic incompetence. In the case of paroxysmal AF, an AV synchronized system may provide protection against deterioration to chronic AF and heart failure and is preferred over VVI pacing, providing that paroxysms are infrequent. Cardioversion should be performed with care in patients with a permanent pacemaker, and certain protective measures must be employed to avoid destruction or malfunction. Drug-pacemaker interaction is rare, but it is recommended that class IC antiarrhythmic agents should not be used in the pacemaker-dependent patient.

Pacemakers, when used according to the strict criteria, constitute an integral part of treatment and may improve quality of life and facilitate the use of necessary drugs in selected patients with AF.

REFERENCES

1. Ector H, Rolies L, DeGeest H. Dynamic electrocardiography and ventricular pauses of 3 seconds and more: etiology and therapeutic implications. *PACE* 1983;6:548–551.
2. Rebello R, Brownlee WC. Intermittent ventricular standstill during chronic atrial fibrillation in patients with dizziness or syncope. *PACE* 1987;10:1271–1276.
3. Pitcher D, Papouchado M, James MA, Rees RJ. Twenty-four hour ambulatory electrocardiography in patients with chronic atrial fibrillation. *Br Med J* 1986;292:594.
4. Saxon LA, Albert BH, Uretz EF, Denes P. Permanent pacemaker placement in chronic atrial fibrillation associated with intermittent AV block and cerebral symptoms. *PACE* 1990;13:724–729.
5. Mazuz M, Friedman HS. Significance of prolonged electrocardiographic pauses in sinoatrial disease: sick sinus syndrome. *Am J Cardiol* 1983;52:485–489.
6. Hilgard JH, Ezri MD, Denes P. Significance of ventricular pauses of three seconds or more detected by twenty-four hour Holter recordings. *Am J Cardiol* 1985;55:1005–1008.
7. Packer DL, Bardy GH, Worley SJ, et al. Tachycardia-induced cardiomyopathy: a reversible form of left ventricular dysfunction. *Am J Cardiol* 1986;57:563–570.
8. Lemery R, Brugada P, Cheriex E, Wellens HJJ. Reversibility of tachycardia-induced left ventricular dysfunction after closed-chest catheter ablation of the atrioventricular junction for intractable atrial fibrillation. *Am J Cardiol* 1987;60:1406–1408.
9. Peters KG, Kienzle MG. Severe cardiomyopathy due to chronic rapidly conducted atrial fibrillation: complete recovery after restoration of sinus rhythm. *Am J Med* 1988;85:242–244.
10. Kay GN, Bubien RS, Epstein AE, Plumb VJ. Effect of catheter ablation of atrioventricular junction on quality of life and exercise tolerance in paroxysmal atrial fibrillation. *Am J Cardiol* 1988;62:741–744.

11. Moreira DAR, Shepard RB, Waldo AL. Chronic rapid atrial pacing to maintain atrial fibrillation: use to permit control of ventricular rate in order to treat tachycardia-induced cardiomyopathy. *PACE* 1989;12:761–775.
12. DeSilva RA, Lown B. Cardioversion for atrial fibrillation—indications and complications. In: Kulbertus HE, Olsson SB, Schlepper M, eds. *Atrial fibrillation.* Molndal, Sweden: AB Hassle, 1984;231–241.
13. Mancini GBJ, Goldberger AL. Cardioversion of atrial fibrillation: consideration of embolization, anticoagulation, prophylactic pacemaker, and long-term success. *Am Heart J* 1982;104:617–621.
14. Falk RH, Zoll PM, Zoll RH. Safety and efficacy of noninvasive cardiac pacing: a preliminary report. *N Engl J Med* 1983;309:1166–1168.
15. Sharkey SW, Chaffee V, Kapsner S. Prophylactic external pacing during cardioversion of atrial tachyarrhythmias. *Am J Cardiol* 1985;55:1632–1634.
16. Feuer JM, Shandling AH, Messenger JC. Influence of cardiac pacing mode on the long-term development of atrial fibrillation. *Am J Cardiol* 1989;64:1376–1379.
17. Rosenqvist M, Brandt J, Schuller H. Long-term pacing in sinus node disease: effects of stimulation mode on cardiovascular morbidity and mortality. *Am Heart J* 1988;116:16–22.
18. Langenfeld H, Grimm W, Maisch B, Kochsiek K. Atrial fibrillation and embolic complications in paced patients. *PACE* 1988;11:1667–1672.
19. Camm AJ, Katritsis D. Ventricular pacing for sick sinus syndrome—a risky business? (editorial). *PACE* 1990;13:695–699.
20. Zanini R, Facchinetti AI, Gallo G, Cazzamalli L, Bonadi L, Dei-Cas L. Morbidity and mortality of patients with sinus node disease: comparative effects of atrial and ventricular pacing. *PACE* 1990;13:2076–2079.
21. Sutton R. Pacing in atrial arrhythmias. *PACE* 1990;13:1823–1826.
22. Griffin JC. Pacemaker selection for the individual patient. In: Barold SS, ed. *Modern cardiac pacing.* Mount Kisco, NY: Futura, 1985;411–420.
23. Fananapazir L, Bennett DH, Monks P. Atrial synchronized ventricular pacing: contribution of the chronotropic response to improved exercise performance. *PACE* 1983;6:601–608.
24. Holmes DR. Hemodynamics of cardiac pacing. In: Furman S, Hayes DL, Holmes DR, eds. A practice of cardiac pacing. Mount Kisco, NY: Futura, 1989;167–191.
25. Furman S. Rate modulated pacing. In: Furman S, Hayes DL, Holmes DR, eds. *A practice of cardiac pacing.* Mount Kisco, NY: Futura, 1989;369–374.
26. Donaldson RM, Fox K, Rickards AF. Initial experience with a physiological, rate responsive pacemaker. *Br Med J* 1983;286:667–671.
27. Shapland JE, MacCarter D, Tockman B, Knudson M. Physiologic benefits of rate responsiveness. *PACE* 1983;6:329–332.
28. Levine PA. Normal and abnormal rhythms associated with dual-chamber pacemakers. *Cardiol Clin* 1985;3:595–616.
29. Levine PA, Seltzer JP. AV universal (DDD) pacing and atrial fibrillation. *Clin Prog Pacing Electrophysiol* 1983;1:275–281.
30. Levine PA. Effect of cardioversion and defibrillation on implanted cardiac pacemakers. In: Barold SS, ed. *Modern cardiac pacing.* Mount Kisco, NY: Futura, 1985;875–886.
31. Levine PA, Barold SS, Fletcher RD, Talbot P. Adverse acute and chronic effects of electrical defibrillation and cardioversion on implanted unipolar cardiac pacing systems. *J Am Coll Cardiol* 1983;1:1413–1422.
32. Preston TA, Fletcher RD, Lucchesi BR, Judge RD. Changes in myocardial threshold. Physiologic and pharmacologic factors in patients with implanted pacemakers. *Am Heart J* 1967;74:235–242.
33. Dohrmann ML, Goldschlager NF. Myocardial stimulation threshold in patients with cardiac pacemakers: effect of physiologic variables, pharmacologic agents and lead electrodes. *Cardiol Clin* 1985;3:527–537.
34. Kubler W, Sowton E. Influence of beta-blockade on myocardial threshold in patients with pacemakers. *Lancet* 1970;2:67–68.
35. Preston TA, Judge RD. Alteration of pacemaker threshold by drugs and physiological factors. *Ann NY Acad Sci* 1969;167:687–692.
36. Creamer JE, Nathan AW, Shennan A, Camm AJ. Acute and chronic effects of sotalol and propranolol on ventricular repolarization using constant-rate pacing. *Am J Cardiol* 1986;57:1092–1096.
37. Falk RH, Knowlton AA, Battinelli NJ. The effect of propranolol and verapamil on external pacing threshold: a placebo-controlled study. *PACE* 1988;11:1439–1443.
38. Gay RJ, Brown DF. Pacemaker failure due to procainamide toxicity. *Am J Cardiol* 1974;34:728–732.
39. Hayler AM, Holt DW, Volans GN. Fatal overdose with disopyramide. *Lancet* 1978;1:968–969.
40. Hellestrand KJ, Nathan AW, Bexton RS, Camm AJ. Electrophysiologic effects of flecainide acetate on sinus node function, anomalous atrioventricular connections, and pacemaker thresholds. *Am J Cardiol* 1984;53:30B–38B.

41. Salel AF, Seagren SC, Pool PE. Effects of encainide on the function of implanted pacemakers. *PACE* 1989;12:1439–1444.
42. Kafka W, Hildebrand U, Stadt WD. Effect of antiarrhythmic agents on chronic pacing and sensing thresholds (abstract). *Circulation* 1985;72(suppl III):III-173.
43. Wittkampf FHM, de Jongste MJL, Lie HI, Meijler FL. Effect of right ventricular pacing on ventricular rhythm during atrial fibrillation. *J Am Coll Cardiol* 1988;11:539–545.
44. Wittkampf FHM, de Jongste MJL. Rate stabilization by right ventricular on-demand pacing in patients with atrial fibrillation. *PACE* 1986;9:1147–1153.
45. Lau CP, Leung WH, Wong CK, Tai YT, Cheng CH. A new pacing method for rapid regularization and rate control in atrial fibrillation. *Am J Cardiol* 1990;65:1198–1203.

Atrial Fibrillation: Mechanisms and Management, edited by
R. H. Falk and P. J. Podrid.
Raven Press, Ltd., New York © 1992.

20

Catheter Ablation in Atrial Fibrillation

*Mårten Rosenqvist and †Melvin M. Scheinman

*Division of Cardiology, Department of Medicine, Karolinska Hospital,
113 22 Stockholm, Sweden; †Department of Medicine, University of California,
San Francisco, San Francisco, California 94143

Atrial fibrillation is a very common rhythm disorder that is usually controlled by antiarrhythmic agents. In some patients, drug therapy alone prevents recurrence of the arrhythmia and/or symptoms related either to the irregular rhythm or to an inordinately rapid rate. A subset of patients with atrial fibrillation will also have either enhanced atrioventricular (AV) nodal conduction or atriohisian bypass tracts. In these patients development of atrial fibrillation may result in a rapid ventricular response that may precipitate ventricular fibrillation (VF). In a recent review of 300 patients with aborted sudden death studied at the University of California–San Francisco (UCSF) Medical Center, approximately 5% had a supraventricular tachycardia that degenerated into VF (1). The most common type of supraventricular tachycardia consisted of patients with organic heart disease and enhanced AV nodal conduction who developed inordinately rapid ventricular response during atrial fibrillation. These patients are typically unresponsive to drugs that act primarily to slow AV nodal conduction.

An additional problem related to drug therapy is that this mode of therapy exposes the patient to potentially dangerous adverse side effects. In a recent meta-analysis of studies utilizing quinidine for control of atrial fibrillation (2), it was demonstrated that while quinidine was associated with a significantly increased incidence of maintenance of sinus rhythm, use of this drug was associated with a higher mortality. It is well appreciated that other drugs in the class IA grouping may produce life-threatening polymorphous ventricular arrhythmias (3). Similar findings have been reported with class IC drugs (4), while IB drugs appear to be ineffective for patients with atrial fibrillation.

Initial nonpharmacologic attempts introduced for control of atrial fibrillation included cardiac electrosurgery, which involved performance of a right atriotomy with either direct dissection or cryodesiccation of the His bundle. In 1982, Scheinman et al. (5) and Gallagher et al. (6) introduced the technique of catheter ablation of the AV junction. This technique is an accepted approach in the management of patients with drug-refractory atrial fibrillation and has virtually obviated the need for cardiac electrosurgery for these patients. The initial power source used for catheter ablation was a high-energy, direct current (DC) electrical discharge. At present, several newer energy sources have been introduced. The purpose of this chapter is to review the technique of catheter ablation of the AV junction with comparison of the available data relative to the diverse energy delivery systems available. In addition, we review the long-term follow-up experience for patients having undergone attempted high-energy DC shocks for catheter ablation of the AV junction in order to place this therapy in the proper clinical context.

ENERGY SOURCES

At present, three different types of energy source have been used clinically for attempted catheter ablation. The advantages and problems of each technique are summarized in Table 1.

Catheter Ablation of the Atrioventricular Junction: Technique

The patient is brought to a cardiac electrophysiology laboratory in the postabsorptive state. A short cannula is inserted into a peripheral artery to allow for continuous monitoring of the systemic pressure. A multipolar electrode catheter is inserted by vein and positioned against the apex of the right ventricle. A new 6F or 7F USCI multipolar electrode catheter is inserted into the femoral vein and positioned across the tricuspid valve to record the largest His bundle potential. The bipolar signal is then processed into two unipolar signals and the electrode with the largest unipolar signal is used for ablation. Recent data from the Percutaneous Cardiac Mapping and Ablation Registry (PCMAR), a worldwide voluntary registry started in 1982 for the purpose of collecting data from patients undergoing ablative procedures, suggest that an unfiltered unipolar His bundle potential of 300 mV or higher is associated with successful ablation. If high-energy, DC electrical energy is used, the electrode with the largest amplitude His potential is made the cathode and a 7-cm R2 patch is positioned over the left scapula and used as the anode (Fig. 1). In addition, the catheter is positioned to record the largest possible atrial deflection in order to avoid delivery of high-energy shocks at the summit of the ventricular septum. The patient is then anesthetized with a short-acting anesthetic agent and one or more shocks are delivered between the electrode catheter and the patch via a standard defibrillator. The available data suggest use of 300 J as the initial shock for maximal success. Many centers use additional shocks even if the initial shock produces complete AV block.

The patient is observed in the catheter laboratory for at least 30 min to be certain that cardiac tamponade due to myocardial perforation does not develop. In addition, rare instances of hypotension requiring pressor support have been noted, but these

TABLE 1. *Differences between various energy sources used for atrioventricular junctional ablation*

	DC-energy	Low-energy DC	Radiofrequency
Barotrauma	+ +	−	−
High voltage	+ +	+	−
Lesion size	+ + +	+ +	+
General anesthesia	+	+	−
Serious complications	+	?	−
Fine-tuning of energy delivery	−	−	+

DC, direct current.

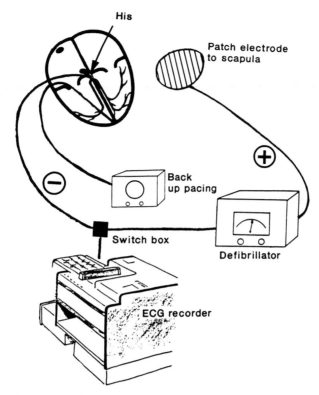

FIG. 1. Schematic illustration of the technique used to ablate the atrioventricular junction with transcatheter direct current shocks. A multipolar electrode catheter is inserted via the femoral vein and positioned across the tricuspid valve to record the His bundle potential. Another catheter is placed in the right ventricular apex for back-up pacing. Once the largest unipolar His bundle potential is recorded, a shock is delivered between the electrode tip acting as a cathode and a back-patch acting as an anode.

episodes are usually transient and likely due to the combination of general anesthesia and acute development of AV block (Fig. 2). Care is taken to provide adequate back-up ventricular pacing with continuous monitoring of the arterial pressure during the monitoring period. The patients are then observed for 24 to 48 hr in a coronary care unit, and if complete AV block persists, a permanent cardiac pacemaker is inserted. The type of pacemaker chosen depends on the nature of the underlying arrhythmia and the type of cardiac disease present.

Histopathologic studies from animals (Fig. 3) and from patients who died soon after DC ablation (7) have shown signs of fibrosis and chronic inflammation with fatty replacement of the conduction system and areas adjacent to it. The extent of the lesion correlates well with the number of shocks delivered. The acute lesion is associated with myofibrillar contraction bands, hemorrhage, and edema.

Low-Energy DC Shock

In order to avoid development of the potentially hazardous barotrauma caused by delivery of DC shocks, it was found (8) that formation of a vapor globe and its as-

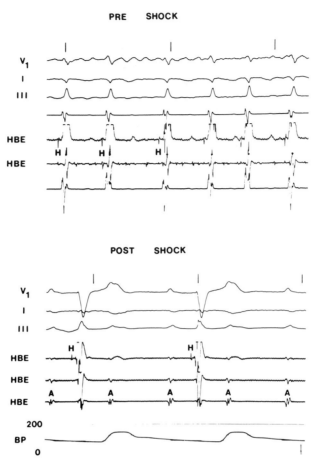

FIG. 2. Simultaneous recordings of surtace leads V$_1$, I, and III together with recordings from the region of the His bundle (HBE) before (**top**) and after (**bottom**) catheter ablation of the atrioventricular (AV) junction. Note that this procedure is associated with complete AV block and a slow ventricular response that requires permanent cardiac pacing.

sociated barotrauma could be reduced by shortening the duration of the shock delivery. It was shown that if shocks were delivered over 10 μsec, as compared to the conventionally used 5 to 6 msec, a higher threshold for globe formation was achieved. It has been further shown that the same degree of tissue injury could be produced using lower energy levels 0.5 to 30 J, without causing significant pressure waves. These findings emphasize that it is the electrical field and not barotrauma that causes tissue injury (9). Further, improved electrode design using a spherical or ellipse-shaped electrode tip seems to further reduce the formation of vapor globes (10). The ablation procedure itself is otherwise the same as for conventional DC ablation, including the need for general anesthesia.

Radiofrequency Energy

High-frequency or radiofrequency energy is usually defined as an electrical current of changing polarities ranging between 30 kHz and 300 mHz. In the clinical setting, unmodulated radiofrequency energy of 350 to 750 kHz has been used to achieve tissue necrosis by heating. Hoyt et al. (11) demonstrated that, *in vitro*, the minimal requirement for tissue damage was a pulse duration of 5 sec with a power of 5 W. Energy is delivered between the electrode tip and a shoulder patch. The energy is delivered over 30 to 100 sec and does not cause any barotrauma. In addition the energy delivery is usually painless and, thus, the procedure can be performed without general anesthesia.

The major determinants for lesion size are the pulse duration, the power, and the degree of tissue contact. Studies using various sizes of electrode tip have shown that the largest lesion size is achieved by using a 4-mm distal electrode tip (12). The main limiting factor for achieving an adequate lesion is due to blood coagulation around the electrode tip inducing an impedance rise. As the power applied depends on the tissue impedance, the actual power delivered varies significantly. It is extremely important to monitor both voltage and current during each application. If there is a sudden rise in voltage and a fall in current, this indicates impedance rise with coagulation over the distal electrode and energy delivery should be stopped. The catheter should then be withdrawn and the coagulum removed. Prolonged energy delivery after impedance rise may increase the risk for catheter fracture due to overheating (13). Monitoring of the catheter tip temperature can be used to avoid impedance rise. Histopathologic studies from animal experiments applying radiofrequency to myocardial tissue have shown well-circumscribed lesions with homogeneous necrosis and minimal inflammatory changes in adjacent areas (7).

A prerequisite for induction of high-grade AV block using radiofrequency energy is adequate tissue contact during energy delivery. It is therefore important to establish a stable catheter position before energy is delivered and to assure that this position is maintained during the procedure. Usually, adequate tissue contact is present if an unfiltered electrogram records an injury potential prior to energy application. From our personal experience it is usually more difficult to achieve high-grade AV block if the patient is in atrial fibrillation during the procedure. Conversion to sinus rhythm by external countershocks may be necessary to record the optimal atrial and His bundle potentials required for catheter ablation.

PATIENT SELECTION

Traditionally, catheter ablation for supraventricular arrhythmias has been reserved for patients with disabling symptoms refractory to drug treatment or for patients who have manifested life-threatening symptoms related to either the arrhythmia or drug therapy. Tables 2 and 3 outline the clinical characteristics of 49 patients with supraventricular arrhythmias who underwent high-energy DC ablation of the AV junction at the UCSF between 1981 and 1988 (14). All our patients were offered amiodarone as an alternative therapy, but they often chose ablative therapy because of the potential side-effect profile of amiodarone. It must be emphasized that virtually all patients considered for ablation failed or had serious side effects related to multiple drug trials and were often not inclined to try additional drugs. It is also important to call attention to the potentially life-threatening complications of drug therapy, which include serious proarrhythmic effects as well as the possibility of serious arrhythmias observed because of drug inefficacy. Drug side effects should be balanced against the potential adverse effects associated with the ablation procedure including the need for chronic pacing after ablation.

TABLE 2. *Clinical characteristics prior to ablation in 49 patients undergoing atrioventricular junctional ablation at the UCSF between 1981 and 1988*

Mean age	54 ± 15 (20–77) years
Sex	27/49 (56%) male
DC conversion	26/49 (53%)
Duration of symptoms	12.6 ± 14 (1–57) years
Ischemic heart disease	11/49 (23%)
Cardiomyopathy	14/49 (29%)
Left ventricular ejection fraction	48 ± 13 (15–65)
Symptoms during tachycardia	
Syncope	14/49 (29%)
Congestive heart failure	15/49 (31%)
Angina	11/49 (23%)
Dizziness	19/49 (38%)
Cardiac arrest	4/49 (8%)
Maximum HR	177 ± 42 (100–300 beats/min)
Failed drugs	
Digitalis	43 (88%)
Calcium channel blockers	43 (88%)
Beta blockers	42 (85%)
Procainamide	39 (79%)
Quinidine	38 (77%)
Disopyramide	17 (35%)
Amiodarone	17 (35%)
Flecainide	8 (16%)

DC, direct current; HR, heart rate.

It is important to remember that all patients undergoing AV junctional ablative procedures require chronic cardiac pacing. Patients with disabling paroxysmal atrial fibrillation may benefit from dual-chambered pacing during the interludes between bouts of atrial fibrillation. Furthermore, patients with recurrent atrial fibrillation not associated with rapid rates would probably not benefit substantially from catheter ablation. In addition, patients with severe cardiomyopathy whose myocardial function is not significantly improved during sinus rhythm as compared to atrial fibrillation would not be expected to benefit from catheter ablation. Preliminary experience from a National Institutes of Health (NIH) sponsored registry suggests that catheter ablation using high-energy DC discharges is associated with excessive procedure-related deaths in patients with severe myocardial dysfunction. The group at risk for death was characterized by an ejection fraction of less than 20% often associated with severe hypotension and/or congestive heart failure (15).

TABLE 3. *Arrhythmia classification and symptom frequency in 49 patients undergoing atrioventricular junctional ablation*

Types of arrhythmias	
Atrial fibrillation/flutter	29 (59%)
AVNRT	13 (26%)
AVRT	6 (12.5%)
Atrial tachycardia	1 (2.5%)
No. of symptomatic episodes per week	
<1 per week	14 (29%)
1–5 per week	20 (40%)
5–10 per week	5 (11%)
>10 per week	10 (20%)

AVNRT, atrioventricular nodal reentry tachycardia; AVRT, atrioventricular reciprocating tachycardia.

Nonresponders usually resume conduction within 24 to 48 hr after the procedure. It is important to emphasize the risk of late progression to high-grade AV block among patients considered early failures. Rosenqvist et al. (14) reported that two of seven patients discharged with intact AV conduction following attempted AV junctional ablation developed high-grade AV block after a follow-up of 4 and 24 months, respectively. These findings support the need for permanent back-up pacing in all patients undergoing ablative procedures.

RESULTS OF ATRIOVENTRICULAR JUNCTION ABLATION— DATA FROM THE PCMAR

The results of catheter ablation of the AV junction have been reported from the PCMAR. Since the first attempted AV junction ablation procedure was performed in March 1982, the PCMAR has collected data on a total of 551 cases of attempted His bundle ablation using DC energy. Of this group, there were 405 cases reported by 47 centers, both in the United States and abroad. There was follow-up of at least 1 week or more in 348 of 405 patients (86%). The average follow-up time in the total group of 405 patients with atrial tachyarrhythmias was almost 2 years. The lack of further long-term follow-up in the remaining 252 patients may significantly affect the true long-term mortality statistics. Atrial fibrillation or flutter was reported in 81% of this group, while the remainder had a variety of other supraventricular arrhythmias.

The escape pacemaker in third-degree AV block was described in 302 patients. It was characterized as supra-His in 33%, sub-His in 52%, and absent in 15%. These determinations were made generally from 24 to 72 hr after ablation. Maximal creatine phosphokinase (CPK) values were reported in 32 patients and averaged 425 ± 443 IU (range 0–2,286 IU). The CPK-MB fraction was reported in 182 patients and averaged 27 ± 32 IU (range 0–205 IU). A permanent pacemaker was implanted in 91% of the 304 patients for whom data were available.

Third-degree AV block developed in 55.6% of 405 patients after the first session, in 34% of the 94 patients who agreed to a second session, in 33.3% of the 12 patients who required a third session, and in the one patient who had five sessions. In the patients for whom data were available, immediate third-degree AV block was produced in 92% of 385 patients at session 1, 80% of the 94 patients at session 2, and 80% of the 12 patients at session 3. Data dating the resumption of conduction were available for 82 patients. The mean time to resumption of conduction was 3.5 ± 11.2 days (range 0–90 days). However, the median time for resumption of conduction was 24 hr. For this reason, investigators in some centers implant permanent pacemakers only after 24 hr of complete third-degree AV block is documented. In four patients, there was late development of third-degree AV block at 3 days, 10 days, 12 months, and 18 months, respectively. Of note, all six patients who had failed catheter ablation and went on to arrhythmia surgery had successful production of third-degree AV block.

Follow-up of at least 1 week or more was available in 348 of the 405 patients (86%), and ranged from 1 week to 78 months. The average follow-up time for the group of 405 patients was 18.9 ± 18.0 months. The median follow-up time was 15 months, and follow-up ranged from 0 days to 78 months. Patients were divided into four outcome classes based on conduction, symptomatology, and need for antiarrhythmic therapy.

Sixty-four percent had third-degree AV block, were reported as asymptomatic of arrhythmia, and were taking no antiarrhythmic drugs. Another 6.2% had resumption of conduction but were asymptomatic and required no antiarrhythmic drug therapy. Twelve percent had resumption of conduction but required antiarrhythmic drug therapy for arrhythmia control. Seventeen percent were unsuccessful. Thus, more than 70% of patients had either third-degree AV block or resumption of conduction and required no antiarrhythmic medication. Another 12% had resumption of conduction and were taking antiarrhythmic medications. Many of these patients who required antiarrhythmic drugs now responded to previously ineffective agents.

In this series, 34 (8.4%) patients died. Seven patients (1.7%) died suddenly, an average of 4.8 months (range 1 week–17 months; median 4 months) after the initial ablation procedure. Procedure-related death was defined as a nonoperative cardiac death occurring within 2 weeks of the ablation procedure, and two patients met these criteria.

The number of patients who have been treated with low-energy DC shock is limited, but data from Rowland's group (10,16) indicate a successful outcome of the same magnitude that has been observed for conventional DC ablation (17). Too few patients have so far been treated in order to identify factors predicting a successful outcome.

The first large-scale clinical series reporting radiofrequency energy for AV junctional ablation used standard electrode catheters and reported a success rate in the range of 60% to 70% (18–21). Langberg et al. (22) recently reported a series of 15 patients undergoing His bundle ablation using a larger catheter tip of 4 mm with a success rate of 83%. Registration of a long HV interval (suggesting a more proximal catheter position) and induction of brief episodes of junctional rhythm during energy application appear to predict a successful outcome (18). As in patients undergoing DC ablation, late progression to high-grade AV block has also been observed using radiofrequency energy both in animal experiments and in the clinical setting (23).

Radiofrequency energy for AV junctional ablation seems to carry a lower risk for severe complications compared to high-energy DC shocks. For example, no episodes of malignant ventricular arrhythmias, hypotension, perforation, or embolic complications have been reported (18,24). Furthermore, Langberg et al. (18) reported that only 7 of 16 patients showed signs of infranodal conduction dysfunction manifested by a new bundle branch block. All these patients showed a stable junctional escape rhythm and an unchanged HV interval probably indicating either nodal or a less extensive infranodal injury.

Lee et al. (25) described three patients, two after DC ablation, and one after radiofrequency ablation, with bradycardia-dependent, nonsustained polymorphous ventricular tachycardia occurring up to 24 hr after the procedure. All responded to an increased paced rate. Pacemaker inhibition to document the underlying rhythm should thus be approached with caution after ablation.

Frohner et al. (13) observed the only significant complication reported in radiofrequency energy delivery for AV junctional ablation. After repeated radiofrequency applications, the catheter fractured and the distal fragment remained in the heart after attempted catheter removal. This was probably caused by an insulation defect caused by overheating and could probably have been avoided if impedance had been cautiously monitored.

Furthermore, chest pain or discomfort during energy delivery has been reported to occur in approximately 40% of patients undergoing radiofrequency ablation. In

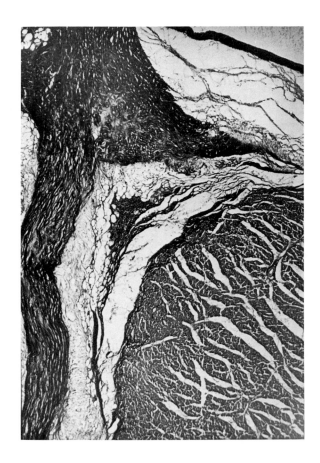

FIG. 3. Histology of the branching portion of the common bundle and bundle branches after direct current catheter ablation. The conduction fibers are replaced by a fibro-fatty infiltrate.

unusual instances, this pain was of sufficient intensity to warrant use of general anesthesia (24).

Caution should be used when applying radiofrequency energy to patients with previously implanted permanent pacemakers. In an animal study, Chin et al. (26) studied the effect of radiofrequency energy on implanted pulse generators. Nineteen pulse generators from seven manufacturers were studied. When radiofrequency energy was applied 4 cm or closer to the pacing electrodes, 16 of the implanted generators showed some change in function, including runaway, false inhibition or reversion to noise mode. No such effect was seen when energy was applied at more remote distances. No pacemaker reprogramming or pacing system malfunction was observed after cessation of radiofrequency application. In order to avoid serious complications, the following precautions are recommended in patients with permanent pacemakers undergoing radiofrequency ablation (26):

1. External sources of ventricular pacing should be available as a standby.
2. In order to avoid pacemaker runaway, permanent pacing systems should be programmed to minimal output or the fixed rate mode if available.
3. A complete pacing analysis should be performed following ablation.
4. Radiofrequency ablation should not be performed in close proximity to permanent leads.

LONG-TERM OUTCOME

In a recent report, we presented our long-term follow-up data for patients undergoing attempted AV junctional ablation. The latter consisted of 49 patients who were followed for a mean of 41 ± 23 months. The long-term course and the survival rate of these patients are shown in Figs. 4 and 5. The objective of this review was to focus on long-term psychosocial as well as objective changes after catheter ablation.

In our experience, 83% of patients report improved well-being and increased activity level after ablation. The improvements were more pronounced in those without evidence of significant cardiac disease (89%) compared to those with cardiac disease (67%). Similar data were reported by Kay et al. (27). Of interest was the finding that 25% of patients with chronic complete AV block described feeling occasional palpitations. Repeated 24-hr Holter monitor recordings showed that palpitations were either correlated with the presence of premature ventricular complexes or associated with regular rhythms. Patients undergoing ablative procedures should be forewarned that palpitations, usually related to premature ventricular complexes, may be perceived after this procedure.

In addition, apart from reports of increased well-being, other advantages were documented. For example, the mean need for hospitalization prior to catheter ablation was 2.4 ± 2 per year as opposed to 0.3 ± 0.5 per year after ablation. In addition, it is important to emphasize that the duration of the hospital stay was usually for 3 to 8 days of monitoring. There was adjustment of antiarrhythmic drugs or dosing, attempted DC cardioversion, and at times initiation of anticoagulant therapy. After

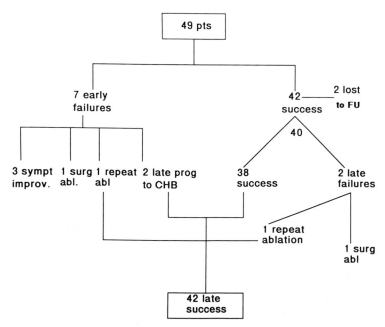

FIG. 4. Long-term course of 49 patients undergoing atrioventricular junctional ablation with direct current shock. CHB, complete heart block; surg abl, surgical ablation; FU, follow-up; prog, progression; sympt improv, symptomatically improved. (From ref. 14, with permission.)

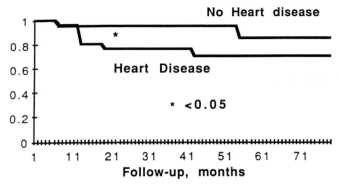

FIG. 5. Actuarial survival curves for patients undergoing atrioventricular junctional ablation. Note that survival was higher among patients without underlying heart disease. (From ref. 14, with permission.)

successful ablation, hospitalization was uncommon and consisted in large measure of pacemaker replacement or adjustments (see below).

The number of antiarrhythmic agents used dropped dramatically after successful ablation. Only 7% of the patients required therapy for bothersome premature ventricular complexes.

In a previous report, Abbott et al. (28) showed that for the group as a whole, catheter ablation of the AV junction was not associated with a significant change in the left ventricular ejection fraction. We extended these findings by analyzing serial echocardiographic studies in the five patients with the poorest left ventricular function (ejection fraction <35%). The left ventricular ejection fraction was unchanged in one but increased significantly in the others. After a median follow-up of 28 months, the preablation ejection fraction rose from 25% to 45%. We interpret these findings as consistent with the superimposition of a tachycardia-induced cardiomyopathy in patients with organic cardiac disease complicated with uncontrolled atrial fibrillation. Rate control as established by catheter ablation appears to (at least in some patients) improve myocardial function.

Also of potential importance was the finding that none of the 27 patients with chronic or paroxysmal atrial fibrillation who were followed for a total of 843 patient-months developed a systemic embolus despite the fact that only one received chronic anticoagulant therapy. The expected incidence for this type of patient cohort would be between 2 and 3 episodes (29). This potentially interesting observation deserves further studies.

CHOOSING THE OPTIMAL PACEMAKER MODE AFTER ABLATION

In patients with chronic atrial fibrillation, ventricular rate adaptive pacing seems to be the most logical choice. This pacing mode is a simple and elegant method for achieving protection against bradycardia while providing the patient with a chronotropic response during physical stress. Kay et al. (27) reported improved exercise capacity after ablation in 12 patients provided with rate adapted ventricular pacemakers who underwent treadmill exercise test before and 6 weeks after ablation. Approximately 30% of our patients originally provided with fixed-rate ventricular pacing had the unit replaced with a rate-responsive unit because of symptoms related to low functional capacity.

In patients with intact sinus node activity between attacks, synchronization between the atrial and the ventricular activity would be of further hemodynamic benefit. However, a common problem in patients with DDD pacemakers and paroxysmal supraventricular arrhythmias is the appearance either of pacemaker-mediated tachycardia or of tracking of fast atrial rhythms during attacks of tachycardia. In our series, four of eight patients provided with AV synchronous units had to have these replaced or reprogrammed because of these complications, underlining the point that AV synchronous pacing alone might not be a first choice in patients who have undergone ablation for supraventricular arrhythmias. In patients with reduced left ventricular compliance (hypertrophic or ischemic heart disease), the preservation of AV synchrony may outweigh these disadvantages.

Two newer principles of AV synchronous pacing might be especially suitable for this patient group. DDI-R pacing with the physiologic sensor driving the atrium, thereby preserving AV synchrony while in sinus rhythm, without sensing the atrial rate is one interesting alternative. Another promising feature is so-called conditional tracking in DDD-R pacing. In this mode, when the atrium senses rapid atrial rates that are not associated with sensor signals indicating increased physical activity, the rhythm is interpreted as supraventricular arrhythmia and the pacemaker automatically switches to a lower rate.

Future studies will determine whether these modifications will be of benefit in these patients.

ALTERNATIVE TECHNIQUES FOR MANAGEMENT OF ATRIAL FIBRILLATION

Another approach to achieve induction of AV nodal destruction or modification in patients with atrial fibrillation has been suggested by Brugada et al. (30). They selectively catheterized the AV nodal artery in seven patients with atrial fibrillation and uncontrollable ventricular rates. After infusion of ice cold saline showed temporary AV block, a small amount of 96% alcohol was given causing complete AV block in five and modification sufficient to control heart rate in two patients. However, in one patient, ethanol infusion caused occlusion of the right coronary artery leading to an inferior wall infarction. Due to the limited experience with this method it should, in our opinion, be used only when catheter ablation has failed.

The previously discussed methods include destruction or modification of the AV nodal conduction to achieve rate control. Levy et al. (31) reported a new method for cardioversion of atrial fibrillation using internal cardioversion. In the initial study of 17 patients severely disabled by chronic atrial fibrillation and resistant to external DC conversion, a 200 to 400-J shock was delivered between the proximal pole of a quadripolar catheter located in the right atrium and a back-plate. Sinus rhythm was restored in 15 patients (88%) and maintained until discharge in 11 patients. During a follow-up of 15 months (range 2–25 months) four patients had recurrence of the atrial fibrillation. A second attempt was successful in one patient. Thus, approximately 50% of the initial group had preserved sinus rhythm by the end of follow-up. The advantage with this method is that it avoids induction of high-grade AV block and permanent pacing, thereby maintaining AV synchronization and a normal ventricular activation sequence. A more comprehensive collaborative study is in progress.

CATHETER ABLATION FOR PATIENTS WITH ATRIAL FIBRILLATION AND WOLFF-PARKINSON-WHITE SYNDROME

It is well recognized that atrial fibrillation occurring in patients with Wolff-Parkinson-White syndrome with short accessory pathway refractory periods may result in life-threatening cardiac arrhythmias (Figs. 6 and 7). Patients with these life-threatening arrhythmias were in the past, generally treated with cardiac surgery, a technique that has proved very effective and safe. More recently, a number of groups have reported using either DC (1) or radiofrequency (2,3) discharges for ablation of accessory pathways in all locations. The left-sided pathways are approached by retrograde left ventricular catheterization and by positioning the ablating catheter at the annulus beneath the mitral valve. Similar techniques have been introduced for right free wall and septal accessory pathways. The initial results of these procedures are excellent (85%–100% success rate) and are associated with minimal adverse effects. The catheter technique promises to become the procedure of choice both for therapy of patients with life-threatening arrhythmias as well as for any symptomatic patient with accessory pathway-mediated arrhythmias.

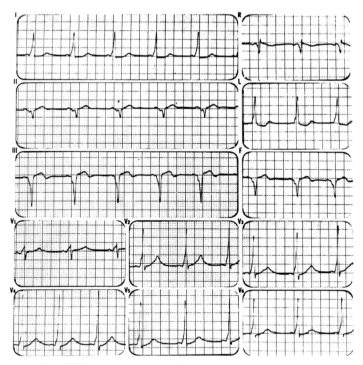

FIG. 6. 12-lead ECG from a patient with a posteroseptal accessory pathway.

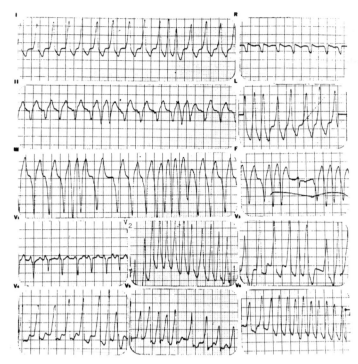

FIG. 7. 12-lead ECG from the patient in Fig. 6 with 12-lead ECG showing atrial fibrillation with extraordinary rapid response.

SUMMARY

Catheter ablation is now considered standard therapy for patients with atrial fibrillation who prove refractory to standard medical therapy. In our practice, we attempt arrhythmia control with standard antiarrhythmic agents and after failure or intolerance to trials of class IA, II, and IV drugs, we offer the patient the option of amiodarone/sotalol or ablation. It is not necessary to expose the patient to every class IA drug or all conceivable combinations of antiarrhythmic drugs. It should be emphasized that drug therapy is not free of adverse risks, including death. The incidence of aborted sudden death in our series was approximately 8% and was related to either inability to control life-threatening arrhythmias or serious adverse drug effects. Precisely when intervention with catheter ablation is proposed is a matter of clinical judgment.

The available experience suggests that radiofrequency application, while somewhat less effective in producing complete AV block compared to high-energy DC shocks, is nevertheless safer and is now considered the initial energy source of choice. If complete AV block is not achieved with radiofrequency application, this does not preclude use of DC shocks at the same session.

Initial experience accumulated for 552 patients undergoing high-energy DC shock ablation from a voluntary registry recorded a 0.4% incidence of procedure-related death and a 1.5% incidence of sudden death from several days to 13 months after ablation. More recent data from an NIH-sponsored prospective registry suggest that the incidence of procedure-related deaths using DC shocks was 5%. It must be emphasized that in the latter study, catheter ablative procedures were extended to some patients who were nearly moribund. More importantly, we are unaware of either procedure-related or late sudden death after radiofrequency applications for attempted AV junctional ablation.

Since catheter ablation of the AV junction was introduced approximately 10 years ago, substantial long-term data are now becoming available. Several studies have documented improved activity status and a sense of well-being after this procedure. In addition, we have intriguing data suggesting that rhythm control after ablation may be associated with an increase in the left ventricular ejection fraction in a selected cohort of patients with atrial fibrillation and that regularization of rate may retard systemic thromboembolism. The latter two points await confirmation from larger study trials.

The reduction of health care costs for patients refractory to standard medical therapy is impressive, since these patients require chronic drug or more frequently combination drug therapy, which is quite expensive when factored over that patient's life. In addition, we found that these patients require very frequent hospital or emergency room visits for arrhythmia control and as emphasized previously, drug therapy may expose the patient to potentially very serious adverse side effects. Finally, impressive advances in catheter ablation of accessory pathways make this procedure the likely technique of choice for treatment of symptomatic patients with arrhythmias related to accessory pathway conduction.

FUTURE DIRECTIONS

Undoubtedly, future efforts will be directed toward the development of catheters with better torque and tip flexion control. A number of investigators are experimenting with laser, cryo-, or microwave energy systems. The importance of these efforts cannot be overemphasized since we believe that future efforts will best be directed at modulating AV nodal conduction without producing complete AV block. If this goal can be achieved by more selective delivery of energy to the AV node, catheter ablative procedures may be more widely applied to those patients with atrial fibrillation who wish to avoid dependence on drug therapy or the need for chronic pacemaker therapy. The ability to predictably modulate AV function would represent an exciting new application of ablative therapy.

REFERENCES

1. Wang YS, Scheinman MM, et al. Incidence, mechanisms and long-term follow-up of patients with supraventricular tachycardia presenting with aborted sudden death (personal communication).
2. Coplen SE, Antman EM, Berlin JA, Hewitt P, Chalmers TC. Efficacy and safety of quinidine therapy for maintenance of sinus rhythm after cardioversion. A meta-analysis of randomized control trials. *Circulation* 1990;82:1106–1116.
3. Kadish AH, Morady F. Torsades de pointes. In: Zipes DP, Jalife J, eds. *Cardiac electrophysiology—from cell to bedside.* Philadelphia: WB Saunders, 1990;605–610.
4. Feld GK, Chen P-S, Nicod P, Fleck P, Meyer D. Possible atrial proarrhythmic effects of class IC antiarrhythmic drugs. *Am J Cardiol* 1990;66:378–383.
5. Scheinman MM, Morady F, Hess DS, Gonzalez R. Catheter induced ablation of the atrioventricular junction to control refractory supraventricular arrhythmias. *JAMA* 1982;248:851–855.
6. Gallagher JJ, Svensen RH, Kasell JH, et al. Catheter technique for closed chest ablation of the

atrioventricular conduction system. A therapeutic alternative for the treatment of refractory supraventricular tachycardia. *N Engl J Med* 1982;306:194–200.

7. Bharati S, Lev M. Histopathologic changes in the heart including the conduction system after catheter ablation. *PACE* 1989;12:159–169.

8. Cunningham D, Rowlands E, Richards AF. A new low-energy power source for catheter ablation. *PACE* 1986;9:1384–1390.

9. Ahsan AJ, Cunningham D, Rowland E, Richards AF. Catheter ablation without fulguration: design and performance of a new system. *PACE* 1989;12:131–135.

10. Ahsan A, Cunningham AD, Richards AF, Rowlands E. Low energy ablation of atrioventricular conduction. *Eur Heart J* 1990;11:233.

11. Hoyt RH, Huang SK, Marcus FI, et al. Factors influencing transcatheter radiofrequency ablation of the myocardium. *J Appl Cardiol* 1986;1:469.

12. Langberg JJ, Lee MA, Chin MC, Rosenqvist M. Radiofrequency catheter ablation: the effect of electrode size on lesion volume in vivo. *PACE* (in press).

13. Frohner K, Podzcek A, Hief C, Nurnberg M, Steinbach KK. Thermal catheter disruption during closed chest radiofrequency ablation of the atrioventricular conduction system. *PACE* 1990; 13:719–723.

14. Rosenqvist M, Lee MA, Moulinier L, et al. Long-term follow-up of patients after transcatheter direct current ablation of the atrioventricular junction. *J Am Coll Cardiol* (*in press*).

15. Evans TG Jr, Huang WH, CAR investigators. In-hospital mortality after direct current catheter ablation of the atrioventricular junction. A prospective international multicenter study. *Circulation* 1990;82:III-691.

16. Rowlands E, Cunningham D, Ahsan A, Richards A. Transvenous ablation of atrioventricular conduction with a low energy power source. *Br Heart J* 1989;62:361–366.

17. Evans GT, Scheinman MM, Zipes DP, et al. The percutaneous cardiac mapping and ablation registry: final summary of results. *PACE* 1988;11:1621–1626.

18. Langberg JJ, Chin MC, Rosenqvist M, et al. Catheter ablation of the atrioventricular junction using radiofrequency energy. *Circulation* 1989;80:1527–1535.

19. Borggrefe M, Podzcek A, Budde T. Catheter ablation of supraventricular tachycardia. *PACE* 1988;11:910.

20. Lavergne TL, Sebag CI, Guize LJ, et al. Transcatheter radiofrequency modification of atrioventricular conduction for refractory supraventricular tachycardia. *Circulation* 1988;78:II-305.

21. Huang SK, Lee MA, Bazgan ID, et al. Radiofrequency catheter ablation of the atrioventricular junction for refractory supraventricular arrhythmias. *Circulation* 1988;78:II-156.

22. Langberg JJ, Chin MC, Lee MA, et al. Ablation of the atrioventricular junction with radiofrequency energy: improved results with a new electrode catheter. *J Am Coll Cardiol* 1990;15:II-133A.

23. Frohner K, Podczeck A, Nürnberg M, Kaltenbrunner W, Steinbach K. Acute and long-term behaviour of AV conduction after radiofrequency ablation. *Eur Heart J* 1990;11:164.

24. Borggrefe M, Hindricks G, Haverkamp W, Budde T, Breithardt G. Radiofrequency ablation. In: Zipes DP, Jalife J, eds. *Cardiac electrophysiology—from cell to bedside*. Philadelphia: WB Saunders, 1990;997–1004.

25. Lee M, Langenberg J, Rosenqvist M, Griffin J, Scheinman M. Polymorphic ventricular tachycardia after high energy direct current or radiofrequency energy ablation of the AV-junction. *Circulation* 1989;80:II-41.

26. Chin M, Lee M, Rosenqvist M, Griffin J, Langberg J. The effect of radiofrequency catheter ablation on permanent pacemakers: an experimental study. *PACE* 1990;13:23–29.

27. Kay GN, Bubien RS, Epstein AE, Plumb VJ. Effect of catheter ablation of the atrioventricular junction on quality of life and exercise tolerance in paroxysmal atrial fibrillation. *Am J Cardiol* 1988;62:741–744.

28. Abbott JA, Schiller NB, Ilvento JB, et al. Catheter ablation of the atrioventricular conduction may improve left ventricular function and cause minimal aortic valve damage. *PACE* 1987;10:411.

29. Wolf PA, Abbott RD, Kannel WB. Atrial fibrillation: a major contribution to stroke in the elderly. *Arch Intern Med* 1987;147:1561–1564.

30. Brugada P, de Swart H, Smeets J, Wellens HJJ. Transcoronary chemical ablation of atrioventricular conduction. *Circulation* 1990;81:757–761.

31. Levy S, Bru PO, Cointe R, Collet F, Metge P, Lacombe P, Gerard R. Cardioversion par choc électricque interne de la fibrillation auricularire permanente. *Arch Mal Coeur* 1989;82:1529–1532.

Atrial Fibrillation: Mechanisms and Management, edited by
R. H. Falk and P. J. Podrid.
Raven Press, Ltd., New York © 1992.

21

Surgical Management of Symptomatic Atrial Fibrillation

James W. Leitch, Gerard M. Guiraudon, George J. Klein, and Raymond Yee

Cardiac Investigation Unit, University Hospital, London, Ontario, Canada N6A 5A5

Atrial fibrillation is probably the most common supraventricular arrhythmia in the community (1–3). Despite its high prevalence, atrial fibrillation is the last of the common supraventricular tachycardias subjected to surgical treatment. There are several reasons for this. Atrial fibrillation is a complex arrhythmia that is difficult to study in humans, even with sophisticated mapping techniques (3,4). Despite extensive basic and clinical research, there are still many uncertainties in the pathophysiology of atrial fibrillation (3). No particular location in the atrium has been shown to be the focus or the necessary substrate for fibrillation. Therefore, standard cardiac electrophysiologic surgical techniques, which rely on either ablation or exclusion of an arrhythmia substrate, have proved difficult to apply to this arrhythmia. In addition, atrial fibrillation is often associated with other cardiac disease that results in diffuse myocardial and electrophysiologic abnormalities. Long-standing atrial arrhythmias may themselves result in atrial dilatation and subsequent electrophysiologic and pathologic abnormalities (5,6). Consequently, there has been some doubt as to whether a surgical technique could restore normal sinus rhythm in patients with long-standing atrial arrhythmias. Finally, the prevalence of atrial fibrillation is closely related to age (7–9), and many otherwise suitable candidates are excluded from operative consideration because of advanced age and associated medical problems.

CANDIDATES FOR SURGICAL THERAPY

Despite the aforementioned limitations, effective operations for atrial fibrillation have been developed (10,11). The most important factor leading to the development of surgery for atrial fibrillation has been a better fundamental understanding of this arrhythmia (3,4). This has allowed a rational approach to operative therapy to be devised. An additional stimulus to the development of surgery has been the often disappointing results of pharmacologic treatment, particularly when used to maintain sinus rhythm (12–17). Usually the best that can be achieved is a decrease in the frequency and severity of fibrillation episodes (17). Even if medication is effective in preventing recurrent fibrillation, side effects and fears of proarrhythmia may limit the use of effective antiarrhythmic agents (13,17–19). An alternative approach is control of the ventricular response without attempting to maintain sinus rhythm. This can be accomplished either pharmacologically or by His bundle ablation (20,21). This is often effective in relieving the symptoms of atrial fibrillation but requires either a life-long commitment to medication or dependence on a ventricular pacemaker.

The ideal candidate for surgical treatment of atrial fibrillation is a relatively young patient, free of other cardiac disease, who does not wish to have either continuous antiarrhythmic medication or a ventricular pacemaker. As will be discussed later, a further important requirement is demonstrably normal sinus node function. Finally, there must be a strong motivation on the patient's part to undertake surgical therapy in an attempt to restore normal sinus rhythm. Thus, although the numbers of patients with atrial fibrillation are large, only a small subset of these patients would be considered at present suitable for a surgical approach. At our institution, of approximately 300 patients with atrial fibrillation, only 11 have undergone surgery in the period from 1985 to 1990. It may be that a greater proportion of patients with atrial fibrillation will be considered for surgical therapy as the current surgical techniques evolve.

THEORETICAL FOUNDATION FOR SURGERY

In 1914, Garrey (22) made the elegant observation that a critical mass of atrial tissue was required to sustain fibrillation. Subsequently, it has become evident that the mechanism for atrial fibrillation is usually continuous multiple intra-atrial reentry (3–5,23–26). The reentrant waves are not confined to any particular location in the atria but vary continuously in size and orientation. This form of reentry has been called reentry without a fixed anatomical obstacle (4). The circulatory wavelets require a certain mass of atrial tissue in which to circulate in order not to extinguish themselves in refractory tissue. The exact amount of tissue required depends on the "wavelength" of the cardiac impulse that is defined as the product of refractory period and conduction velocity (5,27,28). In humans, the mass of atrial tissue required to sustain fibrillation is uncertain and presumably varies individually depending on the extent to which refractoriness and conduction velocity is abnormal. Therefore, although the basic mechanism of atrial fibrillation has been described, there is still substantial uncertainty in the application of this theory to humans. Both of the described surgical approaches to atrial fibrillation were designed with these principles in mind, and their success in preventing atrial fibrillation provides confirming evidence for Garrey's original observations and the current leading circle model of atrial fibrillation.

THE CORRIDOR OPERATION

The corridor operation is designed to maintain sinus rhythm by isolating the sinus node, a small corridor of atrial tissue and the atrioventricular (AV) node from the remaining atrial tissue (11,29–32) (Fig. 1). In designing this operation, it was hypothesized that this small corridor of atrial tissue would not be large enough to sustain atrial fibrillation. Of course, the atria excluded from the corridor might continue to fibrillate, but this atrial activity should not be conducted to the AV node. Sinus node

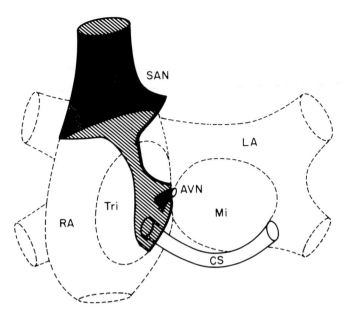

FIG. 1. Schematic anterior view of the atria after the ventricles have been resected. The *dotted lines* outline the right and left atria and the tricuspid and mitral annulus. The *solid line* outlines the corridor (see text). AVN, atrioventricular node; CS, coronary sinus; LA, left atrium; Mi, mitral valve; RA, right atrium; SAN, sinoatrial node; Tri, tricuspid valve. (From ref. 10, with permission.)

depolarization is conducted through the corridor to the AV node and then to the ventricles. This operation would then be expected to maintain normal cardiac chronotropic function but not atrial mechanical function.

Preoperative Evaluation

An electrophysiology study is required preoperatively to determine if there are any other cardiac electrophysiologic abnormalities such as a concealed accessory pathway or AV node reentry that may be a primary trigger for atrial fibrillation. At this study, it is important to evaluate sinus node and AV node function as completely as possible because the results of the operation depend on the integrity of these two structures. Coronary angiography is also required to demonstrate the course of the sinus node artery and to exclude significant coronary artery disease.

Surgical Technique

After median sternotomy and initiation of cardiopulmonary bypass, the aorta is cross-clamped and cold crystalloid cardioplegia infused. The surgical technique comprises two steps (Fig. 2): (a) Left atrial free wall disconnection using a horseshoe incision of the left atrium along its attachment to the atrial septum. (b) The construction of the corridor using a horseshoe incision that starts at the tricuspid annulus in the anterior septal region (right coronary fossa) and ends in the posterior septal re-

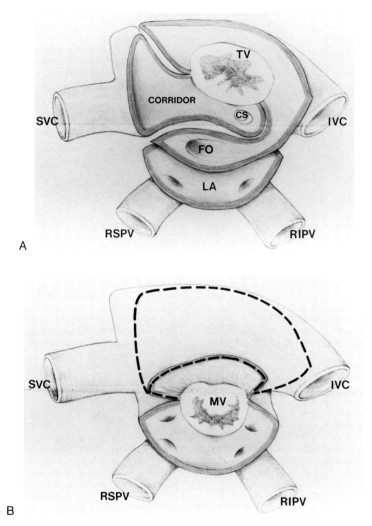

FIG. 2. A: Schematic depiction of the right atrial disconnection. The right atrium is shown after the right atrial incisions have been completed circumscribing the corridor. **B:** Left atrial disconnection. The *dotted lines* indicate the right atrial incisions, which overlie the left atrium in this view. See text for description of operation. CS, orifice of coronary sinus; FO, fossa ovale; IVC, inferior vena cava; LA, left atrium; MV, mitral valve; RIPV, right inferior pulmonary vein; RSPV, right superior pulmonary vein; SVC, superior vena cava; TV, tricuspid valve. (From ref. 10, with permission.)

gion at the tricuspid annulus anterior to the coronary sinus orifice. After dissection of the atria to form the corridor, the two ends of the corridor are cryoablated to ensure that conduction is absent between the excluded left and right atria and the constructed corridor. The atrial incisions are then repaired with sutures, the aorta unclamped, and the patient rewarmed. The corridor is then constructed of a cuff of right atrium around the superior vena cava, a strip of atrial septum anterior to the fossa ovale, and the triangle of Koch with the AV node and the coronary sinus orifice. Electrophysiology testing is performed at completion of surgery to confirm that

TABLE 1. *Clinical features of patients undergoing surgery*

Pt.	Age	Arrhythmia	Heart disease	Symptom duration[a] (years)	Pacemaker implanted	Follow-up (months)	Recurrence of AF
1	54	Paroxysmal AF	Previous arrhythmia surgery[b]	10	AAI	55	Yes
2	45	Chronic AF	Dilated cardiomyopathy	20	VVIR	49	Yes
3	45	Paroxysmal AF		30		44	No
4	40	Paroxysmal AF		10		21	No
5	49	Chronic AF	Mitral stenosis	10	VVIR	15	No
6	25	Chronic AF		5		9	No
7	50	Chronic AF		9		9	No
8	68	Paroxysmal AF		13	VVIR	9	No
9	43	Paroxysmal AF		3		6	No
10	51	Paroxysmal AF	Hypertension	4	VVIR	3	No
11	61	Chronic		20		2	No

[a]From onset of first episode of atrial fibrillation to operation.
[b]Atrial flutter cryoablation and implantation of an atrial antitachycardia pacemaker.
Pt, patient; AF, atrial fibrillation; AAI, atrial demand pacemaker; VVIR, rate-adaptive ventricular demand pacemaker.

atrial segments are electrically independent. Further postoperative testing is carried out prior to discharge 1 to 2 weeks after surgery.

Results of the Corridor Operation

Eleven patients have undergone this operation between 1985 and 1990 (Table 1). Six patients had paroxysmal atrial fibrillation with daily episodes of tachycardia and five patients had chronic atrial fibrillation. The time from the first episode of atrial fibrillation to operation ranged from 3 to 30 years (mean of 12.2 ± 8.2 years) and number of drug trials from 2 to 8 (mean 5 ± 1.5). Nine patients had idiopathic atrial fibrillation, one patient had mitral stenosis, and one patient had mild idiopathic dilated cardiomyopathy (ejection fraction 34%). In the majority of patients it was not possible to accurately measure sinus node recovery times either because sinus rhythm could not be maintained following cardioversion (five patients) or because sustained atrial fibrillation recurred repeatedly during the electrophysiology study (one patient). This is an unfortunate limitation in patients with atrial fibrillation because determination of preoperative sinus node function may be critical in assessing the results of operation. As might be expected, the patients who chose to undergo this operation were severely symptomatic with refractory atrial fibrillation.

Predischarge Electrophysiology Testing

Electrical independence of the atrial segments was achieved in almost all patients (Fig. 3). This is shown in Table 2 in which complete isolation of the corridor was obtained in 10 of the 11 patients. In one further patient there appeared to be atypical

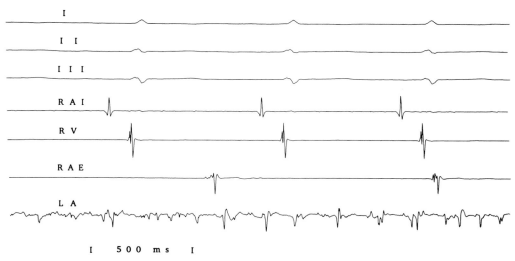

FIG. 3. Recording at predischarge electrophysiologic study showing sinus rhythm in the corridor (RAI), an independent atrial rhythm in the excluded right atrium (RAE), and atrial fibrillation in the excluded left atrium (LA). There was no electrical connection between the atrial segments. I, surface lead 1; II, surface lead 2; III, surface lead 3; LA, left atrium outside corridor; RAE, right atrium outside the corridor; RAI, corridor (included right atrium); RV, right ventricle.

TABLE 2. *Predischarge electrophysiology findings*

Pt.	Sinus node recovery time (msec)	Corridor cycle length (msec)	Excluded right atrium cycle length (msec)	Excluded left atrium cycle length (msec)	Tachycardia in corridor
1	3,000	Flutter/fibrillation	2,000	Fibrillation	Flutter/fibrillation
2	950	880	810	1,010	No
3	840	650	1,600	Fibrillation	No
4	4,660	680	1,000	Fibrillation	No
5	2,700	1,160	2,000	Fibrillation	Atrial tachycardia
6	510	650	720	Quiescent	AV node reentry
7	1,680	990	850	Quiescent	No
8	—[a]	1,120	Quiescent	1,200	No
9	1,310	760	1,980	Fibrillation	No
10	NA	780	2,010	Quiescent	no
11	1,150†	840	Fibrillation	Fibrillation	no

[a]Junctional rhythm.
[b]Secondary pause 3 sec.
Pt., patient; NA, not available because epicardial wires nonfunctional.

slow Wenckebach-like conduction between the excluded right atrium and corridor of minimal functional significance. Reoperation before hospital discharge was required in one patient because of persistent conduction between the left atrium and the corridor. Anterograde conduction from the corridor to the ventricle over the AV node was well maintained (Wenckebach cycle length ranged from 380–620 msec), apart from one patient with Wenckebach block in sinus rhythm (sinus cycle length 760 msec). In the majority of patients, the excluded right atrium demonstrated a regular rhythm from a presumed subsidiary pacemaker. The excluded left atrium was in fibrillation or flutter in six patients and in a regular rhythm from a subsidiary pacemaker in two patients. The corridor was in sinus rhythm in eight patients, in junctional rhythm in one patient (cycle length 1,120 msec), and in atrial tachycardia (cycle length 310 msec) in one patient (Fig. 4) and displayed intermittent nonsustained atrial flutter/fibrillation with sinus bradycardia in the remaining patient.

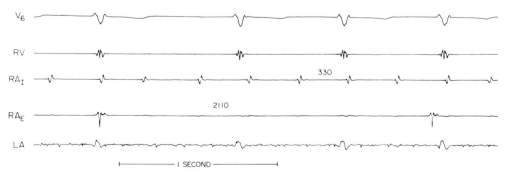

FIG. 4. Atrial tachycardia in the corridor at predischarge electrophysiology testing. There is a regular tachycardia in the corridor with a cycle length of 330 msec. This tachycardia conducts with variable degrees of block to the ventricle. The excluded right atrium has a slow regular rhythm and the left atrium is fibrillating. This tachycardia could be pace terminated and did not recur clinically. V_6, lead V6; other abbreviations as in Fig. 3.

Sinus node recovery times of more than 2 sec were found in three patients with a secondary pause of more than 3 sec in one patient. One patient demonstrated persistent junctional rhythm at a cycle length of 1,120 msec with only intermittent sinus node function. In one patient sustained supraventricular tachycardia with a cycle length of 320 msec was induced in the corridor by ventricular pacing. This tachycardia was believed to be the uncommon form of AV node reentry because it could only be induced by ventricular pacing and could be repeatedly terminated by double ventricular extrastimuli without advancing atrial activation (Fig. 5). This is a surprising finding because there had been no evidence for AV node reentry at the preoperative study, which had been complete. This tachycardia was rendered noninducible following intravenous administration of 5 mg of verapamil and has not recurred clinically. It is intriguing to speculate that this arrhythmia may have either been present before surgery (and perhaps acted as an underlying trigger for fibrillation) or alternatively was a result of the surgery in and around the AV node. Perhaps the most likely explanation is that this was an incidental finding, unrelated to atrial fibrillation and surgery, and of no clinical significance. In no other patient was an atrial arrhythmia, either flutter, fibrillation, or atrial tachycardia, inducible in the corridor, confirming the hypothesis that this small amount of atrial tissue would, in general, not be large enough to sustain fibrillation.

Clinical Outcome

The total follow-up time was 201 patient-months with a mean of 18 months. Only two patients have had a recurrence of atrial fibrillation. One of these patients demonstrated intermittent fibrillation in the corridor at the predischarge electrophysiology study. Induction of fibrillation appeared to be dependent on prolonged sinus pauses. This was the first patient to undergo the corridor operation. Following this clinical failure, the size of the corridor was reduced in subsequent patients. This patient had an atrial demand pacemaker implanted and was maintained on propafenone. With this therapy he has remained asymptomatic over the past 3 years. The

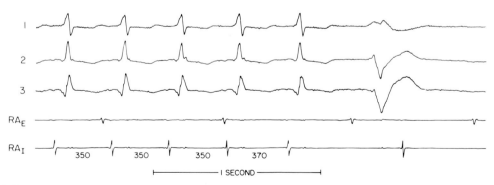

FIG. 5. Inducible atrioventricular (AV) node reentry at predischarge electrophysiology testing. A regular tachycardia (cycle length 350 msec) was induced by ventricular stimulation. This was thought to be atypical AV node reentry because it could be terminated by either ventricular stimulation without advancing atrial activation or by injection of adenosine triphosphate (ATP). This figure shows termination by 8 mg ATP. There is slight slowing of the tachycardia cycle length before termination. After termination, there was transient heart block. Abbreviations as in Figs. 3 and 4.

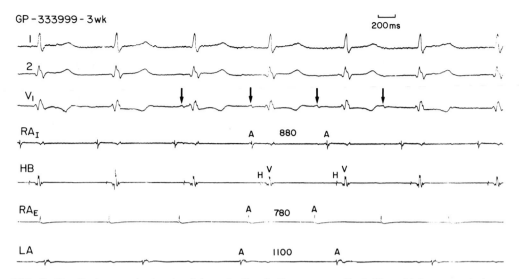

FIG. 6. Predischarge electrophysiology testing in the same patient. The atrial segments have independent atrial rhythms. The corridor (RA$_I$) conducts normally to the ventricles (the patient is in sinus rhythm). An independent rhythm in the excluded right atrium accounts for most of the surface P-wave activity, and it appears on the surface ECG as though there is complete heart block. HB, His bundle recording; other abbreviations as in Figs. 2 and 3.

second patient demonstrated recurrent fibrillation 3 months after discharge. In this patient it was difficult to establish the exact diagnosis of his clinical arrhythmia following surgery because the majority of P-wave activity on the surface ECG was due to activity from the excluded right atrium (Fig. 6). When he presented with clinical fibrillation (Fig. 7), he underwent repeat electrophysiology study in order to deter-

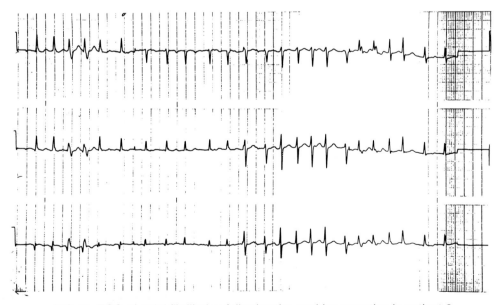

FIG. 7. ECG of atrial fibrillation following the corridor operation in patient 2.

mine the mechanism of this arrhythmia. At electrophysiology study the atrial segments were demonstrated to be completely independent and, furthermore, fibrillation could not be induced in the corridor. However, atrial tachycardia at a cycle length of 400 msec could be induced in the corridor. Whether this tachycardia with an irregular ventricular response was the mechanism for his clinical tachycardia remains uncertain. In any case, in this patient, the operation was not a success because he continued to experience symptomatic episodes of tachycardia. All nine patients operated on after these two patients have remained free of tachycardia. Thus, in the majority of patients, this operation has proved extremely effective in preventing atrial fibrillation.

Pacemaker Implantation

Permanent ventricular pacemakers were implanted in five patients following surgery. In two patients, pacemakers were implanted following symptomatic sinus pauses, and in the third patient a pacemaker was implanted prophylactically when prolonged sinus pauses were demonstrated at the postoperative electrophysiology study. A further patient underwent prophylactic pacemaker implantation because of Wenckebach AV block in sinus rhythm at the predischarge study. One further patient, as mentioned previously, had an atrial pacemaker reimplanted after surgery because of prolonged sinus pauses associated with bradycardia-dependent atrial fibrillation in the corridor. Thus, the main limitation to this operation was a relatively high incidence of postoperative sinus node dysfunction requiring pacemaker implantation.

The reasons for this are uncertain. Because sinus node function could only be measured in a small number of patients preoperatively, it was not possible to determine if sinus node dysfunction postoperatively was a result of previous sinus node disease or a complication of surgery. Atrial arrhythmias and sinus node dysfunction often coexist as different manifestations of the same disease process (32–35). Patients who required pacemakers for sinus node impairment either had associated cardiac disease (cardiomyopathy and mitral stenosis), were elderly (age 68), or had undergone previous cardiac surgery (atrial flutter cryoablation). The extent to which these factors resulted in the need for pacemaker implantation is uncertain.

In order to avoid operative sinus node injury, the atrial incisions were always made at some distance from the anatomical location of the sinus node. However, mapping of the sinus node in humans has demonstrated that its location may be anatomically diverse (36). Subsidiary pacemakers, which may have been excluded from the corridor, may also be important in the maintenance of "sinus rhythm" (37). Because of these problems, our present policy is to recommend this surgery only in those patients in whom it is possible to demonstrate relatively normal sinus node function preoperatively. For this reason patients with chronic atrial fibrillation, in whom it is not possible to restore sinus rhythm preoperatively, are not considered ideal candidates for surgery.

The corridor operation is not designed to restore atrial mechanical function. The excluded atrial segments often continue to fibrillate or remain quiescent. Even when subsidiary pacemaker activity is present, it is dissociated from sinus node depolarization. Despite these theoretical limitations of the operation, patients in this study in sinus rhythm postoperatively did not have any disability. This may be because increases in cardiac output are more dependent on the ability to increase heart rate than on the presence or absence of atrial contraction (38,39) with normal ventricular function. If the corridor operation is successful and normal sinus node function is present, lack of atrial mechanical function should result in minimal or no disability.

The corridor operation may not eliminate the risk of systemic embolization because the left atrium may continue to fibrillate. The necessity for anticoagulation in patients with idiopathic atrial fibrillation and in patients with paroxysmal atrial fibrillation, however, is still uncertain (40). In this series, patients were maintained on anticoagulants for at least 6 months after the operation and thereafter at the discretion of the individual physician.

Another center has performed the corridor operation in 20 patients (30–32). In 16 of 20 patients, complete isolation of the corridor was achieved. Early reoperation to achieve isolation was required in eight patients. Only two patients required pacemakers for sinus node disease, in marked contrast to our results. This difference may be accounted for by patient selection, since only patients with paroxysmal atrial fibrillation underwent operation in this latter series. Preoperative sinus function was evaluated more frequently, and in the absence of chronic fibrillation, there may have been less atrial disease and consequently less sinus node impairment. In agreement with our findings, the 16 patients with an isolated corridor remained free of atrial fibrillation. Atrial flutter occurred in three patients and ectopic atrial tachyarrhythmias in one patient during the mean 20-month follow-up.

These results demonstrate that the corridor operation can maintain sinus rhythm in patients with chronic and paroxysmal atrial fibrillation. At present, at our center, the major limitation to this operation is sinus node dysfunction requiring pacemaker implantation. Patient selection appears to be the critical factor in preventing this outcome. With continuing experience we may be able to select patients with relatively normal sinus node function and thus obviate the need for a pacemaker postoperatively.

THE MAZE OPERATION

This operation, devised by Cox and associates (11) is more ambitious than the corridor operation. In addition to maintaining sinus rhythm, the maze operation is designed to restore atrial mechanical function and obviate the need for anticoagulation. Restoration of sinus rhythm is accomplished by dividing the left and right atria into a continuous strip of atrial tissue. Sinus node depolarization then spreads through the atrium in a variety of directions following the "maze." The maze is constructed sufficiently narrowly so that the conducting wave cannot turn back on itself and allow reentry. In this manner, the operation is designed to allow depolarization of all the atria, apart from the atrial appendages and pulmonary veins, without allowing a reentrant circuit to develop. The operation is performed under cardiopulmonary bypass and a combination of incisions and cryosurgery is used to create the maze.

Only preliminary results are available at present (11). Three patients have been reported to have undergone this operation. All three patients have remained in sinus rhythm following the operation with a normal subjective exercise tolerance. The atria appear to contract normally on noninvasive examination. A further report from this group is in preparation, which should help to determine the relative merits of this procedure.

CONCLUSIONS

Surgery for atrial fibrillation is perhaps the last frontier for the cardiac arrhythmia surgeon. Even with further developments in surgical techniques, it is likely that only a small proportion of patients with atrial fibrillation will be considered suitable for a surgical approach. However, in this subset of suitable patients, the recently developed operations hold the promise of a permanent cure without the need for antiarrhythmic medication or implantation of a pacemaker.

ACKNOWLEDGMENT

We thank Sheila Doan for preparation of the manuscript.

REFERENCES

1. Kannel WB, Abbott RD, Savage DD, McNamara PM. Epidemiologic features of chronic atrial fibrillation. The Framingham study. *N Engl J Med* 1982;306:1018–1022.
2. Selzer A. Atrial fibrillation revisited. *N Engl J Med* 1982;306:1044–1045.
3. Allessie MA, Rensma PL, Brugada J, Smeets JLRM, Penn O, Kirchhof CJHJ. Pathophysiology of atrial fibrillation. In: Zipes DP, Jalife J, eds. *Cardiac electrophysiology. From cell to bedside.* Philadelphia: WB Saunders, 1990;548–559.
4. Allessie MA, Bonke FIM, Schopman FJG. Circus movement in rabbit muscle as a mechanism of tachycardia. III. The "leading circle" concept. A new model of circus movement in cardiac tissue without the involvement of an anatomic obstacle. *Circ Res* 1977;41:9–18.
5. Davies MJ, Pomerance A. Pathology of atrial fibrillation in man. *Br Heart J* 1972;34:520–525.
6. Sanfilippo AJ, Abascal VM, Sheehan M, Oertel LB, et al. Atrial enlargement as a consequence of atrial fibrillation. A prospective echocardiographic study. *Circulation* 1990;82:792–797.
7. Rose G, Baxter PJ, Reid DD, McCartney P. Prevalence and prognosis of electrocardiographic findings in middle-aged men. *Br Heart J* 1978;40:636–643.
8. Cameron A, Schwartz MJ, Kronmal RA, Kosinski AS. Prevalence and significance of atrial fibrillation in coronary artery disease (CASS registry). *Am J Cardiol* 1988;61:714–717.
9. Leitch JW, Thomson D, Baird DK, Harris PJ. The importance of age as a predictor of atrial fibrillation and flutter after coronary artery bypass grafting. *J Thorac Cardiovasc Surg* 1990;100:338–342.
10. Leitch JW, Klein GJ, Yee R, Guiraudon GM. Sinus node-atrio-ventricular node isolation. Long term results with the corridor operation for atrial fibrillation. *J Am Coll Cardiol* 1991;17:970–975.
11. Cox JL, Schuessler RB, Cain ME, et al. Surgery for atrial fibrillation. *Semin Thorac Cardiovasc Surg* 1989;1:67–73.
12. Bauernfeind RA, Welch WJ. New hope in atrial fibrillation. *J Am Coll Cardiol* 1990;15:708–709.
13. Anderson JL, Gilbert EM, Alpert BL, et al. Prevention of symptomatic recurrences of paroxysmal atrial fibrillation in patients initially tolerating antiarrhythmic therapy. *Circulation* 1989;80:1557–1570.
14. Antman EM, Beamer AD, Cantillon C, McGown N, Friedman PL. Therapy of refractory symptomatic atrial fibrillation and atrial flutter: a staged care approach with new antiarrhythmic drugs. *J Am Coll Cardiol* 1990;15:698–707.
15. Connolly SJ, Hoffert DL. Usefulness of propafenone for recurrent paroxysmal atrial fibrillation. *Am J Cardiol* 1989;63:817–819.
16. Horowitz LN, Spielman SR, Greenspan AM, et al. Use of amiodarone in the treatment of persistent and paroxysmal atrial fibrillation resistant to quinidine therapy. *J Am Coll Cardiol* 1985;6:1402–1407.
17. Coplen SE, Antman EM, Berlin JA, Hewitt P, Chalmers TC. Efficacy and safety of quinidine therapy for maintenance of sinus rhythm after cardioversion. A meta-analysis of randomized control trials. *Circulation* 1990;82:1106–1116.

18. Falk RH. Flecainide-induced ventricular tachycardia and fibrillation in patients treated for atrial fibrillation. *Ann Intern Med* 1989;111:107–111.
19. The Cardiac Arrhythmia Suppression Trial (CAST) Investigators. Preliminary report: effect of encainide and flecainide on mortality in a randomized trial of arrhythmia suppression after myocardial infarction. *N Engl J Med* 1989;321:406–412.
20. Langberg JJ, Chin MC, Rosenqvist M, et al. Catheter ablation of the atrioventricular junction with radiofrequency energy. *Circulation* 1989;80:1527–1535.
21. Gallagher JJ, Svensen RH, Kasell JH, et al. Catheter technique for closed-chest ablation of the atrioventricular conduction system. *N Engl J Med* 1982;306:194–200.
22. Garrey WE. The nature of fibrillatory contraction of the heart. Its relation to tissue mass and form. *Am J Physiol* 1914;33:397.
23. Moe GK, Rheinboldt WC, Abildskov JA. A computer model of atrial fibrillation. *Am Heart J* 1964;67:200–220.
24. Moe GK, Abildskov JA. Atrial fibrillation as a self-sustaining arrhythmia independent of focal discharge. *Am Heart J* 1959;58:59–70.
25. Moe GK. On the multiple wavelet hypothesis of atrial fibrillation. *Arch Int Pharmacodyn* 1962;140:183–188.
26. Wiener N, Rosenblueth A. The mathematical formulation of the problem of conduction of impulses in a network of connected excitable elements, specifically in cardiac muscle. *Arch Inst Cardiol Mex* 1945;16:205–265.
27. Rensma PL, Allessie MA, Lammers WJEP, et al. The length of the excitation wave as an index for the susceptibility to reentrant atrial arrhythmias. *Circ Res* 1988;62:395–410.
28. Guiraudon GM, Klein GJ, Sharma AD, Yee R. Surgery for atrial flutter, atrial fibrillation and atrial tachycardia. In: Zipes DP, Jalife J, eds. *Cardiac electrophysiology. From cell to bedside*. Philadelphia: WB Saunders, 1990;915–920.
29. Defauw JJAMT, Guiraudon GM, van Hemel NM, Vermeulen FEE, Kingma JH, de Bakker JMT. Surgical therapy of paroxysmal atrial fibrillation using the "corridor" operation (personal communication).
30. Defauw JJ, van Hemel NM, Vermeulen FE, Kingma JH, Verrostte JM, Guiraudon GM. Short-term results of the "corridor operation" for drug-refractory paroxysmal atrial fibrillation. *Circulation* 1988;8:II-43.
31. Defaux J, van Hemel N, Vermeulen F, Kingma H, Gehlmann G, Guiraudon G. Treatment of paroxysmal atrial fibrillation by surgical protection of sinus impulse formation and conduction (abstract). *Eur Heart J* 1989;10(suppl 92):15.
32. Kaplan BM, Langendorf R, Lev M, Pick A. Tachycardia-bradycardia syndrome (so-called "sick sinus syndrome"). *Am J Cardiol* 1973;31:497–508.
33. Gomes JAC, Kang PS, Matheson M, Gough WB, El-Sherif N. Coexistence of sick sinus rhythm and atrial flutter-fibrillation. *Circulation* 1981;63:80–89.
34. Rubenstein JJ, Schulman CL, Yurchak PM, DeSanctis RW. Clinical spectrum of the sick sinus syndrome. *Circulation* 1972;46:5–13.
35. Boineau JP, Canavan TE, Schuessler RB, Cain ME, Corr PB, Cox JL. Demonstration of a widely distributed atrial pacemaker complex in the human heart. *Circulation* 1988;77:1221–1237.
36. McGuire MA, Johnson DC, Nunn GR, Yung T, Uther JB, Ross DL. Surgical therapy for atrial tachycardia in adults. *J Am Coll Cardiol* 1989;14:1777–1782.
37. Ryden L, Karlsson O, Kristensson BE. The importance of different atrioventricular intervals for exercise capacity. *PACE* 1988;11:1051–1061.
38. Fananapazir L, Bennett DH, Monks P. Atrial synchronized ventricular pacing: contribution of the chronotropic response to improved exercise performance. *PACE* 1983;6:601–607.
39. Kopecky SL, Gersh BJ, McGoon MD, et al. The natural history of lone atrial fibrillation. A population-based study over 3 decades. *N Engl J Med* 1987;10:669–674.
40. Stroke Prevention in Atrial Fibrillation Study Group Investigators. Preliminary report of the stroke prevention in atrial fibrillation study. *N Engl J Med* 1990;323:863–868.

Atrial Fibrillation: Mechanisms and Management, edited by
R. H. Falk and P. J. Podrid.
Raven Press, Ltd., New York © 1992.

22

Management of Atrial Fibrillation— An Overview

*Philip J. Podrid and †Rodney H. Falk

*Arrhythmia Service, University Hospital, Boston, Massachusetts 02118; †Division of
Cardiology, Boston City Hospital, Boston, Massachusetts 02118; *†Boston University
School of Medicine, Boston, Massachusetts 02118*

In the preceding chapters a number of experts have discussed a wide variety of aspects of atrial fibrillation, ranging from experimental observations to surgical therapy. It is the aim of this final chapter to address the overall management of the patient presenting for the first time with atrial fibrillation. A number of issues will be discussed including the initial assessment and therapy of the acute episode, the decision whether to convert the arrhythmia and the choice of therapy, and the management of chronic atrial fibrillation. It is not the purpose of the chapter to give an in-depth analysis of all the management issues—these can be found elsewhere in this volume—but rather to give a practical overview of the treatment of this common clinical entity.

ETIOLOGY

Although establishing the etiology of an episode of atrial fibrillation generally takes second place to the acute management, it is appropriate to review certain specific etiologies at this point, as knowledge of their significance and prevalence may affect the decision-making process.

While a number of primary cardiac disorders are associated with atrial fibrillation, there are also many noncardiac conditions that predispose to the arrhythmia, suggesting that diverse factors may be responsible for its occurrence (Table 1).

A detailed discussion of each of the various etiologies of atrial fibrillation is beyond the scope of this chapter, but certain common conditions warrant some consideration. Elsewhere in this volume, Leather and Kerr discuss the role of noncardiac conditions such as alcohol (1–5) and thyroid disease (6–10) in the genesis of atrial fibrillation. Consequently, our remarks will be limited to a brief discussion of common cardiac conditions, with a short reconsideration of the entity of lone atrial fibrillation.

TABLE 1. *Causes of atrial fibrillation*

Atrial pressure elevation, atrium, secondary to:
   Mitral or tricuspid valve disease
   Myocardial disease (primary or secondary, leading to systolic or diastolic dysfunction)
   Semilunar valvular abnormalities (causing ventricular hypertrophy)
   Systemic or pulmonary hypertension (pulmonary embolism)
   Intracardiac tumors or thrombi
Atrial ischemia
   Coronary artery disease
Inflammatory or infiltrative atrial disease
   Pericarditis
   Amyloidosis
   Myocarditis
Age-induced atrial fibrotic changes
Intoxicants
   Alcohol
   Carbon monoxide
   Poison gas
Increased sympathetic activity
   Hyperthyroidism
   Pheochromocytoma
   Anxiety
   Alcohol
   Caffeine
   Drugs
Increased parasympathetic activity
Primary or metastatic disease in or adjacent to the atrial wall
Postoperative
   Cardiac and pulmonary surgery
   Overhydration
   Pericarditis
   Cardiac trauma
   Hypoxia
   Pneumonia
Congenital heart disease
   Particularly atrial septal defect
Neurogenic
   Subarachnoid hemorrhage
   ? Nonhemorrhagic, major stroke
Idiopathic

Hypertension and Hypertensive Heart Disease

Although the absolute percentage of patients who develop atrial fibrillation purely as a result of systemic hypertension is very small, the very high prevalence of this condition in the general population makes it the single most common cause of the arrhythmia.

While abnormalities of the P wave may be the first electrocardiographic evidence of underlying left ventricular hypertrophy, often ECG evidence of left ventricular hypertrophy may be entirely absent, despite a definite echocardiographically documented increase in left ventricular mass. Estimates of the exact prevalence of left ventricular hypertrophy in hypertension vary (11), but in the Framingham population, left ventricular hypertrophy measured by echocardiography correlated with diastolic blood pressure and was present in 15.5% of men and 21% of women (12). This contrasted to electrocardiographic features of hypertrophy, which were found in only 0.43% and 0.61% of men and women, respectively. As with other conditions, the increased left ventricular mass may be associated with decreased ventricular compliance resulting in an elevated left atrial pressure and left atrial distention—factors that predispose to atrial fibrillation. If left ventricular hypertrophy is severe, overt congestive heart failure may occur, further increasing the risk of atrial fibrillation.

It is uncertain whether an acute elevation of blood pressure in the presence of chronic hypertension and left ventricular hypertrophy will precipitate atrial fibrillation, but clinical observation suggests that this may occur.

Valvular Heart Disease

It is well established that there is a strong association between atrial fibrillation and rheumatic valvular disease, especially when mitral stenosis or regurgitation is present. Indeed in the Framingham study (13), rheumatic heart disease presented the greatest relative risk of any cardiac condition for the development of the arrhythmia (Table 2).

Mitral valve lesions cause an elevation of left atrial pressure resulting in left atrial hypertrophy and dilatation—an appropriate substrate for atrial fibrillation. There may be an association with atrial fibrillation both with left atrial size (14) and with the slowing of intra-atrial conduction as manifest by prolongation of the P-wave duration (Fig. 1). An increased frequency of atrial premature beats, which can act as triggers of arrhythmia, is probably another important factor.

TABLE 2. *Two years age-adjusted risk of chronic or paroxysmal atrial fibrillation in men and women[a]*

	Risk ratio	
	Paroxysmal	Chronic
Coronary artery disease[b]		
Men	2.1	2.2
Women	4.5	0.5
"Pure" coronary artery disease[c]		
Men	2.6[d]	1.4
Women	1.4[d]	1.4
Hypertensive heart disease[e]		
Men	4.4	4.7
Women	4.6	4.0
Rheumatic heart disease		
Men	7.6	9.9
Women	24.3	27.5
Congestive heart failure		
Men	8.2	8.5
Women	20.4	13.7

[a]Data from the Framingham Heart Study (31) showing the risk of chronic or paroxysmal atrial fibrillation in various cardiac conditions. A risk ratio of 1.0 represents the risk of development of the arrhythmia derived from age-matched controls without the underlying cardiac disease.

[b]Including patients with hypertensive heart disease, rheumatic heart disease, and congestive heart failure.

[c]Excluding patients with hypertensive heart disease, rheumatic heart disease, and congestive heart failure.

[d]Includes episodes of atrial fibrillation occurring during an acute myocardial infarction.

[e]Hypertensive heart disease is defined as hypertension with ECG criteria of left ventricular hypertrophy, congestive heart failure, or cardiomegaly on chest x-ray.

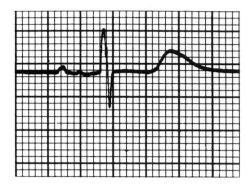

FIG. 1. Lead V_3 of a patient with mitral valve disease and paroxysmal atrial fibrillation. The P wave is 0.20 sec in duration and consists of two distinct peaks. Such an appearance represents markedly prolonged inter- and/or intra-atrial conduction and is frequently a marker of paroxysmal atrial fibrillation.

When atrial fibrillation occurs in mitral stenosis, symptoms are often pronounced, since the shortening of diastole and loss of atrial contraction further elevate left atrial pressure. Rarely atrial fibrillation may go unrecognized, presenting some time after its onset with a devastating stroke.

Atrial fibrillation is less commonly seen with aortic valvular disease and when present suggests the possible coexistence of a mitral valve lesion. However, when severe aortic stenosis results in end-stage myocardial damage or in severe left ventricular hypertrophy, atrial fibrillation may occur. Under these circumstances there is often a rapid hemodynamic deterioration, which may require immediate electrical cardioversion.

Primary isolated right-sided valvular lesions are much less frequently seen than left-sided valve disease, and the prevalence of atrial fibrillation related to right-sided lesions is unknown.

Nonrheumatic valvular disease may also produce changes in the atrial myocardium that predispose to atrial fibrillation. Etiologies of nonrheumatic disease include congenital mitral valve disease, mitral valve prolapse, endocarditis resulting in valvular incompetency and regurgitation, and chordal or papillary muscle rupture.

Pericarditis

The presence of pericarditis is considered an etiologic factor for atrial fibrillation in patients with an acute myocardial infarction, and pericarditis due to other conditions may precipitate the arrhythmia. The presumed cause of atrial fibrillation in pericarditis is inflammation of the sinus node, resulting in sinus node depression, atrial irritability, and changes in membrane excitability (Fig. 2). However, in a prospective review of 100 consecutive cases, Spodick (15) reported that atrial arrhythmia occurred in only seven patients, and in each of these patients, underlying heart disease was present. He proposed that the vulnerability of the sinus node and atrial myocardium to the inflammatory process is insufficient to provoke atrial arrhythmias in the absence of heart disease. A similar observation has also been made in acute myocardial infarction, in which pericarditis was not correlated with the development of atrial fibrillation (16). Thus it is wise to seek out an additional cause of arrhythmia when atrial fibrillation occurs in a patient with pericarditis.

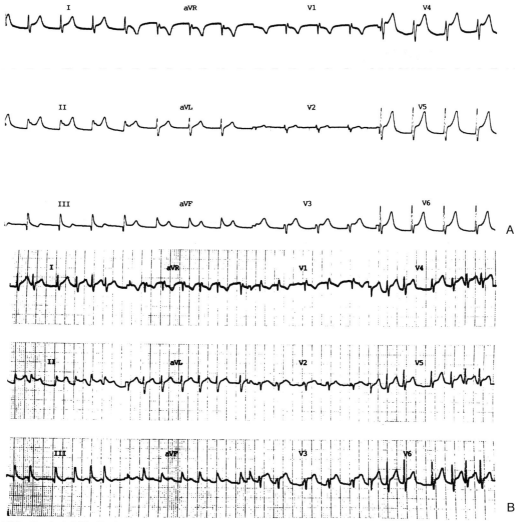

FIG. 2. Atrial fibrillation occurring in a patient with acute viral pericarditis. **A:** ECG at time of presentation with chest pain. Diffuse ST segment elevation typical of pericarditis is present. **B:** One day later atrial fibrillation develops. ST segment elevation is still clearly seen.

Cardiomyopathy

There is a significant incidence of atrial fibrillation in patients with all forms of cardiomyopathy. In most cases of dilated cardiomyopathy, atrial fibrillation is the result of congestive heart failure, which causes an increase in left atrial pressure and in left atrial distention. An additional factor is the development of mitral or tricuspid regurgitation, which often results from ventricular dilatation. The onset of atrial fibrillation in dilated cardiomyopathy may cause a further worsening of congestive heart failure, and correction of the arrhythmia often improves seemingly intractable symptoms of congestion.

Atrial fibrillation occurs in as many as 15% of patients with hypertrophic cardio-myopathy (17–19). In this condition, the factors responsible for the arrhythmia are similar to those in hypertensive heart disease, i.e., reduced left ventricular diastolic compliance and an increase in left ventricular end diastolic pressure. In many patients, mitral regurgitation is also present. The onset of atrial fibrillation in patients with hypertrophic cardiomyopathy may result in a rapid deterioration of hemodynamic status and may cause cardiovascular collapse and pulmonary edema. Rarely the development of ventricular fibrillation precipitated by atrial fibrillation with a rapid ventricular response has been described as a result of myocardial ischemia, despite normal coronary arteries (20) (Fig. 3).

It has been suggested that atrial fibrillation in hypertrophic cardiomyopathy is a marker of poor prognosis, but recent data have shed doubt on this concept. Robinson and co-workers (19) reported on 52 patients with hypertrophic cardiomyopathy who developed paroxysmal or chronic atrial fibrillation and compared them to a matched population with hypertrophic cardiomyopathy who remained in sinus rhythm. The median follow-up was 7 years after the first occurrence of atrial fibrillation. Atrial fibrillation was present in six patients at the time of diagnosis and developed during follow-up in the other 46. The onset of the arrhythmia was associated with a worsening of symptoms in 41 patients (89%), although after therapy (cardioversion or heart rate control), these symptoms generally abated. During the follow-up, 19 patients died from a cardiac cause. The estimated probability of survival at 5, 10, 15, and 20 years was 0.86, 0.71, 0.65, and 0.50, respectively, which was similar to the survival in patients who did not have atrial fibrillation (0.92, 0.82, 0.71, and 0.41, respectively).

Amyloid infiltration of the heart, especially when it involves the atrium is associated with atrial fibrillation (21). Common features are a slow ventricular response, due to concomitant conduction disease, and low-voltage fibrillatory waves, due presumably to replacement of the atrial myocardium by electrically inert amyloid tissue

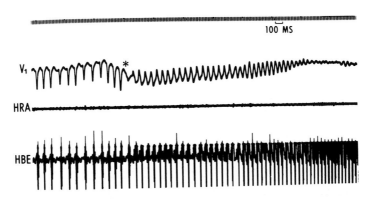

FIG. 3. Development of ventricular fibrillation (*asterisk*) following 1 min 40 sec of atrial fibrillation in a 15-year-old boy with nonobstructive hypertrophic cardiomyopathy and a history of out-of-hospital cardiac arrest. Atrial fibrillation with a ventricular rate of 180 to 190 beats per minute was induced at electrophysiology study and was associated with a systolic blood pressure of 70 mm Hg and ischemic ECG changes. Ventricular stimulation provoked no ventricular arrhythmia. Coronary arteries were normal. HRA, high right atrium; HBE, His bundle electrogram. (From ref. 20, with permission.)

(Fig. 4). Senile amyloid involvement of the atrial myocardium has been proposed as a factor related to the increased incidence of atrial fibrillation in the elderly (22).

Other forms of cardiomyopathy, including Chagas' disease and hemochromatosis, may also cause atrial fibrillation.

Pulmonary Disease

There is a strong association between atrial fibrillation and the presence of pulmonary disease (23–25). In several series, 2% to 3% of patients presenting with atrial fibrillation have underlying pulmonary disease (26,27). The cause of the arrhythmia may be a direct extension of an inflammatory reaction from the lungs to the pericardium, hypoxia, respiratory acidosis (28), increase in circulating catecholamines, the use of sympathomimetic drugs (29), or the development of cor pulmonale. Many patients with lung disease develop frequent atrial premature beats or multifocal atrial tachycardia (Fig. 5). This latter arrhythmia is occasionally indistinguishable from atrial fibrillation or the two arrhythmias may alternate. Often, the treatment of the underlying pulmonary problem is sufficient for reversion of atrial fibrillation to sinus rhythm. However, if atrial fibrillation continues, it is treated in the same manner as in patients without pulmonary disease, except that beta-blocking agents are generally to be avoided.

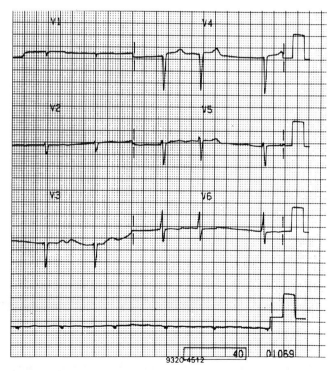

FIG. 4. Tracing of chest leads V₁–V₆ and lead 2 rhythm strip (*bottom line*) in a patient with cardiac amyloidosis and recent-onset atrial fibrillation who was receiving no therapy. Note the low-voltage QRS complexes in lead 2, and pseudoinfarction pattern. The ventricular response is slow and fibrillatory waves are virtually invisible, probably as a result of amyloid infiltration of the atria.

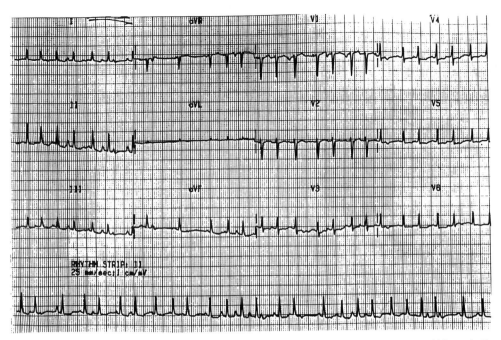

FIG. 5. Multifocal atrial tachycardia (MAT) in a patient with pulmonary disease. Although the rhythm is irregular and may be indistinguishable from atrial fibrillation by palpation of the pulse, examination of the ECG reveals P waves with multiple morphologies, some of which are not conducted. MAT and atrial fibrillation may both occur, at different times, in patients with pulmonary disease.

Other intrathoracic problems, such as tumor, may obstruct pulmonary artery blood flow or directly compress the atrium, resulting in arrhythmia (30).

Coronary Artery Disease

In our experience, a frequently posed question is whether stable patients with recent onset arrhythmia need hospital admission to rule out myocardial infarction. The Framingham study (31) demonstrated an association between prior myocardial infarction and both chronic and paroxysmal atrial fibrillation. However, when subjects were stratified according to the presence or absence of congestive heart failure, rheumatic heart disease, or hypertensive heart disease, it became apparent that it was the presence of one or more of these conditions, rather than the presence of coronary disease, that was the greater predictor of the arrhythmia. In the absence of any of these factors, the relative risk for chronic atrial fibrillation in patients with evidence of coronary heart disease (angina and/or prior infarction) was 1.4 for both men and women. Although transient atrial fibrillation was associated with coronary disease in men, even after correcting for other factors (relative risk 2.6), this was mainly due to atrial fibrillation occurring in the setting of acute infarction. For women, the strong association of transient arrhythmia with coronary heart disease (relative risk 4.5) decreased markedly (to 1.4) after correction for associated factors. Thus, from this epidemiologic study pure coronary disease is seen as an uncommon precursor of atrial fibrillation.

The Framingham data also examined risk factors for atrial fibrillation in another fashion—by examining the "percentage attributable risk" of various cardiovascular diseases to the development of the arrhythmia (31) (Table 3). During the first 24 years of follow-up in 5,209 participants, atrial fibrillation developed in 169 subjects. Overt cardiovascular disease was responsible for only 25% of cases of the arrhythmia (transient or sustained) in men and for 31% in women. The percentages attributable to coronary disease were 8% in men and 3% in women, but it should be emphasized that the coronary disease percentages also include patients with other predisposing conditions. The relatively low overall percentage of cases of atrial fibrillation attributed to cardiovascular disease was probably an underestimate, since hypertensive heart disease was defined as hypertension with cardiomegaly, cardiac failure, or left ventricular hypertrophy by ECG. Subsequent data from Framingham indicate that echocardiographic evidence of left ventricular hypertrophy is far more common than ECG evidence (13), and it is thus highly probable that many cases of atrial fibrillation labeled as not due to cardiovascular disease were, in fact, secondary to undiagnosed hypertensive heart disease.

Further evidence that coronary disease is not a major risk factor for chronic atrial fibrillation comes from a study of more than 18,000 patients with angiographically documented coronary artery disease enrolled in the Coronary Artery Surgical Study (CASS) (32). One hundred and sixteen patients (0.6%) had chronic atrial fibrillation, and the presence of the arrhythmia was associated with age over 60 years ($p<0.0001$), male sex ($p=0.015$), mitral regurgitation ($p<0.001$), and congestive heart failure. There was no association between atrial fibrillation and the number of coronary vessels involved. The presence of atrial fibrillation was also an independent predictor of increased mortality with a relative risk of 1.98 compared to sinus rhythm, and an estimated 7-year probability of survival of 38% for patients with atrial fibrillation versus 80% for those without the arrhythmia ($p<0.001$).

In light of these findings two studies have examined the need for coronary care unit admission in recent-onset atrial fibrillation. Friedman and co-workers (33) reported on 245 patients with atrial fibrillation admitted to a coronary care unit. There were 45 patients in whom atrial fibrillation was of new onset, only five (11%) of whom had elevated levels of MB-CK. All five patients had at least two of the following clinical features: criteria for left ventricular hypertrophy on the ECG ($p<0.01$), an old myocardial infarction on the ECG ($p<0.01$), typical angina pectoris ($p<0.01$), and a duration of symptoms of less than 4 hr ($p<0.05$). In addition, it was unclear whether the myocardial infarction had precipitated the atrial fibrillation or whether

TABLE 3. *Percentage of atrial fibrillation attributed to various etiologies— Framingham Heart Study[a]*

Etiology	Percentage	
	Men	Women
Stroke	3	0
Congestive heart failure	5	88
Rheumatic heart disease	8	28
Coronary artery disease	8	3
Hypertension	13	15
Cardiovascular disease	25	31
Other conditions (including lone atrial fibrillation)	75	69

[a]Percentage of atrial fibrillation (paroxysmal or chronic) attributable to various etiologies, derived from the Framingham Heart Study (Ref 31). Total percentages exceed 100% as individuals may have more than one etiology. See text for details.

atrial fibrillation with a rapid ventricular rate resulted in ischemia and a myocardial infarction. The authors concluded that patients with an acute myocardial infarction only infrequently present with the abrupt onset of atrial fibrillation and that when a patient has new-onset atrial fibrillation, admission to the coronary care unit to rule out a myocardial infarction is unnecessary unless there are symptoms or electrocardiographic changes suggestive of ischemia.

Shlofmitz et al. (27) examined the underlying conditions and hospital course of 97 consecutive patients admitted to a single institution with a first episode of atrial fibrillation. After complete investigation (including cardiac enzymes, thyroid function tests, and echocardiography), 43 patients had no obvious cause found. Of the remainder, 15 were due to valvular disease, 15 to hypertension, nine to chronic ischemic heart disease, and only one to acute myocardial infarction. Miscellaneous causes accounted for the remaining 14 cases. Fifty-two percent of patients reverted to sinus rhythm within 24 hr of admission and an additional 21% reverted within 48 hr. The patient with acute myocardial infarction was clearly identified by ECG changes present on admission, and two other patients had obvious noncardiac indications for hospital admission. The authors concluded that coronary artery disease was an uncommon, but easily identified, cause of atrial fibrillation in their population and that routine intensive care unit admission for investigation of recent-onset atrial fibrillation is not warranted.

The above data indicate that chronic coronary artery disease is an uncommon precipitant of atrial fibrillation unless associated factors such as heart failure or hypertension are present and that the patient who does have the arrhythmia in association with an acute infarction almost always has signs or symptoms suggesting the diagnosis.

It is important to stress that although atrial fibrillation is an uncommon presenting feature of acute myocardial infarction, it is a common complication of this condition occurring in 6% to 23% of cases (16,34–41). Numerous studies have addressed the prognostic significance of atrial fibrillation in association with acute myocardial infarction (16,34–41), and most have found that its presence indicates an adverse prognosis. However, as in chronic coronary disease, atrial fibrillation in acute myocardial infarction is a marker of more extensive infarction and significant ventricular dysfunction. In an analysis of 4,108 patients seen in 16 area hospitals, Goldberg et al. (34) found an overall incidence of new atrial fibrillation of 9.1% and a relative risk of dying in patients who had an episode of atrial fibrillation of 1.7 compared to those with sinus rhythm. When multivariant analysis was applied, atrial fibrillation was not found to be an independent risk factor for in-hospital mortality but rather to be associated with an older age and a higher prevalence of heart failure, shock, or serious ventricular arrhythmias—all factors that are themselves associated with increased mortality risk.

Pulmonary Embolism

Another, often expressed concern is the need to rule out pulmonary embolism as a cause of new-onset atrial fibrillation. Atrial fibrillation in pulmonary embolism may be precipitated by hypoxia, catecholamine release, and/or acute right heart strain. In the National Cooperative Study of Urokinase for Pulmonary Embolism (42), only 3% of patients had atrial fibrillation, despite the fact that many patients had evidence of severe hemodynamic impairment. Since some evidence of significant hemodynamic or pulmonary impairment with pulmonary embolism is probably necessary in the vast majority of patients to produce atrial fibrillation, it is not necessary to exclude pulmonary embolism in patients with atrial fibrillation in whom no clinical suggestion of the condition exists.

Lone Atrial Fibrillation

Among the many etiologies of atrial fibrillation, lone atrial fibrillation is a disorder of exclusion. Originally described as being characterized by a slow resting ventricular response, lack of symptoms, absence of hypertension, and a good prognosis (43), the definition has subsequently varied. Some investigators (44) include all patients without overt heart disease, regardless of age or the presence of hypertension, while others limit the definition to patients under the age of 65, in whom a rigorous examination including echocardiography has excluded organic heart disease (45).

With the recognition of the considerable thromboembolic risk in nonvalvular atrial fibrillation (46–48a), a precise definition of lone atrial fibrillation has assumed new importance since it has been suggested that true lone atrial fibrillation may not require anticoagulation (47,49). This is, however, controversial. The Framingham study (44) found a fourfold increase in stroke risk in patients who had, by their definition, lone atrial fibrillation. In contrast, a study from Olmsted County, Minnesota (49) found no association between lone atrial fibrillation and stroke. This discrepancy may be largely due to differences in definition, since left ventricular hypertrophy may not be apparent on the ECG yet it may be present and result in atrial fibrillation. In the Framingham study 31.5% of patients with lone atrial fibrillation had a history of hypertension without ECG evidence of left ventricular hypertrophy. Studies using echocardiography might have reclassified many of these subjects as having hypertensive heart disease.

True lone atrial fibrillation may be a result of atrial fibrosis (50), a feature of sinus node disease (51), or a manifestation of neurally mediated arrhythmia (see chapter by Coumel). Presumably the low stroke risk is a function of the relatively small atria, the absence of concomitant atherosclerotic disease, and a normal cardiac output. Since, nowadays, virtually everyone with an episode of atrial fibrillation is evaluated by echocardiography, we suggest that the term lone atrial fibrillation be limited to those with a normal echocardiographic study and no other noncardiac cause of arrhythmia (49).

CLINICAL MANAGEMENT OF ATRIAL FIBRILLATION

Having briefly reviewed the significance and prevalence of etiologies of atrial fibrillation, the remainder of the chapter will concentrate on an overview of the clinical management of the patient presenting with a first documented episode of atrial fibrillation (Fig. 6).

Symptoms

Most often the onset of atrial fibrillation is associated with symptoms that cause the patient to seek medical attention. The severity and nature of the symptoms are determined by the heart rate, the nature and extent of underlying heart disease, ventricular systolic and diastolic function, and associated precipitating factors. Minor discomfort may occur such as palpitations, a strange sensation in the chest,

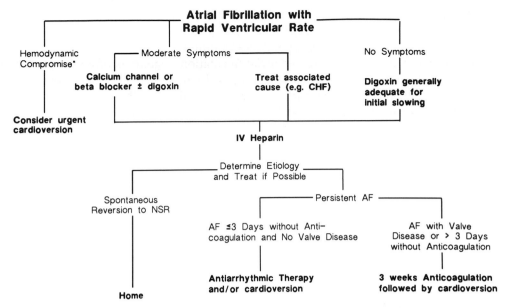

FIG. 6. Outline of the management of the patient presenting with recent-onset atrial fibrillation and a rapid ventricular response. *, acute ischemia, severe heart failure, severe symptomatic hypotension.

increased urination, lightheadedness, or fatigue. More severe problems may also be present such as shortness of breath, congestive heart failure, angina, persistent dizziness, or, rarely, syncope. Occasionally thromboembolism may occur shortly after the onset the arrhythmia, presenting as stroke or systemic embolism. Not infrequently, atrial fibrillation produces no symptoms or ones that are mild and are ignored. In such cases, the patient may not seek medical attention but when examined for some other reason is noted to have the arrhythmia. Alternatively, insidious progressive symptoms of right-sided failure manifest by peripheral edema may develop over the course of days to months, and in such cases it is often unclear whether the heart failure was precipitated by the arrhythmia or vice versa.

When faced with a patient with newly diagnosed atrial fibrillation and a rapid ventricular response, a quick assessment is necessary to detect any associated factors, such as congestive heart failure, and to assess the heart rate and the urgency of heart rate control. While most patients with atrial fibrillation do not present an urgent problem, exceptions exist such as patients with active ischemia, significant valve disease (particularly mitral or aortic stenosis), and preexcitation syndrome with an extremely rapid rate. In these cases, urgent electrical cardioversion may be required. In the majority of patients the first step is usually to control the ventricular rate and correct any associated precipitating factors.

Control of Heart Rate

Initial treatment, directed at slowing the ventricular rate, will frequently improve hemodynamic status and relieve any associated symptoms. As discussed in detail in the chapter by Falk on pharmacologic rate control, a number of agents are effective for this purpose, including verapamil, beta blockers, or digoxin, all of which may be administered intravenously or orally. The agent selected and the route of administration are, in part, dictated by the clinical presentation.

For patients with heart failure and atrial fibrillation, digoxin is often the preferred agent and concomitant treatment with diuretics, by relieving pulmonary congestion, may cause a secondary decrease in heart rate. In addition to the effect of digoxin on the atrioventricular node, the improvement in left ventricular function and hemodynamics may result in a reduction in the ventricular rate and, on occasion, the improved hemodynamics are associated with reversion to sinus rhythm. Since, in the absence of congestive heart failure, the effect of digoxin on heart rate is primarily mediated by its vagotonic effect on the atrioventricular node, significant heart rate slowing may take several hours (52). However, once rate control is achieved by digoxin, its effects are of a long duration, often lasting up to 36 hr.

In many situations verapamil or a beta blocker is the preferred agent for slowing the ventricular response. The onset of their action is rapid, but their effect is of shorter duration than that of digoxin. Caution should be used if these drugs are used in the setting of heart failure. Heart failure is often the result of the rapid ventricular rate, and the slowing of heart rate results in clinical improvement. This is particularly so when diastolic dysfunction predominates, as the rapid ventricular rate impairs ventricular filling. However, in some patients atrial fibrillation is a result of systolic failure, and the negative inotropic effects of beta blockers or calcium channel blockers may worsen left ventricular function. When the arrhythmia is associated with hypotension, similar concerns may exist, i.e., that the negative inotropic and vasodilatory effects of these agents may worsen the clinical status, but as with heart failure, hypotension is most often the result of the rapid heart rate and blood pressure improves when rate slowing is achieved. Nevertheless, the initial dose used should be small and gradually titrated upward based on heart rate slowing, blood pressure, and symptomatic improvement.

If the severity of the symptoms requires a more immediate intervention, electrical cardioversion should be performed in an attempt to restore sinus rhythm (see chapter on direct current cardioversion). If an ongoing process exists that is responsible for the precipitation of atrial fibrillation, sinus rhythm may not be maintained for long, but sufficient time may be gained for other therapies to begin to improve the clinical condition. In certain cases, such as Wolff-Parkinson-White syndrome with preexcited atrial fibrillation and a very rapid ventricular response, cardioversion may be life saving.

For patients in whom the duration of the arrhythmia is more than 3 days or is unknown, the risk of embolization from a left atrial thrombus is increased. This is especially true if the patient has underlying mitral stenosis or a poor cardiac output. In such cases the risks of thromboembolism should be weighed against the benefits of immediate cardioversion. If possible, heart rate should be slowed, anticoagulation with heparin administered, and oral anticoagulation instituted for 2 to 3 weeks before reversion is attempted. During this period, adequate heart rate control is essential.

Which Patients with Newly Diagnosed Atrial Fibrillation Can Be Discharged from the Emergency Room?

Atrial fibrillation per se poses little danger to the patient. Rather it is the hemodynamic effects of the arrhythmia, the presence or absence of associated conditions, and, possibly, the risk of embolization that should dictate whether hospital admission is required. Obviously in a patient with congestive heart failure hospitalization should be strongly considered even if the atrial fibrillation is of indeterminate duration and early conversion is unlikely. However, for a subject with minimal symptoms and arrhythmia of uncertain duration in whom urgent conversion is not a consideration, it is reasonable to arrange outpatient anticoagulation and investigation with a view to later cardioversion, if indicated. Similarly, the patient whose rhythm reverts to sinus shortly after emergency room evaluation rarely needs further in-hospital testing, unless the fibrillation was associated with severe symptoms or hemodynamic compromise and fear exists of a recurrence.

Patients with minimally symptomatic arrhythmia of a few days duration fall into a "gray zone." Many of these patients will spontaneously revert to sinus rhythm within a day of presentation, even in the absence of antiarrhythmic therapy (27,52). Nevertheless, 50% to 60% may remain in atrial fibrillation, and early antiarrhythmic therapy in this group may be effective in terminating the arrhythmia (53,54). Two possible approaches to antiarrhythmic therapy may be used here: in the absence of mitral valve disease or congestive heart failure, pharmacologic therapy can be initiated immediately in the emergency room. An approach found to be effective is the administration of a large loading dose of an antiarrhythmic agent, which often results in the reestablishment of sinus rhythm in 2 to 3 hr at a time of the peak blood level of the drug (54) (Fig. 7). Several medications have been reported to be effective, including quinidine sulfate 600 mg, disopyramide 300 mg, and procainamide 1.5 g.

If a single large dose of an antiarrhythmic agent is not successful in reverting the arrhythmia thereby necessitating the need for another drug, if this approach is not favored, and/or if the patient has significant heart disease that might increase the risks of drug therapy, it is preferable to admit him or her to a monitored floor for observation during the initiation of drug therapy, as aggravation of arrhythmia, although infrequent, is a concern (see chapter on proarrhythmic responses to antiarrhythmic drugs). As there may be a delay of a day or 2 between hospital admission and pharmacologic reversion, it is recommended that therapy with intravenous heparin should be initiated. This permits a more leisurely approach to investigation and therapy, while reducing the risk of thromboembolism.

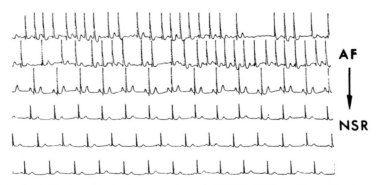

FIG. 7. Acute drug therapy for acute reversion of atrial fibrillation. The patient presented with atrial fibrillation (AF) of 12 hours duration. Two hours after 300 mg of disopyramide, normal sinus rhythm (NSR) was restored.

Since, as discussed previously, occult myocardial infarction or pulmonary embolism are so rarely associated with atrial fibrillation in the absence of other suggestive features, we do not believe that it is necessary to admit all patients with the arrhythmia to rule out these conditions. Rather, the factors outlined above (e.g., uncontrolled rate, heart failure) should dictate whether to admit the patient to the hospital.

Establishing the Etiology

Whether the patient is treated as an inpatient or outpatient, it is important to establish the etiology of the arrhythmia. The history and physical examination are, naturally, of value and may lead to the diagnosis of conditions such as alcohol-induced arrhythmia, thyrotoxicosis, or mitral stenosis. The ventricular response itself may provide some help in directing the differential diagnosis. In general, the mean ventricular rate in an untreated patient with atrial fibrillation is 110 to 160 beats per minute (55,56). When the rate is above this, conditions associated with activation of the sympathetic nervous system should be considered. These include hyperthyroidism, lung disease, uncompensated heart failure, and pulmonary embolism. When the heart rate is slow in the absence of pharmacologic therapy (less than 90 beats per minute), intrinsic atrioventricular nodal disease, often associated with other conduction system abnormalities, should be suspected.

Should At Least One Attempt Be Made to Revert All Patients with Atrial Fibrillation to Sinus Rhythm and If Not All, Then Whom?

While it is preferable to be in sinus rhythm rather than atrial fibrillation, certain factors such as a history of recurrent arrhythmia despite antiarrhythmic therapy, a very large left atrium, or a duration of arrhythmia more than 1 year lower the likelihood of a prolonged period of sinus rhythm after conversion. In addition, subjects with evidence of atrioventricular nodal disease, manifest by a slow ventricular response in the absence of drug therapy may have concomitant sinus node dysfunction resulting in significant pauses after cardioversion. The decision to cardiovert these patients should be taken with care and be based on individual considerations.

Most other patients who remain in atrial fibrillation after heart rate has been controlled deserve an attempt at pharmacologic or electrical cardioversion, as do patients with a recurrent episode of symptomatic arrhythmia. We consider it safe to attempt reversion in nonanticoagulated subjects if the duration of nonanticoagulated arrhythmia is 3 days or less, if no significant valve or myocardial disease exists, and if there is no history of thromboembolism. In patients with arrhythmia of unknown duration or in whom mitral valve disease (especially mitral stenosis) exists, a minimum of 3 weeks anticoagulation adequate to maintain the prothrombin time at an International Normalized Ratio of 2.0 to 2.5 (equivalent to a prothrombin time 1.3–1.5 × control using rabbit brain thromboplastin) prior to attempted cardioversion is recommended.

An exception to waiting 3 weeks is the patient in whom significant arrhythmia-related symptoms persist despite attempts to control heart rate. In such circumstances, if cardioversion is considered, careful examination of the atria with transesophageal echocardiography (57) may help to stratify the embolic risk. If a thrombus is seen cardioversion should be delayed if at all possible pending an adequate level and duration of anticoagulation.

Patients in whom even short-term (3 weeks) warfarin anticoagulation is contraindicated pose a difficult management problem. If cardioversion is considered clinically beneficial, the 1% to 2% short-term embolic risk (58) must be weighed against the approximately 4% per annum embolic risk occurring in the nonanticoagulated patient (46–48). Although the risk-benefit ratio seems to favor cardioversion over the persistence of chronic atrial fibrillation, reversion to atrial fibrillation commonly occurs and with it the resumption of embolic risk. In addition, aspirin therapy for chronic arrhythmia may have some benefit (47), and it is always more difficult for the physician to face the possibility that a procedure (cardioversion) may have provoked a stroke rather than the stroke occurring as part of the natural history of the disease. Thus the decision to cardiovert a patient who is unable to tolerate short-term anticoagulation should be carefully individualized.

Long-Term Anticoagulation

Aspirin therapy prior to cardioversion is of no proven benefit for prevention of thromboembolism related to the procedure and therefore should not be used for this purpose. Its role in preventing thromboembolic events arising from the atria in chronic atrial fibrillation remains controversial with one controlled study (47) finding a reduced stroke risk in patients with chronic, nonvalvular atrial fibrillation who were treated with aspirin compared to those receiving placebo. In contrast, a study of warfarin anticoagulation, uncontrolled for aspirin use, found no benefit of aspirin in the nonwarfarin group when retrospective analysis was performed (48). Based on these equivocal data and the as yet unknown relative value of aspirin and warfarin for reducing stroke risk, we currently favor long-term warfarin anticoagulation in the patient with chronic atrial fibrillation in whom no further cardioversion attempts are considered. Warfarin anticoagulation is mandatory in mitral stenosis and atrial fibrillation, as thromboembolic risk is so great.

A word about the oft-made distinction between valvular and nonvalvular atrial fibrillation in reference to embolic risk is in order at this point. Traditionally, atrial fibrillation has been divided into valvular and nonvalvular disease and the risk of stroke was stratified by the presence or absence of mitral valve disease. This distinction is based on early studies, in which the majority of cases of valvular atrial fibrillation were due to mitral stenosis (59) and the majority of nonvalvular cases to coronary or hypertensive heart disease (59,60). While the distinction between valvular and nonvalvular stroke risk may be valid for groups of patients, multiple factors appear to play a role in thromboembolism, and an individual patient may be at very high thromboembolic risk despite having nonvalvular atrial fibrillation.

The high prevalence of thrombi in mitral stenosis relates to the low flow state across the stenotic valve resulting in considerable atrial enlargement and the potential for intra-atrial stasis. Rheumatic involvement of the atrium may play a role, but this is not considered to be significant (61). Similar, or greater, degrees of left atrial enlargement may occur with severe pure mitral regurgitation compared to mitral stenosis, but thromboembolic risk is said to be less (62). Presumably the "jet" effect of the regurgitant lesion, by producing turbulence, reduces the likelihood of stasis within the atrium (62a). Since stasis is a significant factor in thrombus formation, then nonvalvular conditions with a potential for a high degree of stasis (due either to nonregurgitant atrial enlargement or to a low flow state) might also be at a much increased risk. Such "high-risk" conditions include hypertrophic cardiomyopathy (which produces considerable atrial dilation) and dilated cardiomyopathy (producing both atrial dilation and a low flow state). Unfortunately, no formula exists for predicting which patients with atrial fibrillation are at high or low risk, although low-dose anticoagulation appears to reduce stroke risk in all groups (46–48) except, perhaps, in patients with true lone atrial fibrillation (49).

For the patient with a relative contraindication to long-term anticoagulation, aspirin may offer an alternative to reduce the risk of stroke (47), but generally we reserve aspirin use for patients unwilling or unable to take warfarin or in subjects under age 65 with lone atrial fibrillation. In the latter group embolic events are very rare (although occasional cases are seen), and the potential risks of warfarin seem to outweigh any possible benefits. Although aspirin therapy in these subjects is also unproven, it is minimally inconvenient to the patient and in low doses is well-tolerated.

Recurrent, Paroxysmal Atrial Fibrillation

The recurrence of atrial fibrillation, particularly if it is self-terminating, often poses a management problem especially when symptoms of arrhythmia are troublesome. Although atrial antiarrhythmic therapy may be successful in reducing the frequency of paroxysms, a significant number of treated patients who previously had frequent episodes will continue to have the arrhythmia, albeit less frequently.

Several management strategies may aid in preventing paroxysmal atrial fibrillation and/or controlling symptoms should a paroxysm occur. These include the recognition of the subset of patients with vagally triggered atrial fibrillation, discussed in detail in the chapter by Coumel, in whom digoxin and beta blockers may aggravate the arrhythmia but in whom amiodarone or flecainide (but not propafenone) may be particularly effective.

In subjects with symptomatic, paroxysmal arrhythmia unrelated to vagal triggers and only partially controlled by drugs, the choice of sotalol or a class IC drug, such as propafenone or flecainide, may have advantages over more traditional agents like quinidine as the ventricular rate at the time of recurrence will be slow and symptoms of tachycardia lessened (63,64). This is discussed in detail in the chapter on pharmacologic control. An occasional patient with drug-resistant, symptomatic paroxysmal atrial fibrillation that is preceded by sinus bradycardia may benefit from atrial pacing (see chapters by Coumel and by Pollak and Falk).

Management of Chronic Atrial Fibrillation (Fig. 8)

In the subject with chronic atrial fibrillation heart rate during daily activities may not be reflected by the resting heart rate measured in the office, particularly if digoxin is used as monotherapy (52). The judicious use of calcium channel and beta blockers (discussed in the chapter on pharmacologic control) may be helpful in alleviating tachycardia-mediated symptoms.

If symptoms persist after optimizing other cardiac medications and adequately controlling the heart rate, then, after excluding other causes of persistent symptoms,

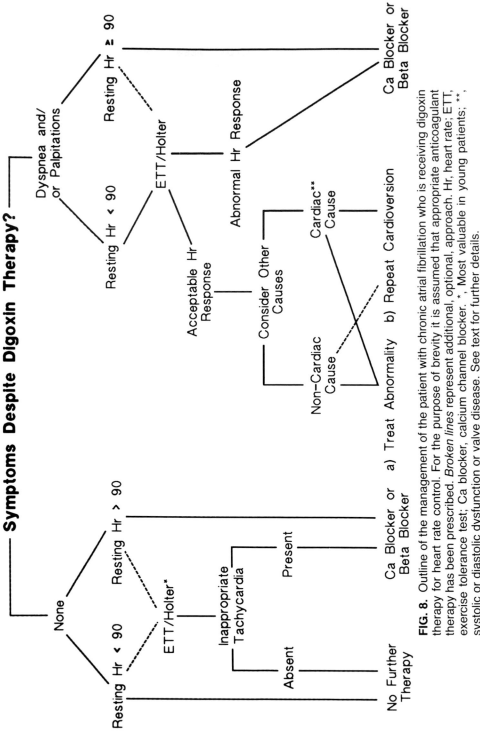

FIG. 8. Outline of the management of the patient with chronic atrial fibrillation who is receiving digoxin therapy for heart rate control. For the purpose of brevity it is assumed that appropriate anticoagulant therapy has been prescribed. *Broken lines* represent additional, optional, approach. Hr, heart rate; ETT, exercise tolerance test; Ca blocker, calcium channel blocker. *, Most valuable in young patients; **, systolic or diastolic dysfunction or valve disease. See text for further details.

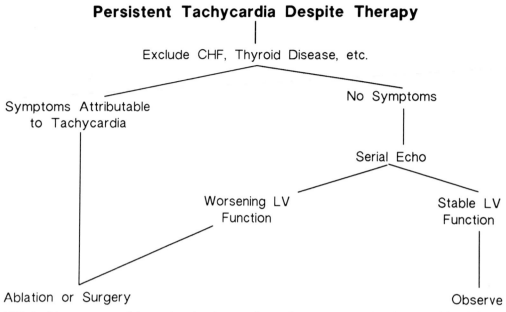

FIG. 9. Management of the patient in whom tachycardia persists despite therapy with calcium-channel blocking or beta-blocking agents.

consideration should be given to a repeat cardioversion attempt using either a previously untried antiarrhythmic agent and/or a combination of agents (64). AV nodal ablation (chapter by Rosenqvist and Scheinman) or surgery (chapter by Leitch et al.) may be required in the patient with symptomatic tachycardia uncontrollable by other means (Fig. 9).

Intermittent Atrial Fibrillation—Pursuit of Elusive Paroxysms

One final consideration is the patient in whom paroxysmal atrial fibrillation has never been documented but in whom it is suspected either because of suggestive symptoms or because of a cryptogenic stroke. The risk of atrial fibrillation increases with age, not only in the normal population, but in virtually every condition associated with the arrhythmia (65,66). Although stroke in mitral stenosis is most highly correlated with the presence of atrial fibrillation, the stroke risk of patients in sinus rhythm increases over the age of 40 (65) and has led to a recommendation by some authors (67) to anticoagulate older patients with all but the mildest mitral stenosis regardless of the rhythm.

The finding of frequent atrial ectopic beats in an asymptomatic patient at high risk for development of atrial fibrillation (e.g., mitral stenosis or hypertrophic cardiomyopathy) may be helpful in the decision to anticoagulate and/or to prescribe atrial antiarrhythmic therapy, since such beats may be precursors of paroxysmal arrhythmia. Similarly, in a patient who has experienced a single episode of atrial fibrillation, the presence of frequent atrial ectopic beats on 24-hr monitoring signals an increased likelihood of recurrence and such a finding may be helpful in planning long-term management.

A more difficult problem is the patient with an embolic event, suspected to be cardiac in origin, who is now in sinus rhythm and in whom no source can be found. How useful are noninvasive tests to detect or predict atrial fibrillation? No study has evaluated this formally, but, in our experience, Holter monitoring rarely demonstrates significant abnormalities. However, certain clues may suggest the possibility of paroxysmal arrhythmia such as an intra-atrial conduction defect on the ECG (Fig. 1), a history of palpitations, or coexistent cardiac lesions associated with atrial fibrillation. In selected patients, transesophageal echocardiography may reveal a previously undetected atrial thrombus (57).

The role of the signal-averaged ECG in predicting patients at risk for ventricular arrhythmias is well established (68) but technical difficulties, mainly related to accurate P-wave triggering, have limited the application of the test for atrial fibrillation (69). Recently, Fukunami et al. (70) reported on P-wave triggered signal averaging to detect patients at risk for atrial fibrillation. They found a 91% sensitivity, 76% specificity, and 83% predictive accuracy for detecting subjects with a prior episode of atrial fibrillation compared to age-matched controls when using the criteria of a filtered P-wave duration of 120 msec or longer in combination with a root mean square voltage of 3.5 μV or less in the last 20 msec of the P wave. Based on this, the authors suggested that the test may be of value for screening patients with suspected paroxysmal arrhythmia. However, application of their data to a broader population than the one studied, while not altering the sensitivity and specificity of the test, would considerably decrease the predictive accuracy to a level unsuitable for guiding clinical decisions. The use of frequency analysis has improved the predictive accuracy of QRS signal averaging for detecting patients at risk of ventricular arrhythmias (71). Whether a similar technique can be developed for the P wave, and if so, whether it would be of value, remains to be determined.

An occasional patient with infrequent recurrent palpitations defies all attempts to document the arrhythmia. If long-term loop ECG recording (72) is unsuccessful in capturing the arrhythmia and symptoms are troublesome, several electrophysiologic techniques have been suggested for deciding whether atrial fibrillation, rather than another etiology, is the cause (73–75). Details of these techniques and their limitations are discussed in the chapter by Simpson.

CONCLUSIONS

Atrial fibrillation is a common problem and the acute, paroxysmal or chronic episode generally presents no obvious management problem. However, as with many conditions, subtle details exist that, if overlooked, may make the difference between adequate and excellent treatment. Despite more than two centuries of available therapy for atrial fibrillation, it is only recently that the exact role of therapy such as digoxin has been defined (52,76) and the value of anticoagulation confirmed (46–48). Presumably, in the coming decade, newer antiarrhythmic agents (77) and further insights into the alternative treatments (78–80) will refine management even more and help to reduce morbidity from this common arrhythmia.

REFERENCES

1. Ettinger PO, Wu CF, De La Cruz C, Weisse AB, Ahmed SS, Regan TJ. Arrhythmias and the "Holiday Heart." Alcohol associated cardiac rhythm disorders. *Am Heart J* 1978;95:555–562.

2. Lownstein SR, Gabow PA, Cramer J, Oliva PB, Ratner K. The role of alcohol in new onset atrial fibrillation. *Arch Intern Med* 1983;143:1882–1885.
3. Rich EC, Siebold C, Campion B. Alcohol related acute atrial fibrillation. A case controlled study and review of 40 patients. *Arch Intern Med* 1985;145:830–883.
4. Koskinen P, Kupair M, Leinonen H, Luomarmaki H. Alcohol and new onset atrial fibrillation in case control study of a current syndrome. *Br Heart J* 1987;57:488–493.
5. Engel TR, Luck JC. Effect of whiskey on atrial vulnerability and "holiday heart." *J Am Coll Cardiol* 1983;1:816–818.
6. Hoffman I, Lowery RD. The electrocardiogram in thyrotoxicosis. *Am J Cardiol* 1968;6:893–904.
7. Sandler G, Wilson GM. The nature and prognosis of heart disease in thyrotoxicosis. *Q J Med* 1959;28:347–369.
8. Iwasaki T, Naka M, Hiramatsu K, et al. Echocardiographic studies on the relationship between atrial fibrillation and atrial enlargement in patients with hyperthyroidism of Grave's disease. *Cardiology* 1989;76:10–17.
9. Fagerberg B, Lindstedt G, Stromblad SO, et al. Thyrotoxic atrial fibrillation: an underdiagnosed or overdiagnosed condition? *Clin Chem* 1990;36:622–627.
10. Tajiri J, Hamasaki S, Shimada T, et al. Masked thyroid dysfunction among elderly patients with atrial fibrillation. *Jpn Heart J* 1986;27:183–190.
11. Black HR, Weltin G, Jaffe CC. The limited echocardiogram: a modification of standard echocardiography for use in the routine evaluation of patients with systemic hypertension. *Am J Cardiol* 1991;67:1027–1030.
12. Levy D, Garrison RJ, Savage DD, Kannel WB, Castelli WP. Prognostic implications of echocardiographically determined left ventricular mass in the Framingham Heart Study. *N Engl J Med* 1990;322:1561–1566.
13. Kannel WB, Abbott RD, Savage DD, McNamara PM. Epidemiologic features of atrial fibrillation. The Framingham study. *N Engl J Med* 1982;306:1018–1022.
14. Henry WL, Morganroth J, Pearlman AS, et al. Relationship between echocardiographically determined left atrial size and atrial fibrillation. *Circulation* 1976;53:273–279.
15. Spodick DH. Arrhythmias during acute pericarditis: a prospective study in 100 consecutive cases. *JAMA* 1976;5:39–41.
16. Sugiura T, Iwasaka T, Takahashi N, et al. Factor associated with atrial fibrillation in Q wave anterior myocardial infarction. *Am Heart J* 1991;121:1409–1412.
17. McKenna WJ, England Doi YL, Deanfield JE, Oakley CM, Goodwin JF. Arrhythmia in hypertrophic cardiomyopathy. I. Influence on prognosis. *Br Heart J* 1981;46:168–172.
18. Gleancy DL, O'Brien KP, Gold HK, Epstein SE. Atrial fibrillation in patients with idiopathic hypertrophic subaortic stenosis. *Br Heart J* 1970;32:652–659.
19. Robinson K, Frenneaux MP, Stockens B, Karatasakes G, Polonieiki JD, McKenna WJ. Atrial fibrillation in hypertrophic cardiomyopathy—a longitudinal study. *J Am Coll Cardiol* 1990;15:1279–1285.
20. Stafford WJ, Trohman RG, Bilsker M, Zaman L, Castellanos A, Myerburg RJ. Cardiac arrest in an adolescent with atrial fibrillation and hypertrophic cardiomyopathy. *J Am Coll Cardiol* 1986;7:701–704.
21. Falk RH. Cardiac amyloidosis. *Prog Cardiol* 1989;2:143–156.
22. Hodkinson HM, Pomerance A. The clinical pathology of heart failure and atrial fibrillation in old age. *Postgrad Med* 1979;55:251.
23. Holford FD, Mithoefer JC, Cardiac arrhythmias in hospitalized patients with chronic obstructive pulmonary disease. *Am Rev Respir Dis* 1973;108:879–885.
24. Incalzi RA, Postelli R, Fuso L. Cardiac arrhythmias and left ventricular function in respiratory failure from chronic obstructive pulmonary disease. *Chest* 1990;97:1092–1097.
25. Grossman J. The occurrence of arrhythmias in hospitalized asthma patients. *J Allerg Clin Immunol* 1976;57:310–317.
26. Hrowsaiva K, Sekiguiki M, Kasanuki H, et al. Natural history of atrial fibrillation. *Heart Vessel Suppl* 1987;2:14–23.
27. Shlofmitz RA, Hirsch BE, Meyer BR. New-onset atrial fibrillation. Is there a need for emergent hospitalization? *J Gen Intern Med* 1986;1:139–142.
28. Flowers NC, Horan LG. Acid-base relationships and the cardiac response to aerosol inhalation. *Chest* 1973;63:74–78.
29. Weinberger M, Hendeles S. Slow release theophylline: rationale and basis for product selection. *N Engl J Med* 1983;308:760–764.
30. Volpi A, Cavalli A, Maggione AP, Pieri-Nerli F. Left atrial compression by a mediastinal bronchogenic cyst presenting with paroxysmal atrial fibrillation. *Thorax* 1988;43:216–217.
31. Kannel WB, Abbott RD, Savage D, McNamara PM. Coronary heart disease and atrial fibrillation: the Framingham study. *Am Heart J* 1983;106:389–396.
32. Cameron A, Schwartz MJ, Kronmal RA, Kosinski AS. Prevalence and significance of atrial fibrillation in coronary artery disease (CASS Registry). *Am J Cardiol* 1988;61:714–717.

33. Friedman HZ, Weber-Bornstein N, Deboe SF, Mancine GB. CCU admission criteria for suspected acute myocardial infarction in now onset atrial fibrillation. *Am J Cardiol* 1987;59:866–869.
34. Goldberg RJ, Seeley D, Becker RC, et al. Impact of atrial fibrillation on the in-hospital and long-term survival of patients with acute myocardial infarction: a community-wide perspective. *Am Heart J* 1990;119:991–1001.
35. Sugiura T, Iwasaka T, Oyawa A, et al. Atrial fibrillation in acute myocardial infarction. *Am J Cardiol* 1985;56:27–29.
36. Cristal N, Scwarcberg J, Gueron M. Supraventricular arrhythmias in acute myocardial infarction. Prognostic importance of clinical setting; mechanism of production. *Ann Intern Med* 1975;82:35–39.
37. Cristal N, Peterberg I, Scwarcberg J. Atrial fibrillation developing in the acute phase of myocardial infarction; prognostic implications. *Chest* 1978;70:8–71.
38. Helmer C, Lundorian T, Morgensen L, Orinias E, Syogren A, Wester DO. Atrial fibrillation in acute myocardial infarction. *Acta Med Scand* 1973;193:39–44.
39. Liem KL, Lie KI, Durrer D, Wellens HJ. Clinical setting and prognostic significance of atrial fibrillation complicating acute myocardial infarction. *Eur J Cardiol* 1976;4:59–62.
40. Klass M, Haywood LJ. Atrial fibrillation associated with acute myocardial infarction. A study of 34 cases. *Am Heart J* 1970;79:752–760.
41. Liberthson RR, Salesbury KW, Hutter AM, DeSanctis RW. Atrial tachyarrhythmias in acute myocardial infarction. *Am J Med* 1976;60:956–960.
42. Urokinase Pulmonary Embolism Trial: Clinical and electrocardiographic observation. *Circulation* 1973;suppl II:60–65.
43. Evans W, Swann P. Lone auricular fibrillation. *Br Heart J* 1954;16:189–194.
44. Brand FN, Abbott RD, Kannel WB, Wolf PA. Characteristics and prognosis of lone atrial fibrillation. 30 year followup in the Framingham study. *JAMA* 1985;254:3449–3453.
45. Roy D, Marchand E, Gagne P, Chabot M, Cartier R. Usefulness of anticoagulation therapy in the prevention of embolic complications of atrial fibrillation. *Am Heart J* 1986;112:1039–1043.
46. Peterson P, Godtfredsen J, Boysen G, Anderson ED, Andersen B. Placebo-controlled, randomized trial of warfarin and aspirin for prevention of thromboembolic complications in chronic atrial fibrillation. *Lancet* 1989;1:175–179.
47. Stroke Prevention in Atrial Fibrillation Investigators. Stroke prevention in atrial fibrillation study: final results: *Circulation* 1991;84:527–539.
48. The Boston Area Anticoagulation Trial for Atrial Fibrillation Investigators. The effect of low dose warfarin on the risk of stroke in patients with nonrheumatic atrial fibrillation. *N Engl J Med* 1990;323:1505–1511.
48a. Connolly SJ, Laupacis A, Gent M, Roberts RS, Cairns JA. Canadian atrial fibrillation (CAFA) study. *J Am Coll Cardiol* 1991;18:349–355.
49. Kopecky SL, Gersh BJ, McGoon MD, et al. The natural history of lone atrial fibrillation. A population base study over 3 decades. *N Engl J Med* 1987;317:669–674.
50. Davis MJ, Pomerance A. Pathology of atrial fibrillation in man. *Br Heart J* 1972;34:520–525.
51. Ferrer MI. The sick sinus syndrome in atrial disease. *JAMA* 1968;206:645–646.
52. Falk RH, Leavitt JI. Digoxin for atrial fibrillation. A drug whose time has gone? *Ann Intern Med* 1991;114:573–575.
53. Suttorp MJ, Kingman H, Lie-A-Huen L, Mast ES. Intravenous flecainide versus verapamil for acute conversion of paroxysmal atrial fibrillation or flutter to sinus rhythm. *Am J Cardiol* 1989;63:693–696.
54. Margolis B, DeSilva RA, Lown B. Episodic drug treatment in the management of paroxysmal arrhythmias. *Am J Cardiol* 1980;45:621–626.
55. Beasley R, Smith DA, McHaffie DJ. Exercise heart rates at different serum digoxin concentrations in patients with atrial fibrillation. *Br Med J (Clin Res)* 1985;290:9–11.
56. Rawles JM, Metcalfe MJ, Jennings K. Time of occurrence, duration and ventricular rate of paroxysmal atrial fibrillation: the effect of digoxin. *Br Heart J* 1990;63:225–227.
57. Mugge A, Daniel WG, Hausmann D, Godke J, Wagenbreth I, Lichtlen PR. Diagnosis of left atrial appendage thrombi by transesophageal echocardiography: clinical applications and followup. *Am J Cardiac Imaging* 1990;4:173–179.
58. Bjerklund C, Orning OM. The efficacy of anticoagulation therapy in preventing embolism related to DC electrical conversion of atrial fibrillation. *Am J Med* 1969;23:208–215.
59. Graham GK, Taylor JA, Ellis LB, Greenberg DJ, Robbins SL. Studies in mitral stenosis: a correlation of postmortem findings with the clinical course in the disease in one hundred and one cases. *Arch Intern Med* 1951;88:532–547.
60. Aberg H. Atrial fibrillation. 1. A study of atrial thrombosis and systemic embolism in a necropsy material. *Acta Med Scand* 1969;185:373–379.
61. Weiss S, Davis D. Rheumatic heart disease III. Embolic manifestations. *Am Heart J* 1933;9:45–52.
62. Daley R, Franks R. Massive dilatation of the left auricle. *Q J Med* 1949;18:81–92.

62a. Black IW, Hopkins AP, Lee LCL, Walsh WF, Jacobson BM. Left atrial spontaneous echo contrast: a clinical and echocardiographic analysis. *J Am Coll Cardiol* 1991;18:398–404.
63. Jull-Moller S, Edvardsson N, Rehnqvist-Alzberg N. Sotalol versus quinidine for the maintenance of sinus rhythm after direct-current cardioversion of atrial fibrillation. *Circulation* 1990;82:1932–1939.
64. Antman EM, Beamer AD, Cantillon C, McGowan N, Friedman PL. Therapy of refractory symptomatic atrial fibrillation and atrial flutter: a staged care approach with new antiarrhythmic drugs. *J Am Coll Cardiol* 1990;15:698–707.
65. Coulshed N, et al. Systemic embolism in mitral valve disease. *Br Heart J* 1970;32:26.
66. Bartels EC. Hyperthyroidism in patients over 65. *Geriatrics* 1965;20:459–462.
67. Dalen JE, Mitral stenosis. In: Dalen JE, Alpert JS, eds. *Valvular heart disease*, 2nd ed. Boston: Little, Brown, 1987;49–110.
68. Winters SL, Stewart D, Targonski A, Gomes JA. Role of signal averaging of the surface QRS complex in selecting patients with nonsustained ventricular tachycardia and high-grade ventricular arrhythmias for programmed ventricular stimulation. *J Am Coll Cardiol* 1988;12:1481–1487.
69. Engel TR, Vallone N, Windle J. Signal averaged electrocardiogram in patients with atrial fibrillation or flutter. *Am Heart J* 1988;115:592–597.
70. Fukunami M, Yamada T, Ohmori M, et al. Detection of patients at risk for paroxysmal atrial fibrillation during sinus rhythm by P wave triggered signal averaged electrocardiogram. *Circulation* 1991;83:162–169.
71. Kelen GJ, Henkin R, Starr AM, Caref EB, Bloomfield D, El-Sherif N. Spectral turbulence analysis of the signal averaged electrocardiogram and its predictive accuracy from inducible sustained monomorphic ventricular tachycardia. *Am J Cardiol* 1991;67:965–975.
72. Linzer M, Pritchett ELC, Pontinen M, McCarthy E, Divine GW. Increased diagnostic yield of loop electrocardiographic recorders in unexplained syncope. *Am J Cardiol* 1990;66:214–219.
73. Tanigawa M, Fukatani M, Konoe A, Isomoto S, Kadena M, Hashiba K. Prolonged and fractionated right atrial electrograms during sinus rhythm in patients with paroxysmal atrial fibrillation and sick sinus node syndrome. *J Am Coll Cardiol* 1991;17:403–408.
74. Simpson RJ, Jr, Foster JR, Gettes LS. Atrial excitability and conduction in patients with interatrial conduction defects. *Am J Cardiol* 1982;50:1331-1337.
75. Simpson RJ Jr, Amara I, Foster JR, Woelfel A, Gettes LS. Thresholds, refractory periods, and conduction times of the normal and diseased human atrium. *Am Heart J* 1988;116:1080–1090.
76. Falk RH, Knowlton AA, Bernard SA, Gotlieb NE, Battinelli NJ. Digoxin for converting recent-onset atrial fibrillation to sinus rhythm. A randomized, double-blind trial. *Ann Intern Med* 1987;106:503–506.
77. Feld GK. Atrial fibrillation—is there a safe and highly effective pharmacological treatment? *Circulation* 1990;82:2248–2250.
78. Rosenqvist M, Lee MA, Moulinier L, et al. Long-term followup of patients after transcatheter direct current ablation of the atrioventricular junction. *J Am Coll Cardiol* 1990;16:1467–1494.
79. Leitch JW, Klein GJ, Yee R, Guiraudon GM. Sinus node atrioventricular node isolation. Long-term results with the corridor operation for atrial fibrillation. *J Am Coll Cardiol* 1991;17:970–975.
80. DiMarco JP. Surgical therapy for atrial fibrillation: a first step on what may be a long road. *J Am Coll Cardiol* 1991;17:976–977.

Subject Index

administration route, 217
exercise heart rate effects, 157
negative inotropic effects, 269
pacemaker effects, 354
pharmacokinetics, 218
as postoperative atrial fibrillation
prophylaxis/therapy, 130,134–135
side effects, 247
sinus rhythm effects, 246–247
ventricular rate effects, 263
Prothrombin time, 403
Pulmonary veins, atrial connection, 16
Purkinje fibers, conduction velocity, 65–66
P wave
fetal, 168
in left ventricular hypertrophy, 390
as postoperative atrial fibrillation
predictor, 129–130
signal-averaging, 408

Q

QRS complex
atrioventricular accessory pathways
and, 335
in cardiac amyloidosis, 395
compensatory pause, 69
in electrical cardioversion, 182–183
fetal, 168
Quinidine
action mechanisms, 198,199
atrial effects, 200
cardioversion and, 172,189
combination therapy, 216
concealed conduction effects, 63
digoxin concomitant therapy, 292–294
drug interactions, 203,204,223
electrophysiologic effects, 53
hemodynamic effects, 203–204
pacemaker use and, 354
as paroxysmal atrial fibrillation therapy,
121
pharmacokinetics, 202–203
as postoperative atrial fibrillation
prophylaxis/therapy, 131,134,139
potassium channel effects, 286
side effects, 204,250,359
mortality, 237,250,285–286
postsurgical, 139
proarrhythmia, 285–286
ventricular rate acceleration,
292–294
sinus rhythm effects, 235–237,238,
243–244,246,249–250,267,275
sodium channel effects, 286
vagolytic activity, 198
ventricular rate effects, 275
verapamil interaction, 221

as Wolff-Parkinson-White syndrome
therapy, 342
Quinidine gluconate, 203,204
Quinidine polygalacturonate, 203,204
Quinidine sulfate, 202–203
atrial fibrillation recurrence and, 237
cardioversion and, 190
as first episode atrial fibrillation therapy,
402
heart rate acceleration effects, 292
ventricular fibrillation, 287

R

Recainam, 199
Refractory period, 109,110
atrial fibrillation induction and,
51–54,55–56
of atrioventricular accessory pathways,
338–342
effective, 324,325,326–327,330
heart rate adaptation, 43
heart weight correlation, 65,66
postpolarization, 43
relative, 324
in sinus node dysfunction, 43–44
total, 323–324
Regurgitation, mitral, 6,7,392–393,397,
404
Rheumatic heart disease, 83,391. *See also*
Atrial fibrillation, rheumatic
anticoagulant therapy, 313
autopsy studies, 3,4,5,7
exercise testing, 152
incidence, 7
mitral regurgitation and, 6
mitral stenosis and, 6
sex factors, 84
stroke and, 307–308

S

Sarcoidosis, 32
Scaling, of ventricular rhythm, 71–73
Sclerosis, endocardial, 18,19,20
Septectomy, atrial procedure, 31
Septum, atrial
age-related changes, 16,17
blood flow, 169–170
defect, 31–32
Sick sinus syndrome
atrial conduction time, 325,326,331
drug-related aggravation, 301
fragmented electrogram, 328–329
pacemaker therapy
as cardioversion back-up, 349–350
dual-chamber pacing, 350
vagal atrial arrhythmia versus, 119